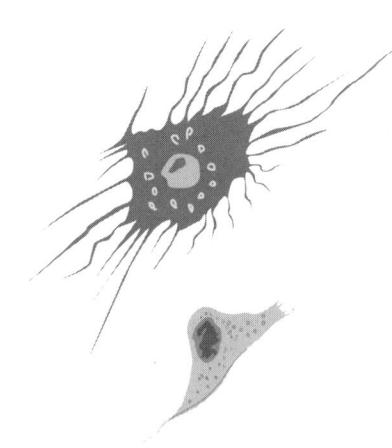

安保徹の原著論文を読む

膠原病、炎症性腸疾患、がんの発症メカニズムの解明

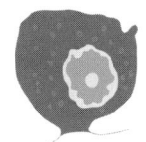

<small>新潟大学大学院医学部教授</small>
安保　徹 著

渡邉まゆみ
富山智香子：日本語訳

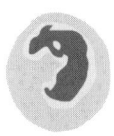

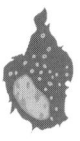

三和書籍

まえがき

　長い間、医学の研究は目の前に起こっている現象の実体や内容を知ることでした。実際に起こっている現象の内容を知ることができれば生命の仕組みがわかり、医学がしだいに体系化されて病気の成り立ちもわかってきます。感染症でも免疫病でも、このような流れで研究が進んできたように思います。

　しかし、1990年頃から少し医学研究の方向性が変わり始めました。遺伝子の構造や反応がわかりだすと、分子生物学が新しい領域として出現したのです。人間の考えで、遺伝子を切ったりつないだりしながらそのできた遺伝子をウイルスやプラスミドなどの微生物に組み込み遺伝子操作をする分野が盛んになりました。

　免疫学の領域にもこの手法が導入され、遺伝子のノックアウト（消去）やトランスジェニック（過剰発現）がマウスで行われ始めたのです。これらの研究で遺伝子とその産物である分子の働きはそれなりに解明できるものの、産み出される事実や論文は全て自然界ではほとんど起こり得ないartifactの世界になってしまいました。

　こういう手法は広く医学研究の領域に入り込み、この流れでiPS細胞をつくり、再生医療をめざす研究も生み出されました。しかし、これもartifactの世界で、自然の摂理からはみ出した医学です。疑問を感じる人も多いでしょう。

　従来行なわれてきた研究のことをdescriptive studyと呼ぶ風潮ができて、自分達が論文を投稿するといやな思いをすることが多くなりました。逆に、人間の考えで組み立てた分子生物学的研究をlogical studyと高く評価しているのです。

　しかし、良く考えてみれば私達人間の頭で考えることはたいしたことはないのです。やはり、生命体の生き様の中に真理が隠れているのです。私は、多くの仲間と共にこういう研究を続け多数の論文をつくってきました。それを抜粋したのがこの論文集です。

　自己免疫疾患は「原因不明の難病で、免疫系の異常で引き起こされる」と考えられています。しかし、マウスやヒトの自己免疫疾患を研究すると原因不明でもなく免疫の異常でもないことがわかります。例えば、自己抗体の出現は自己免疫疾患だけではなく、加齢やマラリア感染でも起こります。そしてこの時、いずれも例外無く、胸腺は萎縮し通常のT細胞やB細胞は激しく抑制されています。

つまり現象の実体や内容を知ると、自己抗体をつくる病態では進化レベルの高い免疫系は抑制され、逆に、自己応答性の古い免疫系が刺激されてくることがわかるのです。ここで、私たちが見い出した発見が役立ちます。胸腺や骨髄でつくられるＴ細胞やＢ細胞は、生物が上陸した後にできた新しい免疫系なのです。外来抗原向けになっています。

　一方、生物が上陸する以前からあった古い免疫系が胸腺外分化Ｔ細胞と自己抗体産生Ｂ-1細胞です。異常自己を監視するinnate immunityとしての役割を果たしています。加齢、細胞内寄生感染症、激しいストレスなどがあるとこの古い免疫系が活性化します。自己免疫疾患の反応を考えると、ストレスで生じた異常自己を排除するための合目的反応です。免疫系の失敗で起こっているわけではありません。

　この論文集を読むと、自己免疫疾患（膠原病）も免疫抑制状態なので、ステロイドや免疫抑制剤を長期間使った治療がむしろ病気を固定したり悪化させたりしてしまうことが理解できます。

　現実に起こっている現象の実体や内容を理解することの大切さは、私達の「新生児の顆粒球増多」neonatal granulocytosisの研究でもわかるでしょう。肺呼吸開始のストレスが交感神経緊張を引き起こし顆粒球増多を誘発していたのです。「白血球の自律神経支配」の法則との組み合わせで理解できるのです。

　こういうストレスによって、交感神経支配下にある顆粒球増多の現象がわかると、炎症性腸疾患のメカニズムも解明できます。ストレス→交感神経刺激→顆粒球増多→粘膜破壊の連鎖です。このようにして、歯周病、胃炎、胃潰瘍、クローン病、潰瘍性大腸炎、痔疾、卵巣嚢腫、突発性難聴などの発症メカニズムが次々と明らかになります。

　「ストレスの正体」や「ガンの発症メカニズム」も現象の理解をかさねることで解明できました。descriptive studyの本当の威力をこの論文集で学んでほしいと思います。

平成24年12月記す
安保　徹

まえがき……………………………………………………………………………………… iii

Chapter 1

放射線照射胸腺摘出マウスへの骨髄移植による、胸腺外である肝臓でT細胞レセプターを中等度に有する細胞が産生された証明 ……………………………………… 3

Evidence for extrathymic generation of intermediate T cell receptor cells in the liver revealed in thymectomized, irradiated mice subjected to bone marrow transplantation. ………… 14

Chapter 2

各免疫臓器におけるTCR^{int}細胞とNK1.1$^+$T細胞の関係：NK1.1$^+$T細胞がTCR^{int}細胞の集団の中に存在する ……………………………………………………………… 25

Relationships between Intermediate TCR cells and NK1.1$^+$T cells in various immune organs: NK1.1$^+$T cells are present within a population of intermediate TCR cells. ………… 38

Chapter 3

胸腺外T細胞は、系統進化的にナチュラル・キラー細胞と胸腺由来T細胞の中間に位置する ………………………………………………………………………………… 53

Extrathymic T cells stand at an intermediate phylogenetic Position between Natural Killer Cells and Thymus-Derived T Cells ………………………………………………… 65

Chapter 4

急性虫垂炎の発症の一因は、交感神経活動増加による顆粒球増多である ……… 83

Granulocytosis induced by increasing sympathetic nerve activity contributes to the incidence of acute appendicitis ……………………………………………………… 93

Chapter 5

成体マウス肝臓におけるc-kit$^+$幹細胞と胸腺前駆細胞 ………………………… 107

c-kit$^+$ stem cells and thymocyte precursors in the livers of adult mice …………… 116

Chapter 6

マウスの胸腺および末梢リンパ球のニコチン性アセチルコリン受容体の同定 … 125

Identification of nicotinic acetylcholine receptors on lymphocytes in the periphery as well as thymus in mice ……………………………………………………………………… 131

Chapter 7

白血球とリンパ球サブセットの日内変動及び自律神経系機能との間の相関関係の可能性 ... 139

Circadian rhythm of leucocytes and lymphocyte subsets and its possible correlation with the function of the autonomic nervous system ... 149

Chapter 8

分娩後、末梢血のみならず肝臓においても新生児顆粒球増多が出現する ... 161

Neonatal granulocytosis is a postpartum event which is seen in the liver as well as in the blood ... 168

Chapter 9

拘束ストレスを与えた齧歯類の胃における潰瘍形成への顆粒球の関与 ... 177

Association of granulocytes with ulcer formation in the stomach of rodents exposed to restraint stress ... 192

Chapter 10

並体結合マウスの肝臓と腸における胸腺外分化T細胞の中にパートナー細胞の混合度は低い:その生物学的意味 ... 209

Low level of mixing of partner cells seen in extrathymic T cells in the liver and intestine of parabiotic mice; its biological implication ... 220

Chapter 11

糖質コルチコイド投与による顕著な骨髄内顆粒球および胸腺外分化T細胞数の増加 ... 233

Administration of glucocorticoids markedly increases the numbers of granulocytes and extrathymic T cells in the bone marrow ... 242

Chapter 12

抗潰瘍剤の顆粒球抑制作用—胃潰瘍発症における顆粒球の役割 ... 253

Suppressive effect of antiulcer agents on granulocytes – a role for granulocytes in gastric ulcer formation ... 259

Chapter 13

T細胞分化の胸腺外経路 ... 267

Extrathymic pathways of T cell differentiation ... 275

Chapter 14

自律神経系による免疫調節:がん、膠原病と炎症性腸疾患治療へのアプローチ ... 287

Immunomodulation by the autonomic nervous system: therapeutic approach for cancer, collagen diseases, and inflammatory bowel diseases ... 298

Chapter 15

アトピー性皮膚炎患者のステロイドホルモン停滞とステロイド軟膏中止後の禁断症状における独特の白血球分画 ... 311

Stagnation of steroid hormones in patients with atopic dermatitis and unique variation of leukocyte pattern ... 318

Chapter 16

ストレス後のナチュラル・キラー T 細胞と顆粒球の機能は加齢に関連して変化する：各ステロイドホルモンと交感神経との相互関係 ... 329

Age-related bias in function of natural killer T cells and granulocytes after stress: reciprocal association of steroid hormones and sympathetic nerves ... 338

Chapter 17

コラーゲン誘導性関節炎のマウスとパラビオーゼ（並体結合）したマウスの関節においてパートナーの顆粒球とリンパ球は混在しない：顆粒球およびリンパ球の局所産生の可能性 ... 349

No mixing of granulocytes and other lymphocytes in the inflamed joints of parabiosis mice with collagen-induced arthritis: possible in situ generation ... 356

Chapter 18

自己免疫疾患における免疫学的状態 ... 365

Immunologic states of autoimmune diseases ... 373

Chapter 19

低蛋白餌が自然免疫によるマラリア防御を強化する ... 387

Protection against malaria due to innate immunity enhanced by low-protein diet ... 397

Chapter 20

αアドレナリン刺激が、体温、血糖、自然免疫におけるストレス適応反応に与える影響 ... 407

Role of α-adrenergic stimulus in stress-induced modulation of body temperature, blood glucose and innate immunity ... 416

Chapter 21

高速水着の着用効果に関するもう一つの重要なメカニズム ... 425

Proposal of alternative mechanism responsible for the function of high-speed swimsuits ... 427

Chapter 22

ストレスによる体温、血糖、自然免疫の変化と糖質コルチコイドとの関連 431

Association of glucocorticoid with stress-induced modulation of body temperature, blood glucose and innate immunity 442

Chapter 23

がん患者の内部環境と提言：発がんは不利な内部状態を克服する解糖系への適応反応である 455

Internal environment in cancer patients and proposal that carcinogenesis is adaptive response of glycolysis to overcome adverse internal conditions. 463

Evidence for Extrathymic Generation of Intermediate T Cell Receptor Cells in the Liver Revealed in Thymectomized, Irradiated Mice Subjected to Bone Marrow Transplantation

放射線照射胸腺摘出マウスへの骨髄移植による、
胸腺外である肝臓でT細胞レセプターを
中等度に有する細胞が産生された証明

The Journal of Experimental Medicine 182: 759-767, 1995

chapter 1

Evidence for Extrathymic Generation of Intermediate T Cell Receptor Cells in the Liver Revealed in Thymectomized, Irradiated Mice Subjected to Bone Marrow Transplantation

放射線照射胸腺摘出マウスへの骨髄移植による、胸腺外である肝臓でT細胞レセプターを中等度に有する細胞が産生された証明

By Kazunari Sato,* Kazuo Ohtsuka,* Katsuhiko Hasegawa,* Satoshi Yamagiwa,* Hisami Watanabe,* Hitoshi Asakura,⁺ and Toru Abo*

From the *Department of Immunology, and the ⁺Third Department of Internal Medicine, Niigata University School of Medicine, Niigata 951, Japan

【要約】

　胸腺内主経路以外に、肝臓と腸に存在する胸腺外経路においてT細胞が分化することが、明らかになった。特に、T細胞レセプターやCD3を中等度に発現する肝臓のT細胞（TCR^{int}細胞）には、常に、自己応答性クローンを含み、また、この細胞は自己免疫疾患における標的組織や、悪性腫瘍部位を含む他の部位にも時々出現する（よく見られる）。本研究の目的は、これらの細胞が、胸腺外で産生されることと、自己応答性を有することを検証することである。そこで、胸腺摘出し、放射線照射した（B6 x C3H/He）F$_1$マウスに、B6マウスの骨髄細胞を移植し、解析した。胸腺が欠損した状態では、末梢免疫臓器で産生されたT細胞は、全てCD3^{int}細胞であることが、明らかになった。胸腺を摘出せずに放射線照射を行ったマウスの場合、CD3^{int}細胞のみならず、CD3^{high}細胞も出現した。新たに産生されたCD3^{int}細胞のフェノタイプは独特であったので（例えば、インターロイキン2レセプターα$^-$/β$^+$CD44$^+$L-セレクチン$^-$）、胸腺由来T細胞との識別が可能であった。骨髄におけるCD3^{int}細胞の前駆細胞は、Thy-1$^+$CD3$^-$であった。CD3^{int}細胞の胸腺外産生を確認するため、以下の組合せの骨髄移植も行った；C3H→C3HおよびB10.Thy1.1→B6.Thy1.2である。高頻度で自己応答性クローンを含んだ肝臓で産生されるCD3^{int}細胞は、内在性スーパー抗原の非主要リンパ球刺激系および抗Vβモノクローナル抗体を用いて、特にB6→（B6 x C3H/He）（移植片対宿主状態）の組合せにて検証された。さらに、これらの自己応答性クローンは、試験管内培養を行うと不応答ではなく、機能した。これらの結果より、CD3^{int}細胞は、実際に胸腺外起源であり、このCD3^{int}細胞だけが自己応答性禁止T細胞クローンで構成されていることが明らかになった。

　T細胞分化の胸腺外経路が肝臓に存在することを、これまで報告してきた (1-4)。これら肝T細胞には、原始リンパ球として独特な特徴がある；（中等度）[1]のTCRを有する細胞（TCR^{int}細胞と名付ける）やダブルネガティブ（DN）CD4$^-$8$^-$細胞が含まれる (5,6)。これらの細胞が、α/βT細胞のみならず高比率のγ/δT細胞で構成され、常に、自己応答性禁止

[1) 本論文における略語：BMT, 骨髄移植；DN, ダブルネガティブ；int, 中等度；MNC, 単核球；mRNA, メッセンジャーRNA; RAG-l, recombination-activating gene 1; Tx(-),胸腺摘出をしない；Tx(+), thmectomized; Tx-RBMT, 胸腺摘出、放射線照射、骨髄移植を行った

クローンを含むことを、内在性スーパー抗原Mls系と抗Vβモノクロナール抗体を用い検証した。他の研究者らも、類似した集団を同定した(7-9)。TCR^{int}細胞は恒常的にIL-2Rβを発現し、NK細胞と類似している。TCR^{int}細胞の大多数を占める$CD8^+$細胞は、CD8抗原のα/αホモ二量体を有する(6)。$CD3^{int}$細胞は、若年期には極少であるが、加齢により著明になる(5,10)。若年期でさえ、$CD3^{int}$細胞の数は、自己免疫疾患の標的臓器(11,12)や、悪性腫瘍局所(13-15)において増加する。胸腺が欠損しているヌードマウスにおいて、腸管以外の末梢臓器のT細胞は、全てTCR^{int}細胞である。故に、ヌードマウスにおけるこれらのT細胞は、胸腺外起源あることが推測される(5)。しかし、これら胸腺が欠損したヌードマウスの場合、遺伝子に異常があるため、胸腺が欠損している通常のマウスにおいて産生されるT細胞が全てTCR^{int}($CD3^{int}$)細胞であるかどうかは、不明である。

この疑問を解決するため、骨髄移植用に胸腺を摘出し、放射線照射したマウス(Tx-RBMT)を用いた。新たに産生されたT細胞の由来を確認するため、胸腺摘出・放射線照射を行った(B6 x C3H/He) F_1マウスに、B6マウス由来の骨髄細胞を移植した(BMT)。T細胞の由来を、H-2K抗原の発現により、レシピエントであるF_1マウス由来($H-2K^{b+k+}$)であるか、ドナーであるB6マウス由来($H-2K^{b+}$)であるか識別できた。このF_1マウスを用いた実験系では、重要な利点が他にも2つあった。近年、胸腺と末梢免疫臓器において中等度のTCRを有する$NK1.1^+$ T細胞が特定された(16-31)。$CD3^{int}$細胞と$NK1.1^+$ T細胞には、共通点が多い(例、TCR発現が中等度でIL-2Rα$^-$/β$^+$且つ$CD44^+$)(32,33)。そこで、本研究では、NK1.1同種抗原を発現するF_1マウスを用いて、直接2種類の細胞$CD3^{int}$細胞と$NK1.1^+$ T細胞の関係を比較した。さらに、B6マウスと遺伝子背景が同一であるB10マウスには、Mls系および抗Vβモノクロナール抗体を用いて測定する自己応答性禁止クローンが存在しない。これらのマウスはI-E抗原が欠損しているため、T細胞にMls抗原が存在する。しかし、F_1マウスは、I-E抗原を有する；特異的に、C3H/He母マウスから、$Mls-1^{b}2^{a}$抗原を受け継いでいるためである。骨髄移植のこの組合せによりGVH病が発症する可能性があるので、他に以下の組み合わせの骨髄移植も行い、$CD3^{int}$細胞の胸腺外産生を確認した：C3H/He → C3H/HeおよびB10Thy1.1 → B6Thy1.2である。

胸腺が欠損した状況では、肝臓や他の臓器で産生されたT細胞は、全て$CD3^{int}$細胞であることが明らかになった。さらに重要なことは、自己応答性禁止クローンは、これらの$CD3^{int}$細胞に限定されていた。特にB6→(B6 x C3H/He) F_1 (GVH状態)の組合せにおいて、新たに発生したクローンは不応答でなくて、機能した。最近の研究成果も合わせて考察すると(32)、胸腺外$CD3^{int}$(またはTCR^{int})細胞には、自己応答性がある故に、多くの免疫学的現象に関係するようである。

材料と方法

マウス

C57BL/6(B6)、B6-nu/nu、C3H/Heおよび(B6x C3H/He) F_1マウス(雄, 7-15週齢)を使用した。F_1マウスの母マウスは雌C3H/He($Mls-1^{b}2^{a}$)(34)であり、F_1マウスは母マウスからスーパー抗原($Mls-1^{b}2^{a}$)を受け継いだ。マウスは、当初、ジャクソン研究所(東京, 日本)より購入し、新潟大学(新潟, 日本)動物飼育施設室内で飼育した。B10.Thy1.1マウス(T. 佐藤博士(放射線医学総合研究, 千葉, 日本)のご厚意による提供)も使用した(35)。B10.Thy1.1

マウスは、B6.Thy1.2マウスと、Thy1.1抗原発現以外、遺伝的に同一だった。

細胞分離.

定法により、肝単核球（MNC）を分離した（36）。略述すると、エーテル麻酔したマウスの心臓から採血し脱血を行った。摘出した肝臓を、200-ゲージステンレススチールメッシュで濾し、PBS(0.1M, pH 7.2)に懸濁させた。PBSで1度洗浄した後、単核球はフィコール・イソパーク液（1.090）で比重遠心分離を行い、肝細胞と肝細胞核から分離した。比重勾配遠心分離時、特定の細胞が選択的に失われないように（37）、濾過した肝臓懸濁液を充分に培養液で希釈した後、肝臓2匹分で30mlを比重液に重層した。中間層より採取した単核球は、2%FCSを添加した培養液に、懸濁した。分離した肝単核球が含有するクッパー細胞は、4%以下であった（36）。胸腺を200-ゲージ・ステンレス・スチール・メッシュで濾過して、胸腺細胞を採取した。脾臓細胞は、フィコール・イソパーク法により採取した。

フローサイトメトリー解析

細胞表面のフェノタイプを、モノクローナル抗体を用いて二重染色または三重染色して、フローサイトメトリー解析を行った（5）。FITC標識抗CD3(145-2C11)モノクローナル抗体は、Pharmingen (San Diego, CA)製である。ビオチン標識抗IL-2Rβ(TM-β1)モノクローナル抗体（38）も使用した（T. 田中博士のご厚意によるご提供，東京都臨床医学総合研究所，東京，日本）。ビオチン標識抗体は、PE標識アビジン(Caltag Laboratories, San Francisco, CA) で発色させた。Vβ$^+$細胞の各集団は、CD3(FITC)、IL-2Rβ(PE)と各Vβ(Red 613)の三重染色を行い検証した（36）。Red 613標識ストレプトアビジンは、Becton Dickinson and Co. (Mountain View,CA)製である。Vβ3,6,8および11に対応する抗Vβモノクローナル抗体のビオチン標識試薬は、全てPharmingen製である。H-2K^k、H-2K^b、IL-2Rα、NK1.1、TCR-α/β、TCR-γ/δ、CD4、CD8、Pgp-1(CD44)、Mel-14(L-セレクチン)、Thy1.1およびThy1.2抗原に対応する他のFITC、または、PE標識モノクローナル抗体もPharmingen製である。蛍光陽性細胞をFACScan®(Becton Dickinson and Co.)を用いて細胞10,000個を解析した。

DNA合成試験

肝臓、脾臓および骨髄より採取した単核球40,000個を，96穴平底ミクロ培養プレートに入れ（2 x 10^{6}個/ml, 0.2ml）、モノクローナル抗体を添加したプレートと無添加のプレートの両方をCO$_2$培養器内で、3日間37℃で培養した。RPMI1640培養液に、1%自己由来マウス血清、5 x 10^{-5} M 2-MEおよび抗生物質を添加して使用した。組換えマウスIL-2（塩野義製薬（株），大阪，日本））濃度10U/mlを添加して、培養を行ったプレートも準備した。定法により、DNA合成を[^{3}H]チミジン取込み分析法により、検証した（1）。0.5μCi [^{3}H]チミジンを培養最後の16時間に添加した。平均値±1SDは、1系列3 wellで実験を行い、算出した。

RT-PCR法によるRAG-1遺伝子メッセンジャーRNA(mRNA)検出

組換活性化遺伝子（RAG-1）のmRNA検出するため、各遺伝子プライマーを用い、RNA逆転写を行った。さらに、cDNAをRAG-1のプライマーを用いて定法によりPCR法で増幅した（9）。略述すると、RNAをチオシアン酸グアニジン・フェノール-クロロホルム法により各臓器の単核球から抽出した。cDNAは10μg RNAを用いモロニーマウス白血病ウイルス逆転写酵素（200U; GIBCO BRL,Gaithersburg,MD)、ランダムプライマー（宝酒造（株），東京，日本）、逆転写酵素緩衝

液（5x; GIBCO BRL）、ジチオスレイトール（1μM）、dNTP、およびリボヌクレアーゼ阻害剤（50 U; 宝酒造（株））を添加し、最終的に20μlで42℃、60分で合成した。

PCR増幅のために、cDNA（5μl）を各チューブに入れた。チューブには、RAG-1のプライマー（10pM）、Taq DNAポリメラーゼ（2.5 U; 東洋紡（株），大阪, 日本）、および10 x PCR緩衝液（東洋紡（株）とMgCl$_2$（2 mM）にdNTP（200μM）を添加したものを入れておいた。RAG-1は、バンドの大きさは603-bpで、5'プライマー=5'-GTCTCCAGnGTTCCAGA (276-294); 3'プライマー=5'-CTAGCCTGAGTTCTCTTG (841-859)を使用した。サンプルをミネラルオイル（Sigma Chemical Co., St. Louis, MO）で覆い、DNA/RNA重合を変性させるため、加熱後（94℃，5分）、以下の30サイクルの増幅をサーマルサイクラー（宝酒造（株））にて行った：94℃（50秒），55℃（30秒）および72℃（2分）。増幅後、PCR産物の33%を用いて、3.0%アガロースゲルで電気泳動を行い、エチジウムブロマイド染色後、紫外線下で視覚化した。β-アクチンプライマーは、RNA精製の完全性の評価にも用いた。

結果

胸腺欠損状況下で産生されたT細胞は、全てCD3^{int}細胞であった

NK細胞、CD3^{int}(TCR^{int})細胞およびCD3^{high}細胞（5,36）を含むリンパ球サブセットを検証するため、CD3とIL-2Rβの二重染色を行った（Fig. 1 A）。対照群B6マウス（9週齢）の肝臓と脾臓の単核球を検証した。CD3$^-$IL-2Rβ$^+$（主にアシアロGM1$^+$ NK）細胞、CD3^{int}$^+$IL-2Rβ$^+$細胞（CD3^{int}細胞）およびCD3^{high}$^+$IL-2Rβ$^-$（CD3^{high}細胞）における顕著なピークを認めた。対照群B6マウスにおいて、CD3$^-$IL-2Rβ$^+$NK細胞とCD3^{int}細胞（矢印）が、脾臓よりも肝臓において豊富であった（Fig. 1 A, 上）。B6マウスの胸腺細胞はCD3$^-$、CD3^{low}およびCD3^{high}細胞で構成されるが、その全てにおいてIL-2Rβの発現が欠損していた。B6ヌードマウスの場合、肝臓と脾臓のT細胞は、全てCD3^{int}細胞であった（Fig. 1 A, 下）。CD3^{high}細胞とCD3^{int}細胞が、それぞれ、胸腺由来、胸腺外由来である可能性を考察した。

この可能性を直接証明するため、(B6 x C3H/He)F$_1$マウスの胸腺を摘出し実験を行った（Fig. 1 B）。7週齢のF$_1$マウスの胸腺摘出を行い、9週齢で放射線照射（10Gy）を行った。この時、胸腺摘出を行わないF$_1$マウスも使用した。これら胸腺を摘出したマウスにも、胸腺を摘出しないマウスにも、放射線照射を行った後、ただちにB6マウスの骨髄細胞（10^7）を移植した。2週後、これら骨髄移植を行ったマウスの肝臓と脾臓より単核球を採取して検証を行った。驚くべきことに、移植2週後、これら骨髄移植マウスの肝臓と脾臓の両方において、胸腺摘出したマウスでも、胸腺摘出しないマウスで、新しく産生されたT細胞は、全てIL-2Rβ$^+$CD3^{int}細胞であった。胸腺を摘出しないマウスの場合（Fig. 1 B, 上）、実験4週後と8週後に、少ないが顕著な比率のCD3^{high}細胞が、肝臓と脾臓に見られた。全く対照的に、胸腺摘出と放射線照射を行ったマウスでは（Fig. 1 B, 2列）、実験後、どの時点でもどの臓器でもこのようなCD3^{high}細胞は見られなかった。移植50週以降も見られなかった（未発表データ）。

骨髄におけるCD3^{int}細胞の前駆細胞のフェノタイプを検証するため、実験を進めた（Fig. 1 B, 3,4列）。そのため、Thy1.2$^+$細胞を除去した骨髄細胞、または、CD3$^+$細胞を除去した骨髄細胞（10^{7}個/匹）をマウスに移入した。興味深いことに、Thy1.2$^+$細胞を除去した骨髄細胞を

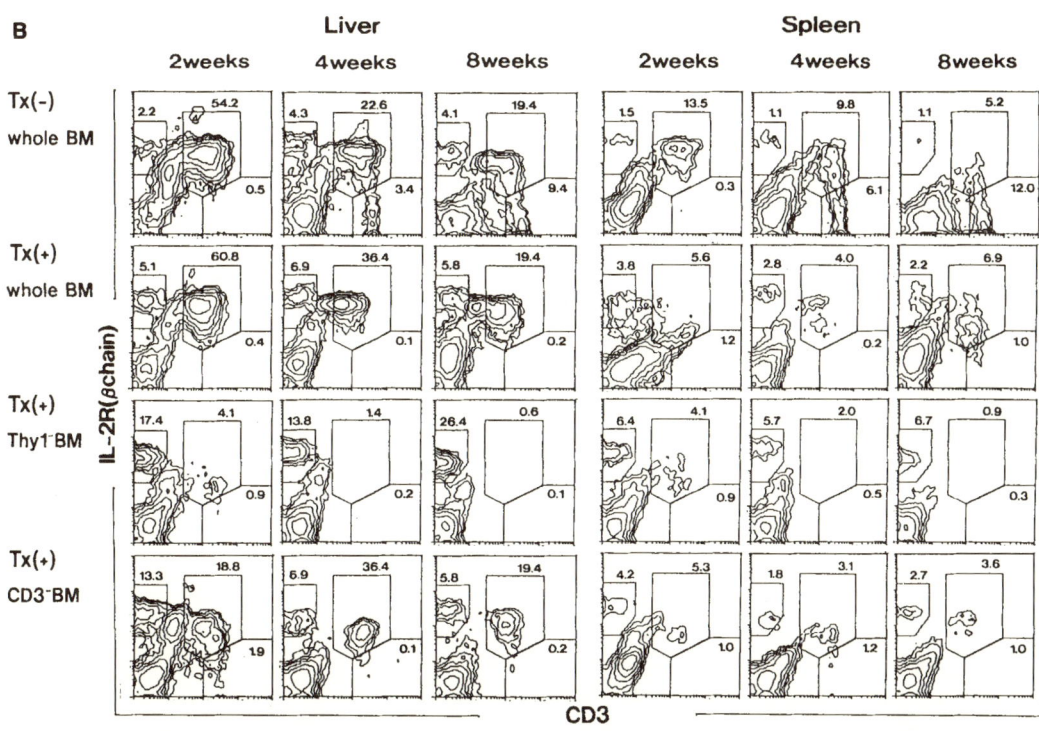

Figure.1

胸腺摘出、放射線照射、そして骨髄移植を行ったマウスにおけるCD3^{int}細胞の増殖。(A) 対照マウスと胸腺欠損ヌードマウスの肝臓においてCD3とIL-2Rβの二重染色を行い、CD3^{int}細胞を同定した。(B) 胸腺摘出、放射線照射、そして骨髄移植を行ったマウスにおけるCD3^{int}細胞の増殖。(C) 肝臓で増殖したCD3^{int}細胞は、ドナー由来である。実験Aでは、C57BL/6(B6)-+/+およびB6-nu/nuマウスを使用した(雄、5週齢)。実験BおよびCでは、(B6 × C3H/He)F$_1$マウス(7週齢)の胸腺摘出を行った。2週後に、これらF$_1$マウスに放射線照射後(10Gy)、B6マウス骨髄細胞(10^7)を、直ちに静脈内移入した。胸腺摘出をしないF$_1$マウスも使用した。骨髄細胞は、骨髄全細胞、Thy1$^+$細胞を除去した細胞およびCD3$^+$細胞を除去した細胞を使用した。CD3^{int}細胞集団を検証するため、CD3とIL-2Rβの二重染色を行った。この染色から、CD3^{int}細胞は、CD3^{int}IL-2Rβ$^+$と考えられた；CD3^{high}細胞(胸腺由来T細胞)は、CD3^{high}IL-2Rβ$^-$と考えられた；また、NK細胞は、CD3$^-$IL-2Rβ$^+$と考えられた。骨髄移植マウスで増殖したT細胞の由来を検証するため、CD3とH-2K^k(またはH-2K^b)の二重染色も行った。各分画内の数値は、蛍光陽性細胞の比率を示す。

移入した場合、8週後でも、CD3^{int}細胞の再構築は見られなかった。一方、CD3$^+$細胞を除去した骨髄細胞を移入した場合、肝臓と脾臓の両方の臓器でCD3^{int}細胞の再構築が見られ、全骨髄細胞を移入した場合に類似していた。その後の研究において、肝単核球、脾細胞およびリン

パ節細胞も使用したところ、胸腺摘出・照射を行ったマウスにおいて、CD3^{int}細胞の再構築が見られた（未発表データ）。

これら細胞のうち、肝単核球を10^7個でなく10^8個を移入すると、CD3^{int}細胞が再構築された。これに対して、脾細胞（10^8）またはリンパ節細胞（10^8）では再構築されなかった。10^7または10^8（個/匹）の脾細胞またはリンパ節細胞を移入したマウスは、実験後4日以内に全て死亡した。

CD3^{int}細胞の由来が、ドナーなのか、レシピエントなのかを確認するため、K^{b+k+}（F_1レシピエント）またはK^{b+}（B6ドナー）に注目して、H-2Kの発現を検証した（Fig.1C）。これらT細胞は、k^-b^+であったので、B6ドナー由来であった。これは骨髄移植マウスの肝単核球の結果であるが、脾細胞の結果も確認した。

新たに産生されたCD3^{int}細胞のフェノタイプの特徴.

骨髄移植（B6→F_1）マウスの肝臓に見られるCD3^{int}細胞のフェノタイプの特徴を、さらに検証した（Fig. 2）。IL-2Rβ^+CD3^{int}細胞は、全てIL-2Rα^-であった。このフェノタイプは、休止もしくは活性化したCD3^{high}細胞のフェノタイプと比較すると、独特であった。休止CD3^{high}細胞は、IL-2Rβ^-IL-2Rα^-であった。これに対して、活性化CD3^{high}細胞は、IL-2Rβ^+IL-2Rα^+であった（36）。CD3^{int}細胞の1/3はNK1.1抗原を共発現しているが、CD3の発現の強度から考えると、NK1.1$^+$ T細胞はCD3^{int}細胞内に限定されていた。産生されたCD3^{int}細胞は、全てTCRα/β^+で、主としてCD8抗原を発現した。CD3（緑）およびCD4とCD8（赤）を用いた二重染色が示すように、CD4$^-$8$^-$細胞の数は極少であった。接着分子は、CD44$^+$(Pgp-1)L-セレクチン(Mel-14)$^-$であった。CD3^{int}細胞表面の接着分子のフェノタイプも、独特だった。その理由は、CD3^{high}細胞はCD44$^-$セレクチン$^+$だからである（33）。

Figure.2

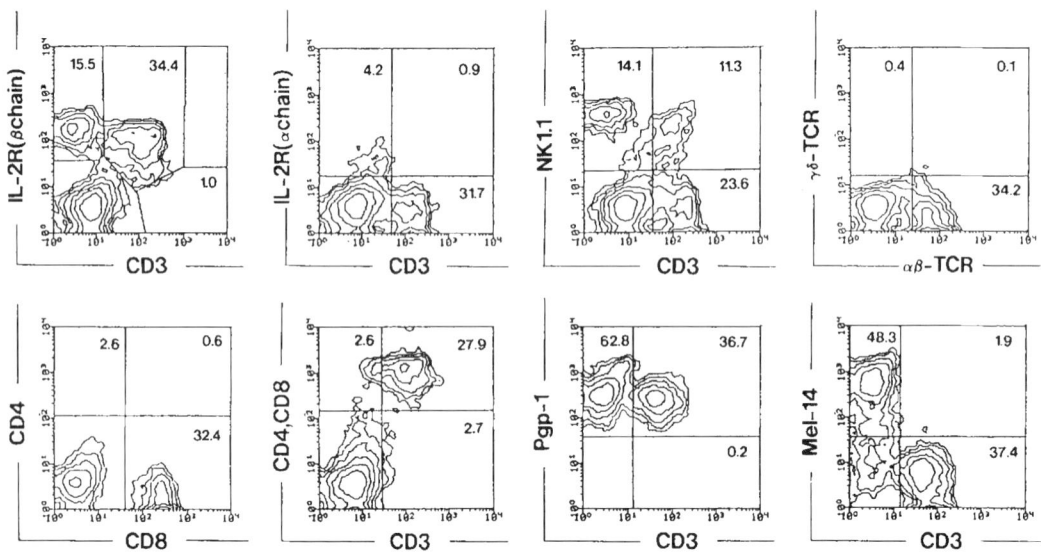

胸腺摘出、放射線照射、そして骨髄移植を行ったマウスの肝臓で増殖したCD3^{int}細胞のフェノタイプのさらなる特徴。多種の組合せで、二重染色を行った。各分画内の数値は、蛍光陽性細胞の比率を示す。CD3^{int}細胞はIL-2Rα^-/β^+と考えられるが、この集団の1/3が、NK1.1抗原を発現した。産生されたCD3^{int}細胞のほぼ全ては、フェノタイプがCD8$^+$とPgp1$^+$Mel-14$^-$であるα/βT細胞であった。

異なる組合せの骨髄移植による CD3^{int} 細胞の胸腺外産生の（立証）

これまでの実験では、骨髄移植（親→F_1）の組合せを使用して、回復したT細胞が、ドナー由来であるか検証した。しかし、この組合せでは、GVH病が誘導される。そこで、さらに異なる以下の組合せの骨髄移植を行い、CD3^{int}細胞の胸腺外産生について検証した：C3H/He→C3H/HeおよびB10.Thy1.1→B6Thy1.2 (Fig.3)。胸腺摘出の有無にかかわらず、全てのレシピエント・マウスに放射線照射後（10Gy）、ドナーの骨髄細胞（10^7個/匹, CD3$^+$細胞を除去）を、直ちに移入した。実験1カ月後、マウスのCD3^{int}細胞およびCD3^{high}細胞の値を測定した。

どちらの組合せでも、胸腺を摘出したマウスでは、CD3^{int}細胞だけが出現した。ところが、胸腺を摘出しないマウスでは、CD3^{int}細胞だけではなく、CD3^{high}細胞も出現した。もう1つの組合せ（B10.Thy1.1→B6.Thy1.2）の結果、胸腺を摘出したマウスで増殖したCD3^{int}細胞は、ドナー由来（Thy1.1$^+$Thy1.2$^-$）であることを確認した。

CD3^{int} 細胞における自己応答性クローンの同定

既報のように（2）、CD3^{int}細胞は、自己反応禁止クローンを含み、内在性スーパー抗原Mls系と抗VβモノクロナールA抗体を用いて測定される。本研究では、骨髄移植マウスにおいて新たに産生されたCD3^{int}細胞が、このような自己応答性クローンを含むかを検証した (Fig.4)。以下、2種の骨髄移植組合せを行った；B6→(B6 x C3H/He)F_1およびC3H/He→C3H/He。

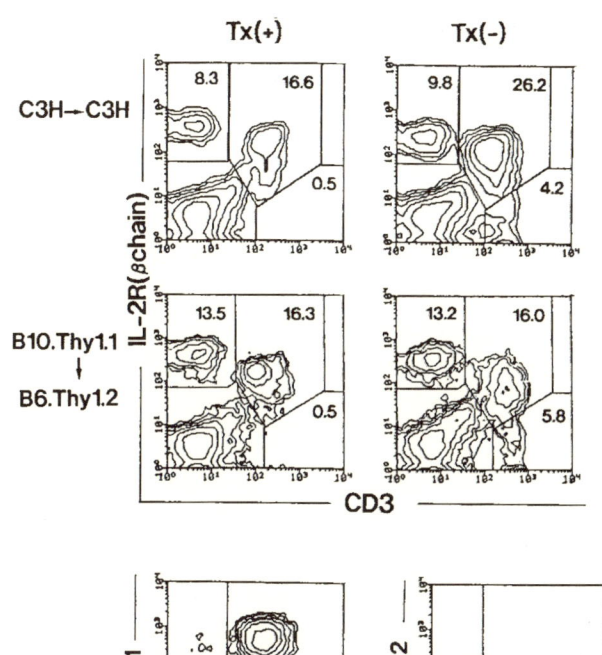

Figure.3

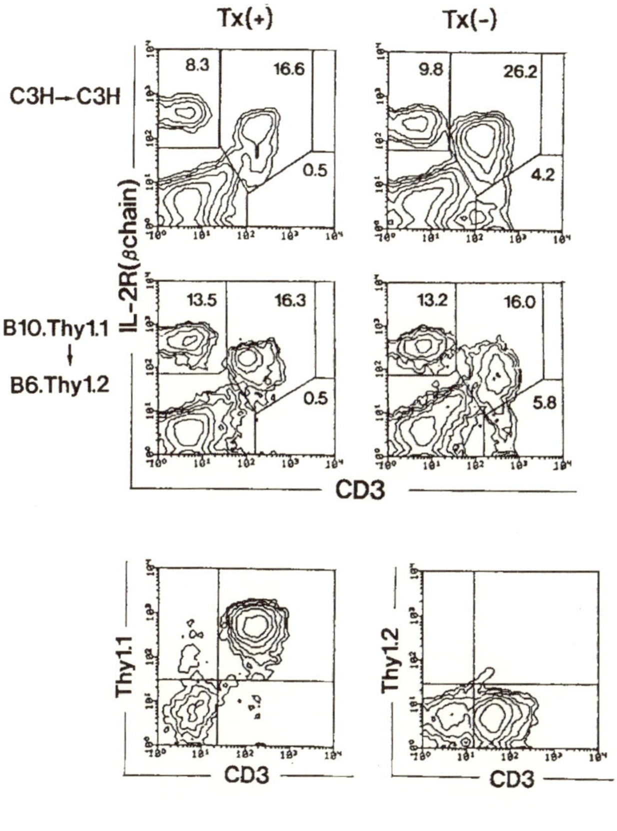

他の組合せの骨髄移植におけるCD3^{int}細胞の胸腺外産生の確認。以下、2種の組み合わせを、胸腺が欠損した状況と胸腺のある状況下で、骨髄移植を行った（C3H/He→C3H/HeおよびB10.Thy1.1→B6.Thy1.2）。実験1カ月後、マウスを検証した。どちらの組合せでも、胸腺を摘出したマウスでは、CD3^{int}細胞だけが産生された。これに対して、胸腺を摘出しないマウスでは、CD3^{int}細胞だけでなく、CD3^{high}細胞も産生された。B10.Thy1.1→B6.Thy1.2の組合せで、産生されるT細胞は、ドナー由来（Thy1.1$^+$1.2$^-$）であることが確認された。

Figure.4

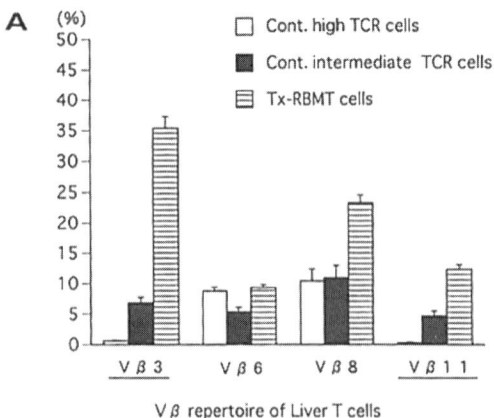

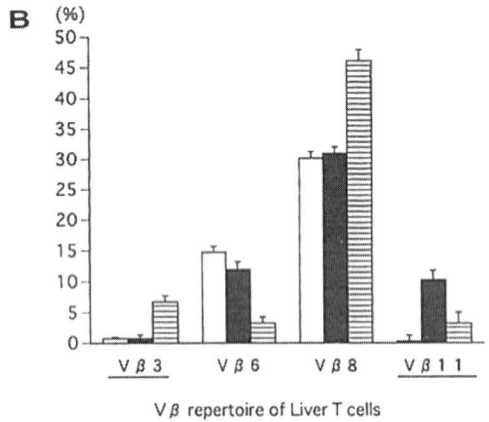

CD3^{int}細胞の自己応答性禁止クローンの同定。(A) B6→(B6 x C3H/He)F1；(B) C3H/He→C3H/He。各Vβ$^+$細胞集団をCD3(FITC)、IL-2Rβ(PE)と対応するVβ(Red 613)の三重染色を行い検証した。Vβ3$^+$とVβ11$^+$細胞（下線）は、自己応答性禁止クローンである。一方、(B6 x C3H/He)F$_1$マウスとC3H/Heマウス(Mls-1^{b}2^a)のVβ6$^+$とVβ8$^+$細胞の非禁止クローンである。平均値±1 SDは、3度実験を行い算出した。

B6マウスには、Mls系と抗Vβモノクロナール抗体を用いて測定される自己応答性禁止クローンは、見られなかった。その理由は、B6マウスは、抗原提示I-E分子を欠損しているからである。しかし、(B6 x 3H/He)F$_1$マウスは、このVβ3$^+$とVβ11$^+$クローンを有する。Mls-1^{b}2^{a}スーパー抗原は、親のC3H/He雌マウスに由来する。

CD3^{high}細胞およびCD3^{int}細胞の対照値は、(B6 x C3H/He)F$_1$とC3H/Heマウスの値である。胸腺摘出、放射線照射、そして骨髄移植を行ったF$_1$マウスの肝臓内のCD3^{int}細胞では、禁止クローンであるVβ3$^+$とVβ11$^+$が非常に顕著であった（Fig. 4 A）。一方、対照F$_1$マウスの肝臓内のCD3^{high}細胞は、自己反応性クローンVβ3$^+$やVβ11$^+$を含まなかった。一方、対照F$_1$マウスの肝臓内のCD3^{int}細胞が含む自己反応性クローンの割合は低かった。非禁止クローンVβ6$^+$およびVβ8$^+$は、検証を行った全細胞分画に分布することが明らかになった。

前述したように、骨髄移植B6→(B6 x C3H/He)F$_1$の組合せでは、GVH病が誘導される。そこで、骨髄移植（C3H/He→C3H/He）の組合せにおいて、Vβ3$^+$およびVβ11$^+$禁止クローンの値を測定した（Fig. 4 B）。この組合せで胸腺摘出、放射線照射、そして骨髄移植を行ったマウスの場合でも、肝臓においてVβ3$^+$およびVβ11$^+$禁止クローンが見られたが、胸腺摘出、放射線照射、そして骨髄移植を行ったマウスB6→(B6 x C3H/He)F$_1$の組合せと比較して、顕著に低値であった。この結果から、F$_1$レシピエント・マウスでは禁止クローンが高値であり、この組合せでのGVH病の原因である可能性が高くなった。

F$_1$レシピエント・マウスの拡大した禁止クローンは、固相化した抗Vβ3モノクロナール抗体に反応できた

B6→(B6 x C3H/He)F$_1$の組合せの骨髄移植マウスで同定したこの自己応答性クローンの状態が、不応答であったのか、非不応答であったかを検証した。骨髄移植F$_1$マウスと対照C3H/Heマウスから分離した肝単核球を、固相化した抗Vβ3モノクロナール抗体で刺激した（Fig. 5）。不応答の状態では、自己応答性Vβ+細胞に低用量IL-2(10U/ml)を添加すると、抗

Figure.5

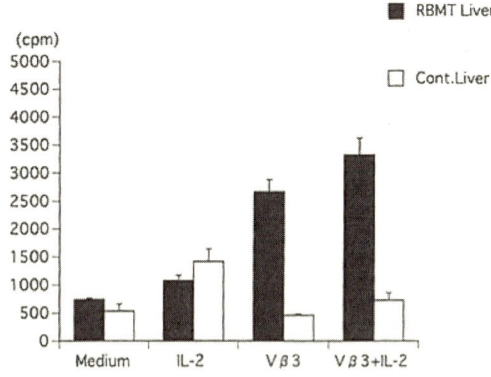

試験管培養（縦軸、[³H]チミジンカウント毎分）において新たに産生されたCD3^{int}細胞の固相化した抗Vβ3モノクロナール抗体に対する増殖応答。B6→(B6 x C3H/He)F$_1$の組合せで骨髄移植を行った1カ月後の胸腺摘出、放射線照射、そして骨髄移植を行ったマウスを使用した。新たに産生されたCD3^{int}細胞の状態が不応答か、非不応答かを検証するため、固相化した抗Vβ3モノクロナール抗体に対する胸腺摘出、放射線照射、そして骨髄移植を行ったマウスと対照マウスの肝単核球の増殖反応を検証した。平均値±1 SDは、1系列当たり3 well培養を行い算出した。

Vβモノクロナール抗体に応答して増殖することが知られているので、この培養も同時に行った。IL-2（非不応答状態）の添加の有無にかかわりなく、骨髄移植マウスから分離した新たに産生された肝T細胞が、抗Vβ3モノクロナール抗体に反応して、活発に増殖することが明らかになった。一方、対照C3H/Heマウスの肝単核球に、IL-2を添加しても抗Vβ3モノクロナール抗体に反応しなかった（顕著な不応答状態）。

骨髄移植マウス肝単核球のRAG-1 mRNA発現

次に、骨髄移植マウスと対照マウスの肝臓と脾臓から採取した単核球がRAG-1 mRNAを発現するか検証した（Fig. 6）。骨髄移植マウスの肝単核球は、おそらく産生が活発であることを反映してRAG-1 mRNAを高度に発現することが明らかになった。この増幅レベル（30サイクル）において、対照マウスの肝単核球におけるRAG-1 mRNAの発現は微弱であった。また、骨髄移植マウスと対照マウスの両方の脾単核球は検出限界以下であった。

考察

本研究では、胸腺を摘出したマウスに放射線照射および骨髄移植を行い、胸腺欠損状況下の肝臓と脾臓において産生されたT細胞の全てが、独特の特徴を持つCD3^{int}(TCR^{int})細胞であることを直接証明した。既報で示したように

Figure.6

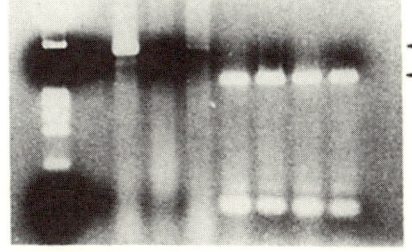

胸腺摘出、放射線照射、そして骨髄移植を行ったマウスから採取した肝単核球のRAG-1 mRNA発現。RAG-1遺伝子mRNAを検証するため、RNAを逆転写してcDNAにし、これをRAG-1のプライマーを用いてPCR法により増幅した。胸腺摘出、放射線照射、そして骨髄移植を行ったマウスの肝単核球において、明瞭にRAG-1のバンドが見られた。

(5,6)、先天的に胸腺が欠損しているヌードマウスにおいては、腸以外の肝臓や他の末梢免疫臓器で見られるT細胞は、全てTCR^{int}細胞である。さらに、RAG-1およびRAG-2のmRNAを対照マウスの肝単核球で検証できた(9)。これら結果より、TCR^{int}細胞は、胸腺外で産生され、主として肝臓において分化する可能性を提示した(5,6)。しかし、以下のような指摘が挙げられた:(a)先天的に胸腺が欠損しているヌードマウスには、胸腺原基があるので、ヌードマウスは胸腺欠損だとは言えない;また、(b)RAG-1とRAG-2の発現は、前駆細胞レベルで高値であるに過ぎない。それ故、T細胞かB細胞のどちらの前駆細胞が、RAG-1とRAG-2のmRNAを発現するのかを推定するのは困難である。

これらの疑問に答えるため、胸腺摘出、放射線照射、そして骨髄移植を行ったマウスを使用した。このように胸腺摘出、放射線照射、そして骨髄移植を行ったマウスを使用すれば、T細胞サブセット産生と骨髄における胸腺外T細胞の前駆細胞のフェノタイプに対して、胸腺が及ぼす影響を検証することもできた。この骨髄移植を行ったマウスは、CD3^{int}細胞だけを産生し、そして、胸腺摘出を行わない骨髄移植マウスではCD3^{int}細胞だけでなく、CD3^{high}細胞も常に産生していた。CD3^{int}細胞は胸腺外由来であり、CD3^{high}細胞は胸腺由来であると考えられる。胸腺外T細胞の前駆細胞のフェノタイプ(Thy-1$^+$CD3$^-$)も、本研究での非常に興味深い発見であった。この方法で実験を行ったところ、胸腺が欠損した状況で産生されたCD3^{int}細胞の特徴は、対照マウスや先天的な胸腺欠損マウスの肝臓に見られるCD3^{int}細胞の特徴と一致した(5,6,32,33)。両方ともCD3^{int}でありフェノタイプはIL-2Rα^-/β^+およびCD44$^+$L-セレクチン$^-$であり、両方とも自己応答性クローンを含んでいた。唯一の違いは、本研究で新たに産生されたCD3^{int}細胞では、CD8$^+$細胞(僅かのCD4$^-$8$^-$細胞)が優位であったことであった。そして、特に親とF$_1$マウスの組み合せにおける自己応答性クローンは、不応答状態ではなかった。最近の研究では、非不応答で活性化した自己応答性T細胞が、慢性GVH病の自己免疫状態におけるエフェクター細胞となると報告した(35)。対照マウスのCD3^{int}細胞は、大概、不応答状態であると報告された(7,39)。同系の組合せ(C3H/He→C3H/He)では、CD3^{int}細胞の自己応答性クローンは、非常に低値で(Fig. 4)、不応答状態であった(未発表データ)。これらのことからも、CD3^{int}細胞の禁止クローンが高値であることは、GVH病の発症を予測する重要な指標である。いずれにせよ、禁止クローンはCD3^{int}細胞のみに限定されるが、CD3^{high}細胞に全く見られなかった。

本研究では、放射線胸腺摘出、放射線照射、そして骨髄移植を行ったマウスで新たに産生されたT細胞のRAG-1 mRNAの発現度を検証した。どのサブセットがmRNAを高度に発現したかは検証できなかったが、実際、これらマウスの肝単核球は対照マウスの肝単核球よりもmRNAを高度に発現した。この状態においては、T細胞またはB細胞の成熟したTCRまたは免疫グロブリンレパートリーが著しく産生されたことが推測できた。CD3^{int}細胞に関する疑問が複数生ずる:例、CD3^{int}細胞は、活性化した胸腺由来T細胞とどのように異なるか? 胸腺由来T細胞は、活性化後IL-2RβおよびCD44抗原を獲得する。しかし、活性化した胸腺由来T細胞は、IL-2Rαを最大限に発現すると同時に、必ずIL-2Rβも有する(36)。NK細胞と胸腺外T細胞だけは、恒常的にIL-2Rβを発現するが、IL-2Rαは欠損している(5)。同様に、その時、活性化した胸腺由来T細胞はCD44抗原を獲得するが、L-セレクチンを失う(33)。さ

らに重要なことは、CD3^{high}細胞が抗原やマイトジェンの刺激により活性化した後、TCRまたはCD3の発現低下は見られなかった (32, 33)。

フェノタイプがCD4$^-$CD8$^-$またはCD4$^+$であるNK1.1$^+$α/βT細胞に注目する研究者も、最近出現した (16-24)。これらの細胞は、本研究におけるTCR^{int}細胞と一致する。本研究で示すように、NK1.1抗原の発現を欠損するCD3^{int}細胞も存在する。そのようなNK1.1$^+$T細胞またはCD3^{int}細胞は胸腺外分化する。しかし、これらの細胞はT細胞の胸腺内分化代替経路でも産生され、胸腺内主経路と呼ばれる主流との依存性はない (21-24)。CD4$^-$8$^-$フェノタイプを持つNK1.1$^+$T細胞の機能に関する研究が多く行われ、この集団は、ハイブリッドレジスタンス (25) や自己応答性 (26-30) が起こるメカニズムを理解するのに、非常に重要であることが明らかになった。NK1.1$^+$T細胞は、優先的に不変鎖Vα14を使用していた (9,31)。B6マウスの各免疫臓器におけるCD3^{int}細胞およびNK1.1$^+$T細胞の関係を現在検証している（投稿準備中）。NK1.1$^+$細胞は全てIL-2Rβ$^+$CD3^{int}細胞に限定され、NK1.1$^+$とNK1.1$^-$サブセットはCD3^{int}細胞集団の中に存在する。NK1.1$^+$サブセットには、主としてCD4$^-$8$^-$細胞とCD4$^+$細胞がある。これに対して、NK1.1$^-$サブセットにはCD4$^-$CD8$^-$とCD4$^+$細胞だけでなくCD8$^+$細胞（優位）もある。

肝臓と胸腺で産生されるTCR^{int}細胞を、T細胞の共通系統として分類しなければならない可能性を提案する。何故ならこの細胞のフェノタイプと機能は原始的であるので、「原始的または原始」T細胞と名付けるべきかもしれない。T細胞分化の原始経路で産生されるこれら原始T細胞（TCR$^-$ → TCR^{int}）は、胸腺内主経路（TCR$^-$ → TCR^{low} → TCR^{high}）よりも系統発生学的に初期に進化した基本的な免疫系である可能性がある。一連の最近の研究において (32,35)、これら原始T細胞が自己免疫疾患の病因または自己応答性クローンが持つ自己応答性が原因である慢性GVH病の自己免疫状態にとって非常に重要であると報告した。

本研究は、TCR^{int}細胞が胸腺が欠損した状況下での正常マウスの肝臓や他の免疫臓器といった胸腺外で産生されるエビデンス（証拠）を示す。しかし、胸腺内代替経路においてCD3^{int}細胞が独立して産生されることを否定するものではない。

渡辺正子氏の原稿準備に深謝する。本研究は、文部科学省およびがん研究補助金による。
Address correspondence to Dr. T. Abo, Department of Immunology, Niigata University School of Medi- cine, Niigata 951, Japan. Received for publication 24 October 1994 and in revised form 30 March 1995.

Evidence for Extrathymic Generation of Intermediate T Cell Receptor Cells in the Liver Revealed in Thymectomized, Irradiated Mice Subjected to Bone Marrow Transplantation

By Kazunari Sato,[*] Kazuo Ohtsuka,[*] Katsuhiko Hasegawa,[*] Satoshi Yamagiwa,[*] Hisami Watanabe,[*] Hitoshi Asakura,[‡] and Toru Abo[*]

From the [*]Department of Immunology, and the [‡]Third Department of Internal Medicine, Niigata University School of Medicine, Niigata 951, Japan

Summary

In addition to the major intrathymic pathway of T cell differentiation, extrathymic pathways of such differentiation have been shown to exist in the liver and intestine. In particular, hepatic T cells of T cell receptors or CD3 of intermediate levels (i.e., intermediate T cell receptor cells) always contain self-reactive clones and sometimes appear at other sites, including the target tissues in autoimmune diseases and the tumor sites in malignancies. To prove their extrathymic origin and self reactivity, in this study we used thymectomized, irradiated (B6 × C3H/He) F_1 mice subjected to transplantation of bone marrow cells of B6 mice. It was clearly demonstrated that all T cells generated under athymic conditions in the peripheral immune organs are intermediate CD3 cells. In the case of nonthymectomized irradiated mice, not only intermediate CD3 cells but also high CD3 cells were generated. Phenotypic characterization showed that newly generated intermediate CD3 cells were unique (e.g., interleukin 2 receptor α^-/β^+ and CD44$^+$L-selectin$^-$) and were, therefore, distinguishable from thymus-derived T cells. The precursor cells of intermediate CD3 cells in the bone marrow were Thy-1$^+$CD3$^-$. The extrathymic generation of intermediate CD3 cells was confirmed in other combinations of bone marrow transplantation, C3H → C3H and B10.Thy1.1 → B6.Thy1.2. The generated intermediate CD3 cells in the liver contained high levels of self-reactive clones estimated by anti-Vβ monoclonal antibodies in conjunction with the endogenous superantigen minor lymphocyte-stimulating system, especially the combination of B6 → (B6 × C3H/He) (graft-versus-host situation). Moreover, these self-reactive clones were not anergic but functional in in vitro cultures. These results reveal that intermediate CD3 cells are truly of extrathymic origin and that only such intermediate CD3 cells comprise self-reactive forbidden T cell clones.

It has been proposed that extrathymic pathways of T cell differentiation exist in the liver (1–4). These hepatic T cells have unique properties as primitive lymphocytes; e.g., they have TCR of intermediate (int)[1] levels (termed int TCR cells) and contain double-negative (DN) CD4$^-$8$^-$ cells (5, 6). They consist of a high proportion of γ/δ T cells as well as of α/β T cells and always contain self-reactive forbidden clones as estimated by anti-Vβ mAbs in conjunction with the endogenous superantigen Mls system. A similar population was also identified by other investigators (7–9). int TCR cells constitutively express IL-2Rβ, similar to NK cells. The majority of CD8$^+$ cells among int TCR cells carry the α/α homodimer of CD8 antigens (6). Although intermediate CD3 cells are very few in youth, they become prominent with aging (5, 10). Even in youth, intermediate CD3 cells increase in number at the target organ in autoimmune diseases (11, 12) and at tumor sites in malignancies (13–15). Since all T cells in the peripheral organs, except the intestine, in athymic nude mice are int TCR cells, we speculate that they are of extrathymic origin (5). However, because of the genetic abnormality of these athymic nude mice, it is unclear whether all T cells generated in normal mice under athymic conditions are int TCR (or CD3) cells.

We used here thymectomized, irradiated mice subjected to bone marrow transplantation (Tx-RBMT) to overcome the above situation. To identify the origin of newly gener-

---

[1] *Abbreviations used in this paper:* BMT, bone marrow transplantation; DN, double negative; int, intermediate; MNC, mononuclear cells; mRNA, messenger RNA; RAG-1, recombination-activating gene 1; Tx(−), nonthymectomized; Tx(+), thymectomized; Tx-RBMT, thymectomized, irradiated, and subjected to bone marrow transplantation.

ated T cells, thymectomized, irradiated (B6 × C3H/He) F_1 mice were subjected to transplantation of bone marrow cells (BMT) of B6 origin. The expression of H-2K antigens enabled us to determine whether they were of recipient F_1 origin ($H-2K^{b+k+}$) or donor B6 origin ($H-2K^{b+}$). The use of these F_1 mice had two other important advantages. Recently, NK1.1$^+$ T cells with TCR of intermediate levels have been identified in the thymus and peripheral immune organs (16–31). Since many properties (e.g., TCR of intermediate levels and the expression $IL-2R\alpha^-/\beta^+$ and $CD44^+$) are shared by intermediate CD3 cells and NK1.1$^+$ T cells (32, 33), we directly compared their relationships in F_1 mice expressing NK1.1 alloantigens in this study. Moreover, B6 mice and B10 congenic mice do not have self-reactive forbidden clones estimated by anti-Vβ mAbs in conjunction with the Mls system. These mice lack I-E molecules, which present Mls antigens to T cells. However, F_1 mice carry I-E molecules; specifically, they receive Mls-1^{b}2^a antigens from their C3H/He mother. Since this combination of BMT has a potential to induce GVHD, the extrathymic generation of int CD3 cells was also confirmed in other combinations: C3H/He → C3H/He and B10.Thy1.1 → B6.Thy1.2.

It was demonstrated that all T cells generated in the liver and other organs under athymic conditions were int CD3 cells. More importantly, self-reactive forbidden clones were confined to these int CD3 cells, and such newly generated clones were not anergic but functional, especially in the combination of B6 → (B6 × C3H/He) F_1 (GVH situation). Taken together with data from recent studies (32), it would appear that extrathymic int CD3 (or TCR) cells are involved in many immunological phenomena because of their autoreactivity.

Materials and Methods

Mice. Male C57BL/6 (B6), B6-*nu/nu*, C3H/He, and (B6× C3H/He) F_1 mice at 7–15 wk of age were used. Mothers of the F_1 mice were female C3H/He (Mls-1^{b}2^a) mice (34) from which the F_1 mice received the superantigen, Mls-1^{b}2^a. They were originally obtained from Jackson Laboratories Japan (Tokyo, Japan) and were maintained in the animal facility of Niigata University (Niigata, Japan). B10.Thy1.1 mice (35), which were kindly provided by Dr. T. Sato (National Institute of Radiological Science, Chiba, Japan), were also used. This strain of mice was genetically identical to B6.Thy1.2 mice except for the expression of Thy1.1 antigens.

Cell Preparations. Hepatic mononuclear cells (MNC) were isolated by a previously described method (36). Briefly, mice anesthetized with ether were killed by total exsanguination by cardiac puncture. To obtain MNC, the liver was removed, pressed through a 200-gauge stainless steel mesh, and suspended in PBS (0.1 M, pH 7.2). After one washing with PBS, MNC were isolated from hepatocytes and hepatocyte nuclei by Ficoll-Isopaque density (1.090) gradient centrifugation. To avoid selective cell loss by the gradient centrifugation method (37), sufficient dilution of mashed liver samples with the medium (i.e., 30 ml for two livers) was important before it was overlaid on the gradient cushion. MNC collected from the interface were then suspended in MEM supplemented with 2% FCS. The preparations of hepatic MNC contained <4% Kupffer cells (36). Spleen cells were also collected by the Ficoll-Isopaque method, while thymocytes were obtained by forcing the thymus through a 200-gauge steel mesh.

Immunofluorescence Test. The surface phenotype of cells was analyzed using mAbs in conjunction with two- or three-color immunofluorescence tests (5). FITC-conjugated anti-CD3 (145-2C11) mAb was obtained from Pharmingen (San Diego, CA). Biotin-conjugated anti–IL-2Rβ (TM-β1) mAb (38) was also used (kindly provided by Dr. T. Tanaka, Tokyo Metropolitan Institute of Medical Science, Tokyo, Japan). Biotin-conjugated reagent was developed with PE-conjugated avidin (Caltag Laboratories, San Francisco, CA). Each population of Vβ^+ cells was identified by three-color staining for CD3 (FITC), IL-2Rβ (PE), and corresponding Vβ (Red 613) (36). Red 613–conjugated streptavidin was obtained from Becton Dickinson and Co. (Mountain View, CA). All biotin-conjugated reagents of anti-Vβ mAbs against Vβ3, 6, 8, and 11 were obtained from Pharmingen. Other FITC- or PE-conjugated mAbs against H-2K^k, H-2K^b, IL-2Rα, NK1.1, TCR-α/β, TCR-γ/δ, CD4, CD8, Pgp-1 (CD44), Mel-14 (L-selectin), Thy1.1, and Thy1.2 antigens were also obtained from Pharmingen. The fluorescence-positive cells were analyzed with a FACScan® (Becton Dickinson and Co.). 10,000 cells were analyzed.

DNA Synthesis Assay. 40,000 MNC from the liver, spleen, and bone marrow (0.2 ml of 2 × 10^6 cells/ml) were cultured for 3 d with or without each immobilized mAb in a 96-well flat-bottomed microculture plate at 37°C in a CO$_2$ incubator. RPMI 1640 medium supplemented with 1% autologous mouse sera, 5 × 10^{-5} M 2-ME, and antibiotics was used. In some cultures, recombinant mouse IL-2 (Sionogi Seiyaku Co., Osaka, Japan) was added at a concentration of 10 U/ml. DNA synthesis was examined by [^{3}H]thymidine uptake assay, as shown previously (1). 0.5 μCi of [^{3}H]thymidine was added in the final 16 h of the culture. The mean ± 1 SD was determined in triplicate cultures.

Reverse Transcription-PCR Assay for the Detection of Messenger RNA (mRNA) of RAG-1 Gene. To detect mRNA of recombination-activating gene 1 (RAG-1) gene, RNA was reversely transcribed using the primers of these genes, and such cDNA was further amplified by the PCR method as previously described (9). Briefly, RNA was prepared from MNC of various organs by an acid guanidinium thiocyanate–phenol-chloroform method. cDNA was synthetized using 10 μg RNA, Moloney murine leukemia virus reverse transcriptase (200 U; GIBCO BRL, Gaithersburg, MD), random primer (Takara Shuzo Co., Tokyo, Japan), reverse transcriptase buffer (5×; GIBCO BRL), dithiothreitol (10 mM), dNTP (1 μM), and RNase inhibitor (50 U; Takara Shuzo Co.) in a final volume of 20 μl for 60 min at 42°C.

For PCR amplification, 5 μl of cDNA was transferred to individual tubes that contained 10 pM of the primers for RAG-1, Taq DNA polymerase (2.5 U; Toyobo Co., Osaka, Japan), and dNTP (200 μM) in 10 × PCR buffer (Toyobo Co.) and MgCl$_2$ (2 mM). For RAG-1, 5' primer = 5'-GTCTCCAGTAGTTCCAGA (276-294); 3' primer = 5'-CTAGCCTGAGTTCTCTTG (841-859), yielding a 603-bp fragment, were used. The samples were overlaid with light mineral oil (Sigma Chemical Co., St. Louis, MO), heated to 94°C for 5 min to denature DNA/RNA duplexes, and then subjected to 30 amplification cycles of 50 s at 94°C, 30 s at 55°C, and 2 min at 72°C, in a thermal cycler (Takara Shuzo Co.). After amplification, 33% of the PCR products were electrophoresed on 3.0% agarose gel, stained with ethidium bromide, and visualized under UV illumination. Primers for β-actin were also used to assess the integrity of the RNA preparation.

Results

All T Cells Generated under Athymic Conditions Are int CD3 Cells. To identify lymphocyte subsets, including NK cells, int CD3 (or TCR) cells, and high CD3 cells (5, 36), two-color staining for CD3 and IL-2Rβ was performed (Fig. 1 A). When MNC in the liver and spleen of control B6 mice (9 wk old) were examined, clear peaks of CD3$^-$IL-2Rβ$^+$ (mainly asialo GM$_1$$^+$ NK) cells, CD3-int$^+$IL-2Rβ$^+$ cells (i.e., int CD3 cells), and CD3-high$^+$IL-2Rβ$^-$ cells (i.e., high CD3 cells) were identified. CD3$^-$IL-2Rβ$^+$ NK cells and int CD3 cells (arrows) were more abundant in the liver than in the spleen of the control B6 mice (Fig. 1 A, upper panels). Thymocytes in the B6 mice consisted of CD3$^-$, CD3-low$^+$, and CD3-high$^+$ cells, all lacking the expression of IL-2Rβ. In the case of B6 nude mice, all T cells in both the liver and spleen were int CD3 cells (Fig. 1 A, lower panels). We postulated that high CD3 cells and int CD3 cells might be of thymic origin and of extrathymic origin, respectively.

To directly prove this possibility, we used thymectomized (Tx(+)) (B6 × C3H/He) F$_1$ mice (Fig. 1 B). These F$_1$ mice were thymectomized at the age of 7 wk and irradiated with 10 Gy 2 wk later. Nonthymectomized (Tx(-)) F$_1$ mice were used in parallel. These Tx(-) or Tx(+) irradiated mice were immediately injected with 10^7 bone marrow cells of B6 mice. 2 wk later, MNC obtained from the liver and spleen of these BMT mice were examined. Surprisingly, all newly generated T cells, both in the liver and spleen of all these BMT mice, were IL-2Rβ$^+$ int CD3 cells at 2 wk after treatment, whether they were Tx(+) or Tx(-). In the case of Tx(-) mice (Fig. 1 B, upper panels), a small but significant proportion of high CD3 cells were generated in the liver and spleen 4 and 8 wk after the treatment. In sharp contrast, Tx(+) irradiated mice did not acquire such high CD3 cells in either organ at any time after treatment (Fig. 1 B, second row). This was true even 50 wk or more after the treatment (data not shown).

To determine the phenotype of the precursors for int CD3 cells in the bone marrow, further experiments were conducted (Fig. 1 B, third and fourth rows). For this purpose, we injected mice with Thy1.2$^+$ cell–depleted or CD3$^+$ cell–depleted bone marrow cells (10^7 cells/mouse). Interestingly, Thy1.2$^+$ cell–depleted bone marrow cells did not reconstitute int CD3 cells even at 8 wk after treatment. On the other hand, CD3$^+$ cell–depleted bone marrow cells reconstituted int CD3 cells in both organs, similar to the case of whole bone marrow cells. In a subsequent study, we also used liver MNC, splenocytes, and lymph node cells to reconstitute int CD3 cells in Tx(+) irradiated mice (data not shown). Among these cells, 10^8 liver MNC, but not 10^7 liver MNC cells, reconstituted int CD3 cells, whereas 10^8 splenocytes or 10^8 lymph node cells did not. All mice injected with 10^7 or 10^8 splenocytes or lymph node cells died within 4 d after treatment.

To determine whether int CD3 cells were of donor or recipient origin, H-2K expression was investigated in terms of K^{b+k+} (F$_1$ recipient) or K^{b+} (B6 donor) (Fig. 1 C). Since these T cells were k$^-$b$^+$, they were of donor B6 origin. This result was derived from the liver of BMT mice, and the result from the spleen confirmed it.

Phenotypic Characterization of Newly Generated int CD3 Cells. Further phenotypic characterization of int CD3 cells appearing in the liver of BMT (B6 → F$_1$) mice was carried out (Fig. 2). IL-2Rβ$^+$ int CD3 cells were all IL-2Rα$^-$. This phenotype was unique when compared with that of resting or activated high CD3 cells. Thus, resting high CD3 cells were IL-2Rβ$^-$IL-2Rα$^-$, while activated high CD3 cells were IL-2Rβ$^+$IL-2Rα$^+$ (36). One-third of the population of int CD3 cells coexpressed NK1.1 antigens, and NK1.1$^+$ T cells were confined to a population of int CD3 cells, concerning their intensity of CD3. All generated int CD3 cells were TCR-α/β$^+$ and expressed mainly CD8 antigens. DN CD4$^-$8$^-$ cells were very few in number, as shown by two-color staining for CD3 (green) and a mixture of CD4 and CD8 (red). The adhesion molecules, were CD44$^+$(Pgp-1)L-selectin$^-$(Mel-14). This phenotype of adhesion molecules on int CD3 cells was also unique, because high CD3 cells are CD44$^-$L-selectin$^+$ (33).

Confirmation of Extrathymic Generation of int CD3 Cells in Different Combinations of BMT. In a previous experiment, we used the combination of BMT, parent → F$_1$, to determine whether the recovered T cells were of donor origin. However, this combination induces GVHD. In this regard, we further examined the extrathymic generation of int CD3 cells in different combinations, i.e., C3H/He → C3H/He and B10.Thy1.1 → B6.Thy1.2 (Fig. 3). All recipient mice with or without thymectomy were irradiated (10 Gy) and were immediately injected with 10^7 bone marrow cells (depleted of CD3$^+$ cells) of the donor. 1 mo after such treatments, mice were examined on the levels of int CD3 cells and high CD3 cells. In both combinations, Tx(+) mice produced only int CD3 cells, whereas Tx(-) mice produced not only int CD3 cells but also high CD3 cells. In the latter combination, we confirmed that the expanding int CD3 cells in Tx(+) mice were of donor origin (i.e., Thy1.1$^+$Thy1.2$^-$).

Identification of Self-reactive Clones among int CD3 Cells. As shown previously (2), int CD3 cells are comprised of self-reactive forbidden clones as estimated by anti-Vβ mAbs in conjunction with the endogenous superantigen Mls system. In this experiment, we investigated whether the newly generated int CD3 cells in BMT mice contained such self-reactive clones (Fig. 4). We used two combinations of BMT, i.e., B6 → (B6 × C3H/He) F$_1$ and C3H/He → C3H/He. B6 mice did not have self-reactive forbidden clones estimated by anti-Vβ mAbs in conjunction with the Mls system, because they lack I-E molecules, which undergo the antigen presentation. However, (B6 × C3H/He) F$_1$ mice have such clones, Vβ3$^+$ and Vβ11$^+$. Mls-1^{b2a} superantigens are derived from parental female C3H/He mice. Control values in high CD3 cells and int CD3 cells were derived from either (B6 × C3H/He) F1 and C3H/He mice. int CD3 cells in the liver of BMT (Tx-RBMT) mice (F$_1$) showed extremely high levels of forbidden clones, both Vβ3$^+$ and Vβ11$^+$ (Fig. 4 A). On the other hand, high CD3 cells seen in the liver of control F$_1$ mice did not contain self-reactive clones Vβ3$^+$ and Vβ11$^+$, while int CD3 cells in the liver of control F$_1$ mice contained a few such clones. The nonforbidden clones Vβ6$^+$ and Vβ8$^+$ were found to be distributed in all cell fractions tested.

As already mentioned, the combination of BMT, B6 → (B6 × C3H/He) F$_1$, induces GVHD. In this regard, we also examined the levels of Vβ3$^+$ and Vβ11$^+$ forbidden

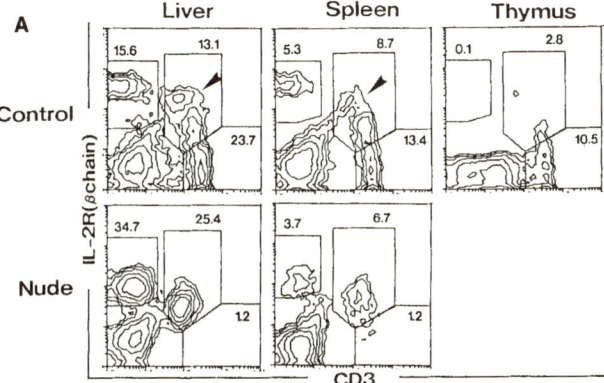

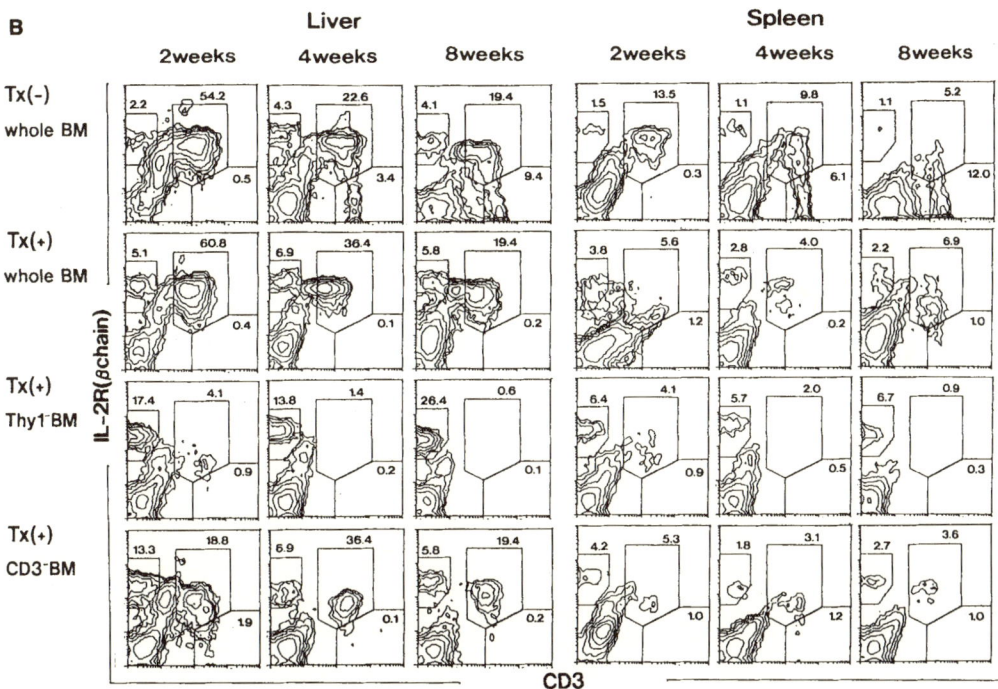

Figure 1. Expansion of int CD3 cells in Tx-RBMT mice. (A) Identification of int CD3 cells in the liver of control and athymic nude mice by two-color staining for CD3 and IL-2Rβ. (B) Expansion of int CD3 cells in Tx-RBMT mice. (C) int CD3 cells expanding in the liver are of donor origin. In experiment A, male C57BL/6 (B6)−+/+ and B6-*nu/nu* mice at the age of 15 wk were used. In experiments B and C, (B6×C3H/He) F$_1$ mice at the age of 7 wk were thymectomized. 2 wk later, these F$_1$ mice were irradiated (10 Gy), and 10^7 bone marrow cells of B6 mice were immediately intravenously injected. Some Tx(−) F$_1$ mice were also used. As sources of bone marrow cells, whole cells, Thy-1$^+$ cell–depleted cells, and CD3$^+$ cell–depleted cells were used. Two-color staining for CD3 and IL-2Rβ was carried out to identify a population of int CD3 cells. By this staining, int CD3 cells were estimated to be CD3-int$^+$IL-2Rβ$^+$; high CD3 cells (i.e., T cells of thymic origin) were estimated to be CD3-high$^+$IL-2Rβ$^-$; and NK cells were estimated to be CD3$^-$IL-2Rβ$^+$. To determine the origin of T cells expanding in BMT mice, two-color staining of CD3 and H-2K^k (or H-2K^b) was also performed. Numbers in the figure indicate the percentages of fluorescence-positive cells in the corresponding area.

clones in the combination of BMT, C3H/He → C3H/He (Fig. 4 B). Although Tx-RBMT mice of this combination also contained Vβ3$^+$ and Vβ11$^+$ forbidden clones in the liver, the levels were extremely low compared with Tx-RBMT mice of B6 → (B6 × C3H/He) F$_1$ combination. This raises the possibility that the high levels of forbidden clones seen in F$_1$ recipient mice might be responsible for the onset of GVHD in this combination.

762   Extrathymic Generation of T Cells

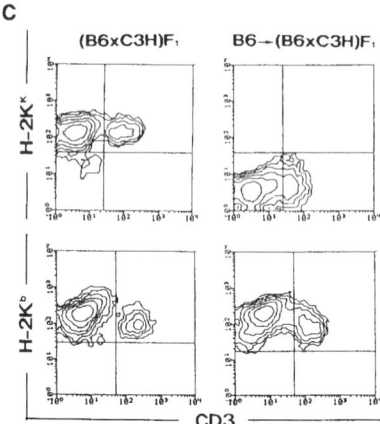

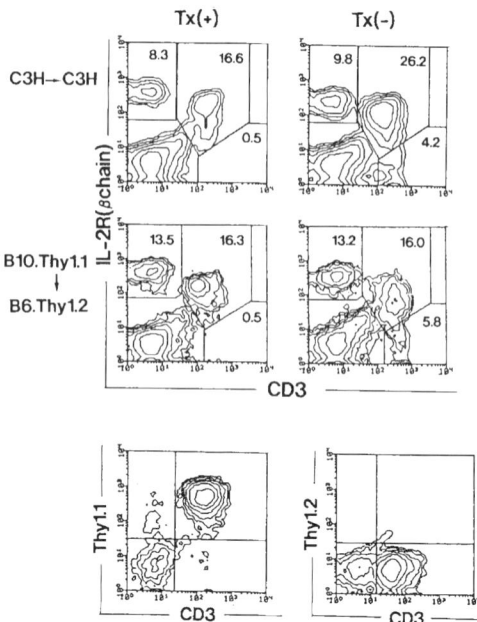

Expanding Forbidden Clones in F_1 Recipient Mice Could Respond to Immobilized Anti-Vβ3 mAb It was then investigated whether such self-reactive clones identified in BMT mice of the combination of B6 → (B6 × C3H/He) F_1 were in anergic states or in nonanergic states. Hepatic MNC isolated from either BMT mice (F_1) or control C3H/He mice were stimulated with immobilized anti-Vβ3 mAb (Fig. 5). Since anergic, self-reactive Vβ^+ cells are known to proliferate in response to anti-Vβ mAb in the presence of a low dose of

Figure 3. Confirmation of the extrathymic generation of int CD3 cells in other combinations of BMT. Two other combinations of BMT, C3H/He → C3H/He, and B10.Thy1.1 → B6.Thy1.2, were performed under athymic and thymic conditions. Mice were examined 1 mo after treatments. In both combinations, only int CD3 cells were generated in Tx(+) mice, whereas not only int CD3 cells but also high CD3 cells were generated in Tx(−) mice. In the combination of B10.Thy1.1 → B6.Thy1.2, the generated T cells were confirmed to be of donor origin (Thy1.1$^+$1.2$^-$).

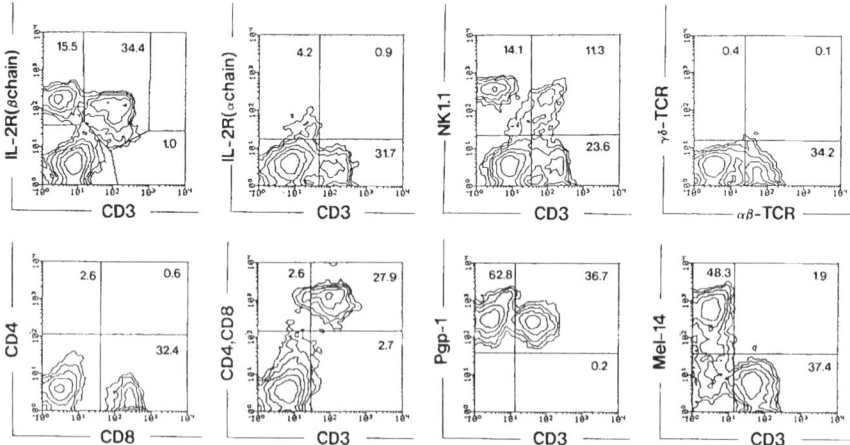

Figure 2. Further phenotypic characterization of int CD3 cells expanding in the liver of Tx-RBMT mice. Two-color stainings for various combinations, as indicated in the figure, were performed. Numbers in the figure indicate the percentages of fluorescence-positive cells in the corresponding area. int CD3 cells were estimated to be IL-2Rα^-/β^+, and one-third of this population expressed NK1.1 antigens. Almost all int CD3 cells generated were α/β T cells with CD8$^+$ and Pgp1$^+$Mel-14$^-$ phenotypes.

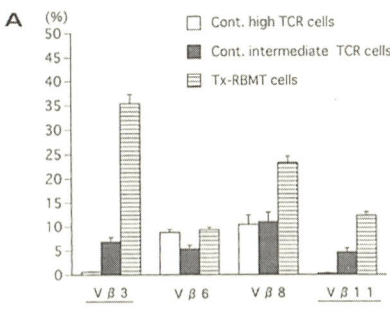

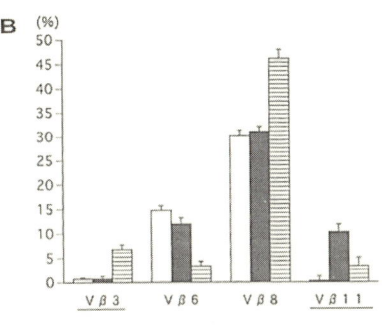

Figure 4. Identification of self-reactive forbidden clones among int CD3 cells. (A) B6 → (B6 × C3H/He) F$_1$; (B) C3H/He→C3H/He. Each population of Vβ+ cells was identified by three-color staining for CD3 (FITC), IL-2Rβ (PE), and corresponding Vβ (Red 613). Vβ3+ and Vβ11+ cells (*underlined*) are self-reactive forbidden clones, while Vβ6+ and Vβ8+ cells are nonforbidden clones in (B6×C3H/He) F$_1$ mice and C3H/He mice (Mls-1^{b}2^a). The mean ± 1 SD was determined from three experiments.

IL-2 (10 U/ml), such culture conditions were applied in parallel. Newly generated hepatic T cells isolated from BMT mice were found to vigorously proliferate in response to anti-Vβ3 mAb, irrespective of the presence of IL-2 (i.e., nonanergic states). On the other hand, hepatic MNC in control C3H/He mice did not respond to anti-Vβ3 mAb even in the presence of IL-2 (i.e., highly anergic states).

The Expression of mRNA of RAG-1 by Liver MNC in BMT Mice. We then examined whether MNC obtained from the liver and spleen of BMT mice and control mice expressed mRNA of RAG-1 (Fig. 6). It was demonstrated that liver MNC in BMT mice highly expressed mRNA of RAG-1, possibly reflecting their active generation. At this amplification level (30 cycles), the expression of mRNA of RAG-1 in liver MNC of control mice was minor, and that in splenic MNC of both BMT and control mice was at an undetectable level.

Discussion

In the present study, using Tx(+) irradiated mice subjected to BMT, we directly demonstrated that all T cells generated

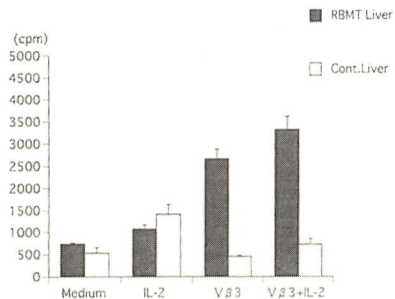

Figure 5. Proliferative response of newly generated int CD3 cells to immobilized anti-Vβ3 mAb in in vitro culture (*ordinate*, counts per minute of [^{3}H]thymidine). Tx-RBMT mice were used 1 mo after BMT of the combination, B6 → (B6 × C3H/He) F$_1$. To examine whether newly generated int CD3 cells were in anergic states or in nonanergic states, the proliferate response of liver MNC in Tx-RBMT mice and control mice to the immobilized anti-Vβ3 mAb was analyzed. The mean ± 1 SD was determined by triplicate cultures.

in the liver and spleen under athymic conditions were int CD3 (or TCR) cells with unique properties. As already shown in our previous studies (5, 6), all T cells seen in the liver and other peripheral immune organs except the intestine in congenitally athymic nude mice are int TCR cells. Moreover, mRNA of RAG-1 and RAG-2 was detectable in liver MNC in control mice (9). In light of these findings, we proposed the possibility that int TCR cells are generated extrathymically and that the liver is the major site of their differentiation (5, 6). However, various criticisms have been raised: (*a*) Congenitally athymic nude mice still have a remnant of the thymus, and these mice are not athymic; and (*b*) the expression of RAG-1 and RAG-2 is only high at the precursor cell level, and, therefore, it is difficult to estimate which type of precursors for T and B cells express mRNA of RAG-1 and RAG-2.

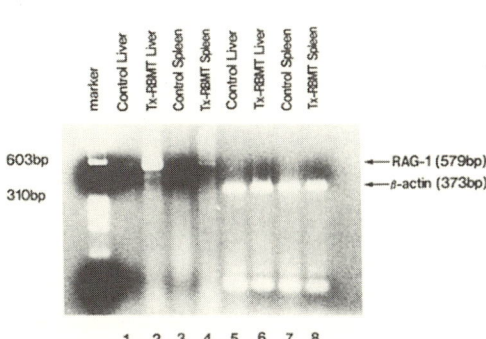

Figure 6. Expression of mRNA of RAG-1 by liver MNC isolated from Tx-RBMT mice. To detect mRNA of RAG-1 gene, RNA was reversely transcribed using the primers of these genes, and cDNA was further amplified by the PCR method. A clear band of RAG-1 was observed in liver MNC of Tx-RBMT mice.

To answer these questions, we used Tx-RBMT mice. By using this protocol, we were also able to investigate the influence of the thymus on the generation of T cell subsets and the phenotype of precursor cells of extrathymic T cells in the bone marrow. Since these BMT mice produced only int CD3 cells, and Tx(−) mice with BMT always produced not only int CD3 cells but also high CD3 cells, we estimate that int CD3 cells are of extrathymic origin and high CD3 cells are of thymic origin. The phenotype of extrathymic T cells, i.e., Thy-1$^+$CD3$^-$, was also a very interesting finding of this study. The properties of int CD3 cells generated under athymic conditions in this experimental protocol coincided with those of int CD3 cells seen in the liver of normal mice and congenitally athymic mice (5, 6, 32, 33). Specifically, both of them expressed CD3 of intermediate levels, both had the phenotype of IL-2Rα^-/β^+ and CD44$^+$L-selectin$^-$, and both contained self-reactive clones. The only difference was that newly generated int CD3 cells in this study showed a predominance of CD8$^+$ cells (very few DN CD4$^-$8$^-$ cells), and self-reactive clones were not in anergic states, especially the combination of parent and F$_1$ mice. In a recent study, we reported that nonanergic, active self-reactive T cells became effector cells for autoimmune states seen in chronic GVHD (35). It has previously been shown that int CD3 cells in normal mice are usually in anergic states (7, 39). In a syngeneic combination (C3H/He → C3H/He), self-reactive clones among int CD3 cells were very low (Fig. 4) and were at anergic state (data not shown). Taken together, the elevated levels of forbidden clones among int CD3 cells are important indicators predicting the onset of GVHD. In any case, forbidden clones were always confined to int CD3 cells but not at all to high CD3 cells.

In this study, we investigated the expression levels of mRNA of RAG-1 of newly generated T cells in Tx-RBMT mice. Although we were not able to determine which subsets expressed high levels of mRNA, it was true that liver MNC in these mice expressed higher levels of mRNA than did liver MNC in control mice. It can be speculated that some T or B cells intensively differentiated to produce a mature repertoire of TCR or immunoglobulins under this condition. Several questions regarding int CD3 cells arise; e.g., how different are int CD3 cells from activated, thymus-derived T cells? Thymus-derived T cells acquire IL-2Rβ and CD44 antigens after activation. However, activated, thymus-derived T cells always acquire IL-2Rβ in parallel with the highest expression of IL-2Rα (36). Only NK cells and extrathymic T cells constitutively express IL-2Rβ but lack IL-2Rα (5). Similarly, activated thymus-derived T cells acquire CD44 antigen but do not lose the expression of L-selectin at that time (33). More importantly, we have not observed that high CD3 cells downregulate their expression of TCR or CD3 after activation by any antigenic and mitogenic stimulations (32, 33).

Several investigators have recently focused attention on NK1.1$^+$ α/β T cells with DN or CD4$^+$ phenotype (16–24). These cells correspond to the int TCR cells in our studies. There are some int CD3 cells lacking the expression of NK1.1 antigens, as shown in this study. Such NK1.1$^+$ T cells or int CD3 cells are generated extrathymically. However, they are also generated through an alternative pathway of T cell differentiation in the thymus, independent from the main stream of the major intrathymic pathway (21–24). Many functional studies on NK1.1$^+$ T cells with DN CD4$^-$8$^-$ phenotype revealed that this population was very important to understanding the mechanism involved in hybrid resistance (25) and autoreactivity (26–30). NK1.1$^+$ T cells preferentially used invariant Vα14 chain (9, 31). We have recently investigated the relationship between int CD3 cells and NK1.1$^+$ T cells in various immune organs of B6 mice in detail (manuscript in preparation). All NK1.1$^+$ cells are confined to IL-2Rβ^+ int CD3 cells, and both NK1.1$^+$ and NK1.1$^-$ subsets are present among intermediate CD3 cells. Such NK1.1$^+$ subsets mainly comprise DN CD4$^-$8$^-$ cells and CD4$^+$ cells, whereas such NK1.1$^-$ subsets comprise CD8$^+$ cells (predominantly) as well as DN and CD4$^+$ cells.

We propose the possibility that int TCR cells generated in the liver and thymus should be categorized as a common lineage of T cells. Because of their primitive phenotype and functions, they may be called "primitive or primordial" T cells. These primitive T cells generated in the primitive pathways of T cell differentiation (TCR$^-$ → TCR^{int}) might be a fundamental immune system phylogenetically developed earlier than the major intrathymic pathway (i.e., TCR$^-$ → TCR^{low} → TCR^{high}). In a series of recent studies (32, 35), we reported that these primitive T cells are quite important to the pathogenesis of autoimmune diseases or autoimmune states induced by chronic GVHD because of their autoreactivity of self-reactive clones. In the present study we provide evidence that int TCR cells are extrathymically generated in the liver and other immune organs of normal mice under athymic conditions. However, we do not deny the independent generation of int CD3 cells in the alternative intrathymic pathway.

We wish to thank Miss Hiroko Karasawa and Mrs. Masako Watanabe for the preparation of the manuscript.

This work was supported in part by a grant-in-aid for cancer research from the Ministry of Education, Science, and Culture, Japan.

Address correspondence to Dr. T. Abo, Department of Immunology, Niigata University School of Medicine, Niigata 951, Japan.

Received for publication 24 October 1994 and in revised form 30 March 1995.

References

1. Ohteki, T., S. Seki, T. Abo, and K. Kumagai. 1990. Liver is a possible site for the proliferation of abnormal CD3$^+$4$^-$8$^-$ double-negative lymphocytes in autoimmune MRL-lpr/lpr mice. *J. Exp. Med.* 172:7–12.
2. Abo, T., T. Ohteki, S. Seki, N. Koyamada, Y. Yoshikai, T. Masuda, H. Rikiishi, and K. Kumagai. 1991. The appearance of T cells bearing self-reactive T cell receptor in the livers of mice injected with bacteria. *J. Exp. Med.* 174: 417–424.
3. Seki, S., T. Abo, T. Ohteki, K. Sugiura, and K. Kumagai. 1991. Unusual $\alpha\beta$-T cells expanded in autoimmune lpr mice are probably a counterpart of normal T cells in the liver. *J. Immunol.* 147:1214–1221.
4. Okuyama, R., T. Abo, S. Seki, T. Ohteki, K. Sugiura, A. Kusumi, and K. Kumagai. 1992. Estrogen administration activates extrathymic T cell differentiation in the liver. *J. Exp. Med.* 175:661–669.
5. Iiai, T., H. Watanabe, S. Seki, K. Sugiura, K. Hirokawa, M. Utsuyama, H. Takahashi-Iwanaga, T. Iwanaga, T. Ohteki, and T. Abo. 1992. Ontogeny and development of extrathymic T cells in mouse liver. *Immunology.* 77:556–563.
6. Ohtsuka, K., T. Iiai, H. Watanabe, T. Tanaka, M. Miyasaka, K. Sato, H. Asakura, and T. Abo. 1994. Similarities and differences between extrathymic T cells residing in mouse liver and intestine. *Cell. Immunol.* 153:52–66.
7. Goossens, P.L., H. Jouin, G. Marchal, and G. Milon. 1990. Isolation and flow cytometric analysis of the free lymphomyeloid cells present in murine liver. *J. Immunol. Methods.* 132:137–144.
8. Murosaki, S., Y. Yoshikai, A. Ishida, T. Nakamura, G. Matsuzaki, H. Takimoto, H. Yuuki, and K. Nomoto. 1991. Failure of T cell receptor Vβ negative selection in murine intestinal intra-epithelial lymphocytes. *Int. Immunol.* 3:1005–1013.
9. Makino, Y., N. Yamagata, T. Sasho, Y. Adachi, R. Kanno, H. Koseki, M. Kanno, and M. Taniguchi. 1993. Extrathymic development of Vα14-positive T cells. *J. Exp. Med.* 177:1399–1408.
10. Ohteki, T., R. Okuyama, S. Seki, T. Abo, K. Sugiura, A. Kusumi, T. Ohmori, H. Watanabe, and K. Kumagai. 1992. Age-dependent increase of extrathymic T cells in the liver and their appearance in the periphery of older mice. *J. Immunol.* 149:1562–1570.
11. Masuda, T., T. Ohteki, T. Abo, S. Seki, M. Nose, H. Nagura, and K. Kumagai. 1991. Expansion of the population of double negative CD4$^-$8$^-$ T$\alpha\beta$-cells in the liver is a common feature of autoimmune mice. *J. Immunol.* 147:2907–2912.
12. Tsuchida, M., H. Hanawa, H. Hirahara, H. Watanabe, Y. Matsumoto, H. Sekikawa, and T. Abo. 1994. Identification of CD4$^-$ CD8$^-$ $\alpha\beta$ T cells in the subarachnoid space of rats with experimental autoimmune encephalomyelitis. A possible route by which effector cells invade the lesions. *Immunology.* 81:420–427.
13. Seki, S., T. Abo, K. Sugiura, T. Ohteki, T. Kobata, H. Yagita, K. Okumura, H. Rikiishi, T. Masuda, and K. Kumagai. 1991. Reciprocal T cell responses in the liver and thymus of mice injected with syngeneic tumor cells. *Cell. Immunol.* 137:46–60.
14. Ohmori, K., T. Iiai, H. Watanabe, T. Tanaka, and T. Abo. 1993. Activation of extrathymic T cells in the liver of mice bearing syngeneic tumors. *Biomed. Res. (Tokyo).* 14:65–79.
15. Iiai, T., H. Watanabe, T. Iwamoto, I. Nakashima, and T. Abo. 1994. Predominant activation of extrathymic T cells during melanoma development of metallothionein/ret transgenic mice. *Cell. Immunol.* 153:412–427.
16. Budd, R.C., G.C. Miescher, R.C. Howe, R.K. Lees, C. Bron, and H.R. MacDonald. 1987. Developmentally regulated expression of T cell receptor β chain variable domains in immature thymocytes. *J. Exp. Med.* 166:577–582.
17. Fowlkes, B.J., A.M. Kruisbeek, H. Ton-That, M.A. Weston, J.E. Coligan, R.H. Schwartz, and D.M. Pardoll. 1987. A novel population of T-cell receptor $\alpha\beta$-bearing thymocytes which predominantly expresses a single Vβ gene family. *Nature (Lond.).* 329:251–254.
18. Crispe, I.N., M.W. Moore, L.A. Husmann, L. Smith, M.J. Bevan, and R.P. Shimonkevitz. 1987. Differentiation potential of subsets of CD4$^-$8$^-$ thymocytes. *Nature (Lond.).* 329: 336–339.
19. Takahama, Y., A. Kosugi, and A. Singer. 1991. Phenotype, ontogeny, and repertoire of CD4$^-$CD8$^-$ T cell receptor $\alpha\beta^+$ thymocytes. Variable influence of self-antigens on T cell receptor Vβ usage. *J. Immunol.* 146:1134–1141.
20. Arase, H., N. Arase-Fukushi, R.A. Good, and K. Onoe. 1993. Lymphokine-activated killer cell activity of CD4$^-$CD8$^-$ TCR$\alpha\beta^+$ thymocytes. *J. Immunol.* 151:546–555.
21. Egerton, M., and R. Scollay. 1990. Intrathymic selection of murine TCR$\alpha\beta^+$CD4$^-$CD8$^-$ thymocytes. *Int. Immunol.* 2:157–162.
22. Suda, T., and A. Zlotnik. 1993. Origin, differentiation, and repertoire selection of CD3$^+$CD4$^-$CD8$^-$ thymocytes bearing either $\alpha\beta$ or $\gamma\delta$ T cell receptors. *J. Immunol.* 150:447–455.
23. Seki, S., D.H. Kono, R.S. Balderas, and A.N. Theofilopoulos. 1994. Vβ repertoire of murine hepatic T cells. Implication for selection of double-negative $\alpha\beta^+$ T cells. *J. Immunol.* 153:637–646.
24. Ohteki, T., and H.R. MacDonald. 1994. Major histocompatibility complex class I related molecules control the development of CD4$^+$8$^-$ and CD4$^-$8$^-$ subsets of natural killer 1.1$^+$ T cell receptor-α/β^+ cells in the liver of mice. *J. Exp. Med.* 180:699–704.
25. Takeda, K., M.W. Moore, and G. Dennert. 1994. Acute rejection of grafts in mice. Dependence on and independence of functional TCR in the rejection process. *J. Immunol.* 152:4407–4416.
26. Prud'homme, G.J., D.C. Boccarro, and E.C.H. Luke. 1991. Clonal deletion and autoreactivity in extrathymic CD4$^-$CD8$^-$ (double negative) T cell receptor-$\alpha\beta$ T cells. *J. Immunol.* 147:3314–3318.
27. Troutt, A.B., and A. Kelso. 1992. Enumeration of lymphokine mRNA-containing cells *in vivo* in a murine graft-versus-host reaction using the PCR. *Proc. Natl. Acad. Sci. USA.* 89:5276–5280.
28. Martínez-A., C., M.A.R. Marcos, I.M. de Alboran, J.M. Alonso, R. de Cid, G. Kroemer, and A. Coutinho. 1993. Functional double-negative T cells in the periphery express T cell receptor Vβ gene products that cause deletion of single-positive T cells. *Eur. J. Immunol.* 23:250–254.
29. Arase, H., N. Arase, Y. Kobayashi, Y. Nishimura, S. Yonehara, and K. Onoé. 1994. Cytotoxicity of fresh NK1.1$^+$ T cell receptor α/β^+ thymocytes against a CD4$^+$CD8$^+$ thymocyte population associated with intact Fas antigen expression on the target. *J. Exp. Med.* 180:423–432.
30. Sakamoto, H., J. Michaelson, W.K. Jones, A.T. Bhan, S. Abhyankar, M. Silverstein, D.E. Golan, S.J. Burakoff, and J.L.M.

Ferrara. 1991. Lymphocytes with a CD4$^+$CD8$^-$CD3$^-$ phenotype are effectors of experimental cutaneous graft-versus-host disease. *Proc. Natl. Acad. Sci. USA.* 88:10890–10894.

31. Lantz, O., and A. Bendelac. 1994. An invariant T cell receptor α chain is used by a unique subset of major histocompatibility complex class I-specific CD4$^+$ and CD4$^-$CD8$^-$ T cells in mice and humans. *J. Exp. Med.* 180:1097–1106.

32. Abo, T., H. Watanabe, T. Iiai, M. Kimura, K. Ohtsuka, K. Sato, M. Ogawa, H. Hirahara, S. Hashimoto, H. Sekikawa, and S. Seki. 1994. Extrathymic pathways of T-cell differentiation in the liver and other organs. *Int. Rev. Immunol.* 11:61–102.

33. Ohtsuka, K., K. Hasegawa, K. Sato, K. Arai, H. Watanabe, H. Asakura, and T. Abo. 1994. A similar expression pattern of adhesion molecules between intermediate TCR cells in the liver and intraepithelial lymphocytes in the intestine. *Microbiol. Immunol.* 38:677–683.

34. Okada, C.Y., B. Holzmann, C. Guidos, E. Palmer, and I.L. Weissman. 1990. Characterization of a rat monoclonal antibody specific for a determinant encoded by the Vβ7 gene segment. Depletion of Vβ7$^+$ T cells in mice with Mls-1^a haplotype. *J. Immunol.* 144:3473–3477.

35. Ikarashi, Y., T. Abo, K. Kawai, T. Iiai, H. Watanabe, K. Suzuki, Y. Matsumoto, S. Omata, and M. Fujiwara. 1994. Expansion of intermediate T-cell receptor cells in mice with autoimmune-like graft-versus-host disease. *Immunology.* 83:205–212.

36. Watanabe, H., T. Iiai, M. Kimura, K. Ohtsuka, T. Tanaka, M. Miyasaka, M. Tsuchida, H. Hanawa, and T. Abo. 1993. Characterization of intermediate TCR cells in the liver of mice with respect to their unique IL-2R expression. *Cell. Immunol.* 149:331–342.

37. Huang, L., K. Sye, and I.N. Crispe. 1994. Proliferation and apoptosis of B220$^+$CD4$^-$CD8$^-$TCR$\alpha\beta^{\text{intermediate}}$ T cells in the liver of normal adult mice: implication for *lpr* pathogenesis. *Int. Immunol.* 6:533–540.

38. Tanaka, T., M. Tsudo, H. Karasuyama, F. Kitamura, T. Kono, M. Hatakeyama, T. Taniguchi, and M. Miyasaka. 1991. A novel monoclonal antibody against murine IL-2 receptor β-chain. Characterization of receptor expression in normal lymphoid cells and EL-4 cells. *J. Immunol.* 147:2222–2228.

39. Tsuchida, M., T. Iiai, H. Watanabe, and T. Abo. 1992. Relative resistance of intermediate TCR cells to anti-CD3 mAb in mice *in vivo* and their partial functional characterization. *Cell. Immunol.* 145:78–90.

Relationships Between Intermediate TCR Cells and NK1.1⁺ T Cells in Various Immune Organs

NK1.1⁺ T Cells Are Present Within a Population of Intermediate TCR Cells

各免疫臓器におけるTCR^{int}細胞とNK1.1$^+$T細胞の関係：
NK1.1$^+$T細胞がTCR^{int}細胞の集団の中に存在する

The Journal of Immunology, 155: 2972-2983, 1995

chapter 2

Relationships Between Intermediate TCR Cells and NK1.1⁺ T Cells in Various Immune Organs
NK1.1⁺ T Cells Are Present Within a Population of Intermediate TCR Cells[1]

各免疫臓器におけるTCR^{int}細胞とNK1.1$^+$T細胞の関係：
NK1.1$^+$T細胞がTCR^{int}細胞の集団の中に存在する

Hisami Watanabe,[2] * Chikako Miyaji,* Uasuyuki Kawachi,* Tsuneo Iiai, *Kazuo Ohtsuka,*
Toshihiko Iwanaga,⁺ Hiromi Takahashi-Iwanaga,⁺ and Toru Abo*

*Department of Immunology and ⁺Third Department of Anatomy, Niigata University School of Medicine, Niigata, Japan

【要約】

　これまでの研究から、マウス肝臓内のT細胞集団には、中等度のTCRを持つ（またはCD3; 以下TCR^{int}, CD3^{int}）細胞が存在し、IL-2Rβ鎖（IL-2Rβ）を発現することが明らかになった。このTCR^{int}細胞は、他の免疫臓器にも、少数ながらも存在する。一方、TCR^{int}を有するNK1.1$^+$T細胞は、胸腺や他の末梢臓器に存在する。2種の細胞の関係を明らかにするために、臓器から採取したCD3^{int}細胞およびNK1.1$^+$T細胞の特徴を、フェノタイプ、Vβレパートリーおよび形態学の観点から検証した。IL-2Rβ$^+$T細胞とNK1.1$^+$T細胞は、いずれもCD3^{int}細胞に分類されるが、NK1.1$^+$T細胞集団は、CD3^{int}細胞集団の中に存在する。肝臓と胸腺のCD3^{int}細胞では、NK1.1$^+$細胞が大多数であった。ところが、脾臓、リンパ節と骨髄におけるCD3^{int}細胞では、NK1.1$^+$細胞は少数であった。CD3^{int}細胞内に存在するNK1.1$^+$サブセットでは、CD4$^-$8$^-$細胞および/またはCD4$^+$が豊富だった。それに対して、NK1.1$^-$サブセットでは、大概、CD8$^+$細胞が豊富だった。Mls系により規定される自己応答性Vβ$^+$クローンは、NK1.1$^+$サブセットにも、NK1.1$^-$サブセット分布すると考えられた。胸腺や他臓器のCD3^{high}細胞には、CD4$^-$CD8$^-$細胞も禁止クローンも見られなかった。CD3^{int}細胞の形態は、パーフォリンを有する顆粒性リンパ球、もしくは、無顆粒性のリンパ球であった。CD3^{int}細胞のうち、NK1.1$^-$サブセットよりも、NK1.1$^+$サブセットのパーフォリン陽性度が高かった。これらの結果は、各臓器におけるTCR^{int}細胞とNK1.1$^+$T細胞の関係を明らかに示している。

　TCR（またはCD3）が中等度で、恒常的にIL-2Rβ鎖（IL-2Rβ）を発現する独特なT細胞集団（TCR$^{int\ 3}$細胞）が、肝臓内に存在することが明らかになった (1-4)。この肝T細胞は、TCRの高発現（TCR^{high}細胞）であるIL-2Rβ$^-$胸腺由来T細胞と容易に区別でき

Received for publication December 19, 1994. Accepted for publication June 30, 1995.
The costs of publication of this article were defrayed in part by the payment of Page Charges. This article must therefore be hereby marked advertisement in accordance with 18 U.S.C. Section 1734 solely Io indicate this fact.

1) This work was supported by a grant-in-aid for Scientific Research from the Ministry of Education, Science and Culture, Japan.
2) Address corresponfence and reprint requests to Dr. Hisami Watanabe of Immunology, Niigata University school of Medicine, Asahimachi, Nilgata 951, Japan.
3) 略語；int, 中等度（細胞；IL-2Rβ, IL-2Rβ 鎖；DN, ダブルネガティブ（CD4$^-$CD8$^-$）；MNC, 単核球；；PE, フィコエリスリン；LGL, 大型顆粒リンパ球；B6 mice, C57BL/6マウス

る。TCR^{int}細胞には、CD4$^+$やCD8$^+$細胞のみならず、CD4$^-$8$^-$細胞がある(1)。またこの細胞は、内因性スーパー抗原Mls系と抗Vβモノクロナール抗体を用いて測定できる自己応答性「禁止」クローンを含む(2)。TCR^{int}細胞には、αβT細胞とγδT細胞がある(4)。先天的に胸腺が欠損しているヌードマウスや、胸腺摘出・放射線照射・骨髄移植を行ったマウスの末梢免疫臓器におけるT細胞は、全てTCR^{int}細胞である。一方、腸のT細胞は例外である。その理由は、腸のT細胞が胸腺外由来である可能性が考えられる(5)。しかし、研究を進めるうち、少数ながらもTCR^{int}細胞が脾臓、リンパ節および胸腺など他の免疫臓器にも存在することが明らかになった(4,5)。

NK1.1抗原を持つCD4$^-$CD8$^-$（またはCD4$^+$）αβT細胞が、胸腺に存在すると多くの研究者らにより報告された(6-15)。既報を詳細に検討したところ、これらNK1.1$^+$T細胞は、通常の成熟T細胞よりもTCRが低発現であることが明らかになった。報告の中には、これらT細胞は、T細胞分化において胸腺内代替経路で発生したと考察するのもあった(16,17)。類似したT細胞集団が、脾臓(18-20)、リンパ節(21,22)および骨髄(23,24)に局在することも示された。フェノタイプおよび機能の特徴のデータから考察すると、IL-2Rβ$^+$TCR^{int}細胞とNK1.1$^+$αβT細胞は、ほぼ同一集団に属するようである。NK1.1$^+$αβT細胞におけるVβレパートリーおよびMHC拘束性について、この概念をサポートするような実験結果がこれまで報告されている(25-27)。

本研究により、フェノタイプ、Vβレパートリーおよび形態学の観点から、各臓器のTCR^{int}細胞とNK1.1$^+$T細胞において、これら集団の特徴が一層明らかになった。これらの細胞は臓器やサブセットによっては小さな差異はあるが、共通点が多いことが明らかになった。これら細胞は、産生については非依存性である可能性はあるが、T細胞集団の類似した系統に属する可能性が考えられる。これら細胞は、肝臓にも胸腺にも存在するので、胸腺外経路もしくは胸腺内代替経路としてのT細胞分化の最終段階ではなさそうだ。原始的特徴に基づいて、これらの細胞を「原始」T細胞と呼ばなければならない；これら細胞は、生体内のあちこちに存在する原始的なT細胞分化の経路において産生されている可能性がある。

材料と方法

マウス

C57BL/6(B6)、SJL、NZBおよび(B6 x 3H/He)F$_1$雌マウス（18-20週齢）、そして老齢B6マウス（116週齢）を使用した。これらのマウスの系統は、全てNK1.1同種抗原を有する。これらのマウスを、日本チャールズ・リバー（神奈川，日本）より購入後、新潟大学動物飼育施設内において特定病原体未感染状態（SPF）下で飼育した。

細胞採取

定法に改良を加え、肝単核球（MNC）を採取した(28)。略述すると、エーテル麻酔下のマウスの心臓より脱血した。単核球採取のため、摘出した肝臓を200-ゲージステンレススチールメッシュで濾し、リン酸緩衝液（PBS）（0.1M, pH7.2）に懸濁した。PBSで洗浄後、フィコール-イソパーク（1.090）の勾配遠心分離法を用いて、単核球を肝細胞と肝細胞核から分離した。特定のサブセットが喪失されるのを避けるため(29)、濾した肝臓サンプルの大幅な希釈を行った（2匹分の肝臓/PBS 30ml）。そして、中間層より採取した単核球を2%仔牛血清を添加したMEM培養液に懸濁した。

脾臓細胞、末梢血リンパ球および骨髄細胞

も、フィコール-イソパーク法を用いて採取した。また、胸腺または鼠径リンパ節を200-ゲージステンレススチールメッシュで濾過して、胸腺細胞とリンパ節細胞を採取した。形態学および組織化学検証を行うため、FITC標識抗CD3モノクロナール抗体およびフィコエリトリン（PE）標識抗IL-2Rβモノクロナール抗体（PharMingen Co, San Diego, CA）による二重染色を行った後、FACStar IIPlus（Becton Dickinson Co., Mountain View, CA）を用いて、IL-2Rβ$^+$CD3^{int}細胞とIL-2Rβ$^-$CD3^{high}細胞の純化採取した実験も行った。抗CD3と抗NK1.1モノクロナール染色後、純化を行い、CD3^{int}細胞集団内のNK1.1$^+$とNK1.1$^-$サブセットを採取した。

フローサイトメトリー解析

細胞表面のフェノタイプ検証には、モノクロナール抗体を用いて一重、二重および三重染色を行いフローメトリー解析を行った（30）。本実験で使用したFITC、PEまたはビオチン標識試薬を含むモノクロナール抗体は、抗CD3(145-2C11)、抗IL-2Rβ鎖（TM-β1）およびNK1.1(PK136)モノクロナール抗体（PharMingen）であった。FITCまたはPE標識抗CD4(L3T4)と抗CD8(Lyt-2)モノクロナール抗体は、Becton Dickinson製である。CD3(FITC)、IL-2RβまたはNK1.1(PE)、および対応するVβ（Red 613）の三重染色を行いVβ$^+$細胞の各集団を検証した。ビオチン標識試薬は、PEまたはRed 613標識ストレプトアビジン（Becton Dickinson）で発色させた。蛍光陽性細胞をFACScan(Becton Dickinson)を用いて解析した。

電子顕微鏡検査

走査型電子顕微鏡検査のため、純化した細胞分画を、2.5%グルタルアルデヒドを添加した0.1M PBS(pH7.4)中で固定した(4)。固定剤に浸した後（2時間）、組織塊を1%四酸化オスミウム添加PBSで後固定して（1.5時間）、エタノールを用い段階的に脱水し、酸化プロピレンを加えたアラルダイトで、包埋した。ウラニルアセテートとクエン酸鉛で染色した極薄の切片を、日立H-7000走査電子顕微鏡（（株）日立，日立，日本）を用いて検証した。

パーフォリン免疫ペルオキシダーゼ染色

純化した分画のサイトスピン（集細胞遠心装置）標本を、空気乾燥させた後、冷アセトン（4分）、および、4%パラホルムアルデヒド添加PBSで固定した(1分)(31)。そして、50mM Tris-HCl(pH 7.6)で洗浄し、0.5% 過ヨウ素酸（10分）と0.3% 過酸化水素メタノールで処理した（15分）。Ca^{2+}不含5%ウシ血清アルブミン0.02%アジ化ナトリウム添加PBSでブロッキングした後（30分）、抗ラット・パーフォリン・モノクロナール抗体（P1-8；奥村康博士（東京，日本）ご提供）で培養（染色）した（60分）。結合抗体を可視化する手順は、以下の通り。洗浄後（Ca^{2+}Mg^{2+}不含PBS）、ビオチン化ヤギ抗ラットIgG(Sigma Chemical Co., St Louis, MO)(60分)で培養（染色）を行った後、Ca^{2+}Mg^{2+}不含PBSで、再洗浄した。そして、エクストラビディン・ペルオキシダーゼ（シグマ）で培養（染色）した後（30分）、再々度洗浄を行い（Ca^{2+}およびMg2$^+$不含PBS）、赤色発色基質（Bio-Makor, Rehovot, Israel）を用いて発色させた細胞を、ヘマトキシリンを用いて対比染色した。

rIL-12のマウスへの全身投与

パーフォリン顆粒を産生させるため、rIL-12（1μg/匹）(Genetic Institute, Andover, MA)の腹腔内投与を複数のマウスに行い、その翌日に細胞を採取した。

結果

各臓器におけるIL-2Rβ⁺ CD3^{int}細胞とNK1.1⁺ T細胞の分布

各臓器におけるCD3^{int}細胞の分布を検証するため、CD3とIL-2Rβの二重染色を行った（Fig.1）。本実験では、NK1.1同種抗原を持つ18週齢B6マウスを使用した。CD3^{high}細胞はIL-2Rβ⁻であるが、CD3^{int}細胞はIL-2Rβ⁺であったため、二重染色を行い、CD3^{int}細胞をCD3^{high}細胞と明確に区別できた（Fig.1,上）。IL-2Rβ⁺CD3^{int}細胞は、肝臓において最も豊富であることが確認できた。しかし、比率は少ないもののCD3^{int}細胞は、検証を行った全臓器で確認された。そして、同じ標本を用いてCD3とNK1.1の二重染色を行った（Fig.1,下）。CD3⁺NK1.1⁺細胞が、検証を行った全臓器で確認され、また、CD3発現が中等度であることが明らかになった。これらのNK1.1⁺細胞は、肝臓でも豊富だったので、IL-2Rβ⁺CD3^{int}細胞とNK1.1⁺T細胞集団とは重複している可能性がある。

各臓器におけるIL-2Rβ⁺CD3^{int}細胞とNK1.1⁺ T細胞の関係

IL-2Rβ⁺CD3^{int}細胞とNK1.1⁺ T細胞の関係を直接比較するため、CD3、IL-2RβとNK1.1の三重染色を行った（Table Ⅰ）。本実験では、NK1.1同種抗原を持つ18週齢のB6マウス、SJLおよびNZBマウス各系統6匹を用いて、平均値±1 SDを算出した。ほぼ全てのNK1.1⁺ T細胞が、IL-2Rβを発現していた（>97%）。それ故、IL-2Rβ⁺CD3^{int}細胞集団内には、NK1.1⁺細胞の比率だけが見られる。肝臓と胸腺においても、両細胞集団は、顕著に重複していた（>50%）。これに対して、脾臓、リンパ節と骨髄ではあまり重複は見られなかった。同様の傾向がマウスの全ての系統に見られた。

*T細胞サブセットにおけるCD4⁻CD8⁻、CD4⁺およびCD8⁺細胞の構成パターン

これまでの実験から、CD3^{int}細胞は全てIL-2Rβ⁺であることが示唆されたが、CD3^{int}細胞には、NK1.1⁺とNK1.1⁻が混在していた。そこで、肝臓、脾臓と胸腺におけるCD3^{int}細胞集団内に

Figure.1

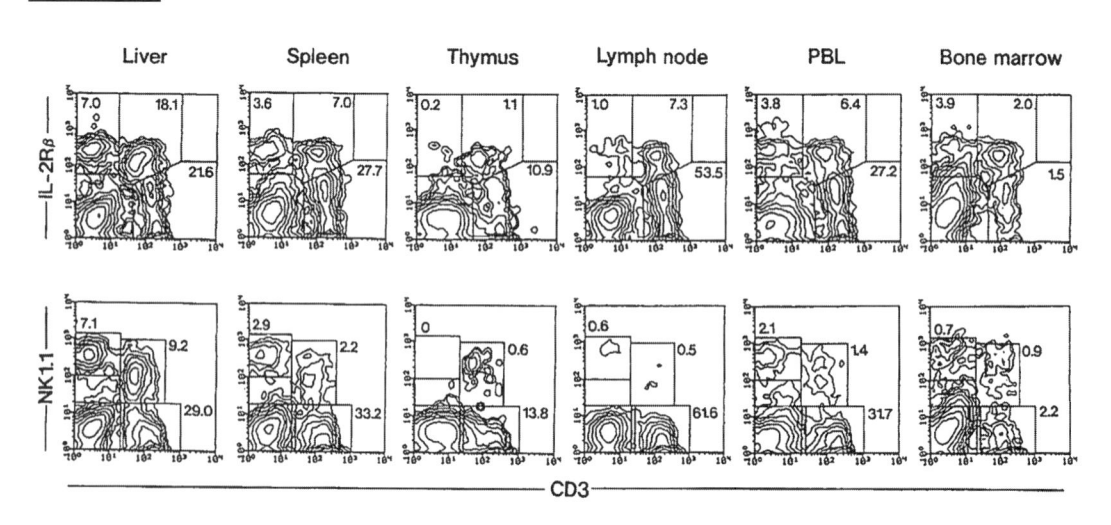

各免疫臓器におけるIL-2Rβ⁺ CD3^{int}細胞とNK1.1⁺ T細胞の同定。18週齢のB6マウスを使用した。IL-2Rβ⁺ CD3^{int}細胞の同定にはCD3とIL-2Rβの二重染色、NK1.1⁺ T細胞の同定にはCD3とNK1.1の二重染色を行った。IL-2Rβ⁺ T細胞もNK1.1⁺ T細胞も、CD3^{int}細胞に属することが明らかになった。各分画内の数値は、蛍光陽性細胞の比率を示す。3度実験を行った典型例を示す。

Table.I

各臓器におけるIL-Rβ$^+$CD3^{int}とNK1.1$^+$ T細胞の関係性の比較^a

Organs	% NK1.1$^+$ Cells Among IL-2Rβ$^+$ int CD3 Cells		
	B6	SJL	NZB
Liver	69.6 ± 11.9	50.9 ± 7.2	56.9 ± 1.9
Spleen	15.8 ± 4.7	22.0 ± 4.3	35.5 ± 0.3
Thymus	56.9 ± 9.2	60.3 ± 8.9	52.6 ± 7.6
Lymph nodes	4.9 ± 2.0	ND	ND
Bone marrow	27.2 ± 6.3	ND	ND

^{a}18週齢のB6、SJLおよびNZBマウスを使用した。CD3(FITC)、IL-2Rβ(PE)とNK1.1(Red 613)の三重染色を行い検証した。平均値±1SDは、各系統6匹のマウスを用いて算出した。

存在するNK1.1$^+$とNK1.1$^-$サブセットは、CD4$^-$8$^-$細胞、およびCD4$^+$細胞またはCD8$^+$細胞をどのように構成しているかを検証した。そこで（検証するため）、CD3(FITC)、NK1.1(またはIL-2Rβ)(PE)およびCD4とCD8(Red 613)の混合液の三重染色を行った（Fig. 2）。B6マウスの肝単核球において、CD3およびNK1.1の発現の観点より3つのサブセット（R1(CD3^{int}NK1.1$^+$)、R2(CD3^{int}NK1.1$^-$)とR3(CD3^{high}NK1.1$^-$)）を同定した。（上記3分画）ゲーティングを行い、肝単核球におけるCD4$^-$CD8$^-$およびCD4$^+$やCD8$^+$の構成パターンを示した（Fig. 2, 下）。CD4$^+$とCD8$^+$細胞を識別するため、CD8の染色強度を高力価抗CD8モノクローナル抗体の添加を行い上昇させた。CD3^{int}NK1.1$^+$細胞には、主としてCD4$^-$8$^-$細胞とCD4$^+$細胞が存在した。これに対し、CD3^{int}NK1.1$^-$細胞には、CD4$^-$CD8$^-$、CD4$^+$およびCD8$^+$細胞が存在することが明らかになった。CD3^{int}細胞表面のCD4とCD8抗原の発現度（染色強度）は、CD3^{high}細胞表面の発現度より若干低かった。

各臓器におけるT細胞サブセットの構成パターンを検証するため、肝臓含む他の臓器まで検証範囲を拡大して、同様の染色を行った（Table Ⅱ）。全てのIL-2Rβ$^-$CD3^{high}細胞およびIL-2Rβ$^+$CD3^{int}細胞の解析をするため、CD3(FITC)、IL-2Rβ(PE)、そしてCD4とCD8(Red 613)との混合液による三重染色を

Figure.2

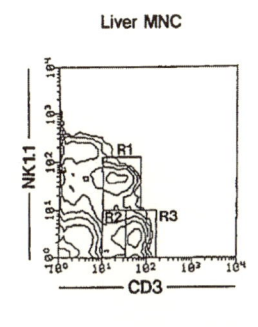

NK1.1$^+$CD3^{int}細胞（R1）、NK1.1$^-$CD3^{int}細胞（R2）およびNK1.1$^-$CD3^{high}細胞（R3）におけるCD4$^-$CD8$^-$、CD4$^+$とCD8$^+$ T細胞の分布。18週齢のB6マウスの肝単核球を使用した。CD3(FITC)、NK1.1(PE)、およびCD4とCD8(Red 613)を混和して三重染色を行った。CD4$^+$とCD8$^+$細胞の分離には、高力価抗CD8モノクローナル抗体を使用した。R1、R2とR3ゲーティングを行い、CD4$^-$CD8$^-$、CD4$^+$とCD8$^+$細胞の比率を測定した。

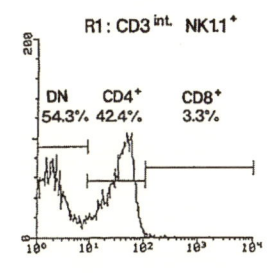

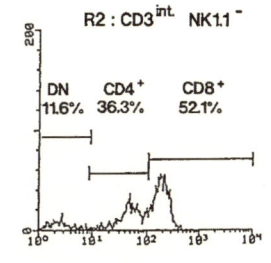

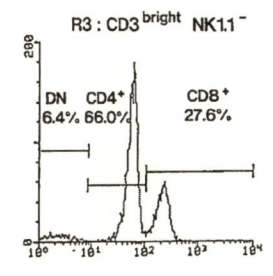

Table.II

各T細胞サブセットにおけるCD4⁻CD8⁻、CD4⁺およびCD8⁺細胞分布のパターン

Organ	T Cell Subset	% Positiv Cells		
		CD4⁻CD8⁻ cells	CD4⁺ cells	CD8⁺ cells
Experiment 1 (B6 mice)				
Liver	Int CD3	45.2	51.9	16.4
	High CD3	6.1	54.1	45.4
Spleen	Int CD3	47.7	27.2	53.4
	High CD3	0.9	61.4	37.5
Tyumus	Int CD3	38.8	40.9	43.9
	High CD3	2.5	84.8	51.4
Experiment 2 (B6 mice)				
Liver	CD3⁺NK1.1⁺	47.2	50.8	3.3
	CD3ⁱⁿᵗNK1.1⁻	16.4	32.5	63.0
	CD3ʰⁱᵍʰNK1.1⁻	3.8	47.8	45.1
Spleen	CD3⁺NK1.1⁺	66.2	22.9	14.9
	CD3ⁱⁿᵗNK1.1⁻	20.5	22.1	62.4
	CD3ʰⁱᵍʰNK1.1⁻	0.3	55.5	42.3
Thymus	CD3⁻NK1.1⁺	42.6	48.2	21.2
	CD3ʰⁱᵍʰNK1.1⁻	2.1	76.3	36.9
Experiment 3 (NZB mice)				
Liver	CD3⁺NK1.1⁺	53.6	32.9	13.5
	CD3ⁱⁿᵗNK1.1⁻	13.2	32.0	54.8
	CDʰⁱᵍʰNK1.1⁻	4.7	70.4	24.8
Spleen	CD3⁺NK1.1⁺	31.9	42.9	25.3
	CD3ⁱⁿᵗNK1.1⁻	9.2	33.3	57.6
	CDʰⁱᵍʰNK1.1⁻	0.8	67.2	32.0
Thymus	CD3⁺NK1.1⁺	66.5	15.6	17.6
	CD3ʰⁱᵍʰNK1.1⁻	<0.1	83.9	22.2

[a] 18週齢のB6およびNZBマウスを使用した。簡略化して3匹のマウスの平均値を示す。

行った（Table II, Expt. 1）。値を標準化し、表を簡素化するため、平均値±SDは3匹のB6マウス（プールした検体）を用いて算出した。既報のように（4, 5）、CD3ⁱⁿᵗ細胞には、CD4⁻8⁻、CD4⁺とCD8⁺細胞が存在するのに対し、CD3ʰⁱᵍʰ細胞にはCD4⁻8⁻細胞が存在しなかった。B6マウスで検証を行った全臓器でも同様であった。CD3ⁱⁿᵗ細胞集団内に存在するNK1.1⁺とNK1.1⁻サブセットの場合、どちらのサブセットも、CD4⁻CD8⁻、CD4⁺およびCD8⁺細胞が、混在していた（experiment 2, B6マウス）。しかし、NK1.1⁺サブセットは、主としてCD4⁻CD8⁻そして/またはCD4⁺細胞であったのに対して、NK1.1⁻サブセットでは、検証した臓器にかかわりなく、大概CD8⁺細胞が優位であった。NZBマウスのデータも同様であった（experiment 3）。

CD3ⁱⁿᵗ細胞集団内に存在するNK1.1⁺とNK1.1⁻サブセットにおけるVβレパートリー

通常系統のB6マウスでも、遺伝子系統が同じでNK1.1同種抗原を有するB10マウスでも、I-E分子発現が欠損している。特定のMls抗原に対応する自己応答性クローンは、I-E分子による負の選択で排除される。故に、B6マウスとB10マウスにはMls系による特異的な自己応答性Vβ⁺クローンは存在しない。その結果、自己応答性禁止クローンの検証に、I-E分子が欠損したマウスの系統は使用できなかった。この問題を克服するため、NK1.1同種抗原を持ち、且つ、I-E分子を発現するNZBマウス（Mls-1²ᵃ⁾）および（B6 x C3H/He）F₁マウス（Mls-1ᵇ²ᵃ/ᵇ⁾）を使用した。どちらの系統のマウスでも、同様の結果が得られたので、本研究では、NZBマウスのデータを示す（Fig. 3）。本研究では、CD3、IL-2Rβ（またはNK1.1）と各Vβ⁺の三重染色を行った。NZBマウスにおいて、Vβ7⁺とVβ11⁺細胞は禁止クローンである。これに対して、Vβ2⁺とVβ8⁺細胞は非禁止クローンである。肝臓の場合（Fig. 3A）、非禁止クローン（Vβ2⁺とVβ8⁺）が、T細胞全サブセット（CD3ʰⁱᵍʰIL-2Rβ⁻、CD3ⁱⁿᵗIL-2Rβ⁺、CD3ⁱⁿᵗ⁺NK1.1⁺とCD3ⁱⁿᵗNK1.1⁻）に分布していることが明らかになった。一方、CD3ⁱⁿᵗ細胞の場合と同様、禁止クローン（Vβ7⁺とVβ11⁺）は、CD3ⁱⁿᵗIL-2Rβ⁺細胞、NK1.1⁺とNK1.1⁻サブセットに限定されていた。

脾臓と胸腺においても、同様の検証を行った（Fig. 3, BとC）。脾臓でさえも、全自己応

Figure.3

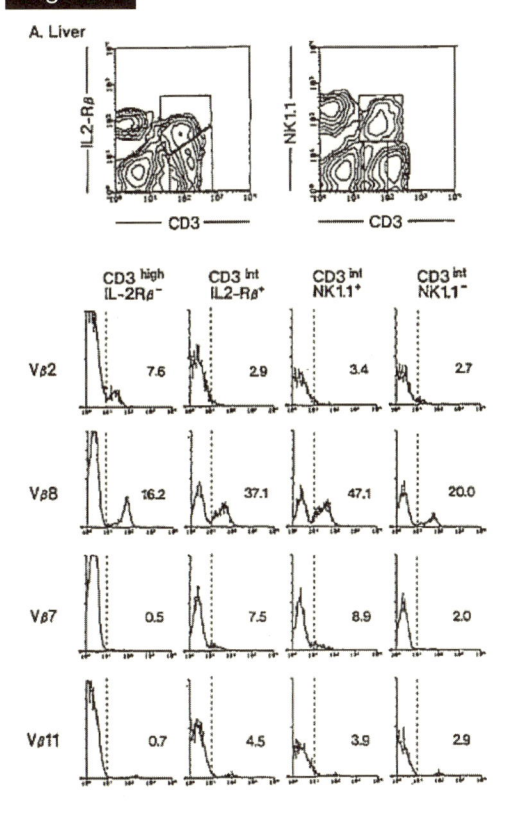

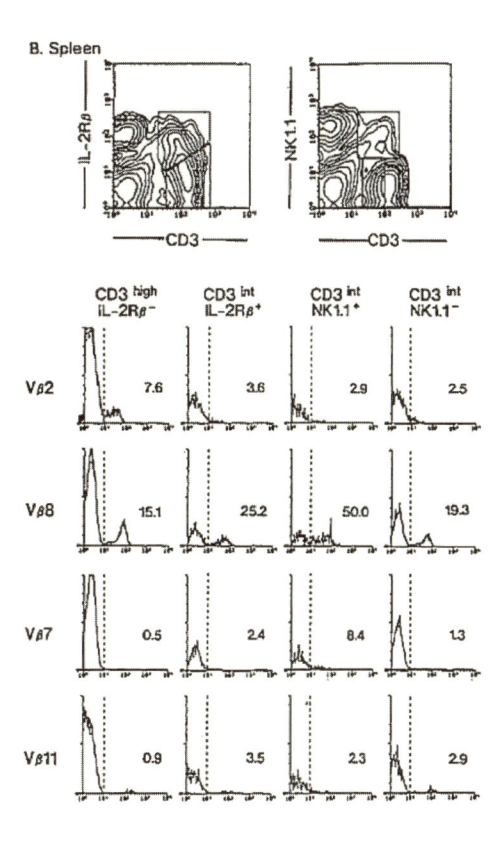

A. Liver

	CD3 high IL-2Rβ−	CD3 int IL2-Rβ+	CD3 int NK1.1+	CD3 int NK1.1−
Vβ2	7.6	2.9	3.4	2.7
Vβ8	16.2	37.1	47.1	20.0
Vβ7	0.5	7.5	8.9	2.0
Vβ11	0.7	4.5	3.9	2.9

B. Spleen

	CD3 high IL-2Rβ−	CD3 int IL2-Rβ+	CD3 int NK1.1+	CD3 int NK1.1−
Vβ2	7.6	3.6	2.9	2.5
Vβ8	15.1	25.2	50.0	19.3
Vβ7	0.5	2.4	8.4	1.3
Vβ11	0.9	3.5	2.3	2.9

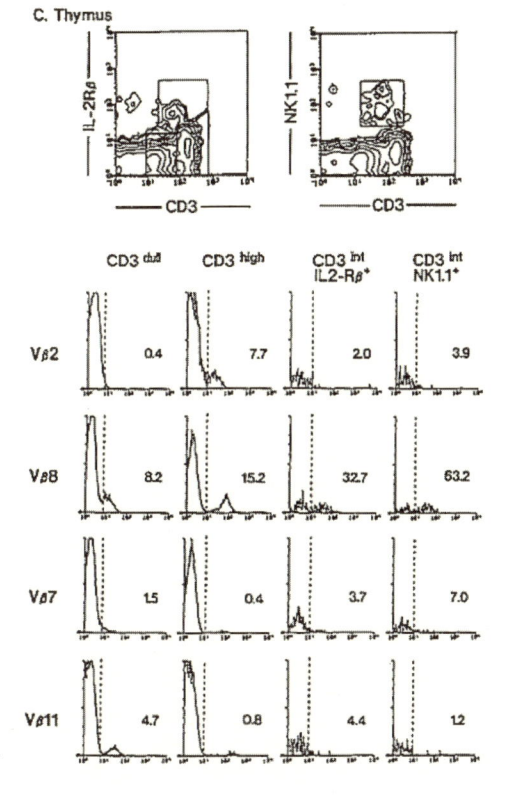

C. Thymus

	CD3 dull	CD3 high	CD3 int IL2-Rβ+	CD3 int NK1.1+
Vβ2	0.4	7.7	2.0	3.9
Vβ8	8.2	15.2	32.7	63.2
Vβ7	1.5	0.4	3.7	7.0
Vβ11	4.7	0.8	4.4	1.2

各免疫臓器における各サブセットの自己応答性禁止T細胞クローンの分布パターン。A. 肝臓；B. 脾臓；C. 胸腺。18週齢のNZBマウスを使用した。CD3(FITC)、IL-2Rβまたは NK1.1(PE)および対応する Vβ(Red 613)の三重染色を行った。CD3^{high}IL-2Rβ−、CD3^{int}IL-2Rβ+、CD3^{int}NK1.1+とCD3^{int}NK1.1−サブセットのゲーティングを行い、各タイプのVβ+細胞の比率を検証した。これらのNZBマウス（Mls-1^{a}2^{a}）において、Vβ2+とVβ8+細胞は非禁止クローンであるが、一方、Vβ7+とVβ11+細胞は禁止クローンである。肝臓と脾臓において、禁止クローンであるVβ7+とVβ11+細胞は、CD3^{int}細胞集団内の全サブセットに見られたが、CD3^{high}IL-2Rβ−サブセットでは見られなかった。胸腺においては、このVβ7+とVβ11+クローンが、CD3^{dull}でもCD3^{int}サブセットでも見られた。どの臓器でも、非禁止クローンが、全サブセットに分布していた。各分画内の数値は、蛍光陽性細胞の比率を示す。3度実験を行った典型例を示す。

chapter 2

Figure.4

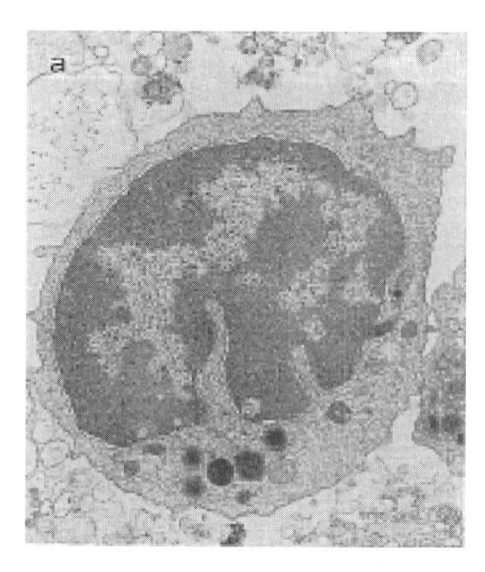

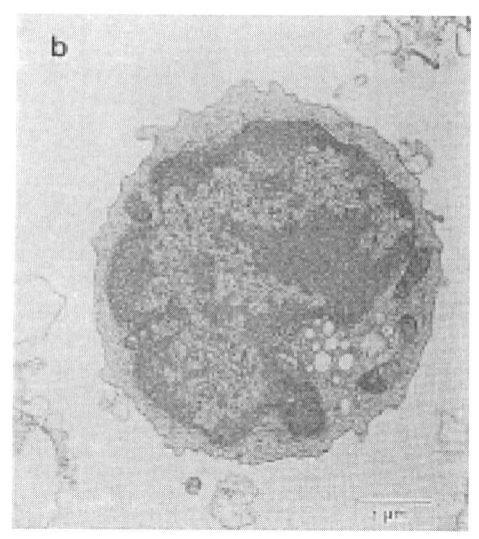

肝臓におけるNK細胞とCD3^{int}細胞の形態学的比較；a, NK細胞；b, CD3^{int}細胞。肝単核球を18週齢のB6マウスから採取した。CD3$^-$IL-2Rβ$^+$NK細胞とIL-2Rβ$^+$CD3^{int}細胞を、CD3とIL-2Rβの二重染色後、ソーターを用いて純化し、電子顕微鏡検査とパーフォリン染色を行った。CD3^{int}細胞の顆粒は僅少だったが、細胞質に液胞が多数あった。

答性クローン（Vβ7$^+$とVβ11$^+$）は、CD3^{int}IL-2Rβ$^+$サブセット、そしてNK1.1$^+$とNK1.1$^-$両サブセットに限定されることが明らかになった。胸腺の場合、CD3^{int}NK1.1$^-$サブセットの位置には、CD3^{dull}NK1.1$^-$細胞（T細胞分化主経路における未熟なT細胞）が見られる。この点から、この染色方法にて胸腺内のCD3^{int}NK1.1$^-$サブセットの解析は行わなかった。胸腺内の自己応答性のクローンは、CD3^{dull}細胞またはCD3^{int}IL-2Rβ$^+$およびCD3^{int}NK1.1$^+$サブセットに見られた。つまり、胸腺または他の臓器において、CD3^{high}細胞には、自己応答性クローンが含まれなかったのである。

本実験の結果から、検証を行った全臓器において、非禁止T細胞クローンであるVβ8$^+$の値がCD3^{int}細胞のNK1.1$^+$サブセットにおいて、非常に高値であることも明らかになった。

CD3int細胞の形態

CD3^{int}細胞の形態的な特徴を示すために、肝臓、胸腺と脾臓からCD3$^-$IL-2Rβ$^+$NK細胞集団とともに、CD3^{int}細胞集団の純化を行った。純化した集団を電子顕微鏡で観察した（Fig. 4）。Fig. 4は、肝臓から採取した細胞の形態を示す。NK細胞分画における細胞の形態は全て大顆粒リンパ球（LGL）であった（Fig. 4a）。一方、CD3^{int}細胞の分画における細胞には、顆粒リンパ球も無顆粒リンパ球もあった（Fig. 4b）。顆粒リンパ球は、CD3^{int}細胞分画の20%未満であった。しかし、顆粒リンパ球の細胞質は非常に大きく、ミトコンドリアや小型の液胞が存在した。脾臓と胸腺の結果も同様であった（未発表データ）。

各リンパ球サブセットにおける
パーフォリン陽性細胞値の比較

NK細胞は、その形態は大型顆粒リンパ球であり、パーフォリンを発現し、細胞質顆粒の中に酵素が局在することが広く知られている（31）。免疫化学染色を行い、パーフォリンを同定した。肝臓より純化採取した以下の各リンパ球サブセットにおけるパーフォリン陽

Table.III

肝臓の各リンパ球サブセットにおけるパーフォリン陽性細胞の比率[a]

Mouse	NK cells	% Perforin+ Cells				High CD3 cells
		Int CD3 Cells				
		IL-2Rβ whole	NK1.1+ subset	NK1.1− subset		
C3H/He	87.0±13.1	55.0±6.6				1.9±0.4
SJL	61.1±7.2	15.7±1.6	21.9±2.3	4.2±0.2		0.6±0.5
B6	62.0±7.2	9.1±2.4	5.7±0.9	1.9±0.4		1.2±0.3
(IL-12 i.p.)	98.2±3.8	25.2±3.2	20.2±3.8	7.9±2.7		2.2±1.5

[a]C57BL/6マウスは、IL-12の投与群と非投与群の両群の数値を示す。平均値±1SDは、三度実験を行い算出した。C3H/Heマウスは、NK1.1同種抗原を持たない。

Figure.5

NK細胞とCD3int細胞集団内に存在するNK1.1+サブセットのパーフォリンの免疫化学染色（×1000）。a, 純化したNK細胞; b, IL-12投与マウスの純化したNK細胞; c, CD3int細胞集団内の純化したNK1.1+サブセット; d, IL-12投与マウスのCD3int細胞集団内の純化したNK1.1+サブセット。各細胞分画をCD3とNK1.1の二重染色を行った後、純化した。

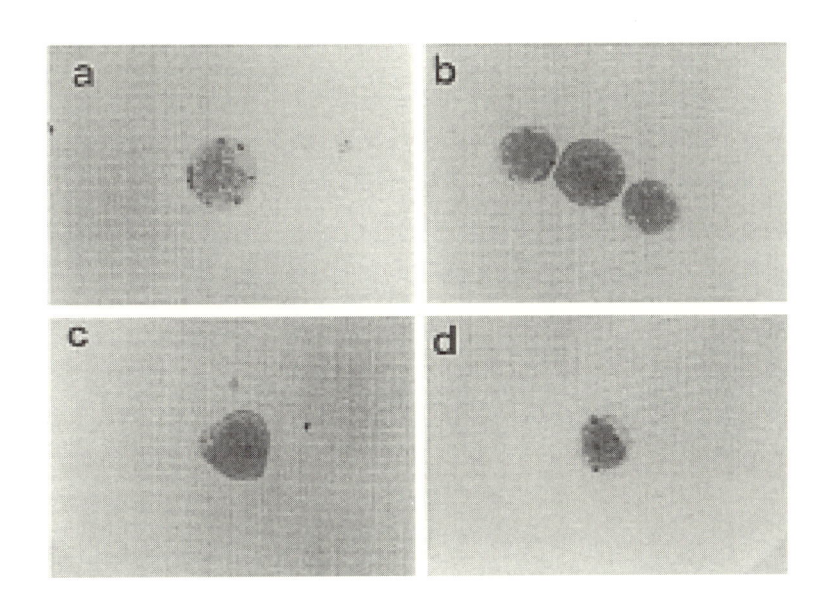

性細胞の比率を比較した；NK(CD3−IL-2Rβ+)細胞、IL-2Rβ+CD3int細胞、CD3int細胞中のNK1.1+とNK1.1−サブセット、IL-2Rβ−CD3high細胞（Table III）。C3H/Heマウス（NK1.1同種抗原−）（NK活性が高い系統である）の場合、NK細胞と全CD3int細胞において、パーフォリン陽性細胞は非常に高値であった。これに対して、CD3high細胞においては顕著に低値であった。B6マウス（NK1.1同種抗原+）でも、同様の傾向が見られた。NK1.1+サブセットは、NK1.1−サブセットよりも、パーフォリン陽性細胞が高値であった。B6マウスのサブセットにおいて、パーフォリン陽性細胞が全般的に低値であることは、B6マウスは、NK活性が低い系統であるという事実と一致する（32）。IL-12をB6マウスに投与すると、全サブセットのパーフォリン陽性細胞の比率が上昇した。

この結果の代表例を、実写真として示す（Fig. 5）。第1に、NK細胞では細胞質にパーフォリン顆粒が多数存在し、そして、パーフォリン陽性細胞の比率が高かった（Fig. 5a）。CD3int細胞集団内のNK1.1+サブセットはほとんどパーフォリン顆粒を含まず、そして、パーフォリン陽性細胞の比率は低かった（Fig. 5c）。IL-12を投与した後、パーフォリン顆粒がNK細胞（Fig. 5b）でもCD3int細胞集団内のNK1.1+サブセッ

ト（Fig. 5d）でも顕著になった。

加齢によるCD3^{int}細胞の増加と、NK1.1$^+$：NK1.1$^-$サブセット比率の減少

老齢マウス場合、肝臓と他の臓器においてCD3^{int}細胞が増加した。老齢マウスにおいてNK1.1$^+$：NK1.1$^-$サブセットの比率が、どのように変化したかを検証した（Fig. 6）。若齢B6マウス（10週齢）も同時に検証した（Fig. 6A）。予想通り、老齢マウス（116週齢）の肝臓と脾臓において、CD3^{int}細胞の比率が増加した（Fig. 6B）。興味深いことに、老齢マウスでは、CD3^{int}細胞集団内のNK1.1$^+$サブセットの比率が減少し、NK1.1$^-$サブセットの比率が増加した。

そこで、CD3^{int}細胞におけるCD4$^+$細胞、CD8$^+$細胞およびCD4$^-$8$^-$細胞の構成パターンを検証した。NK1.1$^+$とNK1.1$^-$サブセットの構成パターンは、対照群である若齢マウスでも基本的に同様であることが、明らかになった（未発表データ）。肝臓と脾臓でも同様の結果であった。

考察

本研究では、多種の免疫臓器におけるCD3^{int}細胞とNK1.1$^+$ T細胞の関係を、直接検証した。NK1.1$^+$ T細胞はCD3^{int}細胞集団に限定され、また、CD3^{int}細胞集団はNK1.1$^+$とNK1.1$^-$サブセットで構成されることが明らかになった。CD3^{high}細胞集団内のNK1.1$^+$IL-2Rβ^-サブセットは僅少であった。最近の研究の結果より（4-15）、TCRint（またはCD3）細胞とNK1.1$^+$ T細胞の共通点は多い（TCR^{int}の発現とCD4$^-$8$^-$細胞の構成）。接着分子の発現も同様に、CD44$^+$L-セレクチン$^-$であった。反対に、胸腺内細胞分化主経路で産生されたT細胞では、接着分子の発現はCD44$^-$L-セレクチン$^+$であった（14, 15, 33）。これら結果の原因は、NK1.1$^+$ T細胞は、全てCD3^{int}細胞集団の中に存在する事実である。肝臓と胸腺におけるCD3^{int}細胞では、かなりNK1.1$^+$サブセットの比率が、高かったが（>50%）、脾臓、リンパ節、末梢血と骨髄では、その比率は低かった（<30%）。

IL-2Rβ^+CD3^{int}細胞は、NK1.1$^+$およびNK1.1$^-$サブセットで構成されているので、CD4$^-$8$^-$とCD4$^+$またはCD8$^+$細胞の構成パターンを比較した。NK1.1$^+$サブセットは、主にCD4$^-$CD8$^-$とCD4$^+$細胞で構成されていた。ところが、NK1.1$^-$サブセットは、CD4$^-$CD8$^-$細胞とCD4$^+$細胞の小集団に加えてCD8$^+$細胞で構成されていた（Fig.7）。NK1.1 T$^+$細胞は、CD4$^-$8$^-$細胞とCD4$^+$細胞で構成されると、Arase（荒瀬）らは以前報告した（15, 34, 35）。そして、本研究の結果より、IL-2Rβ^+CD3^{int}細胞は、CD4$^-$CD8$^-$、CD4$^+$とCD8$^+$細胞が混在していることが明らかになった（30）。現時点では、CD3^{int}細胞集団で、なぜサブセットによってこのような独特の違いが存在するかはわからない。最近の報告では、β_2-ミクログロブリン欠損マウスにおいて、CD4$^-$CD8$^-$とCD4$^+$細胞が同時に減少した（25,26）。この点から、CD4$^-$CD8$^-$細胞とCD4$^+$細胞は、密接に関連している。MRL-lpr/lprマウスのリンパ節において、CD4$^+$細胞が、CD4$^-$CD8$^-$細胞を産生するという報告があった（36）。

本研究においても、NK1.1$^+$とNK1.1$^-$サブセットの自己応答性禁止クローンの分布を検証した。NK1.1同種抗原は、主にB6とB10共通遺伝子系統のマウスに見られるが、この両系統のマウスでは、MHCクラスⅡであるI-E分子が欠損していることが明らかになっている（2）。Mls抗原は、I-E分子により表出される。故に、B6マウスもB10マウスもMls抗原による負の選択が行われないため、自己応答性禁止クローンのVβ^+細胞が存在しないのである。この問題を解決するため、NK1.1同種抗原を発現し、且

Figure.6

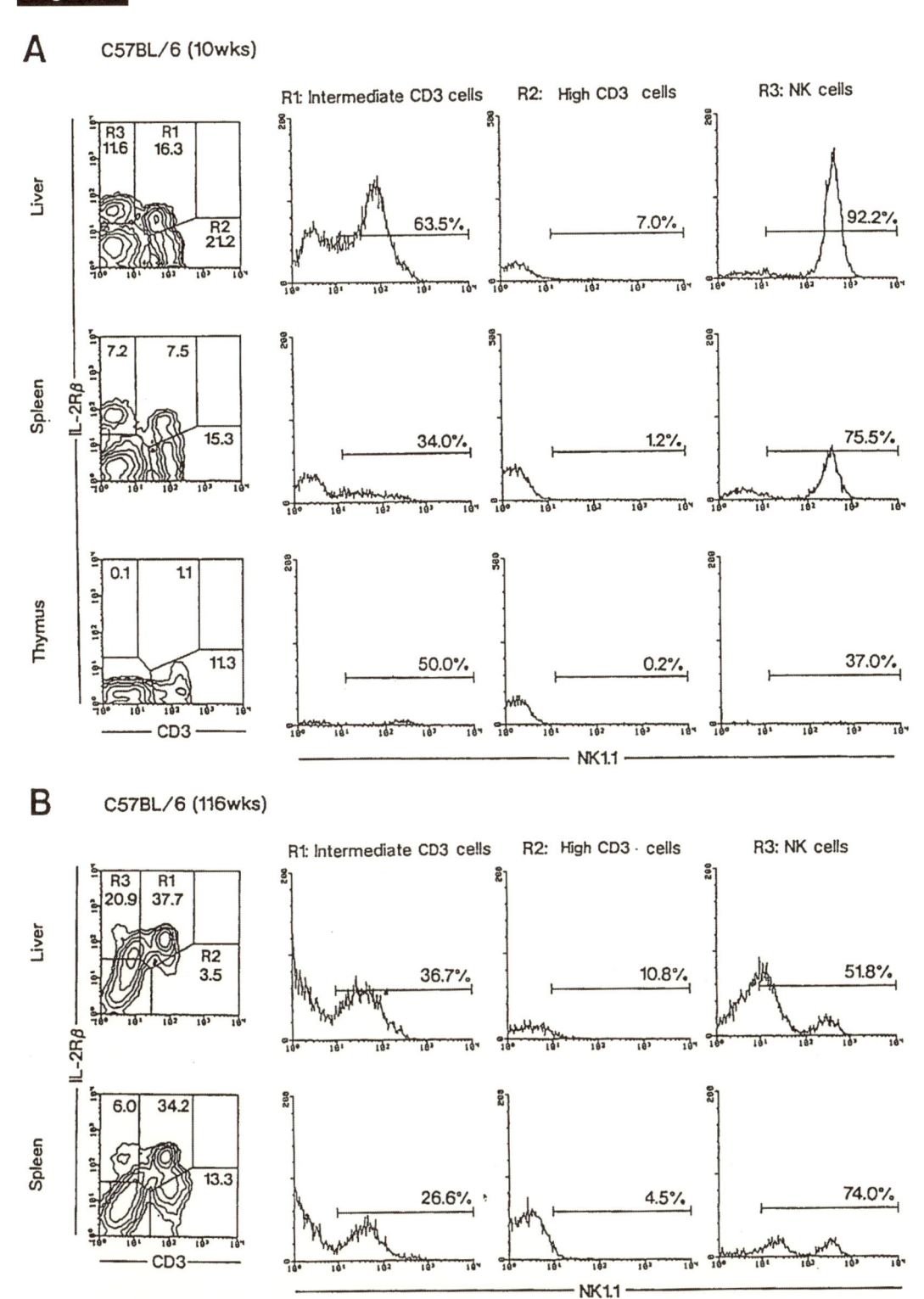

A C57BL/6 (10wks)

B C57BL/6 (116wks)

老齢マウスの肝臓と脾臓におけるCD3^{int}細胞のNK1.1$^+$：NK1.1$^-$サブセット比率の減少を示した。A, 若齢B6マウス；B, 老齢B6マウス。若齢（10週齢）および老齢（116週齢）B6マウスを使用した。CD3、IL-2RβとNK1.1の三重染色には、ゲーティング解析を行い、各分画におけるNK1.1$^+$T細胞の比率を検証した。各分画内の数値は、蛍光陽性細胞の比率を示す。

Figure.7

IL-2Rβ+NK1.1+　IL-2Rβ+NK1.1−

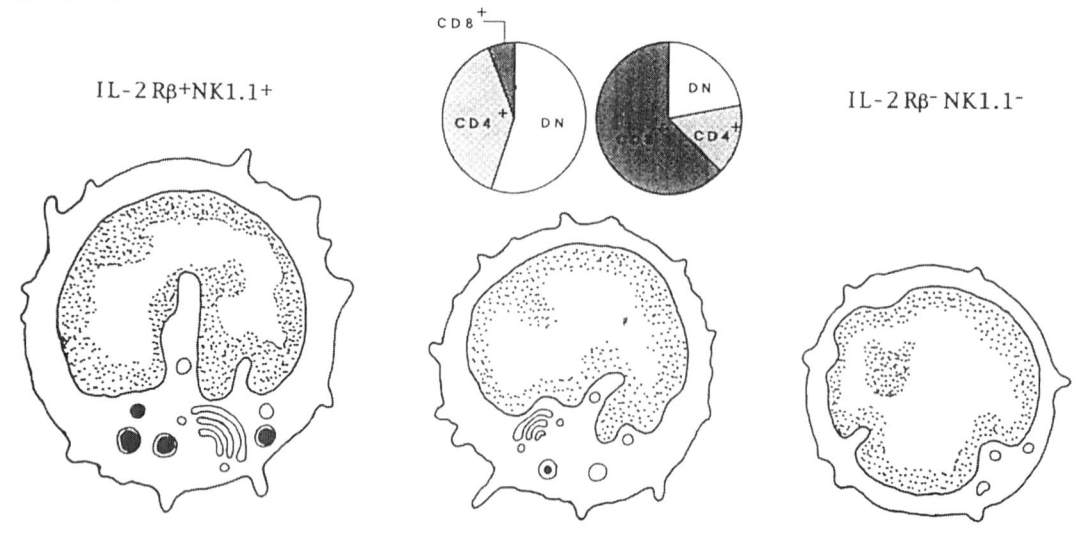

IL-2Rβ+NK1.1+　　　　　　　　　　　　　　　　　IL-2Rβ−NK1.1−

NK細胞、TCR^{int}細胞およびTCR^{high}細胞の特徴を図示する。TCR^{int}細胞のフェノタイプ複数分画から成るので、NK1.1$^+$とNK1.1$^-$サブセットにおけるCD4$^-$CD8$^-$、CD4$^+$、CD8$^+$細胞の分布パターンを示す。

つ、自己応答性禁止クローン持つNZB(Mls-1^{a2a})と(B6 x C3H/He)F$_1$マウス(Mls-1$^{b2a/b}$)を使用した。このようにして、CD3^{int}細胞集団内に存在するNK1.1$^+$とNK1.1$^-$両サブセットのどちらでも自己反応禁止クローンが見られることを明白にした。全く対照的に、NK1.1抗原を持たないCD3^{high}細胞集団では、この自己応答性クローンを含まなかった。換言すると、CD3^{int}細胞分化の経路だけがこのような自己応答性クローンを産生し、末梢臓器へ送るのである。

CD3^{int}細胞集団内では、加齢によりNK1.1$^+$サブセットの比率は減少するが、NK1.1$^-$サブセットの比率は増加する。近年、老齢（>100週齢）マウスにおいて、各サブセットのパーフォリン値とVβ発現の検証を行った。NK1.1$^+$とNK1.1$^-$サブセットのパーフォリン値とVβ発現に加齢による変化は見られなかった。しかしNK1.1$^+$サブセットとNK1.1$^-$サブセットが加齢により変化するため、CD3^{int}細胞集団全体としてパーフォリン値は減少傾向を示した。

現時点では、CD3^{int}細胞が分化する主要部位は、肝臓と胸腺髄質であると考えられる。胸腺髄質にCD3^{int}細胞が存在することを、CD44分子の発現により検証した（37）。このことが事実であるならば、肝臓と胸腺の経路は、独立して存在する可能性がある。そのため、成体において胸腺を摘出しても肝臓のCD3^{int}細胞の値は大きく変化しなかった（4）。同様に、肝硬変では胸腺ではなく、肝臓のCD3^{int}細胞値が減少する（38）。

IL-2Rβ$^+$CD3^{int}細胞が豊富に存在するのは、若齢マウスの肝臓だけある。しかし、加齢により、脾臓、リンパ節と骨髄を含む全臓器で顕著になる（4, 39）。胸腺が欠損しているヌードマウスの場合、T細胞は、肝臓、脾臓とリンパ節を含む全臓器において、全てCD3^{int}細胞であることが明らかになった（4）。このことから、これらのCD3^{int}細胞は、胸腺外で産生されると考えられる；しかし、その後、胸腺内でこのCD3^{int}細胞が、少数ではあるが発見された（5）。本研究では、このCD3^{int}細胞の多くはNK1.1$^+$T細胞と一致することを明らかにしたが、近年、

CD3^{int}細胞は、胸腺内代替経路で産生されることが報告された（16,17）。胸腺の起源は、外胚葉裂孔（えら穴）と初期の呼吸器（えら）に存在する内部上皮リンパ球であるので、進化後も胸腺には原始T細胞の構成要素が僅かに含まれている可能性がある（40）。換言すると、CD3^{int}細胞集団やNK1.1$^+$T細胞集団は、生体の全身部位に存在する原始T細胞である。

形態学的検証から、CD3^{int}細胞は、顆粒リンパ球に属することが明らかになった。しかし、CD3^{int}細胞の電子密度の高い（電子顕微鏡で暗く見える）顆粒とパーフォリンは、NK細胞のものよりも明らかに少なかった。正確には、CD3^{int}細胞の形態は、NK細胞と胸腺由来T細胞の中間に位置する。系統発生の進化の過程において、T細胞の形態が単純化し、休止状態でIL-2Rβを発現しなくなった可能性が考えられた。その結果、最も進化したT細胞（T細胞分化主経路で産生されるT細胞）の場合、形態は休止状態にある小リンパ球で、フェノタイプはIL-2R$\alpha^-\beta^-$である。しかし、抗原刺激すると、形態はリンパ芽球となり、フェノタイプは高親和性のIL-2R$\alpha^+\beta^+$を示す（30）。CD3^{int}細胞の場合、このような活性化は限られている。この結果は、系統発生の進化過程において、細胞の進化の段階をも反映している可能性がある。

パーフォリン陽性細胞の値は、NK細胞に比較して、CD3^{int}細胞では低値である。この結果は、NK機能活性と合致している：CD3^{int}細胞のNK活性は、NK細胞の1/5である（38）。CD3^{int}細胞内にはNK1.1$^+$サブセットとNK1.1$^-$サブセットが存在する。この二つのサブセットのパーフォリン陽性細胞の値を比較すると、NK1.1$^+$サブセットはNK1.1$^-$サブセットよりも、パーフォリン陽性細胞が高値であった。この点について、CD3^{int}細胞のNK機能活性は、主にNK1.1$^+$サブセットが担っている；しかし、だからといって、CD3^{int}細胞またはCD3^{int}細胞内のNK1.1$^-$サブセットの細胞傷害活性が低いことを意味するわけではない。CD3^{int}細胞は、IL-12等の刺激を受け、細胞質内のパーフォリン顆粒や強力な細胞傷害活性を獲得する可能性がある。事実、胸腺由来T細胞の場合は、活性化すると細胞傷害性Tリンパ球として活躍するからである。

最後に、IL-2Rβ^+CD3^{int}細胞およびNK1.1$^+$T細胞が活性化する状況は、加齢、悪性腫瘍（42-44）、遺伝形質が原因である特定の自己免疫疾患（1,45,46）および慢性移植片対宿主病（47）である。このような状況下で、IL-2Rβ^+CD3^{int}細胞は、自己応答性に有益な機能を有する可能性があると考えられる。本研究で示したように、加齢によりCD3^{int}細胞集団が拡大し、NK1.1$^+$：NK1.1$^-$サブセット比が減少した。しかし、両サブセットのCD4、CD8およびCD4$^-$CD8$^-$細胞において構成の比率は変化しなかった。

最近の研究において、マウスにおけるNK1.1$^+$T細胞（48）、または、ヒトにおけるCD4$^-$CD8$^-$$\alpha\beta$T細胞（49, 50）では、V$\alpha$の拘束性があることが、明らかになった。研究をすすめ、これらの集団がどのように自己抗原を認識するのかを検証する必要がある。本研究の結果は、将来、これらの細胞集団の研究にとって、非常に有益である可能性がある。

謝辞

渡辺正子氏の浄書および橋本氏の動物飼育に感謝する。

Relationships Between Intermediate TCR Cells and NK1.1$^+$ T Cells in Various Immune Organs

NK1.1$^+$ T Cells Are Present Within a Population of Intermediate TCR Cells[1]

Hisami Watanabe,[2]* Chikako Miyaji,* Yasuyuki Kawachi,* Tsuneo Iiai,* Kazuo Ohtsuka,* Toshihiko Iwanage,† Hiromi Takahashi-Iwanaga,† and Toru Abo*

*Department of Immunology and †Third Department of Anatomy, Niigata University School of Medicine, Niigata, Japan

Experiments to date have revealed a population of T cells that carry intermediate (int) levels of TCR (or CD3) and express IL-2R β-chain (IL-2Rβ) in mouse liver. Such int TCR cells also reside in other immune organs, although in low numbers. On the other hand, NK1.1$^+$ T cells with int TCR do reside in the thymus and other peripheral organs. To determine the relationship of two types of cells, we characterized int CD3 cells and NK1.1$^+$ T cells throughout the organs in terms of the phenotype, Vβ repertoire, and morphology. Although both IL-2Rβ$^+$ T cells and NK1.1$^+$ T cells are classified as int CD3 cells, NK1.1$^+$ T cells are present within int CD3 cells. The majority of int CD3 cells in the liver and thymus were NK1.1$^+$, whereas the minority of such cells in the spleen, lymph nodes, and bone marrow were NK1.1$^+$. Among int CD3 cells, double-negative (DN) CD4$^-$8$^-$ cells and/or CD4$^+$ were abundant in NK1.1$^+$ subset, whereas CD8$^+$ cells were generally abundant in NK1.1$^-$ subset. Self-reactive Vβ$^+$ clones estimated by the Mls system were distributed to both NK1.1$^+$ and NK1.1$^-$ subsets. High CD3 cells in the thymus and other organs contained neither DN cells nor forbidden clones. Int CD3 cells had the morphology of granular or agranular lymphocytes carrying perforin. Among int CD3 cells, NK1.1$^+$ subset had a higher level of perforin-positive cells than NK1.1$^-$ subset. These results clearly demonstrate the relationship between int TCR cells and NK1.1$^+$ T cells in various organs. *The Journal of Immunology*, 1995, 155: 2972–2983.

A unique population of T cells that carry intermediate levels of TCR (or CD3) (termed intermediate (int)[3] TCR cells) and constitutively express IL-2R β-chain (IL-2Rβ) have been demonstrated to exist in the liver (1–4). These hepatic T cells are easily distinguishable from IL-2Rβ$^-$ thymus-derived T cells with high levels of TCR (i.e., high TCR cells). Intermediate TCR cells comprise double-negative (DN) CD4$^-$8$^-$ cells as well as single-positive CD4$^+$ and CD8$^+$ cells (1), and contain self-reactive "forbidden" clones estimated by anti-Vβ mAbs in conjunction with the endogenous superantigen Mls system (2). Intermediate TCR cells consist of both αβ T cells and γδ T cells (4). Since T cells in the peripheral immune organs of congenitally athymic nude mice and of thymectomized, irradiated, and bone marrow-transplanted mice are all int TCR cells, except for those in the intestine, it is speculated that they might be of extrathymic origin (5). However, our subsequent studies showed that int TCR cells exist in other immune organs, including the spleen, lymph nodes, and thymus, although in low numbers (4, 5).

Many investigators have reported that DN (or CD4$^+$) αβ T cells with NK1.1 Ags exist in the thymus (6–15). Careful study of their data revealed that these NK1.1$^+$ T cells had lower levels of TCR than did usual mature T cells. Some of these authors speculated that these T cells are generated through an alternative intrathymic pathway of T cell differentiation (16, 17). A similar population of T cells was also demonstrated to localize in the spleen (18 to 20), lymph nodes (21, 22), and bone marrow (23, 24). Concerning the data from the phenotypic and functional characterizations, IL-2Rβ$^+$ int TCR cells and NK1.1$^+$ αβ T cells seem to belong largely to the same population. The

---

Received for publication December 19, 1994. Accepted for publication June 30, 1995.

The costs of publication of this article were defrayed in part by the payment of page charges. This article must therefore be hereby marked *advertisement* in accordance with 18 U.S.C. Section 1734 solely to indicate this fact.

[1] This work was supported by a grant-in-aid for Scientific Research from the Ministry of Education, Science and Culture, Japan.

[2] Address correspondence and reprint requests to Dr. Hisami Watanabe, Department of Immunology, Niigata University School of Medicine, Asahimachi 1, Niigata 951, Japan.

[3] Abbreviations used in this paper: int, intermediate (cells); IL-2Rβ, IL-2R β-chain; DN, double-negative; MNC, mononuclear cells; PE, phycoerythrin; LGL, large granular lymphocyte; B6 mice, C57BL/6 mice.

Copyright © 1995 by The American Association of Immunologists   0022-1767/95/$02.00

results of some previous experiments on Vβ repertoire and MHC restriction in NK1.1$^+$ αβ T cells support the above notion (25–27).

In the present study, we further characterized these populations of int TCR cells and NK1.1$^+$ T cells throughout the organs in terms of their phenotype, Vβ repertoire, and morphology. It was demonstrated that they had many properties in common as well as minor district properties, depending on the organs and the subsets. It is presumed that they may be generated independently but belong to a similar lineage of T cell population. Since they exist in both the liver and thymus, the termination of T cell differentiation as either extrathymic pathways or an alternative intrathymic pathway is unlikely. Based on their primordial characteristics, they should be termed "primordial" T cells; they may be generated through the primordial pathways of T cell differentiation at multiple sites in the body.

Materials and Methods
Mice

C57BL/6 (B6), SJL, NZB, and (B6 × C3H/He)F$_1$ female mice were used at the ages of 18 to 20 wk. Older B6 mice aged 116 wk were also used. All of these mouse strains have NK1.1 alloantigens. These mice were originally obtained from Charles River Japan (Kanagawa, Japan) and were maintained at the animal facility of Niigata University. All mice were fed under specific pathogen-free conditions.

Cell preparations

Hepatic mononuclear cells (MNC) were isolated by an improved method as described elsewhere (28). Briefly, mice anesthetized with ether were killed by total bleeding with a cardiac puncture. To obtain MNC, the liver was removed, pressed through 200-gauge stainless steel mesh, and then suspended in PBS (0.1 M, pH 7.2). After washing once with PBS, MNC were isolated from both hepatocytes and the nuclei of hepatocytes by Ficoll-Isopaque density (1.090) gradient centrifugation. To avoid a selective loss of specific subsets (29), the mashed liver samples were diluted intensively (2 livers/30 ml PBS). The MNC from the interface were then suspended in MEM medium supplemented with 2% FCS.

Spleen cells, PBL, and bone marrow cells were also collected by the Ficoll-Isopaque method, whereas thymocytes and lymph nodes were obtained by forcing the thymus or inguinal lymph nodes through 200-gauge steel mesh. In some experiments for morphologic and histochemical studies, purified fractions of IL-2Rβ$^+$ int CD3 cells and IL-2Rβ$^-$ high CD3 cells were sorted after staining with FITC-conjugated anti-CD3 mAb and phycoerythrin (PE)-conjugated anti-IL-2Rβ mAb (PharMingen Co., San Diego, CA) by FACStar IIPlus (Becton Dickinson Co., Mountain View, CA). NK1.1$^+$ and NK1.1$^-$ subsets in int CD3 cells were also sorted after staining with anti-CD3 and anti-NK1.1 mAbs.

Immunofluorescence tests

The surface phenotype of cells was identified by using mAbs in conjunction with either a single-, two-, or three-color immunofluorescence test (30). The mAbs used here included FITC, PE, or biotin-conjugated reagents of anti-CD3 (145-2C11), anti-IL-2Rβ chain (TM-β1), and NK1.1 (PK136) mAbs (PharMingen). FITC or PE-conjugated anti-CD4 (L3T4) and anti-CD8 (Lyt-2) mAbs were obtained from Becton Dickinson. Each population of Vβ$^+$ cells was identified by three-color staining for CD3 (FITC), IL-2Rβ or NK1.1 (PE) and corresponding Vβ (Red 613). Biotin-conjugated reagents were developed with either PE or Red 613-conjugated streptavidin (Becton Dickinson). The fluorescence-positive cells were analyzed by a FACScan (Becton Dickinson).

Electron microscopy

For transmission electron microscopy, the sorted cell fractions were fixed with 2.5% glutaraldehyde in 0.1 M phosphate buffer, pH 7.4 (4). After immersion in the fixative for 2 h, the tissue blocks were postfixed for 1.5 h in 1% OsO$_4$ dissolved in the phosphate buffer, dehydrated through a series of graded ethanol, and embedded in Araldite with propylene oxide. The ultrathin sections were stained with uranyl acetate and lead citrate, and examined under a Hitachi H-7000 transmission electron microscope (Hitachi Seisakusho, Hitachi, Japan).

Immunoperoxidase staining for perforin

Cytospin preparations of sorted fractions were air dried. The preparations were then fixed in cold acetone (4 min) and 4% paraformaldehyde in PBS (1 min) (31). They were then washed with 50 mM Tris-HCl, (pH 7.6) and treated with 0.5% periodic acid (10 min) and 0.3% H$_2$O$_2$ in methanol (15 min). They were blocked with Ca^{2+}-free PBS containing 5% BSA and 0.02% NaN$_3$ (30 min), and incubated with rat anti-mouse perforin mAb (P1-8; kindly provided by Dr. K. Okumura, Tokyo, Japan) (60 min). To visualize Ab binding, the preparations were washed with Ca^{2+}-and Mg^{2+}-free PBS, incubated with biotinylated goat anti-rat IgG (Sigma Chemical Co., St Louis, MO) (60 min), washed again with Ca^{2+}-and Mg^{2+}-free PBS, incubated with extravidin peroxidase (Sigma) (30 min), and washed with Ca^{2+}-free PBS before developing with a substrate mixture kit (Bio-Makor, Rehovot, Israel) to generate the red color. Cells were counter-stained with hematoxylin.

Systemic administration of rIL-12 into mice

To induce perforin granules, some mice were injected with rIL-12 (1 μg/mouse, i.p.) (Genetic Institute, Andover, MA). Cell preparation was performed on day 1 after injection.

Results
Distribution of IL-2Rβ$^+$ int CD3 cells and NK1.1$^+$ T cells in various organs

To determine the distribution of int CD3 cells in various organs, two-color staining for CD3 and IL-2Rβ was carried out (Fig. 1). B6 mice carrying NK1.1 alloantigens at the age of 18 wk were used in this experiment. Int CD3 cells were clearly distinguishable from high CD3 cells by this staining, because int CD3 cells were IL-2Rβ$^+$ while high CD3 cells were IL-2Rβ$^-$ (Fig. 1, *upper columns*). IL-2Rβ$^+$ int CD3 cells were confirmed to be most abundant in the liver. However, int CD3 cells were identified in all tested organs, despite their small proportion.

Two-color staining for CD3 and NK1.1 was then performed using the same materials (Fig. 1, *lower columns*). CD3$^+$NK1.1$^+$ cells were identified in all tested organs and their expression of CD3 was found to be at intermediate levels. Since these NK1.1$^+$ T cells were also abundant in the liver, it is speculated that IL-2Rβ$^+$ int CD3 cells and NK1.1$^+$ T cells are overlapping populations.

Relationship between IL-2Rβ$^+$ int CD3 cells and NK1.1$^+$ T cells in various organs

To directly compare the relationship between IL-2Rβ$^+$ int CD3 cells and NK1.1$^+$ T cells, three-color staining for CD3, IL-2Rβ and NK1.1 was then carried out (Table I). In this experiment, 18-wk-old B6, SJL, and NZB mice having NK1.1 alloantigens were used to produce the mean and 1 SD ($n = 6$ in each strain). Since almost all NK1.1$^+$ T

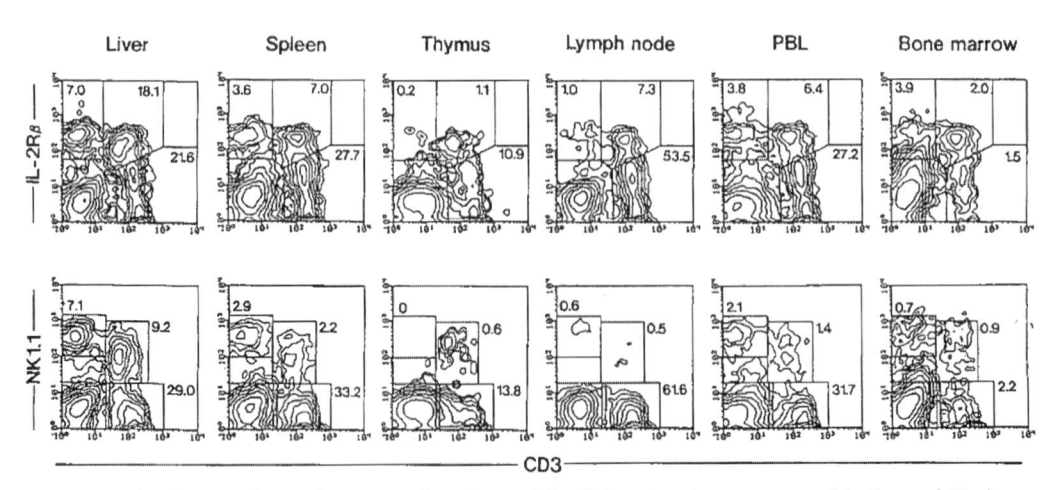

FIGURE 1. Identification of IL-2Rβ⁺ int CD3 cells and NK1.1⁺ T cells in various immune organs. B6 mice aged 18 wk were used. Two-color staining for CD3 and IL-2Rβ was carried out to identify IL-2Rβ⁺ int CD3 cells, whereas that for CD3 and NK1.1 was carried out to identify NK1.1⁺ T cells. Both IL-2Rβ⁺ T cells and NK1.1⁺ T cells were found to belong to int CD3 cells. Numbers in the figure indicate the percentages of fluorescence-positive cells in the corresponding areas. Representative results from three experiments are depicted.

Table I. A comparison of relationship between IL-2Rβ⁺ int CD3 cells and NK1.1⁺ T cells in various organs[a]

Organs	% NK1.1⁺ Cells Among IL-2Rβ⁺ int CD3 Cells		
	B6	SJL	NZB
Liver	69.6 ± 11.9	50.9 ± 7.2	56.9 ± 1.9
Spleen	15.8 ± 4.7	22.0 ± 4.3	35.5 ± 0.3
Thymus	56.9 ± 9.2	60.3 ± 8.9	52.6 ± 7.6
Lymph nodes	4.9 ± 2.0	ND	ND
Bone marrow	27.2 ± 6.3	ND	ND

[a] B6, SJL, and NZB mice at the age of 18 wk were used. The values were obtained by three-color staining for CD3 (FITC), IL-2Rβ (PE), and NK1.1 (Red 613). Mean and 1 SD were produced from six mice of each strain.

cells expressed IL-2Rβ (>97%), only the percentages of NK1.1⁺ cells among IL-2Rβ⁺ intermediate CD3 cells are represented. High levels of the overlapping were seen in the liver and thymus (>50%), whereas lower levels of overlapping were seen in the spleen, lymph nodes, and bone marrow. A similar tendency was observed in all mouse strains.

Composition patterns of DN, CD4⁺, and CD8⁺ cells among T cell subsets

Experiments thus far indicated that all int CD3 cells are IL-2Rβ⁺ while they are a mixture of NK1.1⁺ and NK1.1⁻. It was then examined how NK1.1⁺ and NK1.1⁻ subsets among int CD3 cells in the liver, spleen, and thymus comprised DN CD4⁻8⁻ cells and single-positive CD4⁺ or CD8⁺ cells. For this purpose, three-color staining of CD3 (FITC), NK1.1 (or IL-2Rβ) (PE), and a mixture of CD4 and CD8 (Red 613) was performed (Fig. 2).

When liver MNC of B6 mice are represented in terms of the expression of CD3 and NK1.1, three subsets, including R1(CD3^{int}NK1.1⁺), R2(CD3^{int}NK1.1⁻), and R3(CD3^{high}NK1.1⁻), were identified. To show the composition patterns of DN and single-positive cells among them, the gated analysis is represented (Fig. 2, *lower columns*). To distinguish CD4⁺ and CD8⁺ cells, the staining intensity of CD8 was elevated by the addition of a high titer of anti-CD8 mAb. It was clearly demonstrated that CD3^{int}NK1.1⁺ cells comprised mainly DN CD4⁻8⁻ cells and CD4⁺ cells, whereas CD3^{int}NK1.1⁻ cells comprised a mixture of DN, CD4⁺, and CD8⁺ cells. CD3^{high}NK1.1⁻ cells consisted only of CD4⁺ and CD8⁺ cells. The expression levels of CD4 and CD8 Ags (i.e., staining intensity) on int CD3 cells were slightly lower than those on high CD3 cells.

To determine the composition patterns among T cell subsets in various organs, the same type of staining was extended to other organs including the liver (Table II). The values of total IL-2Rβ⁺ int CD3 cells as well as of IL-2Rβ⁻ high CD3 cells were also analyzed by the three-color staining for CD3 (FITC), IL-2Rβ (PE), and a mixture of CD4 and CD8 (Red 613) (Table II, Expt. 1). To standardize the values and to simplify the table, the mean of three B6 mice (used pooled materials) is presented. As already reported in our previous studies (4, 5), int CD3 cells were confirmed to comprise DN CD4⁻8⁻, CD4⁺, and CD8⁺ cells, whereas high CD3 cells did not contain DN CD4⁻8⁻ cells. This was true in all organs of B6 mice. In the cases of NK1.1⁺ and NK1.1⁻ subsets among int CD3 cells, both subsets were a mixture of DN, CD4⁺, and CD8⁺ cells (experiment 2, B6 mice). However, NK1.1⁺

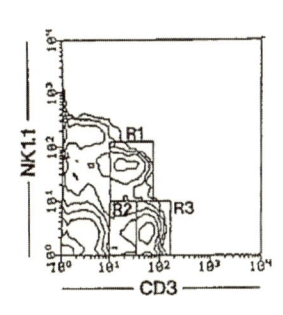

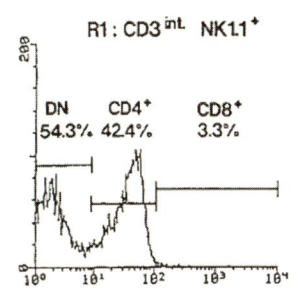

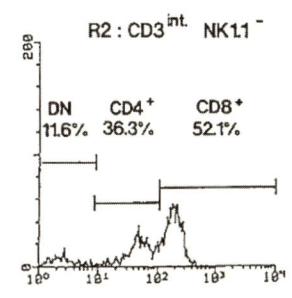

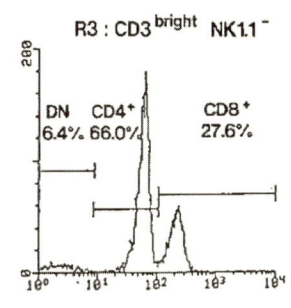

FIGURE 2. Distribution of DN, CD4$^+$, and CD8$^+$ T cells among NK1.1$^+$ int CD3 cells (R1), NK1.1$^-$ int CD3 cells (R2), and NK1.1$^-$ high CD3 cells (R3). Liver MNC of B6 mice aged 18 wk were used. Three-color staining for CD3 (FITC), NK1.1(PE), and a mixture of CD4 and CD8 (Red 613) was performed. To distinguish CD4$^+$ and CD8$^+$ cells, a high titer of anti-CD8 mAb was used. The gated analysis of R1, R2, and R3 was done to determine the proportion of DN, CD4$^+$, and CD8$^+$ cells.

subsets were mainly DN and/or CD4$^+$ cells, whereas NK1.1$^-$ subsets generally predominated CD8$^+$ cells, irrespective of tested organs. Similar data were obtained in NZB mice (experiment 3).

Vβ repertoire among NK1.1$^+$ and NK1.1$^-$ subsets in int CD3 cells

Usual strains of B6 and B10 congenic mice that carry NK1.1 alloantigens lack the expression of I-E molecules. Self-reactive clones corresponding to certain Mls Ags are eliminated by the negative selection in conjunction with I-E. In this regard, such mice do not have specific self-reactive Vβ$^+$ clones estimated by the Mls system. As a result, we were not able to use the mouse strains lacking I-E to estimate self-reactive forbidden clones. To overcome this situation, we used NZB mice (Mls-1^{a2a}) and (B6 × C3H/He)F$_1$ mice (Mls-1$^{b2a/b}$) that carry NK1.1 alloantigens and also express I-E molecules. Since both strains of mice showed similar results, we have herein presented the data of NZB mice (Fig. 3). In these experiments, three-color staining for CD3, IL-2Rβ (or NK1.1), and each Vβ$^+$ was performed. In NZB mice, Vβ2$^+$ and Vβ8$^+$ cells are nonforbidden clones, while Vβ7$^+$ and Vβ11$^+$ cells are forbidden clones. In the case of the liver (Fig. 3A), it was clear that nonforbidden clones, Vβ2$^+$ and Vβ8$^+$, were distributed to all T cell subsets, i.e., CD3^{high}IL-2Rβ$^-$, CD3^{int}IL-2Rβ$^+$, CD3^{int}NK1.1$^+$, and CD3^{int}-NK1.1$^-$. On the other hand, forbidden clones, Vβ7$^+$ and Vβ11$^+$, were confined to CD3^{int}IL-2Rβ$^+$ cells, and to both NK1.1$^+$ and NK1.1$^-$ subsets among int CD3 cells as well.

Similar evaluation was also performed in the spleen and thymus (Fig. 3, B and C). All self-reactive clones, Vβ7$^+$ and Vβ11$^+$, were also found to be confined to CD3^{int}IL-2Rβ$^+$ and both NK1.1$^+$ and NK1.1$^-$ subsets among intermediate CD3 cells, even in the spleen. In the case of the thymus, at the position of the CD3^{int}NK1.1$^-$ subset in the staining figure, CD3^{dull}NK1.1$^-$ cells, which are immature T cells in the main stream of T cell differentiation, are present. In this respect, we did not determine the value of CD3^{int}NK1.1$^-$ subsets in the thymus by this staining method. Self-reactive clones in the thymus were seen in either CD3^{dull} cells or CD3^{int}IL-2Rβ$^+$ and CD3^{int}NK1.1$^+$ subsets. In other words, CD3^{high} cells did not contain self-reactive clones in the thymus or in other organs.

Based on the data of these experiments, the level of nonforbidden T cell clone, Vβ8$^+$ was also found to be

Table II. *Distribution pattern of DN, CD4$^+$, and CD8$^+$ cells among various T cell subsets*[a]

		% Positive Cells		
Organ	T Cell Subset	CD4$^-$CD8$^-$ cells	CD4$^+$ cells	CD8$^+$ cells
Experiment 1 (B6 mice)				
Liver	Int CD3	45.2	51.9	16.4
	High CD3	6.1	54.1	45.4
Spleen	Int CD3	47.7	27.2	53.4
	High CD3	0.9	61.4	37.5
Thymus	Int CD3	38.8	40.9	43.9
	High CD3	2.5	84.8	51.4
Experiment 2 (B6 mice)				
Liver	CD3$^+$NK1.1$^+$	47.2	50.8	3.3
	CD3^{int}NK1.1$^-$	16.4	32.5	63.0
	CD3^{high}NK1.1$^-$	3.8	47.8	45.1
Spleen	CD3$^+$NK1.1$^+$	66.2	22.9	14.9
	CD3^{int}NK1.1$^-$	20.5	22.1	62.4
	CD3^{high}NK1.1$^-$	0.3	55.5	42.3
Thymus	CD3$^+$NK1.1$^+$	42.6	48.2	21.2
	CD3^{high}NK1.1$^-$	2.1	76.3	36.9
Experiment 3 (NZB mice)				
Liver	CD3$^+$NK1.1$^+$	53.6	32.9	13.5
	CD3^{int}NK1.1$^-$	13.2	32.0	54.8
	CD3^{high}NK1.1$^-$	4.7	70.4	24.8
Spleen	CD3$^+$NK1.1$^+$	31.9	42.9	25.3
	CD3^{int}NK1.1$^-$	9.2	33.3	57.6
	CD3^{high}NK1.1$^-$	0.8	67.2	32.0
Thymus	CD3$^+$NK1.1$^+$	66.5	15.6	17.6
	CD3^{high}NK1.1$^-$	<0.1	83.9	22.2

[a] B6 and NZB mice at the age of 18 wk were used. For purposes of simplification, the mean value of three mice is shown.

quite high in the NK1.1$^+$ subset of int CD3 cells in all tested organs.

Morphology of intermediate CD3 cells

To show the morphologic characteristics of int CD3 cells, this population was sorted from the liver, thymus, and spleen in parallel with a population of CD3$^-$IL-2Rβ^+ NK cells. The sorted populations were observed by electron microscopy (Fig. 4). In Figure 4, the morphology of cells isolated from the liver is represented. All cells of the NK cell fraction showed a morphology of large granular lymphocytes (LGL) (Fig. 4a). On the other hand, cells of int CD3 cell fraction contained granular or agranular lymphocytes (Fig. 4b). Lymphocytes with granular lymphocytes comprised less than 20% of the int CD3 cell fraction. However, they had a very wide cytoplasm carrying mitochondrias and small vacuoles. The same results were produced in the spleen and thymus (data not shown).

A comparison of the levels of perforin-positive cells in various lymphocyte subsets

It is well known that NK cells with LGL morphology express perforin, and that its enzyme localizes in the cytoplasmic granules (31). Perforin was identified by immunochemical staining. We compared the proportion of perforin-positive cells in various sorted lymphocyte subsets in the liver, including NK (CD3$^-$IL-2Rβ^+) cells, IL-2Rβ^+ int CD3 cells, their subsets of NK1.1$^+$ and NK1.1$^-$, and IL-2Rβ^- high CD3 cells (Table III). In the case of C3H/He mice (NK1.1 alloantigen$^-$), which is known to be the strain of high NK activity, the levels of perforin-positive cells among NK cells and whole int CD3 cells were very high, while that among high CD3 cells was extremely low. Similarly, such a tendency was also seen in B6 mice (NK1.1 alloantigen$^+$). NK1.1$^+$ subset had a higher level of perforin-positive cells than NK1.1$^-$ subset. The lower levels of perforin-positive cells in the generalized subsets of B6 are coincident to the fact that B6 mice are the strain of low NK activity (32). An in vivo administration of IL-12 increased the proportion of perforin-positive cells in all subsets of B6 mice.

Some of the above results are displayed as actual pictures (Fig. 5). Primarily, NK cells contained many perforin-granules in the cytoplasm, and the proportion of perforin-positive cells was high (Fig. 5a). NK1.1$^+$ subset of int CD3 cells contained few perforin granules and the proportion of such positive cells was low (Fig. 5c). After IL-12 administration, the perforin granules became more prominent in both NK cells (Fig. 5b) and NK1.1$^+$ subset of int CD3 cells (Fig. 5d).

FIGURE 3. Distribution pattern of self-reactive forbidden T cell clones in various subsets of immune organs. A, liver; B, spleen; C, thymus. NZB mice aged 18 wk were used. Three-color staining for CD3 (FITC), IL-2Rβ, or NK1.1 (PE) and corresponding Vβ (Red 613) were performed. Gated analysis of CD3^{high}IL-2Rβ^-, CD3^{int}IL-2Rβ^+, CD3^{int}NK1.1$^+$, and CD3^{int}NK1.1$^-$ subsets was done to identify the proportion of each type of Vβ^+ cell. In these NZB mice (M1s-1^{a}2^a), Vβ2$^+$ and Vβ8$^+$ cells are nonforbidden clones, while Vβ7$^+$ and Vβ11$^+$ cells are forbidden clones. Forbidden Vβ7$^+$ and Vβ11$^+$ clones were found in all subsets of int CD3 cells but not in CD3^{high}IL-2Rβ^- subsets, in the liver and spleen. In the case of the thymus, such Vβ7$^+$ and Vβ11$^+$ clones were found either in CD3^{dull} or CD3^{int} subsets. Nonforbidden clones were distributed to all subsets, irrespective of the organs. Numbers in the figure indicate the percentages of fluorescence-positive cells in the corresponding areas. Representative results from three experiments are depicted.

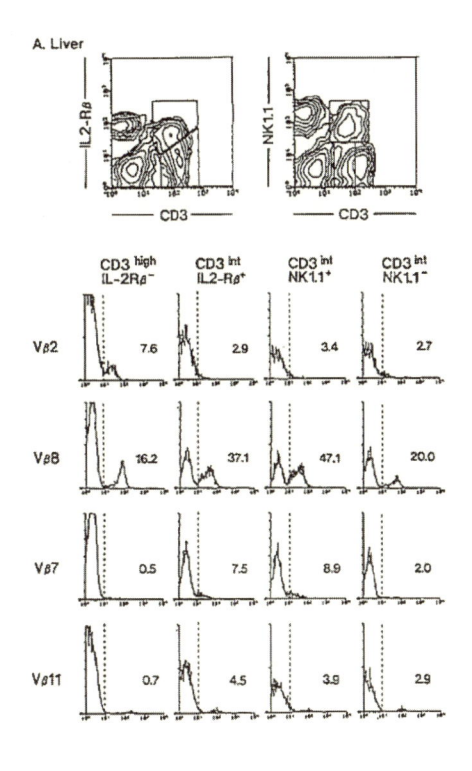

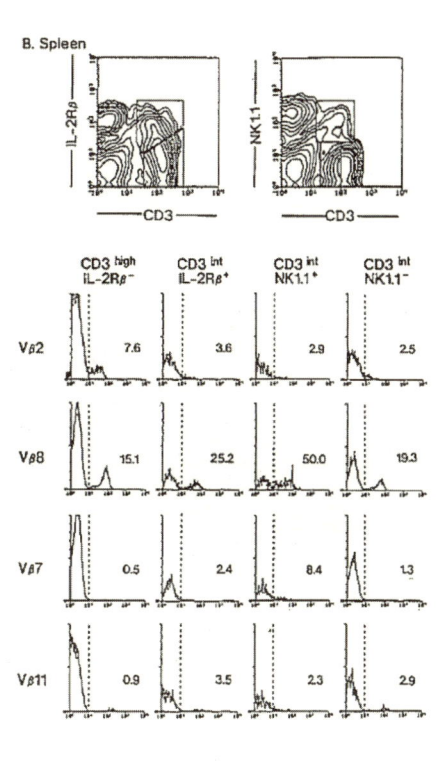

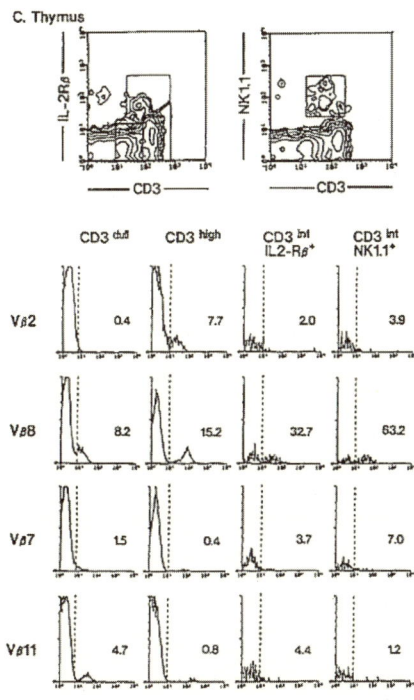

The Journal of Immunology

A. Liver

B. Spleen

C. Thymus

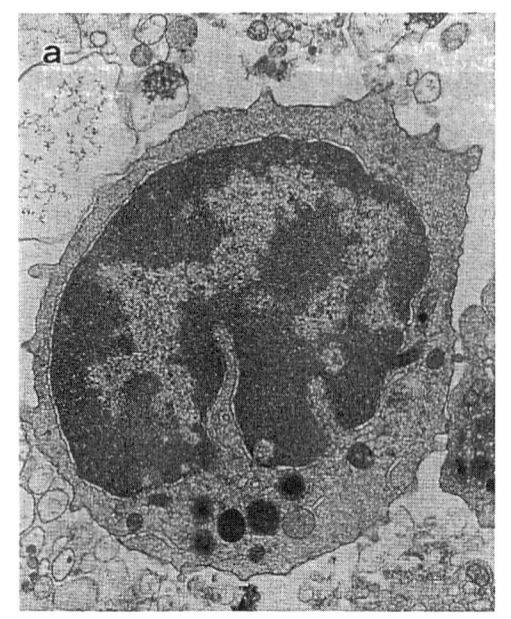

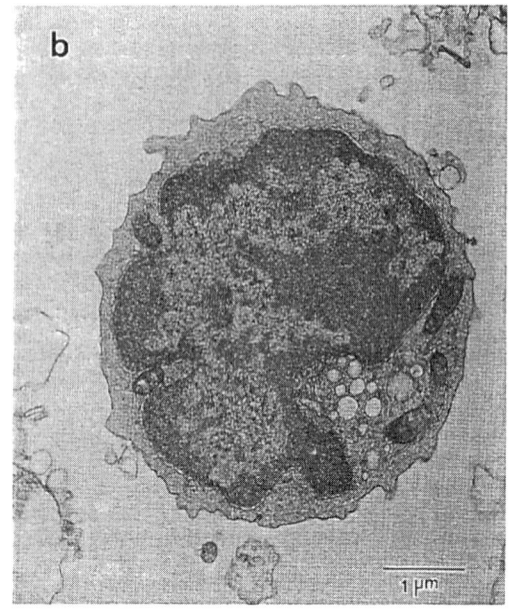

FIGURE 4. A comparison of the morphology between NK cells and int CD3 cells in the liver. *a*, NK cells; *b*, Int CD3 cells. Liver MNC were isolated from B6 mice at 18 wk of age. CD3$^-$IL-2Rβ^+ NK cells and IL-2Rβ^+ int CD3 cells were purified by a cell sorter after two-color staining for CD3 and IL-2Rβ. Electron microscopy and perforin staining was performed. Int CD3 cells had few granules but contained many vacuoles in their cytoplasms.

Table III. *The proportion of perforin-positive cells in various lymphocyte subsets of the liver*[a]

	% Perforin$^+$ Cells				
		Int CD3 Cells			
Mouse	NK cells	IL-2Rβ^+ whole	NK1.1$^+$ subset	NK1.1$^-$ subset	High CD3 cells
C3H/He	87.0 ± 13.1	55.0 ± 6.6			1.9 ± 0.4
SJL	61.1 ± 7.2	15.7 ± 1.6	21.9 ± 2.3	4.2 ± 0.2	0.6 ± 0.5
B6	62.0 ± 7.2	9.1 ± 2.4	5.7 ± 0.9	1.9 ± 0.4	1.2 ± 0.3
(IL-12 i.p.)	98.2 ± 3.8	25.2 ± 3.2	20.2 ± 3.8	7.9 ± 2.7	2.2 ± 1.5

[a] C57BL/6 mice were used with or without administration of IL-12. A mean and 1 SD were produced from three experiments. C3H/He mice lack the expression of NK1.1 alloantigen.

Increase of int CD3 cells with aging accompanied a decrease in the NK1.1$^+$:NK1.1$^-$ subset ratio

Int CD3 cells increase in number in the liver and other organs of older mice. We examined how the NK1.1$^+$:NK1.1$^-$ subset ratio varied in older mice (Fig. 6). Young B6 mice aged 10 wk were examined in parallel (Fig. 6A). As expected, the proportion of int CD3 cells increased in the liver and spleen in older mice (116 wk) (Fig. 6B). Interestingly, the proportion of NK1.1$^+$ subsets decreased and that of NK1.1$^-$ subset increased among int CD3 cells in older mice.

The composition patterns of CD4$^+$ cells, CD8$^+$ cells, and DN CD4$^-$8$^-$ cells among int CD3 cells were then examined. The composition pattern in NK1.1$^+$ and NK1.1$^-$ subsets was found to be essentially the same as that of the control (data not shown). This was true in both the liver and spleen.

Discussion

In this study, we directly examined the relationship between int CD3 cells and NK1.1$^+$ T cells in various immune organs. It was demonstrated that NK1.1$^+$ T cells were confined to a population of int CD3 cells and that int CD3 cells comprised both NK1.1$^+$ and NK1.1$^-$ subsets. The NK1.1$^+$IL-2Rβ^- subset was extremely rare among high CD3 cells. Based on the data from recent studies

FIGURE 5. Immunochemical staining for perforin in NK cells and NK1.1$^+$ subset of int CD3 cells (×1000). *a*, Sorted NK cells; *b*, sorted NK cells from mice treated with IL-12; *c*, sorted NK1.1$^+$ subset of int CD3 cells; *d*, sorted NK1.1$^+$ subset of int CD3 cells from mice treated with IL-12. Each cell fraction was sorted after two-color staining for CD3 and NK1.1.

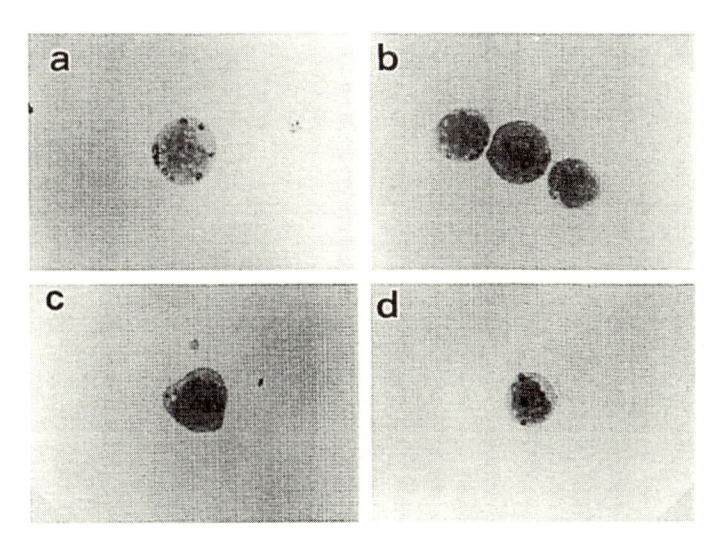

(4–15), int TCR (or CD3) cells and NK1.1$^+$ T cells have many properties in common, e.g., their expression of int TCR and the composition of DN CD4$^-$8$^-$ cells. The expression of adhesion molecules, CD44$^+$L-selectin$^-$, was also the same and this was the reverse of that on T cells derived from the main stream of T cell differentiation in the thymus (i.e., CD44$^-$ L-selectin$^+$) (14, 15, 33). All of these data are derived from the fact that NK1.1$^+$ T cells are present within a population of int CD3 cells. Int CD3 cells in the liver and thymus contained a high proportion of NK1.1$^+$ subsets (>50%), whereas those in the spleen, lymph nodes, blood, and bone marrow contained a low proportion of such subsets (<30%).

Since IL-2Rβ^+ int CD3 cells consisted of both NK1.1$^+$ and NK1.1$^-$ subsets, we compared their composition pattern of DN CD4$^-$8$^-$ and single-positive CD4$^+$ or CD8$^+$ cells. The NK1.1$^+$ subset mainly comprised DN and CD4$^+$ cells, whereas NK1.1$^-$ subsets comprised CD8$^+$ cells as well as a small population of DN cells and CD4$^+$ cells (Fig. 7). In a previous study, Arase et al. reported that NK1.1$^+$ T cells comprised both DN CD4$^-$8$^-$ cells and CD4$^+$ cells (15, 34, 35). On the other hand, we showed that IL-2Rβ^+ int CD3 cells are a mixture of DN, CD4$^+$ and CD8$^+$ cells (30). The present results clarified the above situation. At present, it is unknown why int CD3 cells have such a unique difference depending on the subsets. It was recently reported that DN and CD4$^+$ cells simultaneously decreased in β_2-microglobulin-deficient mice (25, 26). In this regard, DN cells and CD4$^+$ cells are closely related. There was a report that CD4$^+$ cells generate DN cells in the lymph nodes of MRL-*lpr/lpr* mice (36).

We also examined the distribution of autoreactive forbidden clones among NK1.1$^+$ and NK1.1$^-$ subsets. NK1.1 alloantigens are mainly detectable in mice of B6 and B10 congenic strains, and these mouse strains have been shown to lack class II MHC, I-E molecules (2). Since Mls Ag are represented by I-E molecules, none of Vβ^+ cells in these mice are self-reactive forbidden clones due to the lack of negative selection. To overcome this situation, we used NZB (Mls-1^{a}2^a) and (B6 × C3H/He)F$_1$ mice (Mls-1^{b}2$^{a/b}$) that express NK1.1 alloantigens and also have self-reactive forbidden clones. By using this protocol, we directly proved that both NK1.1$^+$ and NK1.1$^-$ subsets among int CD3 cells contained self-reactive forbidden clones. In sharp contrast, high CD3 cells lacking NK1.1 Ags did not contain any such self-reactive clones. In other words, only the pathways of int CD3 cell differentiation produce and send such self-reactive clones into the peripheral organs.

Among int CD3 cells, NK1.1$^+$ subset decreases while NK1.1$^-$ subset increases in proportion with aging. In aged mice (>100 wk), we have recently examined the perforin level and Vβ expression in each subset. The perforin level and Vβ expression among NK1.1$^+$ and NK1.1$^-$ subsets were unchanged with aging. However, because of the age-dependent variation of NK1.1$^+$ and NK1.1$^-$ subsets, the perforin level tended to decrease in whole int CD3 cells.

At present, we consider that the major sites for int CD3 cell differentration are the liver and the thymic medulla. The existence of int CD3 cells in the thymic medulla was determined by their expression of CD44 molecules (37). If this is the case, these pathways in the liver and thymus might be present independently. Thus, adult thymectomy did not change significantly the level of int CD3 cells in the liver (4). Similarly, hepatic cirrhosis decrease the levels of int CD3 cells in the liver but not in the thymus (38).

As for IL-2Rβ^+ int CD3 cells, they are abundant only in the liver of young mice. However, with aging they become prominent throughout the organs, including the spleen,

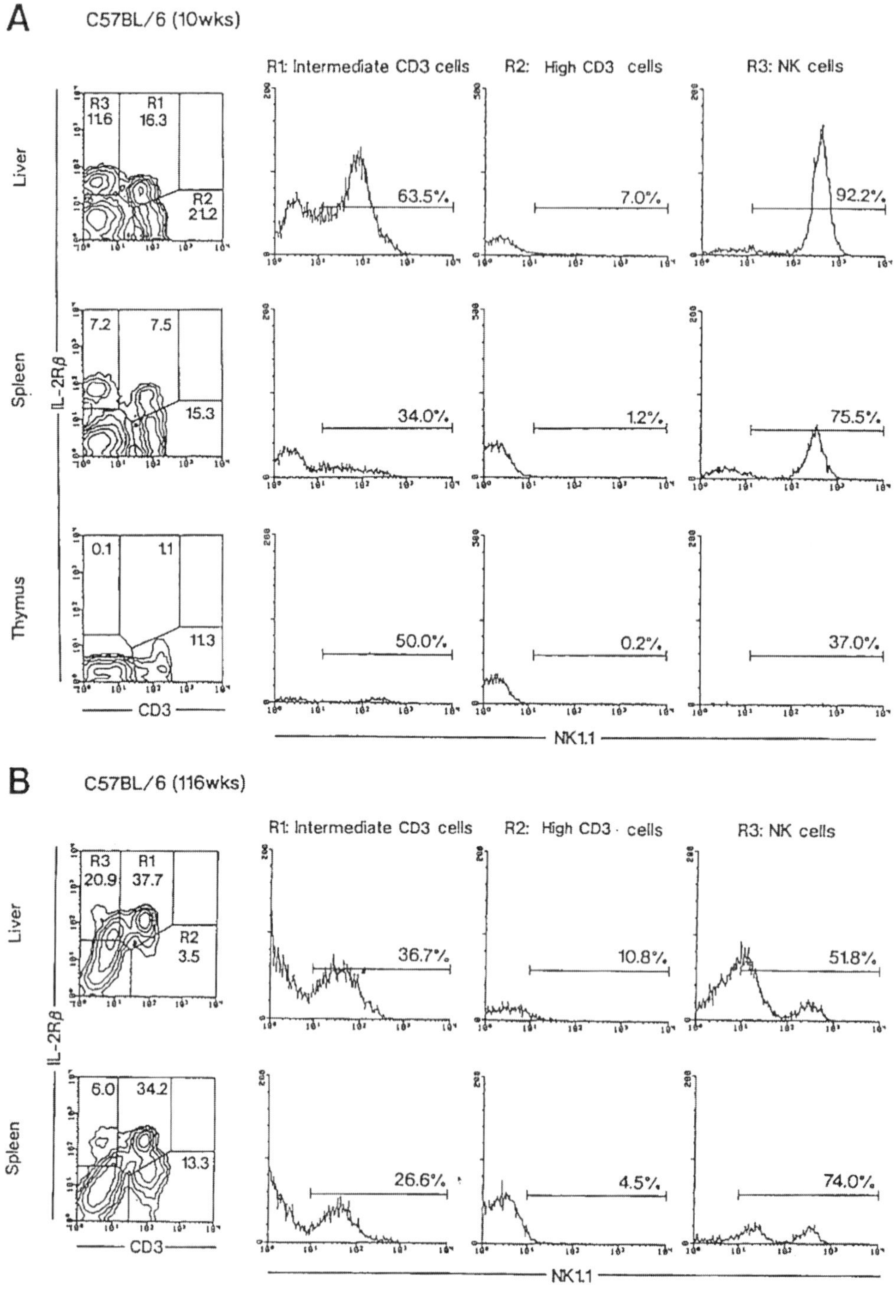
A
C57BL/6 (10wks)
R1: Intermediate CD3 cells
R2: High CD3 cells
R3: NK cells
Liver
Spleen
Thymus
IL-2Rβ
CD3
R3 11.6
R1 16.3
R2 21.2
7.2
7.5
15.3
0.1
1.1
11.3
63.5%
7.0%
92.2%
34.0%
1.2%
75.5%
50.0%
0.2%
37.0%
NK1.1
B
C57BL/6 (116wks)
R1: Intermediate CD3 cells
R2: High CD3 cells
R3: NK cells
Liver
Spleen
IL-2Rβ
CD3
R3 20.9
R1 37.7
R2 3.5
6.0
34.2
13.3
36.7%
10.8%
51.8%
26.6%
4.5%
74.0%
NK1.1

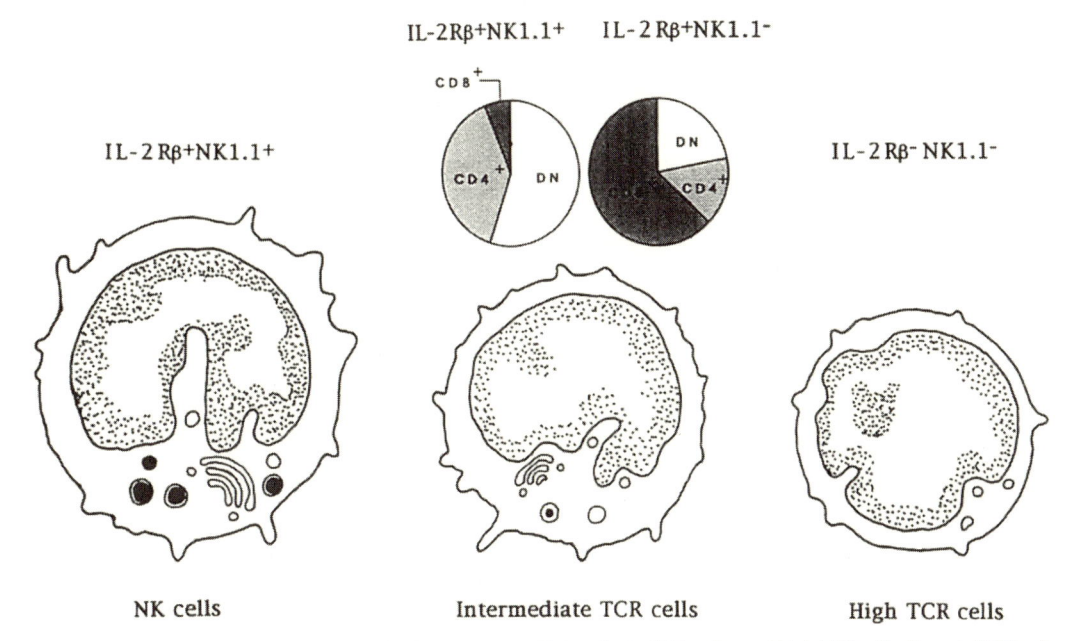

FIGURE 7. Schematic representation of the characteristics of NK cells, int TCR cells, and high TCR cells. Since int TCR cells are heterogeneous in terms of the phenotype, the distribution pattern of DN, CD4$^+$, and CD8$^+$ cells in NK1.1$^+$ and NK1.1$^-$ subsets among them is also represented.

lymph nodes, and bone marrow (4, 39). All T cells in athymic nude mice were found to be int CD3 cells in all organs, including the liver, spleen, and lymph nodes (4). In this regard, we speculate that these int CD3 cells are generated extrathymically; however, such int CD3 cells were subsequently found in the thymus, although in low numbers (5). It was demonstrated in the present study that many of them correspond to NK1.1$^+$ T cells, which were recently proposed to be generated through an alternative intrathymic pathway (16, 17). Since the thymus originates from the intraepithelial lymphocytes in early respiratory organs (i.e., gills) in conjuction with the ectodermal cleft (i.e., gill holes), the developed thymus may still contain a minor component of primordial T cells (40). In other words, a population of int CD3 cells or NK1.1$^+$ T cells are primordial T cells existing at generalized sites in the body.

In a morphologic study, it was demonstrated that int CD3 cells apparently belong to a family of granular lymphocytes. However, their electron dense granules and perforin were apparently fewer than those of NK cells. More precisely, the morphology of int CD3 cells is at an intermediate position between NK cells and thymus-derived T cells. We speculated that T cells may simplify their morphology and lose the expression of IL-2Rβ at conditions of rest in phylogenetic development. As a result, the most developed T cells (i.e., T cells generated through the main stream of T cell differentiation) have the morphology of small resting lymphocytes and an IL-2R$\alpha^-\beta^-$ phenotype. However, after antigenic stimulation, they acquire the lymphoblastic morphology and the high affinity of IL-2R$\alpha^+\beta^+$ (30). Such activation is limited in the case of int CD3 cells. These findings might reflect their stages of phylogenetic development as well.

The levels of perforin-positive cells is lower in int CD3 cells than in NK cells. This is in good agreement with the NK functional activity; namely, the NK activity of int CD3 cells is one-fifth that of NK cells (38). When compared with the level of perforin-positive cells between NK1.1$^+$ and NK1.1$^-$ subsets among int CD3 cells, NK1.1$^+$ subset contained a higher level of perforin-positive cells than NK1.1$^-$ subset. In this regard, the NK functional activity mediated by int CD3 cells is mainly performed by NK1.1$^+$

FIGURE 6. Int CD3 cells showed a decreased level of NK1.1$^+$:NK1.1$^-$ subset ratio both in the liver and spleen of mice with aging. *A*, young B6 mice; *B*, Old B6 mice. Young (10-wk) and old (116-wk) B6 mice were used. Three-color staining for CD3, IL-2Rβ, and NK1.1 was carried out and gated analysis was performed to know the proportion of NK1.1$^+$ T cells among each fraction. Numbers in the figure indicate the percentages of fluorescence-positive cells in the corresponding areas.

subset; However, these situations do not always mean the lower cytotoxic activity of int CD3 cells or of their subset of NK1.1$^-$ cells. There is a possibly that after some activation process (e.g., IL-12) (41), int CD3 cells acquire perforin granules in the cytoplasm and potent cytotoxic activity, as it is the case that thymus-derived T cells act as CTL after activation.

Finally, IL-2Rβ^+ int CD3 cells and NK1.1$^+$ T cells are activated with aging and under conditions of malignancies (42–44), certain autoimmune diseases induced by genetic traits (1, 45, 46), and chronic graft-vs-host disease (47). It is speculated that IL-2Rβ^+ int CD3 cells may have a beneficial function under these conditions due to their autoreactivity. With aging, as shown in this study, expanding int CD3 cells showed a decreased level of NK1.1$^+$:NK1.1$^-$ subset ratio, without a change in the composition of CD4, CD8, and DN cells among the subsets. In recent studies, NK1.1$^+$ T cells in mice (48) or DN $\alpha\beta$ T cells in humans (49, 50) manifested restricted use of Vα. Further experiments are required to determine how these populations recognize the self-Ag. The present results may also be very useful for dealing with these populations in future studies.

Acknowledgments

The authors thank Mrs. Masako Watanabe for manuscript preparation and Mr. Tetsuo Hashimoto for animal maintenance.

References

1. Seki, S., T. Abo, T. Ohteki, K. Sugiura, and K. Kumagai. 1991. Unusual $\alpha\beta$-T cells expanded in autoimmune *lpr* mice are probably a counterpart of normal T cells in the liver. *J. Immunol. 147:1214*.
2. Abo, T., T. Ohteki, S. Seki, N. Koyamada, Y. Yoshikai, T. Masuda, H. Rikiishi, and K. Kumagai. 1991. The appearance of T cells bearing self-reactive T cell receptor in the livers of mice injected with bacteria. *J. Exp. Med. 174:417*.
3. Okuyama, R., T. Abo, S. Seki, T. Ohteki, K. Sugiura, A. Kusumi, and K. Kumagai. 1992. Estrogen administration activated extrathymic T cell differentiation in the liver. *J. Exp. Med. 175:661*.
4. Iiai, T., H. Watanabe, S. Seki, K. Sugiura, K. Hirokawa, M. Utsuyama, H. Takahashi-Iwanaga, T. Iwanaga, T. Ohteki, and T. Abo. 1992. Ontogeny and development of extrathymic T cells in mouse liver. *Immunology 77:556*.
5. Ohtsuka, K., T. Iiai, H. Watanabe, T. Tanaka, M. Miyasaka, K. Sato, H. Asakura, and T. Abo. 1994. Similarities and differences between extrathymic T cells residing in mouse liver and intestine. *Cell. Immunol. 153:52*.
6. Budd, R. C., G. C. Miescher, R. C. Howe, R. K. Lees, C. Bron, and H. R. MacDonald. 1987. Developmentally regulated expression of T cell receptor β chain variable domains in immature thymocytes. *J. Exp. Med. 166:577*.
7. Crispe, I. N., M. W. Moore, L. A. Husmann, L. Smith, M. J. Bevan, and R. P. Shimonkevitz. 1987. Differentiation potential of subsets of CD4$^-$8$^-$ thymocytes. *Nature 329:336*.
8. Fowlkes, B. J., A. M. Kruisbeek, H. Ton-That, M. A. Weston, J. E. Coligan, R. H. Schwartz, and D. M. Pardoll. 1987. A novel population of T-cell receptor $\alpha\beta$-bearing thymocytes which predominantly expresses a single Vβ gene family. *Nature 329:251*.
9. Papiernik, M., and C. Pontoux. 1990. In vivo and in vitro repertoire of CD3$^+$CD4$^-$CD8$^-$ thymocytes. *Int. Immunol. 2:407*.
10. Egerton, M., and R. Scollay. 1990. Intrathymic selection of murine TCR$\alpha\beta^+$CD4$^-$CD8$^-$ thymocytes. *Int. Immunol. 2:157*.
11. Levitsky, H. I., P. T. Golumbek, and D. M. Pardoll. 1991. The fate of CD4$^-$8$^-$ T cell receptor-$\alpha\beta^+$ thymocytes. *J. Immunol. 146:1113*.
12. Takahama, Y., A. Kosugi, and A. Singer. 1991. Phenotype, ontogeny, and repertoire of CD4$^-$CD8$^-$ T cell receptor $\alpha\beta^+$ thymocytes: variable Influence of self-antigens on T cell receptor Vβ usage. *J. Immunol. 146:1134*.
13. Zlotnik, A., D. I. Godfrey, M. Fischer, and T. Suda. 1992. Cytokine production by mature and immature CD4$^-$CD8$^-$ T cells. $\alpha\beta$-T cell receptor$^+$ CD4$^-$8$^-$ T cells produce IL-4. *J. Immunol. 149:1211*.
14. Goff, L. K., and R. D. J. Huby. 1992. Characterization of constitutive and strain-dependent subsets of CD45RA$^+$ cells in the thymus. *Int. Immunol. 4:1303*.
15. Arase, H., N. Arase, K. Ogasawara, R. A. Good, and K. Onoe. 1992. An NK1.1$^+$ CD4$^+$8$^-$ single-positive thymocyte subpopulation that expresses a highly skewed T-cell antigen receptor Vβ family. *Proc. Natl. Acad. Sci. USA 89:6506*.
16. Budd, R. C., M. Schreyer, G. C. Miescher, and H. R. MacDonald. 1987. T cell lineages in the thymus of *lpr/lpr* mice: evidence for parallel pathways of normal and abnormal T cell development. *J. Immunol. 139:2200*.
17. Suda, T., and A. Zlotnik. 1993. Origin, differentiation, and repertoire selection of CD3$^+$CD4$^-$CD8$^-$ thymocytes bearing either $\alpha\beta$ or $\gamma\delta$ T cell receptors. *J. Immunol. 150:447*.
18. Reimann, J., A. Bellan, and P. Conradt. 1988. Development of autoreactive L3T4$^+$T cells from double-negative (L3T4$^-$/Ly-2$^-$) Thy-1$^+$ spleen cells of normal mice. *Eur. J. Immunol. 18:989*.
19. Prud'homme, G. J., D. C. Bocarro, and E. C. H. Luke. 1991. Clonal deletion and autoreactivity in extrathymic CD4$^-$8$^-$ (double negative) T cell receptor-α/β T cells. 1991. *J. Immunol. 147:3314*.
20. Kikly, K., and G. Dennert. 1992. Evidence for extrathymic development of T$_{NK}$ cells. NK1.1$^+$CD3$^+$ cells responsible for acute marrow graft rejection are present in thymus-deficient mice. *J. Immunol. 149:403*.
21. Guidos, C. J., I. L. Weissman, and B. Adkins. 1989. Developmental potential of CD4$^-$8$^-$ thymocytes: peripheral progeny include mature CD4$^-$8$^-$ T cells bearing $\alpha\beta$ T cell receptor. *J. Immunol. 142:3773*.
22. Huang, L., and I. N. Crispe. 1992. Distinctive selection mechanisms govern the T cell receptor repertoire of peripheral CD4$^-$CD8$^-$ α/β T cells. *J. Exp. Med. 176:699*.
23. Palathumpat, V., S. Dejbakhsh-Jones, B. Holm, H. Wang, O. Liang, and S. Strober. 1992. Studies of CD4$^-$CD8$^-$ $\alpha\beta$ bone marrow T cells with suppressor activity. *J. Immunol. 148:373*.
24. Martinez-A., C., M. A. R. Marcos, I. M. de Alboran, J. M. Alonso, R. de Cid, G. Kroemer, and A. Coutinho. 1993. Functional double-negative T cells in the periphery express T cell receptor Vβ gene products that cause deletion of single-positive T cells. *Eur. J. Immunol. 23:250*.
25. Coles, M. C., and D. H. Raulet. 1994. Class I dependence of the development of CD4$^+$CD8$^-$NK1.1$^+$ thymocytes. *J. Exp. Med. 180:395*.
26. Ohteki, T., and H. R. MacDonald. 1994. Major histocompatibility complex class I related molecules control the development of CD4$^+$8$^-$ and CD4$^-$8$^-$ subsets of natural killer 1.1$^+$ T cell receptor-α/β^+ cells in the liver of mice. *J. Exp. Med. 180:699*.
27. Seki, S., D. H. Kono, R. S. Balderas, and A. N. Theofilopoulos. 1994. Vβ repertoire of murine hepatic T cells. Implication for selection of double negative $\alpha\beta^+$ T cells. *J. Immunol. 153:637*.
28. Watanabe, H., K. Ohtsuka, M. Kimura, Y. Ikarashi, K. Ohmori, A. Kusumi, T. Ohteki, S. Seki, and T. Abo. 1992. Details of an isolation method for hepatic lymphocytes in mice. *J. Immunol. Methods 146:145*.
29. Huang, L., K. Sye, and I. N. Crispe. 1994. Proliferation and apoptosis of B220$^+$CD4$^-$CD8$^-$TCR-$\alpha\beta^{intermediate}$ T cells in the liver of normal adult mice: implication for *lpr* pathogenesis. *Int. Immunol. 6:533*.
30. Watanabe, H., T. Iiai, M. Kimura, K. Ohtsuka, T. Tanaka, M. Miyasak, M. Tsuchida, H. Hanawa, and T. Abo. 1993. Characterization of intermediate TCR cells in the liver of mice with respect to their unique IL-2R expression. *Cell. Immunol. 149:331*.

31. Kawasaki, A., Y. Shinkai, H. Yagita, and K. Okumura. 1992. Expression of perforin in murine natural killer cells and cytotoxic T lymphocytes in vivo. *Eur. J. Immunol. 22:1215.*

32. Itoh, H., T. Abo, S. Sugawara, A. Kanno, and K. Kumagai. 1988. Age-related variation in the proportion and activity of murine liver natural killer cells and their cytotoxicity against regenerating hepatocytes. *J. Immunol. 141:315.*

33. Ohtsuka, K., K. Hasegawa, K. Sato, K. Arai, H. Watanabe, H. Asakura, and T. Abo. 1994. A similar expression pattern of adhesion molecules between intermedite TCR cells in the liver and intraepithelial lymphocytes in the intestine. *Microbiol. Immunol. 38: 677.*

34. Arase, H., N. Arase-Fukushi, R. A. Good, and K. Onoe. 1993. Lymphokine-activated killer cell activity of CD4$^-$CD8$^-$ TCR-$\alpha\beta^+$ thymocytes. *J. Immunol. 151:546.*

35. Arase, H., N. Arase, K. Nakagawa, R. A. Good, and K. Onoe. 1993. NK1.1$^+$CD4$^-$CD8$^-$ thymocytes with specific lymphokine secretion. *Eur. J. Immunol. 23:307.*

36. Laouar, Y., and S. Ezine. 1994. In vivo CD4$^+$ lymph node T cells from *lpr* mice generate CD4$^-$CD8$^-$B220$^+$TCR-β^{low} cells. *J. Immunol. 153:3948.*

37. Kimura, M., H. Watanabe, K. Ohtsuka, T. Iiai, M. Tsuchida, S. Sato, and T. Abo. 1993. Radioresistance of intermediate TCR cells and their localization in the body of mice revealed by irradiation. *Microbiol. Immunol. 37:641.*

38. Kawachi, Y., T. Iiai, T. Moroda, T. Watanabe, M. Haga, H. Watanabe, K. Hatakeyama, and T. Abo. 1994. Profound suppression of the differentiation and functions of intermediate TCR cells in the liver of mice with liver injury induced by carbon tertrachloride. *Biomed. Res. 15:325.*

39. Ohteki, T., R. Okuyama, S. Seki, T. Abo, K. Sugiura, A. Kusumi, T. Ohmori, H. Watanabe, and K. Kumagai. 1992. Age-dependent increase of extrathymic T cells in the liver and their appearance in the periphery of older mice. *J. Immunol. 149:1562.*

40. Abo, T., H. Watanabe, T. Iiai, M. Kimura, K. Ohtsuka, K. Sato, M. Ogawa, H. Hirahara, S. Hashimoto, H. Sekikawa, and S. Seki. 1994. Extrathymic pathways of T-cell differentiation in the liver and other organs. *Int. Rev. Immunol. 11:61.*

41. Hashimoto, W., K. Takeda, R. Anzai, K. Ogasawara, H. Sakihara, K. Sugiura, S. Seki, and K. Kumagai. 1995. Cytotoxic NK1.1 Ag$^+$ $\alpha\beta$ T cells with intermediate TCR induced in the liver of mice by IL-12. *J. Immunol. 154:4333.*

42. Seki, S., T. Abo, K. Sugiura, T. Ohteki, T. Kobata, H. Yagi ta, K. Okumura, H. Rikiishi, T. Masuda, and K. Kumagai. 1991. Reciprocal T cell responses in the liver and thymus of mice injected with syngeneic tumor cells. *Cell. Immunol. 137:46.*

43. Ohmori, K., T. Iiai, H. Watanabe, T. Tanaka, M. Miyasaka, and T. Abo. 1993. Activation of extrathymic T cells in the liver of mice bearing syngeneic tumors. *Biomed. Res. 14:65.*

44. Iiai, T., H. Watanabe, T. Iwamoto, I. Nakashima, and T. Abo. 1994. Predominant activation of extrathymic T cells during melanoma development of metallothionein/ret transgenic mice. *Cell. Immunol. 153:412.*

45. Ohteki, T., S. Seki, T. Abo, and K. Kumagai. 1990. Liver is a possible site for the proliferation of abnormal CD3$^+$4$^-$8$^-$ double-negative lymphocytes in autoimmune MRL-lpr/lpr mice. *J. Exp. Med. 172:7.*

46. Masuda, T., T. Ohteki, T. Abo, S. Seki, M. Nose, H. Nagura, and K. Kumagai. 1991. Expansion of the population of double negative CD4$^-$8$^-$ T $\alpha\beta$-cells in the liver is a common feature of autoimmune mice. *J. Immunol. 147:2907.*

47. Ikarashi, Y., T. Abo, K. Kawai, T. Iiai, H. Watanabe, K. Suzuki, Y. Matsumoto, S. Omata, and M. Fujiwara. 1994. Expansion of intermediate T-cell receptor cells in mice with autoimmune-like graft-versus-host disease. *Immunology 83:205.*

48. Makino, Y., N. Yamagata, T. Sasho, Y. Adachi, R. Kanno, H. Koseki, M. Kanno, and M. Taniguchi. 1993. Extrathymic development of Vα 14-positive T cells. *J. Exp. Med. 177:1399.*

49. Lantz, O., and A. Bendelac. 1994. An invariant T cell receptor α chain is used by a unque subset of major histocompatibility complex class I-specific CD4$^+$ and CD4$^-$8$^-$ T cells in mice and humans. *J. Exp. Med. 180:1097.*

50. Dellabona, P., E. Padovan, G. Casorati, M. Brockhaus, and A. Lanzavecchia. 1994. An invariant Vα24-JαQ/Vβ11 T cell receptor is expressed in all individuals by clonally expanded CD4$^-$8$^-$ T cells. *J. Exp. Med. 180:1171.*

EXTRATHYMIC T CELLS STAND AT AN INTERMEDIATE PHYLOGENETIC POSITION BETWEEN NATURAL KILLER CELLS AND THYMUS-DERIVED T CELLS

胸腺外T細胞は、系統進化的にナチュラル・キラー細胞と胸腺由来T細胞の中間に位置する

Natural Immunity, 14: 173-187, 1995

chapter 3

Extrathymic T Cells Stand at an Intermediate Phylogenetic Position between Natural Killer Cells and Thymus-Derived T Cells

胸腺外T細胞は、系統進化的にナチュラル・キラー細胞と胸腺由来T細胞の中間に位置する

Toru Abo, Hisami Watanabe, Kazunari Sato, Tuneo Iiai, Tetsuya Moroda, Kazuyoshi, Takeda, Shuhji Seki

Department of Immunology, Niigata University School of Medicine, Niigata, Japan

【キーワード】

胸腺外分化T細胞、NK細胞、胸腺由来T細胞、肝臓、腸

【要約】

　最近一連の研究において、T細胞分化の胸腺外経路がマウスとヒトにおける多くの部位に存在することが明らかになった。胸腺外T細胞の特徴は、系統進化においてナチュラル・キラー（NK）細胞と胸腺由来T細胞の中間に位置する可能性がある。NK細胞や胸腺外T細胞のような原始リンパ球は、腸、皮膚そして肝臓の上皮に存在した原始マクロファージから進化したと推測される。一方、骨髄と胸腺の免疫系は比較的新しく、両生類など生物の上陸開始後に進化した。胸腺内T細胞分化主経路において自己応答性T細胞クローンは完全に除去される。自己応答性T細胞クローンは、胸腺外経路において持続的に産生される。従って、胸腺由来T細胞は外来抗原を処理するのに効率的である。これに対して、胸腺外T細胞は異常な自己細胞を認識する。若年期は、胸腺由来T細胞が主役である。これに対して、胸腺外T細胞は、加齢、悪性腫瘍、細胞内感染、妊娠や自己免疫疾患においてむしろ重要な役割を果たす可能性がある。

はじめに

　長い間、T細胞が産生されるのは胸腺内に存在するT細胞分化主経路であると考えられてきた。しかし、腸上皮内T細胞は、胸腺外で産生されると示唆した報告も少ないながら存在する[1,2]。抗T細胞レセプター（TCR）$\gamma\delta$や抗TCR$\alpha\beta$モノクロナール抗体（mAbs）が使用されるようになってから、胸腺外でT細胞が産生されるというエビデンス（証拠）が相当量蓄積されている。例えば、$\gamma\delta$T細胞は、先天的に胸腺が欠損しているヌードマウス[3,4]に存在すること、そして、CD4$^-$8$^-$ $\alpha\beta$T細胞が、MRL-lpr/lprマウスの肝臓で産生されることが明らかになった[5,6]。その後、腸[7-10]、大網[11,12]、皮膚[13,14]と子宮[15,16]において、上皮内T細胞が局所的に胸腺外産生されることが明らかなった。

　これらの研究とともに、多数の研究者が胸腺におけるCD4$^-$8$^-$（またはCD4$^+$）、TCR$\alpha\beta^+$ [17-25]細胞でNK1.1抗原を発現する独特なT細胞集団を発見した。このT細胞集団は、後にCD4$^+$8$^+$となるCD4$^-$8$^-$フェノタイプの未熟T細胞とは、区別される。その後の研究により、NK1.1抗原を発現するこのCD4$^-$8$^-$ $\alpha\beta$T細胞は、末梢の各免疫臓器（脾臓[27-31]，骨

髄［32］, リンパ節［33,34］）にさえも、存在することが明らかになった。

肝臓と他の末梢免疫臓器に存在する胸腺外T細胞と胸腺に存在するNK1.1⁺T細胞は、類似系統の原始T細胞である可能性も明らかになった［35,36］。これら細胞には、以下のように原始T細胞として共通点が多い；TCRを中等度発現していること（TCR^{int}）、インターロイキン（IL）-2レセプターβ鎖（IL-2Rβ）を本質的に発現すること、そして、持続的に自己応答性クローンを産生することである。さらに、接着分子についてはCD44⁺L-セレクチン⁻である。本総説では、胸腺外T細胞およびNK1.1⁺T細胞の最新データを紹介し、この2種類の細胞の系統発生における関係を明らかにする。

マウスの胸腺外T細胞としてTCR^{int}細胞を同定する

マウス（おそらくヒトも）において、胸腺外T細胞分化は主に2つの部位（腸と肝臓）で行われる。一般に腸上皮内T細胞は産生された部位で働く。しかし、TCR^{int}細胞が産生されるのは肝臓であるが、加齢マウスの他の臓器［37-39］、悪性疾患における腫瘍部位［40-43］、そして、自己免疫疾患［5,6,44,45］または、慢性移植片対宿主（GVH）病における標的器官［46, 47］にも出現する。先ずマウスのTCR^{int}細胞に注目した。

先天的に胸腺が欠損しているヌードマウスの特徴として、検証を行った全臓器においてT細胞は全てTCR^{int}細胞であることが判明した

Figure.1

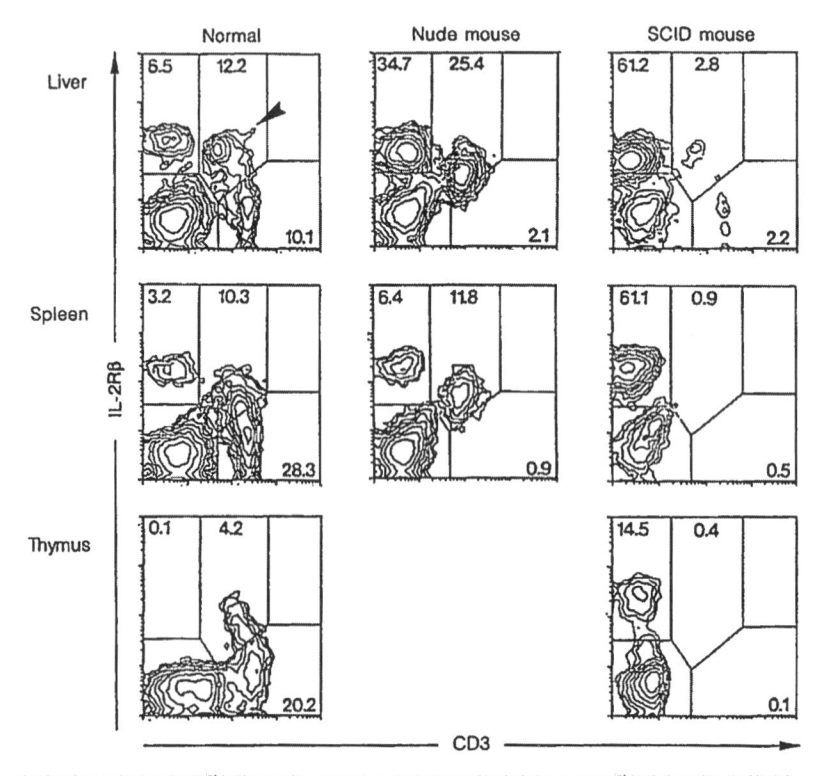

各種マウスにおけるCD3^{int}細胞の同定。CD3とIL-2Rβの二重染色を行い、CD3^{int}細胞を同定した（矢印）。SCID＝重症複合免疫不全。

(fig. 1)。このことが示唆するのは、TCR^{int}細胞はT細胞の前駆細胞であるというよりは、むしろ成熟T細胞であることである。ヌードマウスでは、TCR^{int}細胞はIL-2Rβの発現が若干低く、CD3は若干高かった。この理由は正常マウスの場合、TCR^{int}細胞は、CD4$^+$が大部分であるが、ヌードマウスの場合、TCR^{int}細胞の大部分がCD8$^+$であるからだ。その理由は、CD8$^+$細胞に比較してCD4$^+$T細胞が発現するIL-2Rβは高く、CD3は低いからである。

先天的に胸腺を欠損したマウスでも、胎児期には胸腺が残存していると指摘する研究者も存在する。故に、TCR^{int}細胞は、胸腺外T細胞ではない可能性がある。そこで、以下の実験を、TCR^{int}細胞が胸腺外で産生されることを示すため行った(fig.2)。本研究では、胸腺を摘出した(Tx)マウス、照射・骨髄移植を行った(BMT)マウスを使用した。

胸腺摘出を行わないTx(−)マウスの場合でも、BMTの2週後までは新たに産生されたT細胞は、IL-2Rβ^+TCR^{int}細胞であった。しかし、BMTの4週後、Tx(−)マウスの肝臓と脾臓において、IL-2Rβ^-TCR^{high}細胞が出現した。対照的に、BMTを行った後の時間にかかわりなく、Tx(+)マウスではTCR^{int}細胞だけが出現した。結論として、胸腺が欠損した状態で産生されるT細胞は、全てIL-2Rβ^+TCR^{int}細胞である。この実験の際に、興味深い現象に遭遇した:骨髄細胞のうち、CD3$^+$細胞除去でなく、Thy-1$^+$細胞のみを除去した場合、TCR^{int}細胞は産生されなかったのである。故に、TCR^{int}細胞の前駆細胞は、Thy-1$^+$CD3$^-$である可能性がある[48]。この前駆細胞が、骨髄のみならず肝臓にも存在することが最近明らかになった(未発表データ)。もう1つの可能性は、Thy-1$^+$細胞の中には(サイトカインを産生して)TCR^{int}細胞の胸腺外産生を助ける細胞が存在する可能性である。

2種のサブセット、TCR^{int}におけるNK1.1$^+$とNK1.1$^-$

TCR^{int}細胞とNK1.1$^+$T細胞(またはT$_{NK}$細胞)の特徴には共通点が多い。両者の関係を明確にするため、TCR^{int}細胞とNK1.1$^+$T細胞とを直接比較した(fig. 3)。TCR^{int}細胞同様、NK1.1$^+$T細胞は、CD3(およびTCR)発現が中等度であるT細胞の小数集団であった。しかし、検証を行った全臓器において、TCR^{int}細胞の比率と比較して、NK1.1$^+$T細胞の比率は、常に小さかった。実験を進めるうち、TCR^{int}細胞集団の中にNK1.1$^+$T細胞が存在することが明らかになった[36]。換言すると、TCR^{int}細胞を構成する細胞は、NK1.1$^+$とNK1.1$^-$サブセットである。

この特徴から、さらに興味深い結果を得た。NK1.1$^+$サブセットを構成するのは、CD4$^-$8$^-$細胞とCD4$^+$細胞であった。これに対して、NK1.1$^-$サブセットの大多数をCD8$^+$細胞が構成していた(fig. 4)。この図は、ナチュラル・キラー(NK)細胞、TCR^{int}細胞および胸腺由来T細胞において、もう1つの重要な関係を示す。CD3とIL-2Rβの二重染色を行い、セルソーターで分画を純化したものを用いて、形態学的観察をイラスト化した。NK細胞が、大顆粒リンパ球(LGL)であることは広く知られている。しかし、TCR^{int}細胞はNK細胞より小型で、NK細胞ほど細胞内に顆粒を含まない。

胸腺由来T細胞は、形態学的に最も単純である。胸腺由来T細胞は、休止状態でIL-2Rを発現しない(IL-2R$\alpha^-\beta^-$)が、抗原刺激を受け活性化すると、高親和性IL-2R(IL-2R$\alpha^+\beta^+$)となる。特異的クローンが刺激された(活性化した)時、機能を発揮するのである。全く対照的に、恒常的にIL-2Rβを発現するTCR^{int}細胞は、活性化後でも、生体内ではIL-2Rαを発現できない[49];IL-2R(IL-2R$\alpha^-\beta^+$)の発現は、中親

Figure.2

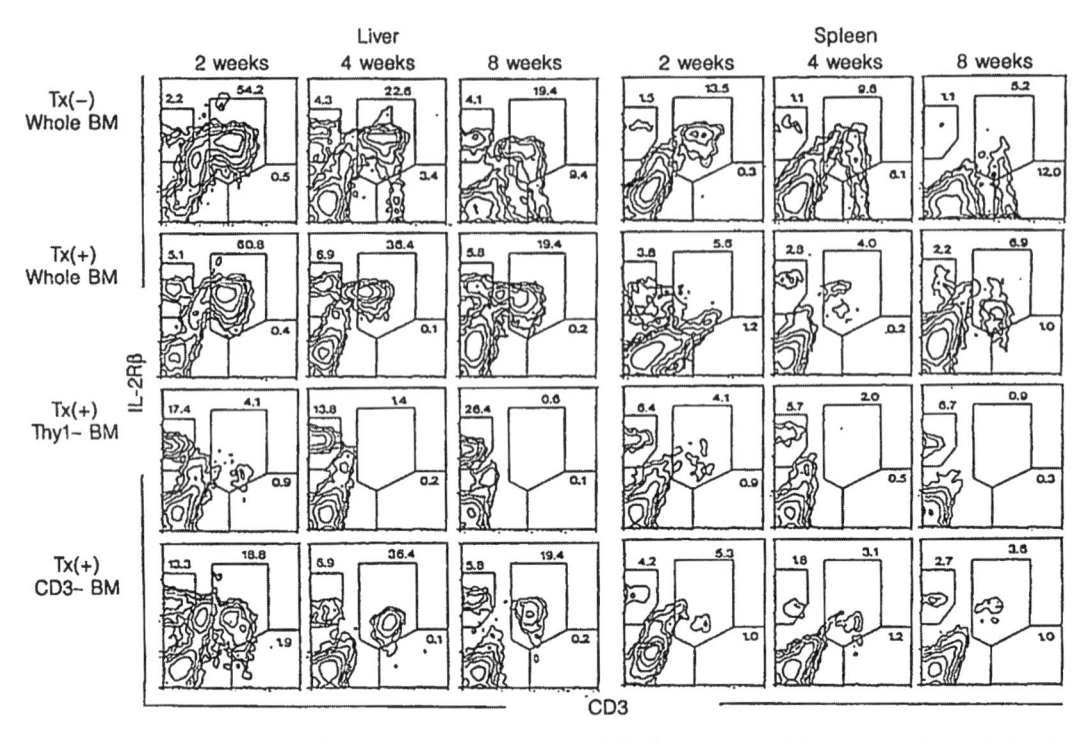

Tx(−) Whole BM / Tx(+) Whole BM / Tx(+) Thy1− BM / Tx(+) CD3− BM

Liver (2 weeks, 4 weeks, 8 weeks) / Spleen (2 weeks, 4 weeks, 8 weeks)

軸：IL-2Rβ（縦軸）、CD3（横軸）

胸腺が欠損するとCD3^{int}細胞のみが産生される。胸腺摘出(Tx)(−)マウスおよびTx(+)マウスの両実験群に、放射線照射（9Gy）と骨髄移植（BM）を行った。

Figure.3

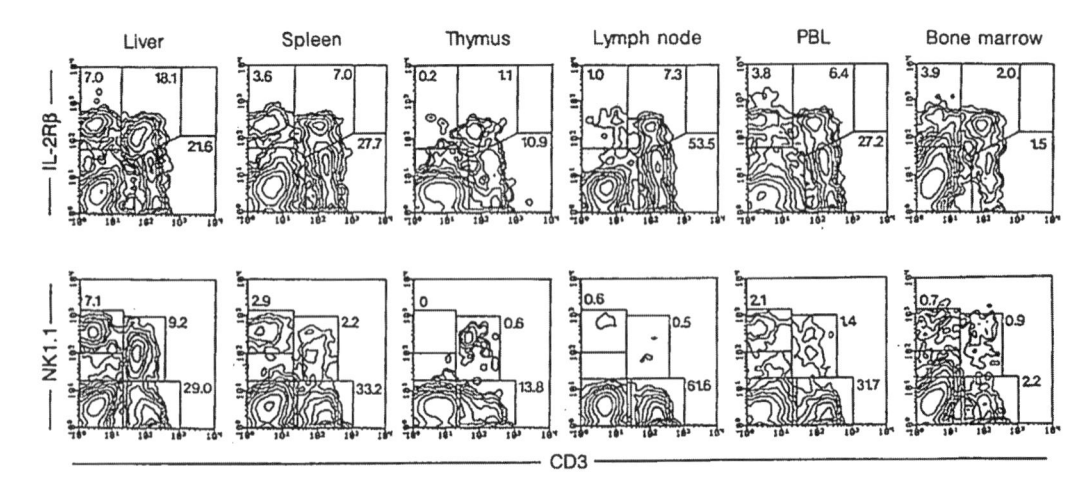

Liver / Spleen / Thymus / Lymph node / PBL / Bone marrow

軸：IL-2Rβ（上段縦軸）、NK1.1（下段縦軸）、CD3（横軸）

C57BL/6 (B6)マウスの各免疫臓器におけるCD3^{int}細胞とNK1.1$^+$ T細胞の比較。検証した全臓器において、CD3^{int}細胞の比率と比較してNK1.1$^+$ T細胞の比率は常に少なかった。PBL＝末梢血リンパ球。

Figure.4

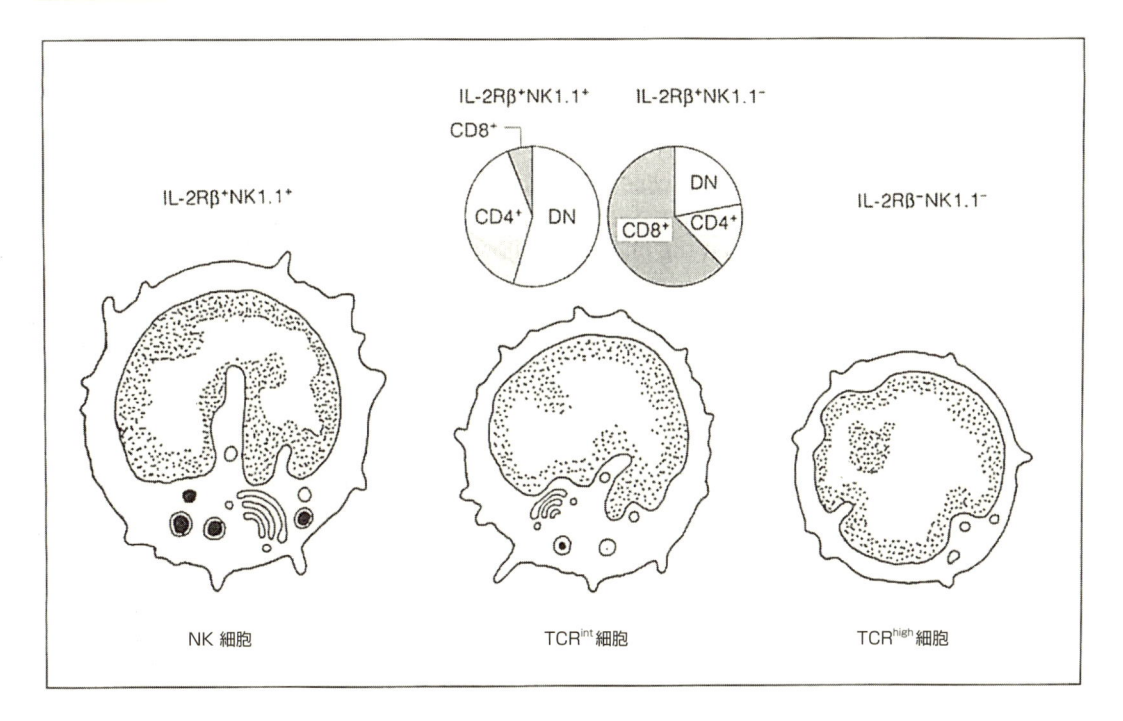

ナチュラル・キラー（NK）細胞、TCR^{int}細胞とTCR^{high}細胞の形態の略図とフェノタイプ。

和性に留まる。

NK細胞、TCR^{int}細胞と胸腺由来T細胞の形態的および機能的な特性は、系統進化における位置を反映するようである。最近の研究により、TCR^{int}細胞のフェノタイプは、ほぼ全て所謂メモリーT細胞であることが明らかになった（投稿中）。

小リンパ球として休止状態にある胸腺由来T細胞に見られるナイーブT細胞のフェノタイプは、形態学的に十分に進化した特徴である可能性がある。対応する特異抗原を認識するまでエネルギーを節約するので、寿命が延びる。NK細胞やTCR^{int}細胞のような特異性を持たないリンパ球は、常に活性化した状態にある。NK細胞やTCR^{int}細胞は、エネルギーを消費し寿命が短い傾向がある。

以下のように、リンパ球活性化には独特の順番がある；何らかの抗原刺激 → NK細胞 → TCR^{int}細胞 → 胸腺由来T細胞である［50］。最近の研究において、マウスの場合、NK1.1$^+$ T細胞（TCR^{int}細胞内に存在するNK1.1$^+$サブセット）は、不変鎖（インバリアント）Vα14を利用することが明らかになった［51,52］。しかし、TCR^{int}細胞内に存在するNK1.1$^-$サブセットの場合には、このようなインバリアントVα14の限定した利用は見られない［未発表データ］。Vα14$^+$ T細胞は、単様性MHC抗原（例、CD1b）により、最終的に選択されるようである。マウスVα14$^+$細胞に対応する細胞は、ヒトにおいてはVα24$^+$である［53-55］。

NK1.1$^+$ T細胞が、同系腫瘍細胞に対する主要な攻撃（エフェクター）細胞であることも知られている。その細胞傷害性（NK細胞の細胞傷害性と同様）は、IL-12を生体に投与すると

chapter 3 57

効率的に増大する [56]。その理由は、細胞質におけるパーフォリン量が増加するからである [36]。抗CD3モノクロナール抗体が存在する場合には、NK細胞傷害活性耐性を持つ同系の標的（腫瘍細胞）に対してさえ、細胞傷害性を発揮するのである [35]。

自己応答性禁止クローンは、TCR^{int}細胞分化によってのみ産生される

自己応答性禁止T細胞クローンが産生される原因は、胸腺内主経路の失敗であると考えていた研究者は多い。しかし、この概念が真実だとは考えられない。胸腺細胞は、CD3$^-$、CD3^{low}およびCD3^{high}である胸腺内主経路の細胞（すべてIL-2Rβ$^-$）とIL-2Rβ$^+$TCR^{int}（またはCD3^{int}）細胞で構成されている。そこで、CD3、IL-2Rβおよび各Vβの三重染色を行い、内因性スーパー抗原Mls系の自己応答性クローンを同定した（tableⅠ）。つまり、自己応答性クローンが存在するのは、どのT細胞サブセットであるかを検証した。

本研究では、C3H/Heマウス（Mls-1^{b}2^a）とAKR/Jマウス（Mls-1^{a}2^b）を使用した；自己応答性クローンを表では太字で示した。当初、行った二重染色ではIL-2Rβ抗体を使用せず、CD3^{low}とCD3^{high}細胞のみが同定できた。既報では、自己応答性クローンはCD3^{low}分画において同定される。しかし、三重染色を行ったところ、CD3^{low}、CD3^{high}とIL-2Rβ$^+$CD3^{int}細胞分画でも同定することができた。自己応答性クローンの大多数は、CD3^{int}分画に存在することが明らかになったのである。従って、CD3^{int}細胞の分化経路では、自己応答性クローンが産生される。ところが、胸腺におけるT細胞分化主経路は、この自己応答性クローンを効率よく排除する。

同様に、肝臓と脾臓のリンパ球の三重染色を行った（未発表データ）。どちらの種類のマウスでも、自己応答性クローンは肝臓と脾臓ではCD3^{int}細胞のみであった。胸腺でも肝臓でも自己応答性T細胞クローンは、CD3^{int}細胞分化によってのみ産生された。胸腺外経路と胸腺内代替経路は、自己応答性クローンを持続的に産生すると結論される（fig. 5）。TCR^{int}細胞の中に存在するTCRまたはCD3複合体が中等度であるため、自己応答性クローンの存在を（おそらく負の選択が不完全であるため）許容しているのである。その結果、これらクローンの自己応答性が適度に活性化して、異常な自己細胞の排除に役立つ可能性がある。

Table.I

胸腺T細胞の禁止クローンの分布

	Vβ	Positive cells(%)among		
		CD3^{dull}	CD3^{bright}	CD3^{int}
Two-color staining(CD3/Vβ)				
C3H/He	Vβ2	4.4	6.9	—
	Vβ3	2.8	0.2	—
	Vβ6	5.2	11.9	—
	Vβ8	7.7	31.9	—
	Vβ11	5.4	0.7	—
AKR/J	Vβ2	3.5	9.6	—
	Vβ3	4.2	6.4	—
	Vβ6	2.0	0.1	—
	Vβ8	14.2	24.3	—
	Vβ11	4.2	0.3	—
Three-color staining(CD3/IL-2Rβ/Vβ)				
C3H/He	Vβ2	2.0	6.8	3.9
	Vβ3	0.1	0.2	5.3
	Vβ6	4.8	11.3	2.4
	Vβ8	7.2	29.1	52.5
	Vβ11	0.7	0.3	13.8
AKR/J	Vβ2	2.9	10.1	5.5
	Vβ3	2.7	2.3	30.0
	Vβ6	0.9	0.2	4.3
	Vβ8	14.8	22.8	38.1
	Vβ11	3.3	0.1	9.5

表を簡単にするためにC3H/HeマウスとAKR/Jマウス各1匹のデータを示す。各マウスの禁止クローンは、太字で示す。

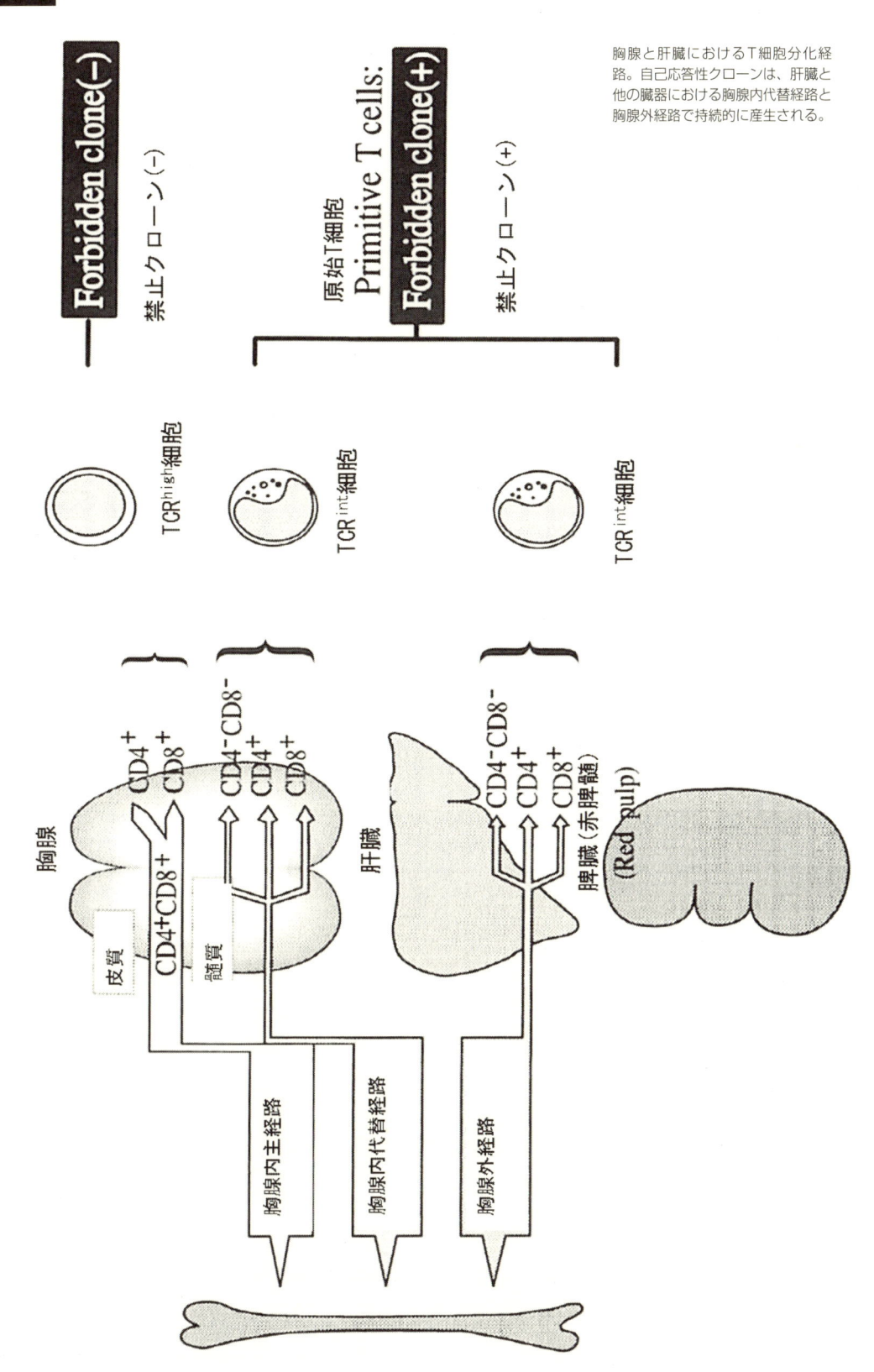

Figure.5

胸腺と肝臓におけるT細胞分化経路。自己応答性クローンは、肝臓と他の臓器における胸腺内代替経路と胸腺外経路で持続的に産生される。

chapter 3

Figure.6

各免疫臓器における単核球のフェノタイプの特徴。CD3とIL-2Rβの二重染色を行った。腸の単核球の染色パターンは、独特だった。PBL＝末梢血リンパ球；IEL＝上皮内リンパ球；LPL＝粘膜固有層リンパ球。

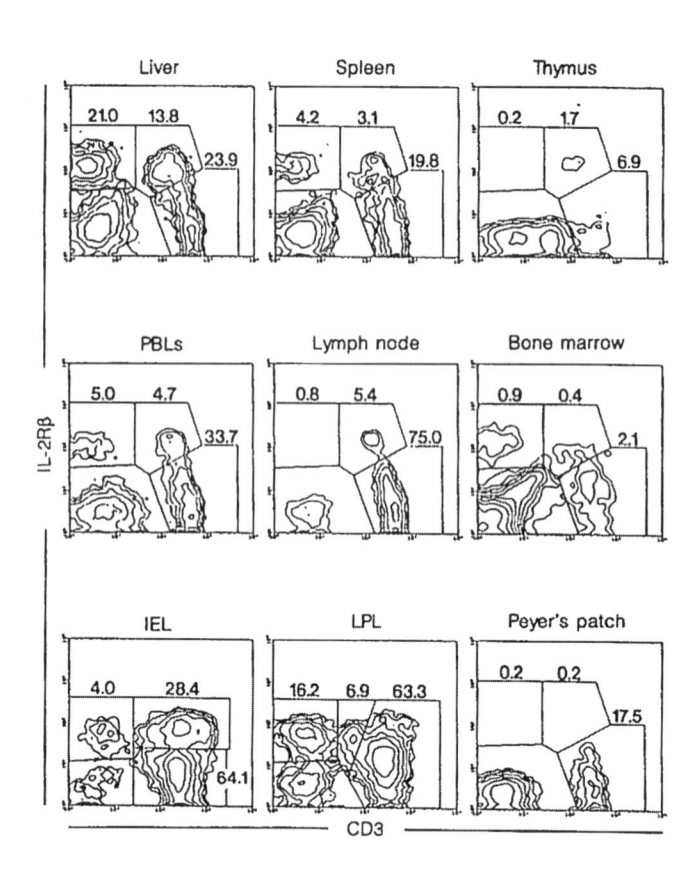

腸、肝臓と他の免疫臓器における胸腺外T細胞の特徴の比較

各免疫臓器に存在する胸腺外T細胞の特性を比較するため、各免疫臓器より採取した単核球（MNC）を使用してCD3とIL-2Rβの二重染色を行った（fig. 6）。腸の単核球以外の全ての臓器にIL-2Rβ$^+$CD3^{int}細胞が少量ながらも見られた。一方、上皮内（IEL）、粘膜固有層（LPL）およびパイエル板から採取した単核球には、採取した部位特有の特徴が見られた。

上皮内には、2種類のT細胞集団（IL-2Rβ$^+$とIL-2Rβ$^-$）があった。IL-2Rβ$^+$ T細胞は、ほとんどがγδT細胞である。これに対して、IL-2Rβ$^-$細胞はαβT細胞である。これらT細胞は、全てCD3（またはTCR）の発現量は最高値であった。粘膜固有層も独特であった。CD3$^+$細胞の大多数において、IL-2Rβ$^+$は中等度でCD3は高値を示した。また、IL-2Rβ$^+$CD3^{int}細胞も粘膜固有層に少量存在した。パイエル板の単核球は、リンパ節の単核球に類似したパターンを示した；パイエル板のT細胞は、大概胸腺由来である。

最新の研究では、特に炎症時、肺や腎臓にもIL-2Rβ$^+$TCR^{int}細胞が見られることがあることが明らかになった（投稿中）。非炎症時、IL-2Rβ$^+$TCR^{int}細胞は、これら臓器にはほとんど見られなかった。このことから、肝臓または胸腺で産生されるIL-2Rβ$^+$TCR^{int}細胞が、炎症時に肺や腎臓に移動できる可能性が高まる。もう1つの可能性は、少数のIL-2Rβ$^+$TCR^{int}細胞が局所で産生され、炎症時に増大することである。

肝臓と腸の胸腺外T細胞に、なぜ類似点と相違点が存在するかという疑問がある。原始肝臓は腸から進化したので肝臓上皮と腸上皮の原始リンパ球は同一である（fig. 7）。しかし、その後、腸と肝臓は別の過程をたどり進化したため、

Figure.7

肝臓と腸の胸腺外T細胞はもともと同じ状況下で進化した。

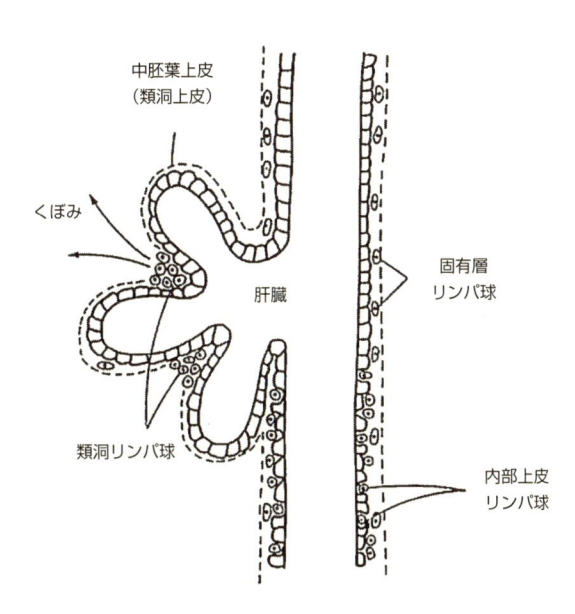

中胚葉上皮
(類洞上皮)

くぼみ

肝臓

類洞リンパ球

固有層リンパ球

内部上皮リンパ球

特徴が異なる胸腺外T細胞を有するに至った。いずれにせよ、呼吸器（えら）のみならず消化管は生物の胸腺外T細胞産生にとって重要な部位であった。

高等脊椎動物では、T細胞分化の胸腺内主経路と胸腺内代替経路がどのように進化したか？

T細胞分化の胸腺外経路は、腸、肝臓、皮膚と子宮などの生体の多部位に見られる。一方、胸腺にはT細胞分化主経路とT細胞分化代替経路がある。胸腺内代替経路で産生されたT細胞も、共通して原始的特性を有する点において、胸腺外分化T細胞とむしろ類似している。そこで、これらの細胞を原始T細胞と呼ぶ。

次に、どのようにして異なる2種の経路が胸腺で存在するようになったか考察する（fig. 8）。初期の胸腺は上皮内リンパ球とえら上皮から拡散し、胸腺として進化したことが知られている。呼吸孔（えら穴）が進化した時、外胚葉裂隙の構成要素の中には、拡散した胸腺を包むものもあった[57]。この外胚葉組織は、発達して胸腺のうち胸腺被膜と胸腺髄質になる。外胚葉組織には、主として原始T細胞が存在するので、

胸腺髄質にもこの原始T細胞が存在する。一方、呼吸器上皮下で産生されるT細胞は、MHC発現が高い外胚葉組織と相互作用する。故に、自己応答性クローンの正の選択や負の選択といった進化したシステムが生まれた。

腸上皮には、$CD4^+8^+$細胞が存在する[7-10]。同様に、この$CD4^+8^+$細胞は、えら上皮から進化した可能性がある。しかし、えら上皮は、常時刺激を受け、機能が進化し続けて危険な存在となった。この危険（自己応答性）から免れるために、選択システムが生まれた可能性がある。胸腺外細胞には、いまだにT細胞の最初の形態（原型）が残存しているようだ。

ヒト胸腺外T細胞

ヒトにおいて胸腺外T細胞に相当する細胞は、$CD56^+$ T細胞および$CD57^+$ T細胞のようである；これらT細胞は、いくつかのNKマーカーを発現している[58,59]。これら$CD56^+$ T細胞および$CD57^+$ T細胞の特徴は、マウスの胸腺外T細胞の特徴と全て類似している。例えば、$CD56^+$ T細胞および$CD57^+$ T細胞には、$CD4^+$細胞、$CD8^+$細胞と同様$CD4^-8^-$細胞が存在し、$\gamma\delta$ T細胞（最高30%）を含み、生体内において

Figure.8 胸腺の系統進化

Figure.9 ヒト胸腺外分化T細胞CD57⁺(a)およびCD56⁺(b) T細胞の分布

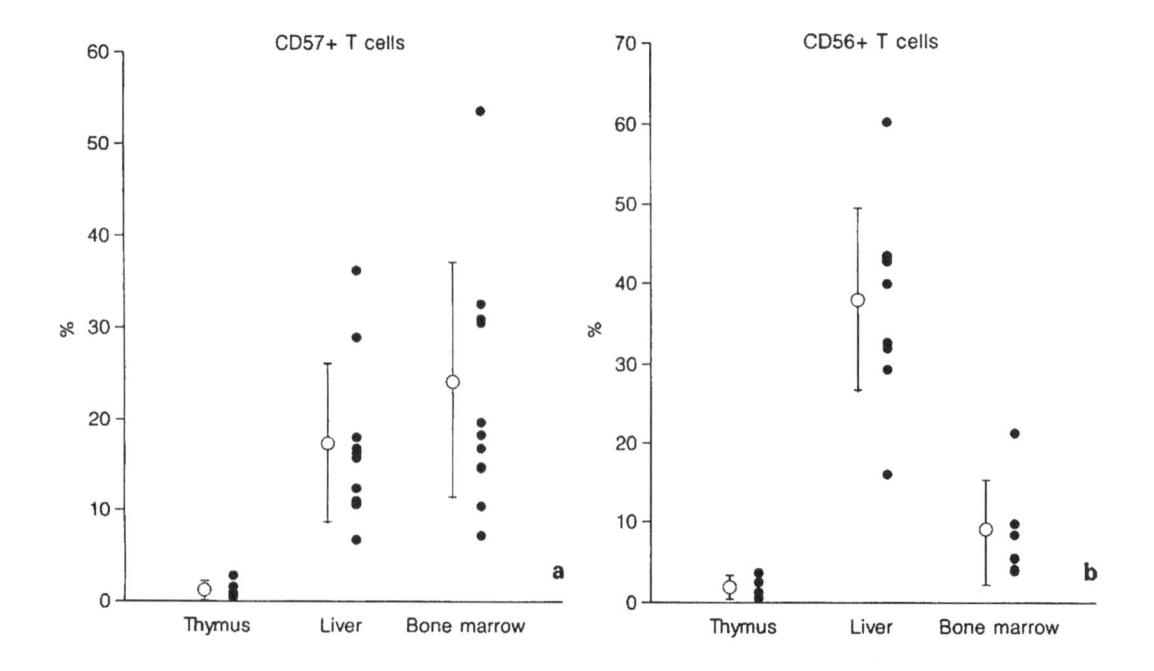

独特な部位に存在する。

興味深いことに、CD56$^+$T細胞は、肝臓に豊富に存在する。一方、CD57$^+$T細胞は骨髄に豊富に存在する(fig. 9)。末梢血や末梢免疫臓器では、CD56$^+$T細胞とCD57$^+$T細胞は少量のみ存在している。

前述したが、マウスにおいて、全てではないが大部分の胸腺外分化T細胞はNKマーカ(NK1.1抗原)を有する。従って、胸腺外分化T細胞にNKマーカーが発現している点において、マウスと類似する。系統進化の途上において、胸腺外分化T細胞はNK細胞と胸腺由来T細胞の間に位置するが故に、このような結果が得られた可能性がある。

マウスにおいて、胸腺外分化T細胞が生体内の複数部位で産生されることを明らかにした。ヒトの胸腺外分化T細胞(CD56$^+$T細胞およびCD57$^+$T細胞)には、臓器により独特な特徴があることは、マウスに見られる状態を反映している。

胸腺外分化T細胞における生理的および病理学的機能

マウスでもヒトでも、胸腺外分化T細胞の出現は誕生時には稀であるが、加齢とともにその数が増加する [37-39]。この現象は胸腺退縮に伴って出現する。100週齢マウスでは、CD3^{int}細胞が肝臓のみならず、他の臓器でも顕著になった (fig. 10)。老齢マウスの脾臓とリンパ節でも、CD3^{high}細胞に比較してCD3^{int}細胞の比率が大概圧倒的に多い。胸腺外分化T細胞の概念なしでは、加齢による免疫現象を理解できなかったのである。

若齢期でも、胸腺外分化T細胞の値が急性胸腺萎縮に伴い増加することがある。このような状況には、細胞内病原体(リステリアまたはウイルス感染)[50]、悪性腫瘍 [40-43] や妊娠 [15,16] がある。胸腺外分化T細胞は、生体内で発生する異常な自己細胞の排除に役立つ可能性がある。しかし、胸腺外分化T細胞が過剰に活性化すると、自己免疫疾患発症の原因となる

Figure.10

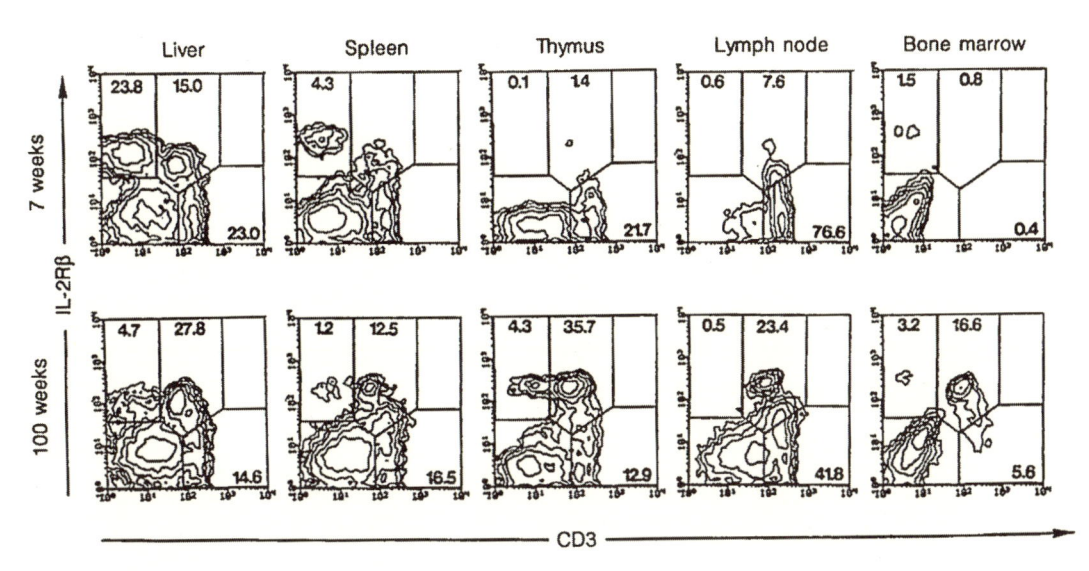

老齢マウスの各免疫臓器ではCD3^{int}細胞が顕著である。

可能性もある [5,6,44,45]。もう一つの例が、慢性移植片対宿主病である [46, 47]。自己免疫疾患や慢性移植片対宿主病の標的組織に浸潤するT細胞のほとんどはTCR^{int}細胞である。

　結論を記す。胸腺外T細胞の概念がなければ、多くの難病（例、悪性腫瘍、自己免疫疾患）に関係するメカニズム、そして、加齢や妊娠に見られる免疫学的現象を適切に理解できないのである。

Natural Immunity
Editor-in-Chief: R.B. Herberman, Pittsburgh, Pa.

Reprint
Publisher: S. Karger AG, Basel
Printed in Switzerland

Review

Toru Abo
Hisami Watanabe
Kazunari Sato
Tsuneo Iiai
Tetsuya Moroda
Kazuyoshi Takeda
Shuhji Seki

Department of Immunology,
Niigata University School of
Medicine, Niigata, Japan

Extrathymic T Cells Stand at an Intermediate Phylogenetic Position between Natural Killer Cells and Thymus-Derived T Cells

Key Words
Extrathymic T cells
NK cells
Thymus-derived T cells
Liver
Intestine

Abstract

A series of recent studies have revealed that extrathymic pathways of T cell differentiation exist at multiple sites in mice and humans. In terms of their properties, extrathymic T cells may stand at an intermediate position between natural killer (NK) cells and thymus-derived T cells in phylogenetic development. It is speculated that primitive lymphocytes such as NK cells and extrathymic T cells develop from primordial macrophages in intraepithelial regions of e.g., the intestine, skin and liver. In this regard, the immune system of the bone marrow and thymus is relatively recent, developing after the emergence of living beings onto the land (i.e., amphibia). A complete elimination of self-reactive T cell clones occurs in mainstream intrathymic T cell differentiation and a consistent generation of such clones occurs through the extrathymic pathways. Therefore, thymus-derived T cells are efficient for processing foreign antigens, whereas extrathymic T cells recognize abnormal self-cells. Although thymus-derived T cells play the major role in youth, extrathymic T cells may play rather a pivotal role with aging and under conditions of malignancy, intracellular infections, pregnancy, and autoimmune diseases.

Introduction

For a long time, T cells were believed to be generated only by the intrathymic pathway of T cell differentiation. However, a few investigators suggested that some intraepithelial T cells in the intestine are generated extrathymically [1, 2]. After the introduction of anti-T cell receptor (TCR)γδ and anti-TCRαβ monoclonal antibodies (mAbs), considerable evi-

Toru Abo
Department of Immunology
Niigata University School of Medicine
Niigata 951 (Japan)

© 1996
S. Karger AG, Basel
1018–8916/95/
0144–0173$10.00/0

dence for the extrathymic generation of T cells has accumulated. For example, it was demonstrated that γδ T cells exist in congenitally athymic nude mice [3, 4] and that double-negative (DN) CD4⁻8⁻ αβ T cells are generated in the liver of MRL-*lpr/lpr* mice [5, 6]. Subsequently, it was revealed that some intraepithelial T cells in the intestine [7–10], omentum [11, 12], skin [13, 14], and uterus [15, 16] are generated extrathymically in situ.

In parallel with these studies, many investigators encountered a unique population of T cells, namely, DN CD4⁻8⁻ (or CD4⁺), TCRαβ⁺ cells expressing NK1.1 antigens in the thymus [17–25]. This population of T cells is distinguished from immature T cells with DN phenotype which later enter the stage of a double-positive (DP) CD4⁺8⁺ phenotype. Subsequent studies revealed that such DN αβ T cells with NK1.1 antigens exist even in peripheral immune organs such as the spleen [27–31], bone marrow [32], and lymph nodes [33, 34].

It has also been demonstrated that extrathymic T cells in the liver and other peripheral immune organs and NK1.1⁺ T cells seen in the thymus may be primordial T cells of a similar cell lineage [35, 36]. They share many properties as primordial T cells, including the intermediate intensity TCR (TCR^{int}), constitutive expression of interleukin (IL)-2 receptor β chain (IL-2Rβ), and a consistent generation of self-reactive clones. With respect to adhesion molecules they are CD44⁺ L-selectin⁻. In this review, recently acquired data on extrathymic T cells and NK1.1⁺ T cells are introduced to demonstrate their relationship and their phylogenetic position.

Identification of TCR^{int} Cells as Extrathymic T Cells in Mice

There are two major sites of extrathymic T cell differentiation in mice (and possibly in humans), namely, the intestine and the liver. In general, intraepithelial T cells in the intestine work at the site where they are originally generated. However, TCR^{int} cells, which are generated in the liver, also appear in other organs with aging [37–39], at tumor sites during malignant conditions [40–43], and in target organs during autoimmune diseases [5, 6, 44, 45] or chronic graft-versus-host (GVH) disease [46, 47]. We first focus our attention on TCR^{int} cells in mice.

When congenitally athymic nude mice were characterized, all T cells were found to be TCR^{int} cells, irrespective of the organs tested (fig. 1). It is suggested that TCR^{int} cells are mature T cells rather than precursors of T cells. In the case of nude mice, TCR^{int} cells showed a slightly lower intensity of IL-2Rβ and a slightly higher intensity of CD3. This is because TCR^{int} cells in normal mice are mainly CD4⁺ but those in nude mice are mainly CD8⁺, and CD4⁺ T cells express a higher level of IL-2Rβ and a lower level of CD3 than CD8⁺ cells.

It has been pointed out by some investigators that congenitally athymic mice have remnants of the thymus in the fetal stage and, therefore, that TCR^{int} cells may not be extrathymic T cells. The following experiment was therefore conducted to prove the extrathymic generation of TCR^{int} cells (fig. 2). In this study, thymectomized (Tx), irradiated mice subjected to bone marrow transplantation (BMT) were used. Even if mice were Tx(⁻), newly generated T cells were IL-2Rβ⁺ TCR^{int} cells up to 2 weeks after BMT. However, IL-2Rβ⁻ TCR^{high} cells appeared from 4 weeks after BMT in both the liver and spleen of Tx(⁻) mice. In contrast, Tx(⁺) mice acquired

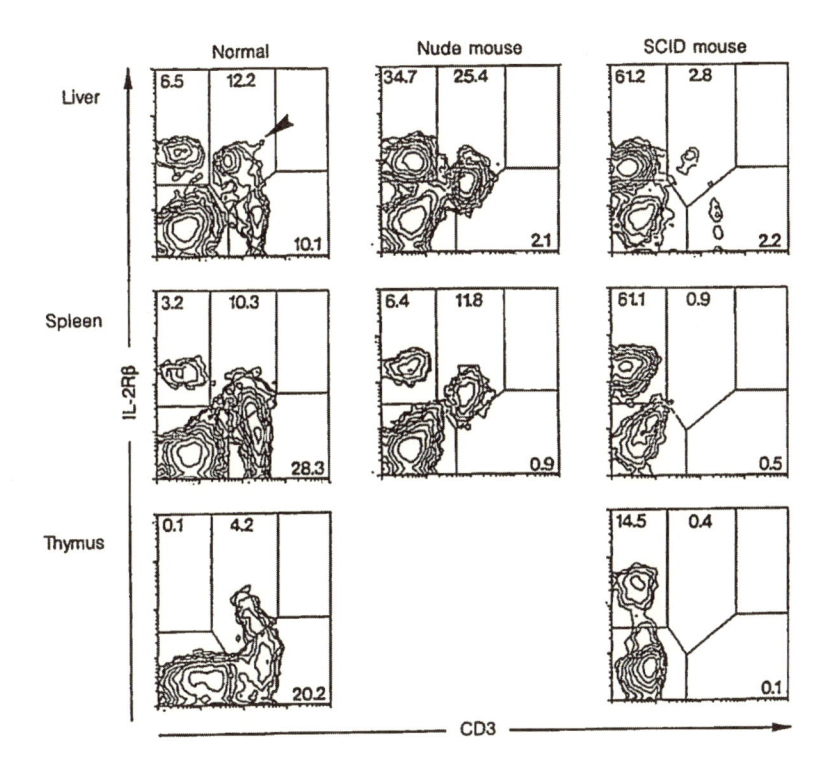

Fig. 1. Identification of CD3^{int} cells in mice of various strains. Two-color staining for CD3 and IL-2Rβ identified CD3^{int} cells (indicated by an arrowhead in the liver of normal mice). SCID = Severe combined immunodeficiency.

only TCR^{int} cells, irrespective of the time after BMT. It is concluded that all T cells generated under athymic conditions are IL-2Rβ$^+$ TCR^{int} cells. During this experiment, we encountered an interesting phenomenon: Thy-1+-cell-depleted, but not CD3$^+$-cell-depleted, bone marrow cells were not able to produce TCR^{int} cells. Therefore, the precursors of TCR^{int} cells might be Thy-1$^+$ CD3$^-$ [48]. Such a precursor population was recently found to exist not only in the bone marrow, but also in the liver [our unpubl. obs.]. An alternative possibility is that some Thy-1$^+$ cells support (by the production of cytokines) the extrathymic generation of TCR^{int} cells.

Two Subsets, NK1.1+ and NK1.1– of TCR^{int} Cells

Intermediate TCR cells and NK1.1$^+$ T cells (or T$_{NK}$ cells) have many properties in common. To definitely determine their relationship, a direct comparison between TCR^{int} cells and NK1.1$^+$ T cells was performed (fig. 3). It was obvious that, similar to TCR^{int}

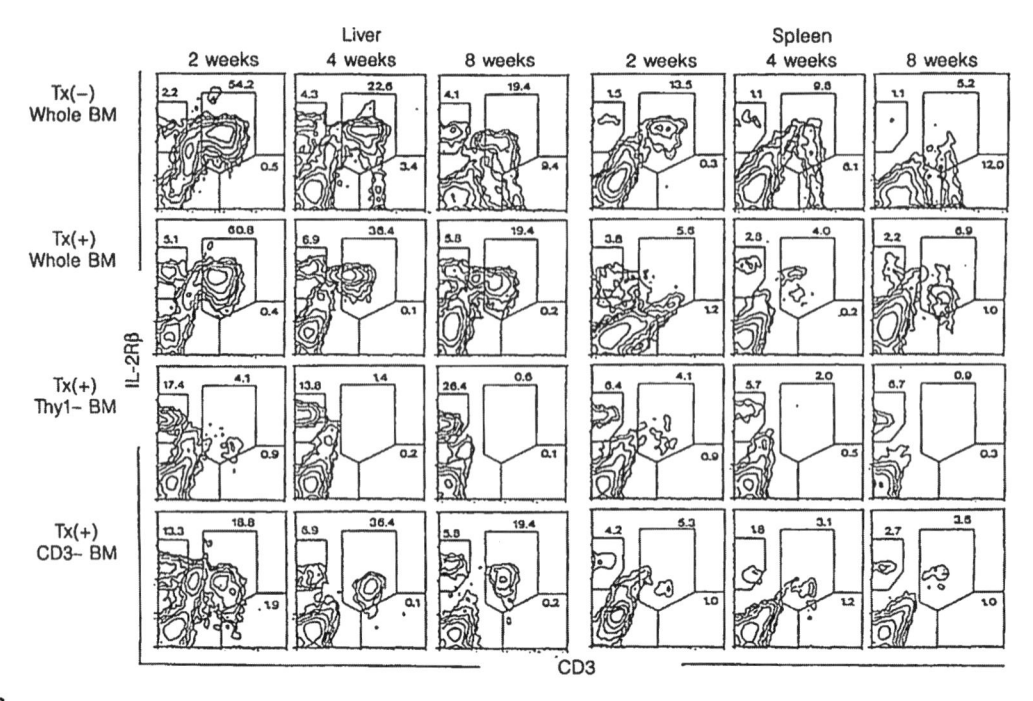

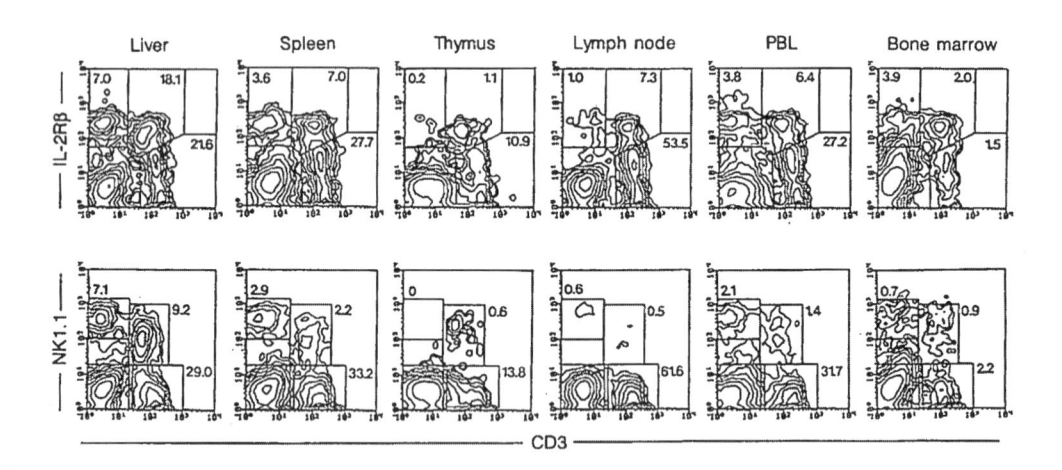

Fig. 2. Only CD3^{int} cells are generated under athymic conditions. Both thymectomized (Tx) (⁻) and Tx (⁺) mice were irradiated (9 Gy) and subjected to bone marrow (BM) transplantation.

Fig. 3. A comparison of CD3^{int} cells and NK1.1⁺ T cells in various immune organs of C57BL/6 (B6) mice. The proportion of NK1.1⁺ T cells was always smaller than that of CD3^{int} cells in all organs tested. PBL = Peripheral blood lymphocyte.

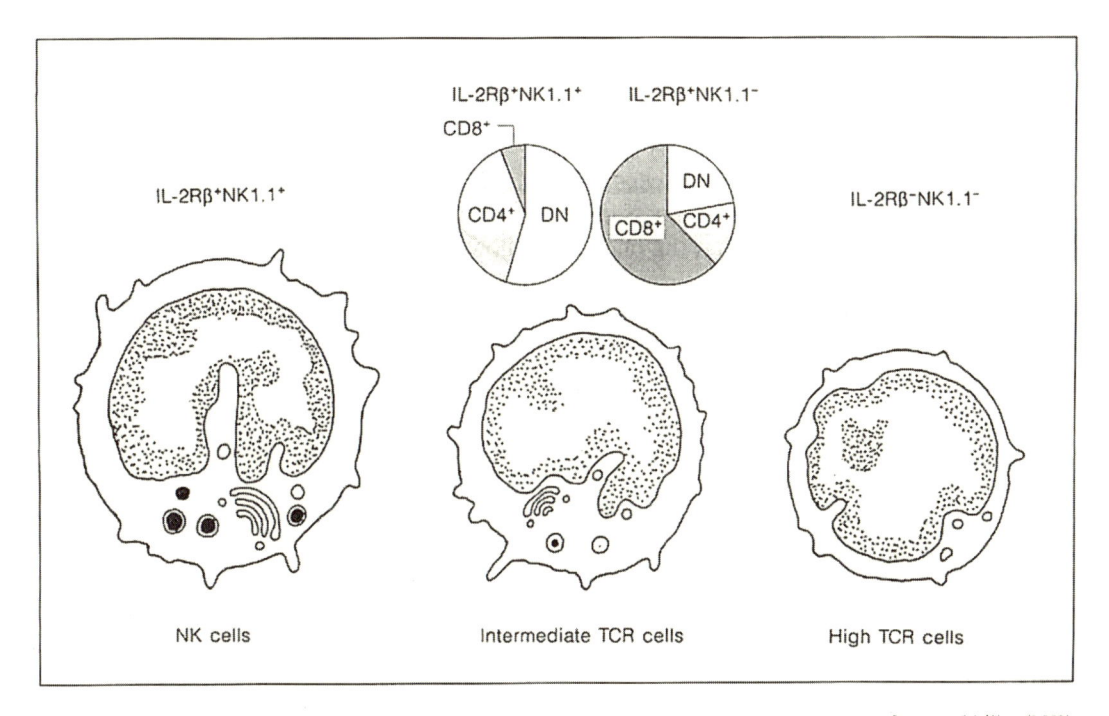

Fig. 4. Schematic representation of the morphology and phenotype of natural killer (NK) cells, TCR^{int} cells, and TCR^{high} cells.

cells, NK1.1$^+$ T cells were a minor population of T cells expressing intermediate levels of CD3 (and TCR). However, the proportion of NK1.1$^+$ T cells was always smaller than that of TCR^{int} cells in every organ tested. Subsequent experiments revealed that NK1.1$^+$ T cells are within a population of TCR^{int} cells [36]. In other words, TCR^{int} cells consist of NK1.1$^+$ and NK1.1$^-$ subsets.

This characterization provided an even more interesting result. The NK1.1$^+$ subset was found to comprise mainly DN CD4$^-$8$^-$ and CD4$^+$ cells, whereas the NK1.1$^-$ subset comprises mainly CD8$^+$ cells (fig. 4). This scheme also shows another important relationship among natural killer (NK) cells, TCR^{int} cells, and thymus-derived T cells. The morphological study illustrated was carried out using fractions purified by the cell sorter after staining for CD3 and IL-2Rβ. As well established, NK cells are large granular lymphocytes (LGLs). However, TCR^{int} cells are smaller and contain fewer cytoplasmic granules than do NK cells.

Thymus-derived T cells have the simplest morphology. They lack the expression of IL-2R (i.e., they are IL-2Rα$^-$β$^-$) under resting conditions but acquire high-affinity IL-2R (i.e., become IL-2Rα$^+$β$^+$) after antigenic activation. They function only when their specific clones are stimulated. In sharp contrast, TCR^{int} cells which constitutively express IL-2Rβ are not able to acquire IL-2Rα in vivo, even after activation [49]; they remain at a level of intermediate-affinity expression of IL-2R (IL-2Rα$^-$β$^+$).

These morphological and functional properties seen in NK cells, TCR^{int} cells, and thymus-derived T cells seem to refect their position in phylogenetic development. A recent study revealed that almost all TCR^{int} cells carry the phenotype of so-called memory T cells [submitted]. It is conceivable that the phenotype of naive T cells seen in thymus-derived T cells as small lymphocytes under resting conditions is a well-developed characteristic of the morphology. Prior to the recognition of corresponding specific antigens, they can conserve energy and increase their lifespan. Less specific lymphocytes such as NK cells and TCR^{int} cells are always in activated states. They tend to lose energy and have a limited lifespan. Thus, there is a certain order of lymphocyte activation, i.e., NK cells → TCR^{int} cells → thymus-derived T cells after any antigenic stimuli [50].

In recent studies, NK1.1$^+$ T cells (i.e., the NK1.1$^+$ subset of TCR^{int} cells) were found to use an invariant V$_\alpha$14 chain in mice [51, 52]. However, such limited usage of an invariant V$_\alpha$14 chain is not seen in the NK1.1$^-$ subset of TCR^{int} cells [our unpubl. obs.]. V$_\alpha$14$^+$ T cells seem to be positively selected by monomorphic MHC antigens (e.g., CD1b). There is a counterpart of mouse V$_\alpha$14$^+$ cells, namely, V$_\alpha$24$^+$ cells, in humans [53–55].

NK1.1$^+$ T cells are also known to be the major effector cells against syngeneic tumor cells. Their cytotoxicity, as well as the cytotoxicity of NK cells, is efficiently augmented by in vivo administration of IL-12 [56]. This is due to the augmentation of perforin levels in their cytoplasm [36]. They become cytotoxic even against NK-resistant syngeneic targets in the presence of anti-CD3 mAb [35].

Self-Reactive Forbidden Clones Are Generated Only through TCR^{int} Cell Differentiation

Many investigators have believed that self-reactive forbidden T cell clones are generated following the failure of the mainstream intrathymic pathway. However, this concept does not appear to be true. Since even thymocytes comprise IL-2Rβ^+ TCR^{int} (or CD3^{int}) cells as well as mainstream cell populations (CD3$^-$, CD3^{low}, and CD3^{high}, all lacking IL-2Rβ expression), three-color staining for CD3, IL-2Rβ, and each V$_\beta$ was applied to identify self-reactive clones in the endogenous superantigen Mls system (table 1). In other words, we examined what type of T cell subsets carried self-reactive clones.

In the experiment, C3H/He mice (Mls-1^{b}2^a) and AKR/J mice (Mls-1^{a}2^b) were used; self-reactive clones are italicized in the table. When two-color staining (no use of IL-2Rβ) was first applied, we identified only CD3^{low} and CD3^{high} cells. Self-reactive clones were identified in the CD3^{low} fraction as already reported. However, when three-color staining was applied, we were able to identify CD3^{low}, CD3^{high}, and IL-2Rβ^+ CD3^{int} cells. The majority of self-reactive clones were found to exist in the CD3^{int} fraction. Therefore, the pathway of CD3^{int} cell differentiation can be seen to consistently produce self-reactive clones, whereas mainstream T cell differentiation in the thymus efficiently eliminates such self-reactive clones.

Similarly, three-color staining was performed using lymphocytes in the liver and spleen (data not shown). In both types of mice, self-reactive clones were confined to CD3^{int} cells in these organs. Irrespective of the thymus and liver, self-reactive T cell clones were generated by CD3^{int} cell differentiation. It is concluded that the extrathymic pathways and an alternative intrathymic pathway consistently produce self-reactive clones (fig. 5). The intermediate levels of TCR or CD3 complex in TCR^{int} cells permit the existence of self-reactive clones (possibly because of the incompleteness of the interaction for negative selection). As a result, these clones may be beneficial for the elimination of abnormal self-cells due to the moderate activity of self-reactivity.

Comparison of Characteristics among Extrathymic T Cells in the Intestine, Liver, and Other Immune Organs

To compare the properties of extrathymic T cells located in various immune organs, two-color staining for CD3 and IL-2Rβ was performed using mononuclear cells (MNCs) isolated from various organs (fig. 6). Except for MNCs in the intestine, all organs contain IL-2Rβ$^+$ CD3^{int} cells, although in small proportions. On the other hand, MNCs isolated from the intraepithelium (IEL), lamina propria (LPL), and Peyer's patches in the intestine were unique, depending on the sites.

In the case of the IEL, there were two T cell populations IL-2Rβ$^+$ and IL-2Rβ$^-$ The majority of IL-2Rβ$^+$ T cells are γδ T cells, whereas IL-2Rβ$^-$ T cells are αβ T cells. All these T cells carried the highest levels of CD3 (or TCR). The LPL was also unique, the majority of CD3 cells having intermediate levels of IL-2Rβ$^+$ and high levels of CD3. A small population of IL-2Rβ$^+$ TCR^{int} cells was also present at this site. MNCs in the Peyer's patches showed a pattern similar to that of lymph nodes: almost all T cells in Peyer's patches are derived from the thymus.

In our most recent study, we demonstrated that the lungs and kidneys also sometimes contain IL-2Rβ$^+$TCR^{int} cells, especially when inflammation is evoked [submitted]. Under noninflammatory conditions, IL-2Rβ$^+$ TCR^{int} cells were extremely rare in these organs. This raises the possibility that IL-2Rβ$^+$ TCR^{int} cells generated in the liver or thymus can migrate into the lungs and kidneys under conditions of inflammation. Alternatively, a small population of IL-2Rβ$^+$ TCR^{int} cells are generated in situ and expand under condition of inflammation.

There is the question as to why extrathymic T cells in the liver and those in the intestine

Table 1. Distribution of forbidden T cell clones in the thymus

	$V_β$	Positive cells (%) among		
		CD3^{dull}	CD3^{bright}	CD3^{int}
Two-color staining (CD3/$V_β$)				
C3H/He	$V_β2$	4.4	6.9	–
	$V_β3$	**2.8**	**0.2**	–
	$V_β6$	5.2	11.9	–
	$V_β8$	7.7	31.9	–
	$V_β11$	**5.4**	**0.7**	–
AKR/J	$V_β2$	3.5	9.6	–
	$V_β3$	4.2	6.4	–
	$V_β6$	**2.0**	**0.1**	–
	$V_β8$	14.2	24.3	–
	$V_β11$	**4.2**	**0.3**	–
Three-color staining (CD3/IL-2Rβ/$V_β$)				
C3H/He	$V_β2$	2.0	6.8	3.9
	$V_β3$	**0.1**	**0.2**	**5.3**
	$V_β6$	4.8	11.3	2.4
	$V_β8$	7.2	29.1	52.5
	$V_β11$	**0.7**	**0.3**	**13.8**
AKR/J	$V_β2$	2.9	10.1	5.5
	$V_β3$	2.7	2.3	30.0
	$V_β6$	**0.9**	**0.2**	**4.3**
	$V_β8$	14.8	22.8	38.1
	$V_β11$	**3.3**	**0.1**	**9.5**

To simplify the table, the data of a single C3H/He mouse and a single AKR/J mouse are represented. Forbidden clones for each mouse are in bold type.

5

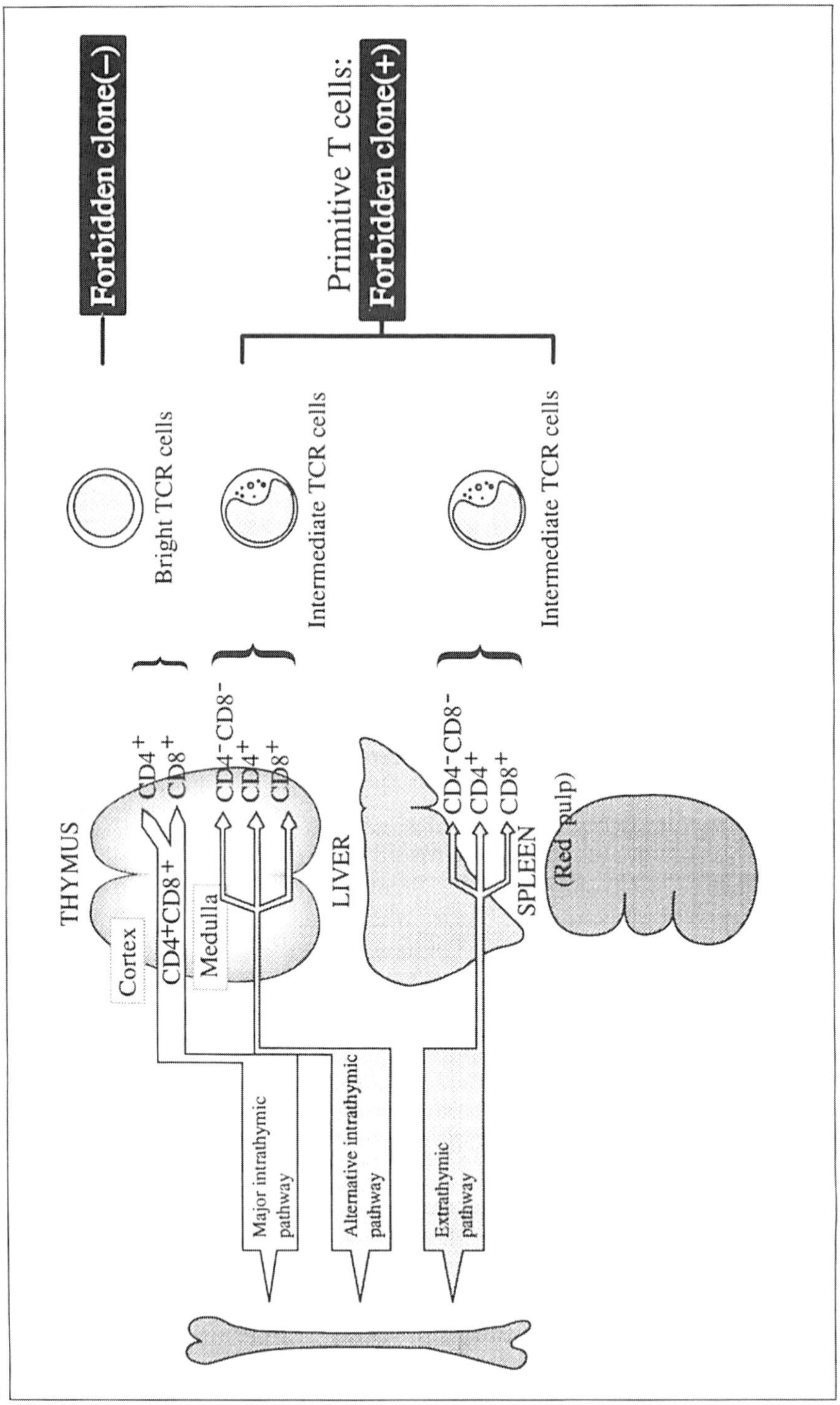

Forbidden clone(−)
Primitive T cells:
Forbidden clone(+)
Bright TCR cells
Intermediate TCR cells
Intermediate TCR cells
THYMUS
Cortex
Medulla
CD4+CD8+
CD4+
CD8+
CD4−CD8−
CD4+
CD8+
LIVER
CD4−CD8−
CD4+
CD8+
SPLEEN
(Red pulp)
Major intrathymic pathway
Alternative intrathymic pathway
Extrathymic pathway

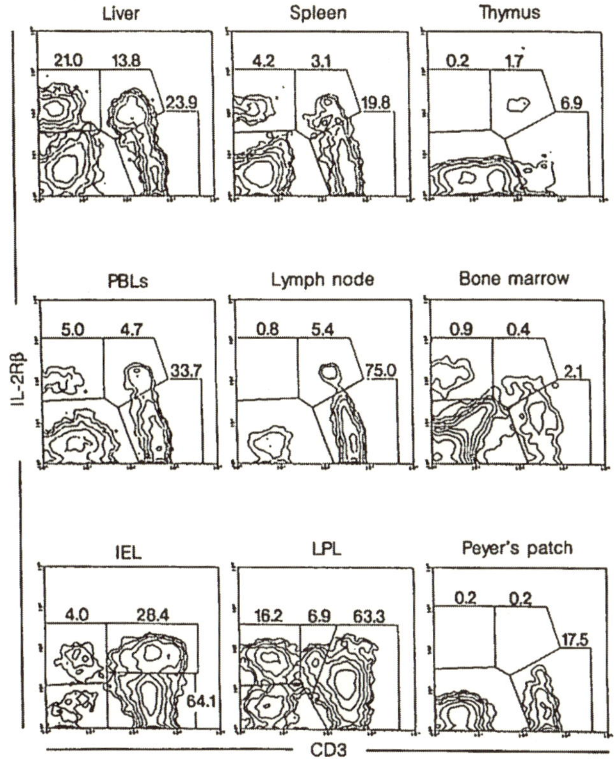

Fig. 6. Phenotypic characterization of MNCs in various immune organs. Two-color staining for CD3 and IL-2Rβ was carried out. The staining patterns of MNCs in the intestinal sites were unique. PBL = Peripheral blood lymphocyte; IEL = intraepithelium lymphocyte; LPL = lamina propria lymphocyte.

have both similar and distinct properties. Since the primordial liver originally developed from the intestine, both the epithelium of the liver and that of the intestine comprise the same primitive lymphocytes (fig. 7). However, because of their subsequent different courses of development, the liver and intestine came to have extrathymic T cells with distinct properties. In any case, the digestive organs as well as the respiratory organs (i.e., gills) would have been important sites for the generation of extrathymic T cells in living organisms.

Fig. 5. Pathways of T cell differentiation in the thymus and liver. Self-reactive clones are consistently generated through an alternative intrathymic pathway and the extrathymic pathways in the liver and other organs.

How Did the Major Intrathymic Pathway and an Alternative Intrathymic Pathway of T Cell Differentiation Develop in Higher Vertebrates?

The extrathymic pathways of T cell differentiation occur at multiple sites in the body, including the intestine, liver, skin, and uterus. On the other hand, the thymus comprises

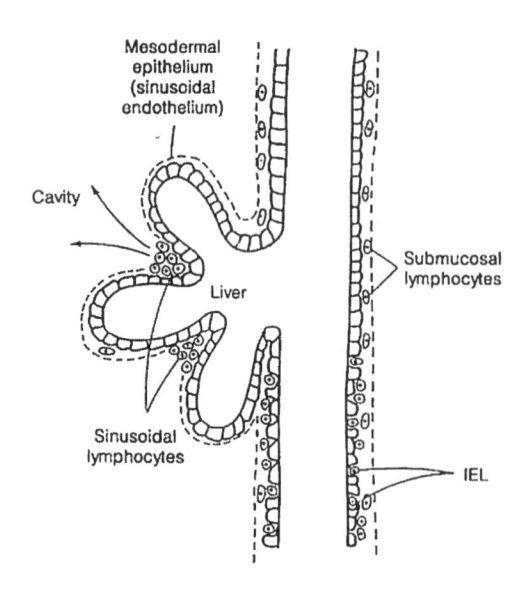

Fig. 7. Extrathymic T cells in the liver and intestine originally developed under the same circumstances.

both the major pathway of T cell differentiation (the mainstream) and an alternative pathway of T cell differentiation. T cells generated by the latter pathway are rather similar to extrathymic T cells in terms of their common primordial properties. We therefore term them primordial T cells.

We next speculate on how two different pathways came to be present in the thymus (fig. 8). It is known that the early thymus develops as a diffuse thymus from intraepithelial lymphocytes and the epithelium in the gills. When respiratory holes (i.e., gill holes) develop, some components of the ectodermal cleft wrap around the diffuse thymus [57]. Such ectodermal tissues develop into the capsule and medulla of the complete thymus. Since the ectodermal tissue primarily contains primordial T cells, the thymic medulla still contains such primordial T cells. On the other hand, T cells developed under the respiratory epithelia interact with the ectodermal tissue with a high expression of MHC and, therefore, produce a developed system with positive and negative selection of self-reactive clones.

DP $CD4^+8^+$ cells are seen in the IEL of the intestine [7–10]. Similarly, such DP cells may be developed in the IEL of gills. However, the IEL of gills becomes dangerous with successive functional development caused by continuous stimuli. It may acquire a selection system to escape danger (i.e., autoreactivity). It seems that extrathymic T cells still retain their earliest form (i.e., the prototype) of T cells.

Extrathymic T Cells in Humans

Counterparts in humans to extrathymic T cells seem to be $CD56^+$ T cells and $CD57^+$ T cells, namely, T cells expressing some NK markers [58, 59]. All properties carried by these $CD56^+$ T cells and $CD57^+$ T cells are similar to those ascribed to extrathymic T cells in mice. For example, they comprise DN $CD4^-8^-$ cells as well as single-positive cells, contain $\gamma\delta$ T cells (up to 30%), and exist at unique sites in the body.

Interestingly, $CD56^+$ T cells are abundant in the liver, whereas $CD57^+$ T cells are abundant in the bone marrow (fig. 9). Only small populations of $CD56^+$ and $CD57^+$ T cells appear in the peripheral blood and peripheral immune organs.

As already mentioned, most if not all extrathymic T cells in mice carry a NK marker, NK1.1 antigen. Therefore, the expression of NK markers on extrathymic T cells resembles the situation in mice. These results may be derived from the fact that extrathymic T cells stand at an intermediate phylogenetic position between NK cells and thymus-derived T cells.

Fig. 8. Phylogenetic development of the thymus.

Fig. 9. Distribution of extrathymic, CD57$^+$ (**a**) and CD56$^+$ (**b**) T cells in humans.

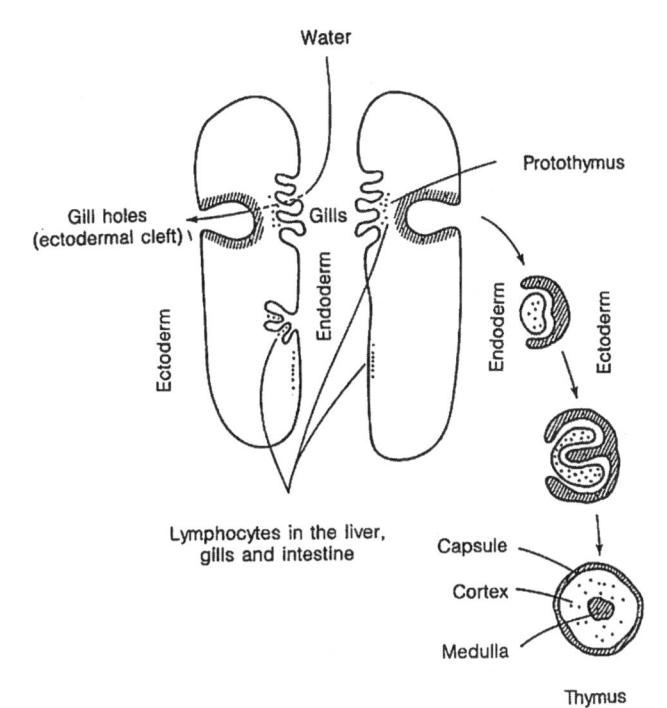

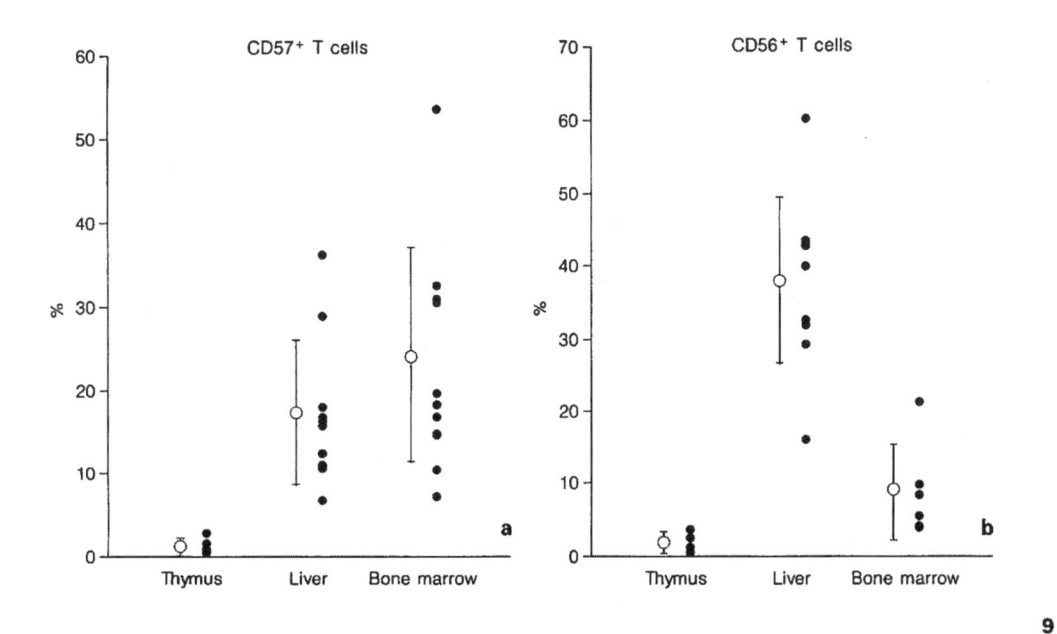

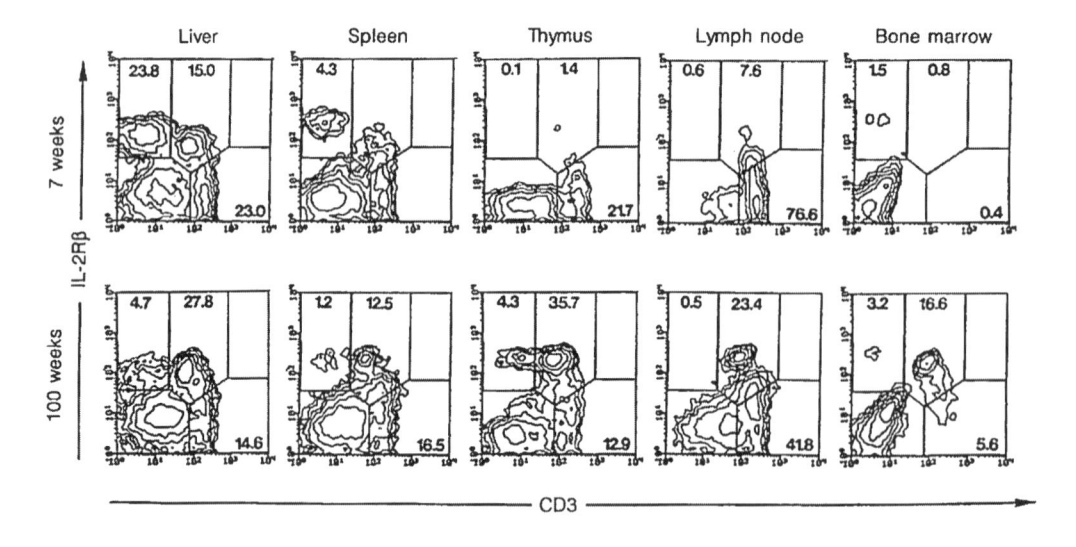

Fig. 10. Predominance of CD3^{int} cells in various immune organs of aged mice.

In the case of mice, we revealed that extrathymic T cells are generated at multiple sites in the body. The existence in humans of extrathymic T cells with unique properties (i.e., CD56$^+$ and CD57$^+$ T cells), depending on the organ, reflects the situation seen in mice.

Physiological and Pathological Functions of Extrathymic T Cells

Extrathymic T cells are extremely rare at birth in mice and humans. They increase in number with age [37–39]. This phenomenon occurs in parallel wit thymic involution. In mice, CD3^{int} cells became prominent in not only the liver but in other organs also at the age of 100 weeks (fig. 10). The proportion of CD3^{int} cells almost overcomes that of CD3^{high} cells even in the spleen and lymph nodes in aged mice. Without the concept of extrathymic T cells, we could not understand the immune phenomenon in aging.

Even in youth, the levels of extrathymic T cells sometimes increases, accompanying acute thymic atrophy. Such conditions include infections by intracellular pathogens (e.g., listerial or viral infection) [50], malignancies [40–43], and pregnancy [15, 16]. It is conceivable that extrathymic T cells are beneficial for the elimination of abnormal self-cells generated in the body. However, an overactivation of extrathymic T cells might be responsible for the onset of some autoimmune diseases [5, 6, 44, 45]. Another example of such events is chronic GVH disease [46, 47]. The majority of T cells infiltrating the target tissues in autoimmune diseases and chronic GVH diseases are TCR^{int} cells.

It is concluded that, without introduction of the concept of extrathymic T cells, the mechanisms involved in various incurable diseases (e.g., malignancies and autoimmune diseases) and the immunologic phenomena seen with aging and in pregnancy cannot be properly understood.

References

1 Ferguson A, Parrott DM: The effect of antigen deprivation on thymus-dependent and thymus-independent lymphocytes in the small intestine of the mouse. Clin Exp Immunol 1972; 12:477–488.
2 Guy-Grand D, Griscelli C, Vassalli P: The gut-associated lymphoid system: Nature and properties of the large dividing cells. Eur J Immunol 1974;4:435–443.
3 MacDonald HR, Lees RK, Bron C, Sordat B, Miescher G: T cell antigen receptor expression in athymic (*nu/nu*) mice: Evidence for an oligoclonal β chain repertoire. J Exp Med 1987;166:195–209.
4 Kishihara K, Yoshikai Y, Matsuzaki G, Mak TW, Nomoto K: Functional α and β T cell chain receptor messages can be detected in old but not young athymic mice. Eur J Immunol 1987;17:477–482.
5 Ohteki T, Seki S, Abo T, Kumagai K: Liver is a possible site for the proliferation of abnormal $CD3^+4^-8^-$ double-negative lymphocytes in autoimmune MRL-*lpr/lpr* mice. J Exp Med 1990;172:7–12.
6 Seki S, Abo T, Ohteki T, Sugiura K, Kumagai K: Unusual $αβ^-$ T cells expanded in autoimmune *lpr* mice are probably a counterpart of normal T cells in the liver. J Immunol 1991; 147:1214–1221.
7 De Geus B, Van den Enden M, Coolen C, Nagelkerken L, Van den Heijden P, Rozing J: Phenotype of intraepithelial lymphocytes in euthymic and athymic mice: Implications for differentiation of cells bearing a $CD3^-$associated γδ T cell receptor. Eur J Immunol 1990;20:291–298.
8 Mosley RL, Styre D, Klein JR: $CD3^+CD8^+$ murine intestinal intraepithelial lymphocytes. Int Immunol 1990;2:361–365.
9 Bandeira A, Itohara S, Bonneville M, Burlen-Defranous O, Mota-Santos T, Countinho A, Tonegawa S: Extrathymic origin of intestinal intraepithelial lymphocytes bearing T-cell antigen receptor γδ. Proc Natl Acad Sci USA 1991;88:43–47.

10 Guy-Grand D, Cerf-Bensussan N, Malissen B, Malassis-Seris M, Briottet C, Vassalli P: Two gut intraepithelial $CD8^+$ lymphocyte populations with different T cell receptors: A role for the gut epithelium in T cell differentiation. J Exp Med 1991: 173:471–481.
11 Ishikawa H, Saito K: Congenitally nu/nu) mice have Thy-1⁻ bearing immunocompetent helper T cells in their peritoneal cavity. J Exp Med 1980;151:965–968.
12 Andreu-Sanchez JL, de Alboran IM, Marcos MAR, Sanchez-Movilla A, Martinez-A C, Kroemer G: Interleukin 2 abrogates the nonresponsive state of T cells expressing a forbidden T cell receptor repertoire and induces autoimmune disease in neonatally thymectomized mice. J Exp Med 1991;173:1323–1329.
13 Elbe A, Kilgus O, Strohal R, Payer E, Schreiber S, Stingl G: Fetal skin: A site of dendritic epidermal T cell development. J Immunol 1992;149: 1694–1701.
14 Ogimoto M, Matsuzaki G, Yoshikai Y, Tauchi Y, Nomoto K: Appearance of $TCR-αβ^+$ $CD4^-CD8^-$ skin intraepithelial lymphocytes in radiation bone marrow chimeras. J Immunol 1993;151:3000–3006.
15 Saito S, Nishikawa K, Morii T, Enomoto M, Narita N, Motoyoshi K, Ichijo M: Cytokine production by $CD16^-CD56^{bright}$ natural killer cells in the human early pregnancy decidua. Int Immunol 1993;5:559–563.
16 Kimura M, Hanawa H, Watanabe H, Ogawa M, Abo T: Synchronous expansion of intermediate TCR cells in the liver and uterus during pregnancy. Cell Immunol 1995;162: 16–25.
17 Budd RC, Miescher GC, Howe RC, Lees RK, Bro C, MacDonald HR: Developmentally regulated expression of T cell receptor β chain variable domains in immature thymocytes. J Exp Med 1987;166:577–582.

18 Fowlkes BJ, Kruisbeek AM, Ton-That H, Weston MA, Coligan JE, Schwartz RH, Pardoll DM: A novel population of T-cell receptor $αβ^-$ bearing thymocytes which predominantly expresses a single $V_β$ gene family. Nature 1987;329:251–254.
19 Crispe IN, Moore MW, Husmann LA, Smith L, Bevan MJ, Shimonkevitz RP: Differentiation potential of subsets of $CD4^-8^-$ thymocytes. Nature 1987;329:336–339.
20 Takahama YA, Kosugi A, Singer A: Phenotype, ontogeny, and repertoire of $CD4^-CD8^-$ $TCRαβ^+$ thymocytes. J Immunol 1991;156:1134–1141.
21 Arase H, Arase-Fukushi N, Good RA, Onoe K: Lymphokine-activated killer cell activity of $CD4^-CD8^-$ $TCRαβ^+$ thymocytes. J Immunol 1993;151:546–555.
22 Egerton M, Scollay R: Intrathymic selection of murine $TCRαβ^+$ $CD4^-CD8^-$ thymocytes. Int Immunol 1990;2:157–162.
23 Suda T, Zlotnik A: Origin, differentiation, and repertoire selection of $CD3^+$ $CD4^-CD8^-$ thymocytes bearing either αβ or γδ T cell receptors. J Immunol 1993;150:447–455.
24 Seki S, Kono DH, Balderas RS, Theofilopoulos AN: $V_β$ repertoire of murine hepatic T cells: Implication for selection of double-negative $αβ^+$ T cells. J Immunol 1994;153:637–646.
25 Ohteki T, MacDonald HR: Major histocompatibility complex class I related molecules control the development of $CD4^+8^-$ and $CD4^-8^-$ subsets of natural killer 1.1+ T cell receptor-α/β⁺ cells in the liver of mice. J Exp Med 1994;180:699–704.
26 Kikly K, Dennert G: Evidence for extrathymic development of TNK cells: $NK1^+$ $CD3^+$ cells responsible for acute marrow graft rejection are present in thymus-deficient mice. J Immunol 1992;149:403–412.
27 Mieno M, Suto R, Obata Y, Udono H, Takahashi T, Shiku H, Nakayama E: $CD4^-8^-$ T cells responsible for acute marrow graft rejection are present in thymus-deficient mice. J Immunol 1991;174:193–201.

28 Zlotnik A, Godfrey DI, Fischer M, Suda T: Cytokine production by mature and immature CD4⁻CD8⁻ T cells: αβ-T cell receptor⁺ CD4⁻CD8⁻ T cells produce IL-4. J Immunol 1992;149:1211-1225.
29 Skinner MA, Sambhara SR, Benveniste P, Miller RG: Characterization of αβ⁺ CD4⁻ CD8⁻ CTL lines isolated from mixed lymphocyte cultures of adult mouse spleen cells. Cell Immunol 1992;139:375-385.
30 Reimann J, Bellan A, Conradt P: Development of autoreactive L3T4⁺ T cells from double-negative (L3T4⁻/Ly-2⁻) Thy-1⁺ spleen cells of normal mice. Eur J Immunol 1988;18:989-999.
31 Prud'Homme GJ, Bocarro DC, Luke ECH: Clonal delection and autoreactivity in extrathymic CD4⁻CD8⁻ (double negative) T cell receptor-α/β T cells. J Immunol 1991;147:3314-3318.
32 Plathumpat V, Jones DS, Holm B, Wang H, Liang O, Strober S: Studies of CD4⁻ CD8⁻ αβ bone marrow T cells with suppressor activity. J Immunol 1992;148:373-380.
33 Guidos CJ, Weissman IL, Adkins B: Developmental potential of CD4⁻8⁻ thymocytes: Peripheral progeny include mature CD4⁻8⁻ T cells bearing αβ T cell receptor. J Immunol 1989;142:3773-3780.
34 Huang L, Crispe IN: Distinctive selection mechanisms govern the T cell receptor repertoire of peripheral CD4⁻CD8⁻α/β T cells. J Exp Med 1992;176:699-706.
35 Kawachi Y, Watanabe H, Moroda T, Haga M, Iiai T, Hatakeyama K, Abo T: Existence of self-reactive T cell clones in a restricted population of IL-2Rβ⁺ intermediate T cell receptor cells in the liver and other immune organs. Eur J Immunol 1995;25:2272-2278.
36 Watanabe H, Miyaji C, Kawachi Y, Iiai T, Ohtsuka K, Iwanaga T, Takahashi-Iwanaga H, Abo T: Relationships between intermediate TCR cells and NK1.1⁺ T cells in various immune organs: NK1.1⁺ T cells are present within a population of intermediate TCR cells. J Immunol 1995;155:2972-2983.

37 Ohteki T, Okuyama R, Seki S, Abo T, Sugiura K, Kusumi A, Ohmori T, Watanabe H, Kumagai K: Age-dependent increase of extrathymic T cells in the liver and their appearance in the periphery of older mice. J Immunol 1992;149:1562-1570.
38 Iiai T, Watanabe H, Seki S, Surgiura K, Hirokawa K, Utsuyama M, Takahashi-Iwanaga H, Iwanaga T, Ohteki T, Abo T: Ontogeny and development of extrathymic T cells in mouse liver. Immunology 1992;77:556-563.
39 Ohtsuka K, Iiai T, Watanabe H, Tanaka T, Miyasaka M, Sato K, Asakura H, Abo T: Similarities and differences between extrathymic T cells residing in mouse liver and intestine. Cell Immunol 1994;153:52-66.
40 Seki S, Abo T, Masuda T, Ohteki T, Kanno A, Takeda K, Rikiishi H, Nagura H, Kumagai K: Identification of activated T cell receptor γδ lymphocytes in the liver of tumor-bearing hosts. J Clin Invest 1990;86:409-415.
41 Seki S, Abo T, Sugiura K, Ohteki T, Kobata T, Yagita H, Okumura K, Rikiishi H, Masuda T, Kumagai K: Reciprocal T cell responses in the liver and thymus of mice injected with syngeneic tumor cells. Cell Immunol 1991;137:46-60.
42 Ohmori K, Iiai T, Watanabe H, Tanaka T, Miyasaka M, Abo T: Activation of extrathymic T cells in the liver of mice bearing syngeneic tumors. Biomed Res 1993;14:65-79.
43 Iiai T, Watanabe H, Iwamoto T, Nakashima I, Abo T: Predominant activation of extrathymic T cells during melanoma development of metallothionein/ret transgenic mice. Cell Immunol 1994;153:412-427.
44 Masuda T, Ohteki T, Abo T, Seki S, Nose M, Nagura H, Kumagai K: Expansion of the population of double negative CD4⁻8⁻ Tαβ-cells in the liver is a common feature of autoimmune mice. J Immunol 1991;147:2907-2912.
45 Iiai T, Kimura M, Kawachi Y, Hirokawa K, Watanabe H, Hatakeyama K, Abo T: Characterization of intermediate TCR cells expanding in the liver, thymus and other organs in autoimmune lpr mice: Parallel analysis with their normal counterparts. Immunology 1995;77:601-608.

46 Ikarashi Y, Abo T, Kawai K, Iiai T, Watanabe H, Suzuki K, Matsumoto Y, Omata S, Fujiwara M: Expansion of intermediate TCR cells of mice with autoimmune-like graft-versus-host disease. Immunology 1994;83:205-212.
47 Osman Y, Watanabe T, Kawachi Y, Sato K, Ohtuska K, Watanabe H, Hsahimoto S, Moriyama Y, Shibata A, Abo T: Intermediate TCR cells with self-reactive clones are effector cells which induce syngeneic graft-versus-host disease in mice. Cell Immunol 1995;166:172-186.
48 Sato K, Ohtsuka K, Hasegawa K, Yamagiwa S, Watanabe H, Iwanaga T, Tahahashi-Iwanaga H, Asakura H, Abo T: Evidence for extrathymic generation of intermediate TCR cells in the liver revealed in thymectomized, irradiated mice subjected to bone marrow transplantation. J Exp Med 1995;182:759-767.
49 Watanabe H, Iiai T, Kimura M, Ohtsuka K, Tanaka T, Miyasaka M, Tsuchida M, Hanawa H, Abo T: Characterization of intermediate TCR cells in the liver of mice with respect to their unique IL-2R expression. Cell Immunol 1993;149:331-342.
50 Ohtsuka K, Sato K, Watanabe H, Kimura M, Asakura H, Abo T: Unique order of the lymphocyte subset induction in the liver and intestine of mice during *Listeria monocytogenes* infection. Cell Immunol 1995;161:112-124.
51 Makino Y, Yamagata N, Sasho T, Adachi Y, Kanno R, Koseki H, Kanno M, Taniguchi M: Extrathymic development of $V_\alpha 14$⁻positive T cells. J Exp Med 1993;177:1399-1408.
52 Adachi Y, Koseki H, Zijlstra M, Taniguchi M: Positive selection of invariant $V_\alpha 14$⁺ T cells by non-major histocompatibility complex-encoded class I-like molecules expressed on bone marrow-derived cells. Proc Natl Acad Sci USA 1995;92:1200-1204.

53 Lantz O, Bendelac A: An invariant T cell receptor α chain is used by a unique subset of major histocompatibility complex class I-specific CD4$^+$ and CD4$^-$8$^-$ T cells in mice and humans. J Exp Med 1994;180: 1097–1106.

54 Dellabona P, Padovan E, Casorati G, Brockhaus M, Lanzavecchia A: An invariant V$_\alpha$24-J$_\alpha$Q/V$_\beta$11 T cell receptor is expressed in all individuals by clonally expanded CD4$^-$8$^-$ T cells. J Exp Med 1994;180:1171–1176.

55 Sumida T, Sakamoto A, Murata H, Makino Y, Takahashi H, Yoshida S, Nishioka K, Iwamoto I, Taniguchi M: Selective reduction of T cells bearing invariant V$_\alpha$24J$_\alpha$Q: Antigen receptor in patients with systemic sclerosis. J Exp Med 1995;182: 1163–1168.

56 Hashimoto W, Takeda K, Anzai R, Ogasawara K, Sakihara H, Sugiura K, Seki S, Kumagai K: Cytotoxic NK1.1 Ag$^+$ αβ T cells with intermediate TCR induced in the liver of mice by IL-12. J Immunol 1995; 154:4333–4340.

57 Haynes BF: Human thymic epithelium and T cell development: Current issues and future directions. Thymus 1990;16:143–157.

58 Takii Y, Hashimoto S, Iiai T, Watanabe H, Hatakeyama K, Abo T: Increase in the proportion of granulated CD56$^+$ T cells in patients with malignancy. Clin Exp Immunol 1994;97:522–527.

59 Okada T, Iiai T, Kawachi Y, Moroda T, Takii Y, Hatakeyama K, Abo T: Origin of CD57$^+$ T cells which increase at tumor sites in patients with colorectal cancer. Clin Exp Immunol 1995;102:159–166.

GRANULOCYTOSIS INDUCED BY INCREASING SYMPATHETIC NERVE ACTIVITY CONTRIBUTES TO THE INCIDENCE OF ACUTE APPENDICTIS

急性虫垂炎の発症の一因は、
交感神経活動増加による顆粒球増多である

Biomedical Research, 17: 171-181, 1996

chapter 4

GRANULOCYTOSIS INDUCED BY INCREASING SYMPATHETIC NERVE ACTIVITY CONTRIBUTES TO THE INCIDENCE OF ACUTE APPENDICTIS

急性虫垂炎の発症の一因は、交感神経活動増加による顆粒球増多である

MINORU FUKUDA[1], TETSUYA MORODA[2], SHINICHI TOYABE[2], TSUNEO IIAI[2], YASUYUKI KAWACHI[2], HIROMI TAKAHASHI-IWANAGA[3], TOSHIHIKO IWANAGA[3], MASAHIKO OKADA[4], and TORU ABO[2]

[1]Sakamachi Hospital, Arakawamachi, Niigata 959-31, Department of Immunology, [3]Trhird Department of Anatomy, and
[4]Department of Diagnostics, Niigata University School of Medicine, Niigata 951, Japan

【要約】

　急性虫垂炎発症には、天候の影響を受けるようであるが、そのメカニズムを検証した。虫垂を切除した患者（112人）を、発症時の気圧により3群に分類した。高気圧時は、壊疽性症例（顆粒球高浸潤）の頻度が、カタル性症例（顆粒球浸潤なし）の頻度よりも顕著に高かった。低気圧時は、その反対であった。健常被験者において、末梢血中の顆粒球およびリンパ球の変動を気圧と心拍数との関連から検証した。顆粒球増多は、高気圧時の交感神経緊張（高心拍数）ともに出現した、一方、リンパ球増加は、低気圧時の副交感神経優位（低心拍数）とともに出現した。壊疽性症例において、末梢血や虫垂に顆粒球増多が見られ、カタル性症例において、末梢血や虫垂にリンパ球増加が見られた。これら患者データの結果と健常被験者の実験結果とを総合的に考察すると、交感神経緊張による顆粒球増多が、壊疽性虫垂炎の発症と関連していると仮定できる。ヒトおよびマウスを対象とした実験結果が示すのは、アドレナリン受容体を介したカテコラミンによる顆粒球増多が出現することである。壊疽性症例における虫垂の電子顕微鏡検査を行ったが、顆粒球周囲に細菌は見られなかった。本研究の結果は、化膿性疾患の病因の重要な手がかりとなる可能性がある。

　天候の影響で病態が悪化する患者が存在するという臨床医は多い（2, 3, 5-7, 32, 35, 39）。しかし、気候的要因と関連する生体防御系の基礎メカニズムを検証することは困難である。本研究の共著者の1人は、過去10年間、重症虫垂炎（穿孔を含む）発症は、晴天（高気圧）時であるという傾向を発見した。この経験が偶然に過ぎないのかを検討すべく、虫垂炎（112症例）を虫垂炎の種類と発症時の気圧について検証した。虫垂炎自体は、いかなる気圧状況下でも発症するが、壊疽性虫垂炎は高気圧時に発症する頻度が顕著に高くなる。

　本研究では生体防御系に着目した。特に、健常被験者群と患者群で、虫垂および末梢血における顆粒球とリンパ球の比率が気圧によりどのように変動したかに着目した。

　高気圧時には、顆粒球増多が出現する頻度が多いが、低気圧時にはリンパ球増加が出現する頻度が増加することが明らかになった。患者群の末梢血および虫垂においても気圧に伴い類似した変動が見られた。晴天（高気圧）時、交感神経緊張が出現する結果、感情が高揚する（9, 21, 35）。

　この状況下では、アドレナリン受容体を有する顆粒球がカテコラミン分泌の増加により活性化している可能性がある（19, 25, 34）。これに

対し、悪天候（低気圧）時は、副交感神経優位が出現する結果、抑鬱感が頻出するが（17, 24, 31, 35, 39）、この時、顆粒球値はむしろ減少している可能性がある。

本論文では、交感神経緊張により生理的に顆粒球増多が出現することと、重症急性虫垂炎の発症増加との関連性の可能性について提案する。交感神経緊張は他の要因（例、ストレス、過剰飲酒や過重労働）でも容易に出現する（10, 18-20, 22）。故に、顆粒球増多が多くの化膿性疾患（例、中耳炎、歯周炎、胃炎、潰瘍性大腸炎、肝膿瘍、肛門周囲膿瘍等）の原因である可能性である。さらに重要なのは、細菌がない場合でも過度な顆粒球浸潤が出現して、おそらくフリーラジカルや超酸化物分泌により周辺組織が破壊される可能性がある。

材料と方法

患者と健常被験者

本研究は、虫垂炎患者112例（虫垂を切除した患者：男性=58例、女性=54例、年齢5-58歳、平均=28.6歳）を対象とした。肉眼および顕微鏡観察により、虫垂炎を3群（カタル性症例、蜂巣炎性症例および壊疽性症例）に分類した。患者は、荒川町在住（新潟市の北約50km）、調査期間は、1992年2月-1994年2月であった。平均発症年齢と虫垂炎の種類の関係は、以下の通り；カタル性症例24.1歳、蜂巣炎性症例25.6歳、壊疽性症例37.6歳であった。

右下腹部または上腹部での疼痛発生を虫垂炎の発症と考え、この時点での気圧を測定した。本研究では手術前に3日以上抗生物質を投与した患者を除外した。

健常人群のデータは、健康診断の外来症例を用いた（n=146、年齢28-79歳、平均=37.0歳）。採血時の気圧により、健常人を以下2群に分類した；高気圧群（平均=1,019hPa）（35.3 ± 9.4歳）群および低気圧群（平均=1,009hPa）（40.2 ± 10.2歳）。

気圧測定

大気圧は、百葉箱に設置したアネロイド気圧計と温湿度記録計で計測した。

顆粒球とリンパ球の数と割合

抗凝固剤を添加した末梢血を新潟大学医学部検査診断学教室に委託して、臨床的定法により白血球分画の測定を行った。

顆粒球採取

ヘパリン化した末梢血をFicoll-Isopaque勾配（1.077）による遠心分離により、単核細胞（MNC）と混和物（顆粒球と赤血球）に分離した（37）。混和物（1ml）を、0.17M Tris緩衝液（9ml、0.83%NH_4Cl添加）を用いて溶血した。RPMI 1640培養液（10% 非動化FCSを添加）で2度洗浄後、顆粒球を培養液中に懸濁させた。

細胞解析のための虫垂からの細胞採取

虫垂より単核球を採取して、フローサイトメトリー解析を行った（38）。検体をハサミで細切し、200-ゲージのステンレススチールメッシュで濾過後、細胞を培養液の中に懸濁した。最後に、Ficoll-Isopaque勾配（1.077）遠心分離を行い、単核球を採取した。

フローサイトメトリーよる細胞表現型の解析

FTTC、PEまたはPer-CP標識したモノクローナル抗体を添加し、虫垂より採取した単核球を染色した（16）。使用した抗体を以下示す；CD3（NU-T3；（株）ニチレイ、東京、日本）、CD8（NU-Ts/c；（株）ニチレイ）、CD4（Leu3a）、CD56（Leu-19）、TCR$\alpha\beta$（TCR-1）（Becton-Dickinson, Mountain View, CA）とTCR$\gamma\delta$（TCRδ1）（T Cell Sciences, Cambridge, MA）(2)。FACScan（Becton-Dickinson）による二重染色のフローサイトメトリー解析を行った。1万個の細胞を解析に用いた。

電子顕微鏡検査

3%グルタルアルデヒドによりサンプルを

迅速固定後、1% OsO_4による後固定を行った(15)。Epon 812に包埋した極薄切片をJEOL 100B電子顕微鏡（JEOL, Peabody, MA）で検証した。

Ca^{2+}流入の測定

フルオ-3-アセトシメシイ・エステル（Flue-3-AM）、プルロニックF-127、ホルミル-メチオニル-ロイシル-フエニルアラニン（fMLP）およびイオノマイシン（Sigma, St. Louis, MO）を使用した（26, 33）。ヒト顆粒球（2 x 10^6）をflue-3（3%プルロニックF-127および18%DMSO添加、最終濃度$2\mu M$）と、培養標識後（弱光, 37℃, 30分）、2度洗浄した。その後、フローサイトメトリーを用い解析した。前培養後（暗所, 37℃, 10分）、基礎蛍光測定を行い、その後、細胞をfMLP、イオノマイシンまたはアドレナリンで刺激した。

マウスへのアドレナリン投与と顆粒球数測定

仮説（交感神経緊張により顆粒球が増多する）の有効性を検証するため、マウスの実験を以下のように行った。注入ポンプ（Model 1007D, Alza, Palo Alto, CA）を用いて、アドレナリンを1週間持続性投与した（0.2mg/匹／週）。そして、マウスの各免疫臓器より単核球を採取した。FITC標識抗顆粒球モノクロナール抗体（PharMingen, San Diego, CA）を用いて、顆粒球の免疫蛍光染色を行った。

統計分析

有意差検定にはAnova検定とDuncan法を用いた（$p<0.05$）。顆粒球とリンパ球の日内変動リズムの検定には、Rogers法を用いた。

結果

高気圧時、急性虫垂炎の壊疽性型の発症率が高い

急性虫垂炎（虫垂を切除）患者112人を発症時の気圧により3群に分類した（Fig. 1A）。各群の患者数は以下の通り；1群（1,001-1,010hPa；42人（38%））、2群（1,011-1,020hPa；42人（38%））、3群（1,021-1,030hPa；28人（23%））。虫垂炎の種類に着目すると、気圧が上昇すると壊疽性虫垂炎が増加するが、反対に、カタル性虫垂炎は減少する傾向があった。高気圧時、蜂巣炎性虫垂炎は、減少を示した。

気圧の影響を受け、急性虫垂炎の種類が変化したとしても、気圧が唯一の関連要因であるとは考えにくい。この点を検証するため、虫垂炎の種類を別の観点から（発症が昼間であるか夜

Figure.1

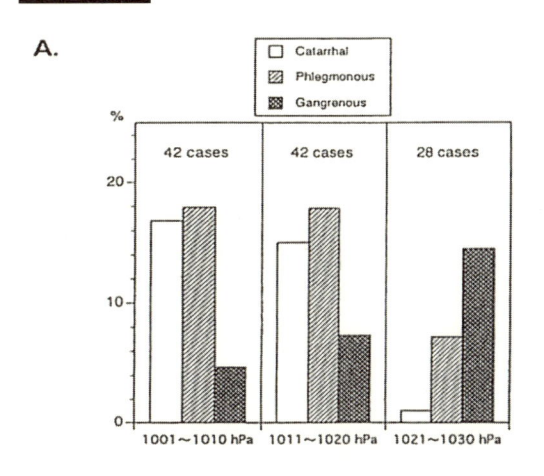

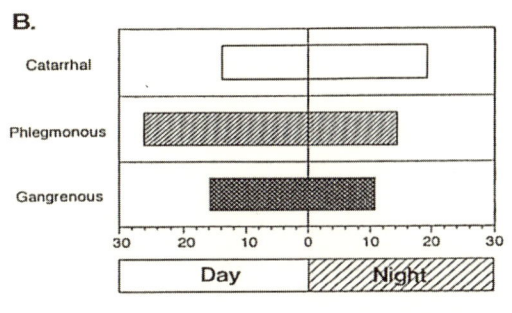

気圧（A）と時刻（B）別による虫垂炎の種類（カタル性、蜂巣炎、壊疽性）の発症率変化。急性虫垂炎（症例数：112）発生率を、気圧と時刻の観点より検証した。壊疽性症例に着目すると、発症は、高気圧時と昼間に集中していることが判明した。カタル症例では、その反対であった。発生率を百分率で示す（100%＝合計112症例）。昼間は8:00a.m.-8:00p.m、夜間は8:00p.m-8:00a.mである。

間であるか）再分類した（Fig. 1B）。蜂巣炎性虫垂炎および壊疽性虫垂炎（穿孔例を含む）の発症率は昼間に高く、一方、カタル性虫垂炎の発症率が夜間に比較的高かった。

ヒトは、晴天（高気圧）時、活動的である。反対に、雨天（低気圧）時、活動的ではなく、抑鬱感を抱く傾向がある。このように、自律神経系が交感神経緊張であるか副交感神経優位であるかにより、体調は変動する。その影響で感情が揺れ動く。つまり、体調は天候の影響のみならず、昼間（交感神経緊張）であるか夜間（副交感優位）であるかで変動する。

健常被験者群における白血球分画の気圧による変化

気圧と疾病の発症率の基礎メカニズムを確認するため、顆粒球とリンパ球の比率が気圧の影響を受けて変動するか検証を行った（Fig. 2A）。「壊疽性虫垂炎（虫垂への顆粒球高浸潤）では、生理的な顆粒球の増多が出現し、その原因は気圧である」という仮説を検証する。健常被験者群における顆粒球とリンパ球の比率を1か月間分析した。気圧と末梢血の白血球分画値を図に示す。低気圧ではリンパ球増加が、高気圧では顆粒球増多が出現した（約70％一致）。心拍数は高気圧で増加した（63.0 ± 3.2/分）一方、低気圧で減少した（61.0 ± 2.7/分）ことも確認できた（$P<0.05$）。白血球分画や心拍数には日内変動があるので、本研究では毎日午前11時に測定を行った。

つまり、交感神経緊張により顆粒球が増多するという本仮説が真であるならば、簡易な実験を行えば末梢血における白血球分画の変動を確認できるのである。この点について、上記実験と同じ被験者群に同様の日内変動が見られるか検証した（Fig. 2B）。リンパ球増加は夜間（副交感神経優位）、そして、顆粒球増多は昼間（交感神経緊張）出現することが明らかになった。

この顆粒球とリンパ球の変化について、統計学的に有意差が得られた（$P<0.0001$）。換言すると、白血球分画は、気圧以外にも複数の影響を受け変動するのである。

更に厳密に、気圧と末梢血における白血球分画との関連性を検証するため、健常被験者（n=146）のデータを分析した（Fig. 2C）。高気圧時に採血した被験者の末梢血における顆粒球比率は、低気圧時に採血したものに比較して顕著に高値であった（$P<0.01$）。一方、末梢血のリンパ球比率は、完全に逆であった（$P<0.01$）。

壊疽性虫垂炎患者組織と同時に末梢血顆粒球も増加していた

高気圧時、健常被験者の末梢血において、顆粒球増多が見られたことから、このような顆粒球増多が患者組織に誘導され、壊疽性虫垂炎を招くことが推測できる。壊疽性虫垂炎では、顆粒球の虫垂浸潤の計測は重要である。発症時における白血球分画と虫垂炎の種類を示す（Fig. 3）。壊疽性虫垂炎の末梢血では、顆粒球高値が出現することが明らかになった。反対に、カタル性虫垂炎（リンパ球のみの炎症）の末梢血では、リンパ球高値が見られた。換言すると、末梢血と組織における顆粒球値とリンパ球値も影響を受けているのである。

患者の虫垂より採取した白血球のフローサイトメトリー解析

病理学的診断により、カタル性、蜂巣炎性、壊疽性虫垂炎を分類したものを、さらにフローサイトメトリーを用いて確認を行った。カタル性虫垂炎および壊疽性虫垂炎の代表例を示す（Fig. 4）。光散乱分析により、カタル性虫垂炎の場合、顆粒球は僅少（1.8％）で、壊疽性虫垂炎の場合、顆粒球多数（24.7％）であった（Region 2）。壊疽性虫垂炎症例（Fig. 4A）より採取した単核球（Region 1）の表面フェノタイプをモノクローナル抗体染色により解析し

Figure.2

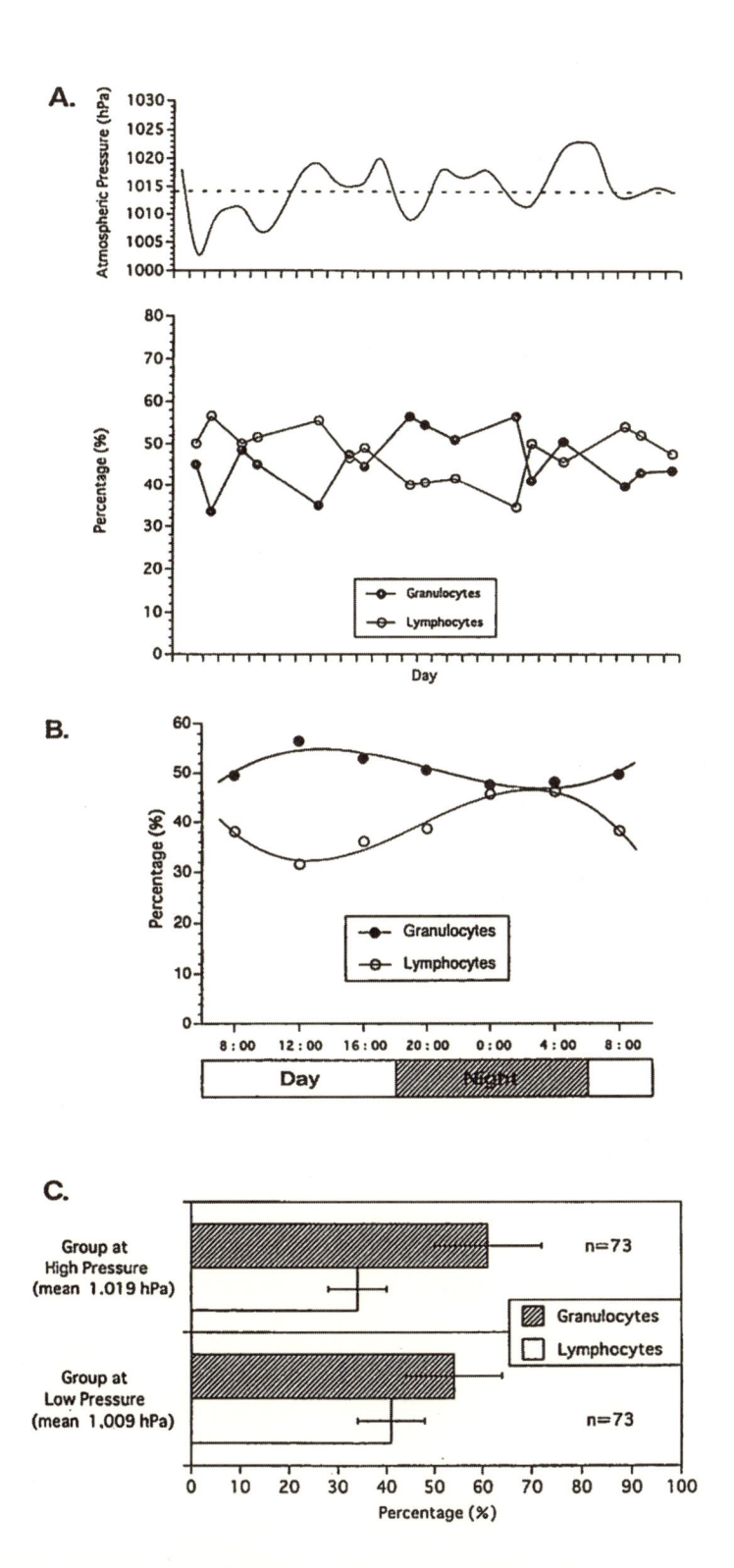

気圧と白血球の比率の関係。A：健常被験者における月内変動。B：健常被験者における白血球比率の日内変動。C：高気圧時および低気圧時における健常被験者の白血球比率データ。健常被験者（男性，47才）の末梢血中の顆粒球とリンパ球の比率を検証した。この被験者の白血球の総数は、観察期間中（1995年1月-2月）、6,000-6,500/mm^{3}であった。健康診断ために来院した健常被験者（n=146）のデータも使用した。データは採血時の気圧により、2群に分類した。

chapter 4　87

Figure.3

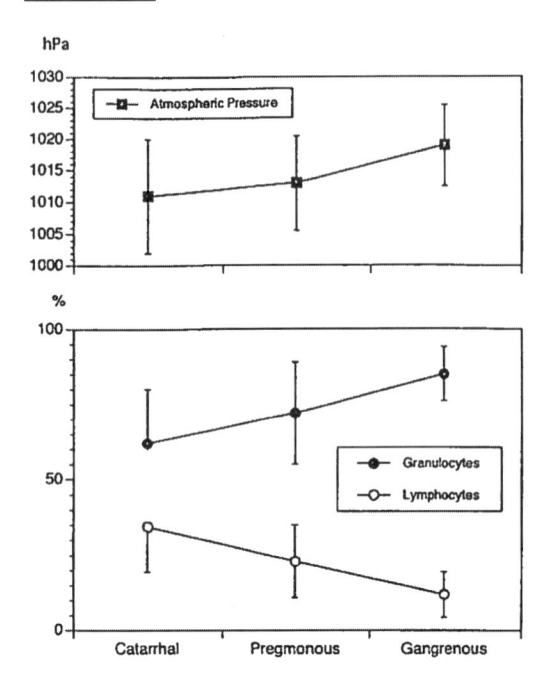

気圧、白血球比率と急性虫垂炎の種類；3つのパラメータ間の関係。虫垂炎の112の症例を3群（カタル性（n=35）、蜂巣炎（n=47）、壊疽性（n=30））に分類して、気圧と発症時の顆粒球とリンパ球の比率を示す。カタル性と壊疽性間の有意差検定にAnovaとDuncan法を用いて、有意差を得た（P<0.01）。

Figure.4

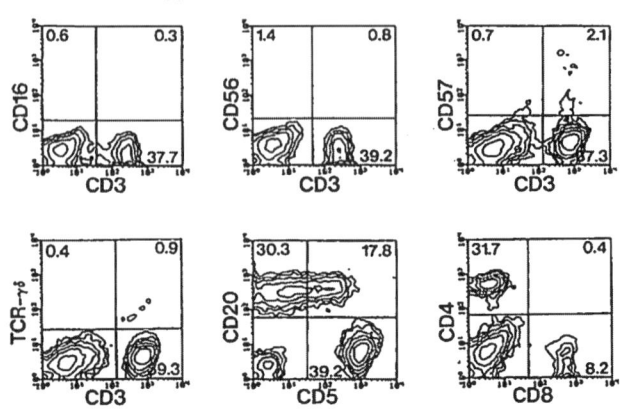

虫垂より採取した単核球のフローサイトメトリー解析による特徴。A：光散乱により単核球を、顆粒球とリンパ球に識別した。B：単核球用リンパ球マーカーを用い、T、BおよびNK細胞を同定した。各分画内の数値は、蛍光陽性細胞の比率を示す。結局、壊疽性（病理学的診断による）には顆粒球が多いことが確認された。虫垂（壊疽例のRegion1）の単核球のリンパ球サブセット分布は独特であり、$\alpha\beta$T細胞およびCD5$^+$B細胞が大量に見られた。

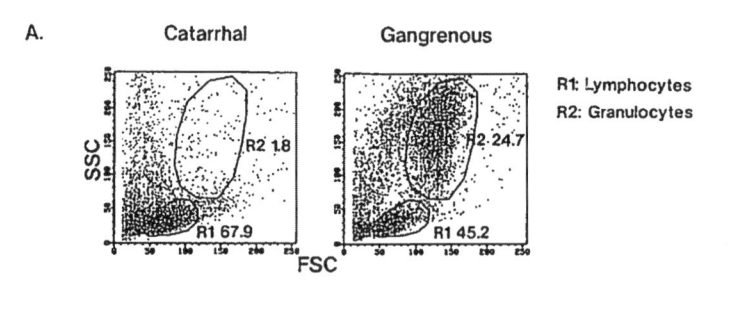

た（Fig. 4B）。CD16、CD56とCD57を用い同定したNK細胞は僅少（<2.0％）で、CD3を用いて同定したT細胞は相当量だった（39％）。T細胞はすべて$\alpha\beta$T細胞で、CD4$^+$細胞が多数を占めた（31.7％）。結果で興味深いのは、虫垂リンパ球の大多数はB細胞であったことと、そのB細胞の多数（37％）が、自己抗体を産生するCD5$^+$B細胞であったということである（37）。顆粒球浸潤の程度にかかわらず、このリンパ球の結果は基本的に同じであった。小腸や大腸の単核球の大部分は、$\gamma\delta$T細胞であり、この虫垂炎症例におけるデータは独特である（23）。虫垂のリンパ球サブセット局在パターンは、むしろ、扁桃腺のものに類似している（未発表データ）。

壊疽性症例組織での細菌の不在

本研究では、蜂巣炎性虫垂炎および壊疽性虫垂炎の検体の電子顕微鏡検査を行った。壊疽性

Figure.5

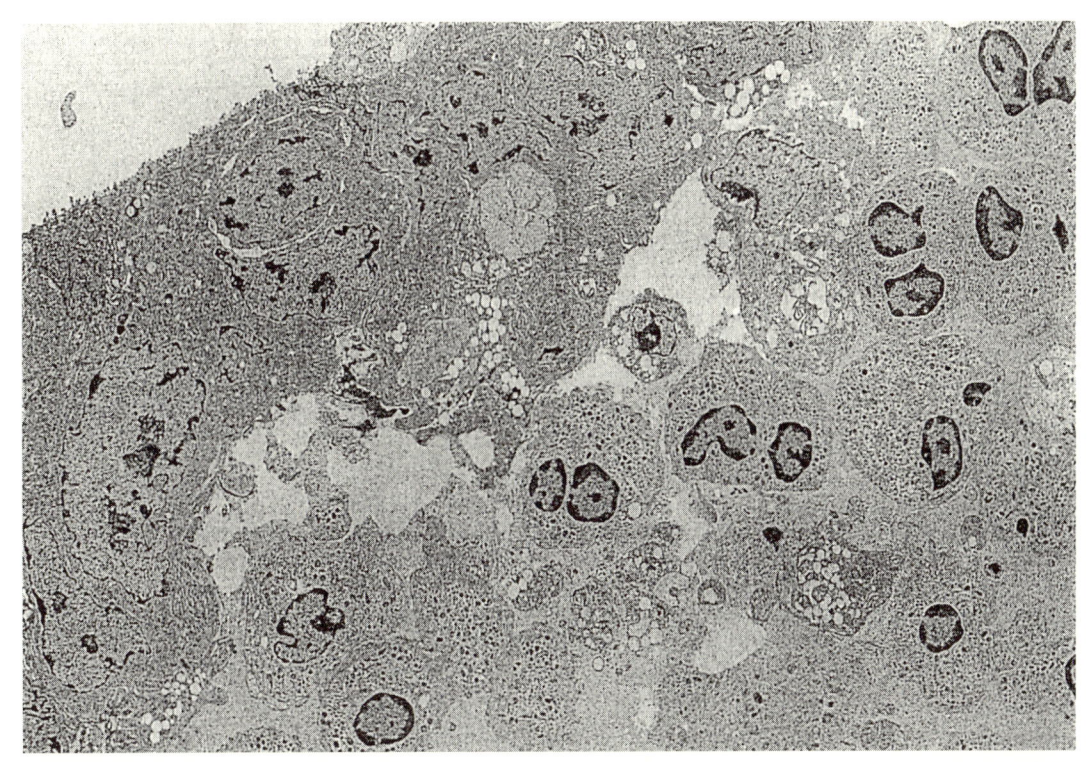

急性虫垂炎の壊疽性より採取した虫垂の電子顕微鏡検査（×2,000）。顆粒球が大量に浸潤し組織を破壊した。しかし、組織にも顆粒球の細胞質にも、細菌は全く見られなかった。顆粒球は、明らかな細菌感染がなくとも組織を損傷（例、フリーラジカルと超酸化物産生による）する可能性が高くなった。

虫垂炎の典型的症例を示す（Fig. 5）。顆粒球が、虫垂上皮下に大量に浸潤し、組織破壊が見られた。驚くべきことに、顆粒球周囲にもまた、顆粒球の細胞質にも全く細菌は見られなかった。このことから、細菌感染が主な要因ではなく、活性化した顆粒球による組織破壊が原因である可能性が高まった。

カテコールアミンが、リンパ球でなく、顆粒球のCa^{2+}インフラックスを誘導する

高気圧や昼間といった状態における基本的な共通点は、身体活動が活発なことである。この状態は、交感神経緊張が高まると出現する可能性がある。交感神経が緊張すると顆粒球の活性化が見られるかを検証するため、ヒト末梢血より採取した顆粒球またはリンパ球に、アドレナリン刺激を与える培養実験を行った（Fig. 6）。Ca^{2+}インフラックスを活性化の指標とした。陽性対照（イオノマイシン（$1\mu M$））では、顆粒球でもリンパ球でもCa^{2+}インフラックスが見られたが、アドレナリン（$5-50\mu g/ml$）では、顆粒球のみにCa^{2+}インフラックスが見られた。

アドレナリン連続投与がマウスに顆粒球増多を誘導する

カテコールアミンにより顆粒球増多が出現するかを直接検証するため、注入ポンプを用いてアドレナリンをマウスに投与する実験（0.2mg/マウス/週）を行った（Fig. 7）。予備実験を行い、マウスが死亡することなく白血球数が変化する投与量を決定した（データ未発表）。アドレナリンを連続投与すると、最終的には検証を行ったすべての臓器で顆粒球増多が誘導されたことが明らかになった。

Figure.6

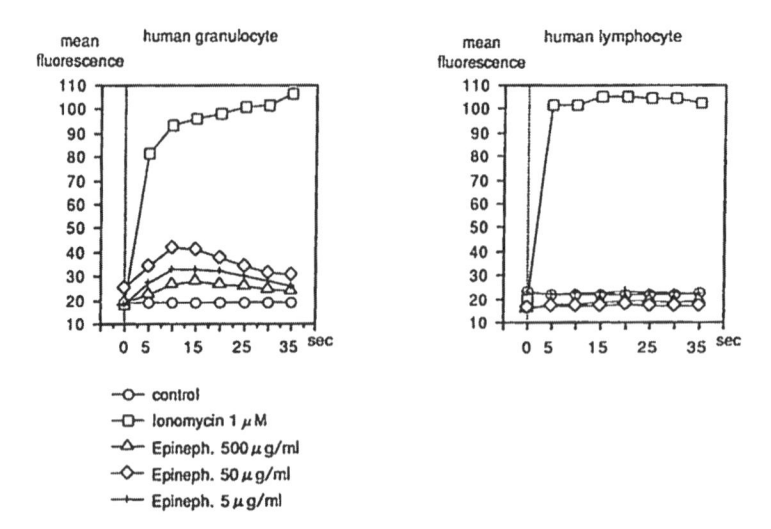

human granulocyte / human lymphocyte

- control
- Ionomycin 1 μM
- Epineph. 500 μg/ml
- Epineph. 50 μg/ml
- Epineph. 5 μg/ml

アドレナリンによりCa^{2+}が顆粒球に流入する。顆粒球とリンパ球をヒト末梢血より分離した。アドレナリンにより、リンパ球ではなく顆粒球にCa^{2+}が流入した。陽性対照(イオノマイシン)では、顆粒球でもリンパ球でもCa^{2+}が流入した。3度実験を行った典型的な結果を示す。

Figure.7

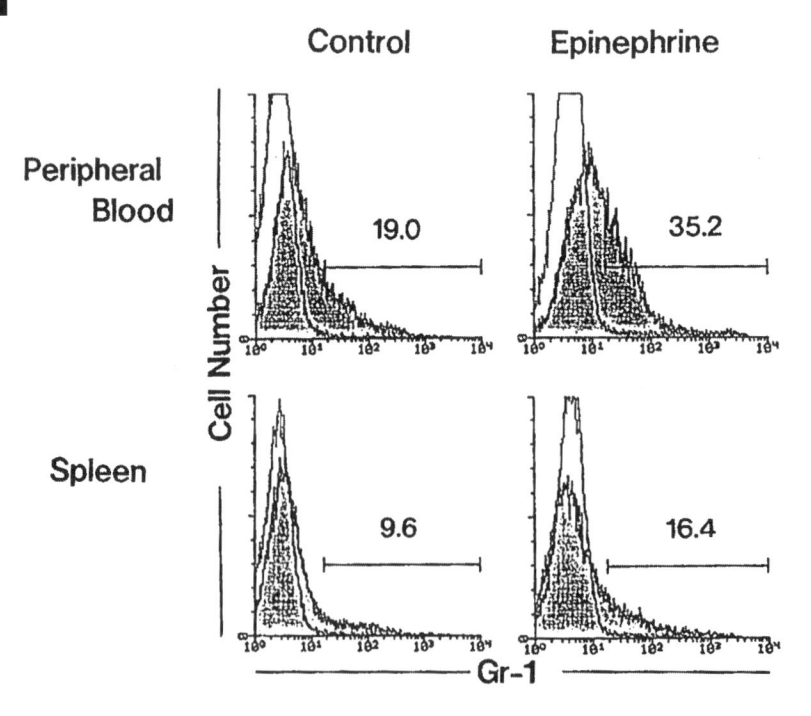

Control / Epinephrine

Peripheral Blood: 19.0 / 35.2
Spleen: 9.6 / 16.4

Cell Number / Gr-1

マウスに注入ポンプを用いてアドレナリンを持続的に注入した。すると末梢血と脾臓はじめとする各臓器において顆粒球増多が出現した。本仮説(交感神経緊張により顆粒球が増多する)が正しいか証明するために、マウスに一週間(0.2mg/匹/週)アドレナリンを投与し、各臓器における顆粒球値を測定した。測定を行った臓器では、顆粒球値が上昇していた。この時、脾臓における顆粒球絶対数も増加を示し、処置後1週間に40%の脾腫が見られた。細線は、FITC標識コントロール抗体を用いた陰性対照を示す。

考察

急性虫垂炎患者における外部環境、体調および発症の基礎メカニズムを検証した。顆粒球とリンパ球の比率の変化が要因の1つであり、上記のメカニズムと関連すると仮定できた。このことが、体調と疾病の発症を結びつける主要因である可能性がある。この概念を極端に単純化して以下に示す: 高気圧 → 交感神経緊張 → 顆粒球増多 → 化膿性疾患発症率上昇である。疾病の発症に、天候が影響することもあると考える臨床医は多いが (2, 3, 5-7, 32, 35, 39)、諸原因の関係を総合的に解明する研究はこれまで報告されていない。顆粒球とリンパ球の比率が、体調（自律神経系の活動状態）の影響を受けている可能性があることも考慮すると、外部環境と疾病の発症との関係が明らかになる。

虫垂切除した患者を、虫垂への顆粒球浸潤程度により3群に分類すると、末梢血中の顆粒球値は、組織中への顆粒球浸潤に比例して変化することが明らかになった。一例を挙げると、壊疽性虫垂炎患者の末梢血においては、顕著な顆粒球増多とリンパ球減少が見られた。交感神経緊張による顆粒球増多は、全身的な現象である可能性が考えられる。本研究では、虫垂炎の種類の病理学診断に細胞解析による検証を加えた。

先ず、気圧と虫垂炎発症の基礎メカニズムを検証するため、気圧の変化が患者群と健常者群の末梢血中における顆粒球とリンパ球値に影響するか検証した。本研究では、斎藤章の既報に則っているが、斎藤は、交感神経緊張では顆粒球増多が、また、副交感神経優位ではリンパ球増加が見られると報告した (27-30)。昼間（交感神経緊張）は、顆粒球増加が一般的であるのに対し、夜間（副交感神経優位）はリンパ球増加が、一般的であることが十分に証明された (1, 4, 8)。晴天時（高気圧）には、ヒトは活動的で、雨天時（低気圧）には、ヒトは不活発で抑鬱的であることはよく見られる (9, 17, 24, 25, 31, 35)。

高気圧時、顆粒球増多が出現したのに対し、低気圧時、リンパ球増加が出現した（Fig. 2）。しかし、この発見の重要性を無視することはできないが、限定的である (9)。その理由は気圧以外の多くの要因が体調調節に関与するためである。

興味深い疑問は、交感神経系緊張により顆粒球増多がどのように誘導されるかということである。この点について顆粒球表面上に存在するアドレナリン受容体が想起される (19, 25)。この受容体の存在について、多数報告があるものの、その生理的重要性は不明なままであった。カテコールアミンが、顆粒球とマクロファージの酵素の細胞外輸送を抑制する効果を示す培養実験に関する報告も複数存在する (12-14)。本研究では、アドレナリン刺激により、ヒト顆粒球内へCa^{2+}が流入することが明らかになった。

注入ポンプを用いてマウスにアドレナリンを投与したところ、末梢血および脾臓において顆粒球増多が出現することが明らかになった。この時、胸腺萎縮とT細胞の顕著な減少が出現した（未発表データ）。これまで類似した結果も報告されていた (11)。このような研究方針（カテコールアミン値と生体防御機構）が、これからの研究に重要であるようである。ヒトとマウスを対象とした本研究の結果と総合的に考察すると、交感神経緊張により全身における顆粒球値が上昇するようである。

もう1つの疑問は、このように出現した顆粒球増多が原因で、どのように疾病が発症するのかということである。壊疽性虫垂炎症例の虫垂において顆粒球浸潤部位を検証したところ、多くの細動脈が拡張しており、そのような広範囲部位で大量に顆粒球（主に好中球）が浸潤して

いたことが明らかになった（Fig. 5）。驚くべきことに、細菌は顆粒球周囲および顆粒球の細胞質に見られなかった。活性化され、アポトーシスを起こした顆粒球が組織（例、虫垂上皮）を破壊することが推測できる。近年、明らかになったのは、主としてマクロファージ（TNFα）とリンパ球（TNFβ）が産生する腫瘍壊死因子（TNF）が引き金となって、顆粒球がフリーラジカルと超酸化物を分泌することである（36, 40）。閾値を超えると、顆粒球はこのフリーラジカルや超酸化物を用いて組織を損傷することができる。

虫垂炎の組織の電子顕微鏡写真の中には、虫垂上皮にアデノウイルス（最も一般的な風邪ウイルス）が見られることもあった（未発表データ）。虫垂炎症例の中には、ウイルス感染が原因であるものもある可能性がある。そうであるならば、初期反応はリンパ球反応であるカタル性である可能性がある。顆粒球反応は、最終段階で起こる可能性がある。風邪の鼻炎には、類似した連続反応が見られる。つまり、最初はカタル性鼻汁であるが、その後化膿性鼻汁が見られるのである。このような顆粒球反応が閾値を超えた時、急性虫垂炎が出現する可能性がある。上述した発見に関連するが、虫垂と扁桃腺のリンパ球サブセット分布には類似性が見られることは大変興味深い。

本研究では、気圧と急性虫垂炎発症との関係に注目した。これらの関係を説明するため、自律神経系が組織における顆粒球およびリンパ球比率の変化と、緊密に関連している可能性を提案する。現在でも、病因不明の化膿性疾患は多い；この中には、潰瘍性大腸炎、胃切除（迷走神経切除を伴う）後の胆嚢炎、ストレス性胃炎（胃潰瘍）と肛門周囲膿瘍を含む。これら化膿性疾患における共通点は、組織への顆粒球浸潤であるが、明らかな細菌感染が見られる場合も見られない場合もある。高気圧、心身ストレス、手術後の迷走神経切断、アルコール過剰摂取、過労などの体調が原因で、交感神経緊張が出現し、顆粒球増多が出現する可能性がある（17, 24, 31, 35, 39）。顆粒球増多を誘導する生体生理により化膿性疾病が発症する可能性がある。

渡辺正子氏の原稿作成に深謝する。本研究は、文部科学省およびがん研究補助金による。

GRANULOCYTOSIS INDUCED BY INCREASING SYMPATHETIC NERVE ACTIVITY CONTRIBUTES TO THE INCIDENCE OF ACUTE APPENDICITIS

Minoru Fukuda[1], Tetsuya Moroda[2], Shinichi Toyabe[2], Tsuneo Iiai[2], Yasuyuki Kawachi[2], Hiromi Takahashi-Iwanaga[3], Toshihiko Iwanaga[3], Masahiko Okada[4] and Toru Abo[2]

[1]Sakamachi Hospital, Arakawamachi, Niigata 959-31, [2]Department of Immunology, [3]Third Department of Anatomy, and [4]Department of Diagnostics, Niigata University School of Medicine, Niigata 951, Japan

ABSTRACT

Since the incidence of acute appendicitis seems to vary with weather, we investigated the underlying mechanism. When 112 patients who had undergone appendectomy were classified into three groups according to atmospheric pressure at the time of onset, gangrenous cases (high infiltration of granulocytes) were much greater in frequency than catarrhal cases (no infiltration of granulocytes) at high pressure. At low pressure, the situation was the reverse. The variation of granulocytes and lymphocytes in the blood as related to atmospheric pressure and heart rate was examined in healthy donors. Granulocytosis was seen with increased sympathetic activity (high heart rate) at high pressure, whereas lymphocytosis was seen with increased parasympathetic activity (low heart rate) at low pressure. Taken together with the results from patients, in which gangrenous cases showed granulocytosis in the blood as well as in the appendix while catarrhal cases showed lymphocytosis in the blood and appendix, it is presumed that granulocytosis induced by increased sympathetic activity might be related to the onset of gangrenous appendicitis. Experimental results using human and mouse materials indicated that catecholamines induce granulocytosis via their adrenergic receptors. Even in gangrenous cases, bacteria were not detected in the vicinity of granulocytes in the appendix by electron microscopy. The present results seem to shed important light on the etiology of suppurative diseases.

Many clinicians have observed that the disease state in some patients deteriorates under the influence of weather (2, 3, 5–7, 32, 35, 39). However, it is difficult to determine the mechanism underlying the host defence system related to climatic factors. One of the authors in this study has noticed for the past 10 years that severe cases of appendicitis, including perforation, tend to occur at high atmospheric pressure accompanying fine weather. To determine whether this experience is more than just incidental, 112 cases of appendicitis were examined in terms of the type of appendicitis and atmospheric pressure at the onset of disease: Although appendicitis itself occurs under conditions of any atmospheric pressure, gangrenous cases of appendicitis occur much more frequently at the time of high atmospheric pressure.

We also focused our attention on the host defense system, especially on how the ratio of granulocytes and lymphocytes in the peripheral blood as well as in the appendix varies depending on atmospheric pressure in healthy donors and patients. It was demonstrated that granulocytosis occurred more frequently under high atmospheric pressure, whereas lymphocytosis occurred more frequently under low atmospheric pressure. A similar variation depending on atmospheric pressure was also seen in the blood and the appendix of patients.

When we are exposed to high atmospheric pressure which accompanies fine weather, sympathetic activity becomes high and this results in heightened feelings (9, 21, 35). Under such conditions, granulocytes carrying adrenergic receptors might be activated by the increased secretion of catecholamines (19, 25, 34). On the other hand, feelings of depression are more common (high parasympathetic activity) under conditions of bad weather accompanied by low atmospheric pressure (17, 24, 31, 35, 39), in which case there may be a rather decreased level of granulocytes.

In this paper, we propose the possibility that granulocytosis physiologically induced by high sympathetic nerve activity may be related to the high incidence in severe cases of acute appendicitis. Since the sympathetic nervous system is easily activated by other factors such as stress, heavy drinking of alcohol, and overwork (10, 18–20, 22), consequently induced granulocytosis might be responsible for many suppurative diseases, e.g., otitis media, periodontitis, gastritis, ulcerative colitis, liver abscess, periproctal abscess, ets. More importantly, even in the absence of bacteria, over-infiltrating granulocytes seem to destroy the surrounding tissues, possibly by their subsequent release of free radicals and superoxides.

MATERIALS AND METHODS

Patients and Healthy Individuals

One hundred and twelve patients with appendicitis, who had undergone appendectomy, were included in this study. They consisted of 58 men and 54 women, aged from 5 to 58 years, with the average age being 28.6 years. The appendicitis was classified into three groups, namely, catarrhal, phlegmonous, and gangrenous, by macroscopic and microscopic observations. The patients lived in Arakawa-machi, which is located about 50 km north of Niigata City. The survey period was from February 1992 to February 1994. As to the relationship between age of onset and the types of appendicitis, it was 24.1 years old for catarrhal-type, 25.6 years for phlegmonous-type, and 37.6 years for gangrenous-type appendicitis.

The onset of appendicitis was considered to occur when pain developed in the right lower abdomen or in the upper abdomen; atmospheric pressure was measured at this point. The subjects who were treated with antibiotics for more than 3 days before surgery were excluded from this study.

The data from normal individuals (n = 146), aged from 28 to 79 years (mean = 37.0), who visited the hospital for health checks were also used. They were classified into two groups according to the atmospheric pressure at the time when blood samples were taken: a group under conditions of high atmospheric pressure (mean = 1,019 hPa) (35.3 ± 9.4 years old) and a second group under conditions of low atmospheric pressure (mean = 1,009 hPa) (40.2 ± 10.2 years old).

Measurement of Atmospheric Pressure

The atmospheric pressure was measured by using an aneroid manometer and a thermohygrograph barometer placed in an instrument shelter.

Enumeration of the Numbers and Proportions of Granulocytes and Lymphocytes

Peripheral blood with anti-coagulants were sent to the Department of Diagnostics of Niigata University for enumeration of the ratio of leukocytes. The regular method used in the clinic was applied.

Preparation of Granulocytes

Heparinized blood was separated into mononuclear cells (MNC) and a mixture of granulocytes and erythrocytes by Ficoll-Isopaque gradient (1.077) centrifugation (37). One ml of the mixture was used and erythrocytes were disrupted by adding 9 ml of 0.17 M Tris buffer supplemented with 0.83% NH_4Cl. After being washed twice with RPMI1640 medium supplemented with 10% heat-inactivated FCS, granulocytes were suspended in the medium.

Cell Preparation from the Appendix for Cell Analysis

MNC were isolated from the appendix to characterize them by means of a cell analyzer (38). To prepare MNC, the samples were cut into small pieces with scissors and then passed through 200-gauge stainless steel mesh. Cell pellets were suspended in the medium. MNC were finally isolated by Ficoll-Isopaque gradient (1.077) centrifugation.

Phenotyping of Cells by Flow Cytometry

MNC obtained from the appendix were incubated with FITC-, PE-, or Per-CP-labelled mAbs (16). These mAbs were CD3 (NU-T3; Nichirei, Tokyo, Japan), CD8 (NU-Ts/c; Nichirei), CD4 (Leu-3a), CD56 (Leu-19), TCR $\alpha\beta$ (TCR-1) (Becton-Dickin-

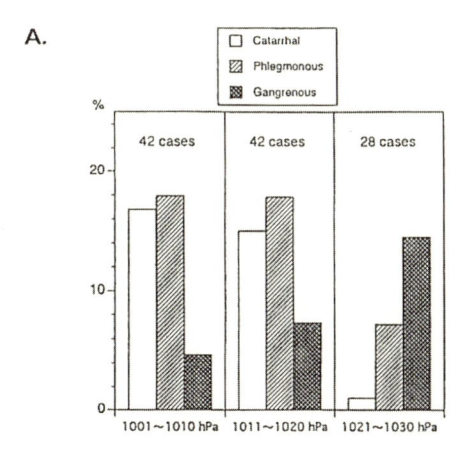

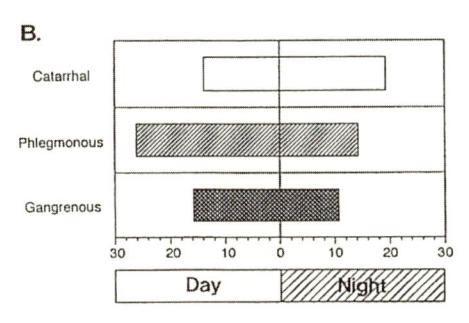

Fig. 1 Variation of the incidence of catarrhal, phlegmonous, and gangrenous types of appendicitis with atmospheric pressure (A) and time of day (B). The incidence of 112 cases of acute appendicitis was studied in terms of atmospheric pressure and time of day. When attention was focused on the gangrenous type, the incidence was found to be concentrated during high atmospheric pressure and daytime. In the case of catarrhal type, the situation was the reverse. The incidence is represented as the percentages (100% = total 112 cases). Daytime is 8:00 a.m. to 8:00 p.m. and night is 8:00 p.m. to 8:00 a.m.

son, Mountain View, CA), and TCR γδ (TCR δ 1) (T Cell Sciences, Cambridge, MA) (2). Two-color flow cytometric analysis was performed using a fluorescence-activated cell analyser (FACScan; Becton-Dickinson). Ten thousand cells were analysed.

Electron Microscopy

Specimens were quickly fixed in 3% gultaraldehyde, followed by postfixation in 1% OsO_4 (15). They were embedded in Epon 812, and ultrathin sections were examined with a JEOL 100B electron microscope (JEOL, Peabody, MA).

Measurement of Ca^{2+} Influx

Fluo-3-acetoxymethy ester (Fluo-3-AM), pluronic F-127, formyl-methionyl-leucyl-phenylalanine (fMLP) and ionomycin were purchased from Sigma, St. Louis, MO (26, 33). Human granulocytes (2×10^6 cells) were labelled with fluo-3 (final concentration, $2\,\mu M$) containing 3% pluronic F-127 and 18% DMSO by incubating them in subdued light for 30 min at 37°C and washed twice before analysis. Thereafter, cells were analyzed by FACS. Cells were preincubated at 37°C in the dark for 10 min. After the basal fluorescence was measured, cells were stimulated with fMLP, ionomycin, or epinephrine.

Epinephrine Injection into Mice and Enumeration of Granulocytes

To determine whether our hypothesis (i.e., increasing sympathetic activity induces granulocytosis) is valid, the following mouse study was attempted. By using a perfusion pump (Model 1007D, Alza, Palo Alto, CA), a continuous injection of epinephrine was carried out for 1 week (0.2 mg/mouse/week). After treatment, mice were sacrified and MNC were isolated from various immune organs. Immunofluorescence staining for granulocytes was performed by using FITC-conjugated anti-granulocyte mAb (PharMingen, San Diego, CA).

Statistical Analysis

The data were analyzed by the Annova and Duncan method with a level of significance of 5%. The rhythmicity in the circadian variations of granulocytes and lymphocytes was analyzed by the Rogers' method.

RESULTS

High Incidence of Gangrenous Type in Acute Appendicitis under High Atmospheric Pressure

One hundred and twelve patients with acute appendicitis, who underwent appendectomy, were divided into three groups according to the atmospheric pressure under which they had noticed the onset of disease (Fig. 1A). The number of patients in each group was 42 patients (38%) in the 1,001 to 1,010 hPa group, 42 patients (38%) in 1,011 to 1,020 hPa

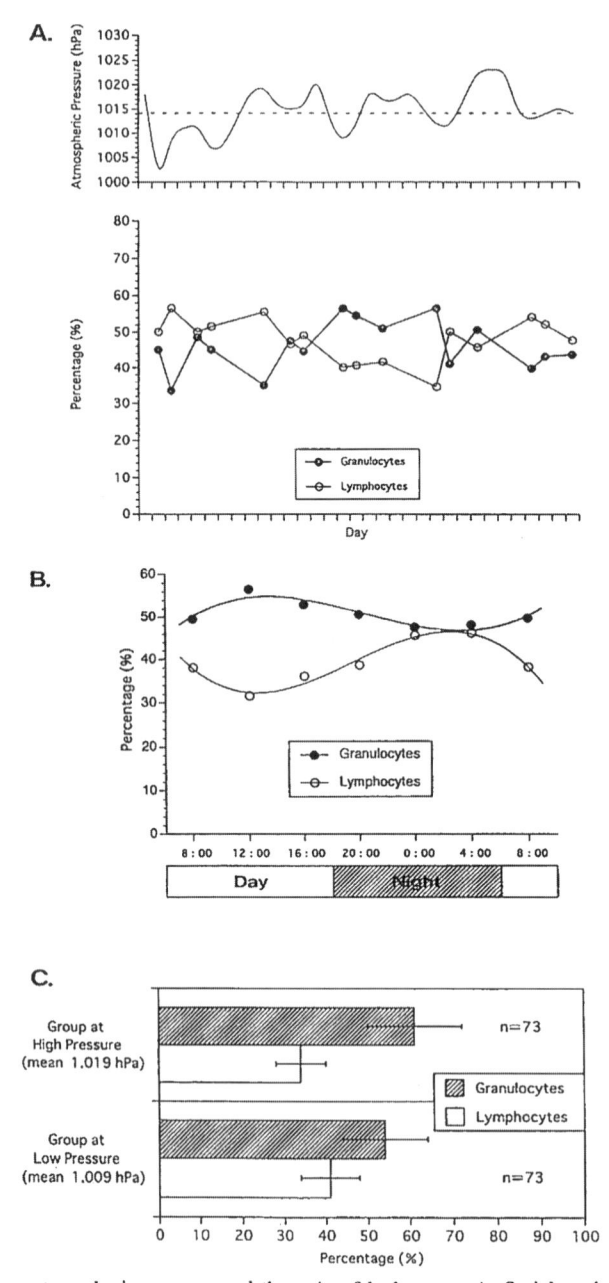

Fig. 2 Relationship between atmospheric pressure and the ratio of leukocytes. A: Serial study for one month in a healthy subject. B: Circadian rhythm in the ratio of leukocytes in a healthy subject. C: Data from normal individuals on the ratio of leukocytes at high atmospheric pressure and at low atmospheric pressure. A healthy subject (male, 47 years old) was examined as to the ratio of granulocytes and lymphocytes in the blood. The total number of leukocytes in this subject ranged from 6,000 to 6,500/mm^3 during this period, January 1995 to February 1995. Data from normal individuals (n = 146) who visited the hospital for health checks were also used. They were classified into 2 groups according to the atmospheric pressure at which their bloods were taken.

group, and 28 patients (23%) in 1,021 to 1,030 hPa group. When attention was focused on the type of appendicitis, there was a tendency for gangrenous-type appendicitis to increase in parallel with the increase in atmospheric pressure while catarrhal-type appendicitis decreased inversely. The variation of phlegmonous-type appendicitis decreased under conditions of high pressure.

Even if the type of acute appendicitis varied under the influence of atmospheric pressure, it is unlikely that atmospheric pressure is the only factor involved. In this regard, the types of appendicitis were subdivided as to another factor, daytime or night (Fig. 1B). It appeared that the incidence of catarrhal-type appendicitis was relatively higher at night while the phlegmonous and gangrenous types (including cases of perforation) were higher in the daytime.

One tends to feel energetic under conditions of high atmospheric pressure accompanying fine weather. In contrast, under low pressure accompanying bad weather, one tends to feel inactive or depressed. These feelings reflect our physical conditions which are regulated by the autonomic nervous system, such as sympathetic nerve dominance or parasympathetic nerve dominance. Namely, physical conditions are influenced by daytime (sympathetic dominance) and night (parasympathetic dominance), as well as under the influence of weather.

Variation in the Ratio of Leukocytes in Healthy Donors by Atmospheric Pressure

To determine the mechanism underlying the relationship between the atmospheric pressure and the incidence of diseases, we then investigated whether the ratio of granulocytes and lymphocytes varied as a function of atmospheric pessure (Fig. 2A). The working hypothesis is that gangrenous-type appendicitis (high infiltration of granulocytes into the appendix) is accompanied by physiological granulocytosis, and that one of the factors inducing this might be atmospheric pressure. A healthy subject was analyzed as to the ratio of granulocytes and lymphocytes for one month. The atmospheric pressure and the ratio of leukocytes in the blood are depicted in the figure. Granulocytosis was induced at high pressure while lymphocytosis was induced at low pressure (the coincidence is approximately 70%). It was also confirmed that heart rates increased at high pressure (63.0 ± 3.2/min) but decreased at low pressure (61.0 ± 2.7/min) ($P < 0.05$). Since the ratio of leukocytes and heart rate

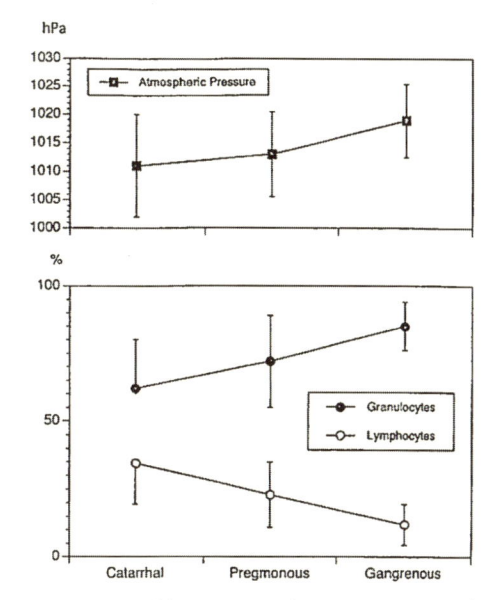

Fig. 3 Relationship among three parameters, i.e., atmospheric pressure, the ratio of leukocytes, and the types of acute appendicitis. One hundred and twelve cases of appendicitis were classified into three groups, i.e., catarrhal (n = 35), phlegmonous (n = 47) and gangrenous types (n = 30), and the atmospheric pressure and the ratio of granulocytes and lymphocytes at the onset of disease are depicted. When these factors between the catarrhal and gangrenous types were statistically analyzed by the Annova and Duncan methods, the differences were shown to be significant ($P < 0.01$).

varies with circardican rhythm, the analysis was perfomed at 11 00 a.m. every day.

If our hypothesis, namely, increasing sympathetic nervous system activity induces granulocytosis, is true, a simpler experiment would show variation in the ratio of leukocytes in the blood. In this regard, we examined such variation during one day in the same subject as above (Fig. 2B). It was demonstrated that granulocytosis occurred in the daytime (increasing sympathetic activity) while lymphocytosis was seen at night (increasing parasympathetic activity). These variations of granulocytes and lymphocytes were statistically significant ($P < 0.0001$). In other words, the ratio of leukocytes varies under the influence of multiple factors other than atmospheric pressure.

To determine more definitely the relationship between atmospheric pressure and the ratio of blood leukocytes, data from normal individuals (n

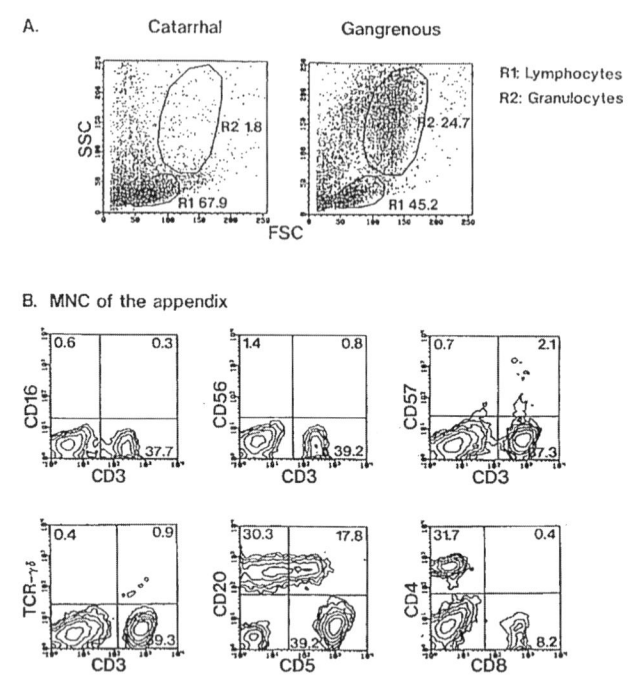

Fig. 4 Characterization of MNC isolated from the appendix by cell analyzer. A: Light scatter of MNC for the identification of granulocytes and lymphocytes. B: Lymphocyte markers on MNC for the identification of T, B and NK cells. Numbers in the figure indicate the positive cells in corresponding areas. It was confirmed that the gangrenous type, as determined by pathological criteria, eventually contained many granulocytes. MNC in the appendix (Region 1 of the gangrenous case) displayed a unique distribution of lymphocytes subsets, showing an abundance of $\alpha\beta$T cells and CD5$^+$B cells.

= 146) were used (Fig. 2C). The percentages of granulocytes in subjects whose blood was taken under conditions of high atmospheric pressure were significantly higher than those of subjects whose blood was taken at low pressure ($P < 0.01$), while the percentages of lymphocytes in the blood were completely the reverse ($P < 0.01$).

Parallel Increase of Granulocytes in the Blood with Those in the Tissue of Patients with Gangrenous Appendicitis

Since granulocytosis is induced in the blood of healthy donors at high atmospheric pressure, it is speculated that such granulocytosis is also induced in the tissue of patients and results in gangrenous appendicitis. The gangrenous type is primarily determined by the criterion of the infiltration of granulocytes into the appendix. The ratio of leukocytes at the onset of disease is depicted according to the type of appendicitis in Fig. 3. It was clearly demonstrated that there was a higher level of granulocytes in the blood in cases of the gangrenous type. In contrast, in the catarrhal type (inflammation of only lymphocytes), there was a high level of lymphocytes in the blood. In other words, the levels of granulocytes and lymphocytes between the blood and the tissue are co-regulated.

Characterization of Leukocytes Isolated from the Appendix of Patients by Cell Analyzer

The types of catarrhal, phlegmonous, and gangrenous appendicitis were determined in light

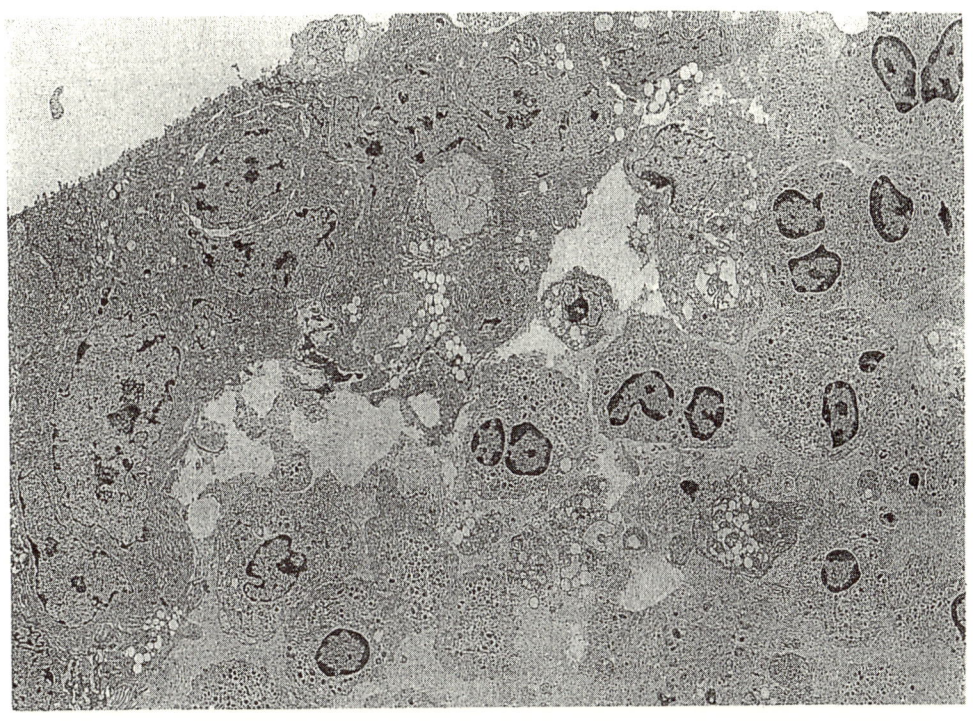

Fig. 5 Electron microscopy of the appendix isolated from the gangrenous type of acute appendicitis (× 2,000). Many granulocytes infiltrated and destroyed the tissue. However, we did not detect any bacteria in the tissue nor in the cytoplasma of granulocytes. This raises the possibility that granulocytes damage the tissue (e.g., by their production of free radicals and superoxides) without apparent bacterial infection.

microscopic study by pathologists. This identification was also confirmed by means of a cell analyzer. Representative cases of catarrhal and gangrenous appendicitis are shown in Fig. 4. The existence of only a few granulocytes (1.8%) in the case of catarrhal appendicitis and the existence of numerous granulocytes (24.7%) in the case of gangrenous appendicitis were demonstrated by light scatter analysis (see Region 2). The surface phenotype of MNC (Region 1), which were derived from the gangrenous case of Fig. 4A, was characterized after staining with corresponding mAbs (Fig. 4B). NK cells identified with CD16, CD56, and CD57 were extremely few (<2.0%), whereas T cells identified with CD3 were substantial (39%). All T cells were $\alpha\beta$ T cells, showing a predominance of CD4$^+$ cells (31.7%). An interesting result was that the majority of lymphocytes in the appendix were B cells, and a large proportion (37%) of such B cells were CD5$^+$ B cells which are known to produce autoantibodies (37). These results on lymphocytes were essentially the same, irrespective of infiltration levels of granulocytes. The data from these cases of appendicitis are unique because MNC isolated from the small and large intestines comprise a large proportion of $\gamma\delta$ T cells (23). Rather, the distribution pattern of lymphocyte subsets in the appendix is similar to that of the tonsil (our unpublished observation).

Absence of Bacteria in the Tissue of Gangrenous Cases

In this experiment, some samples of phlegmonous and gangrenous appendices were exmained by electron microscopy. A typical case of gangrenous appendicitis is represented (Fig. 5). Many granulocytes infiltrated the site under epithelia of the appendix and destroyed the tissue. Surprisingly, we were unable to detect any bacteria in the vicinity of

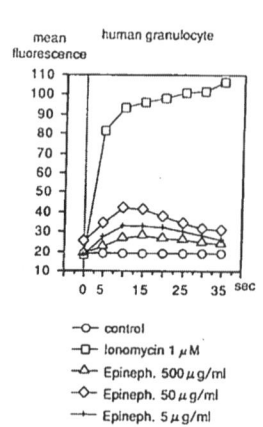

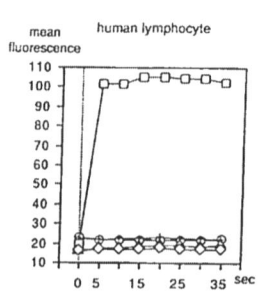

Fig. 6 Epinephrine induces an influx of Ca^{2+} for granulocytes. Granulocytes and lymphocytes were isolated from human peripheral blood. Epinephrine induced an influx of Ca^{2+} for granulocytes but not for lymphocytes. A positive control, ionomycin, induced an influx of Ca^{2+} for both granulocytes and lymphocytes. Representative results from three experiments are depicted.

granulocytes nor in the cytoplasma of granulocytes. This raises the possibility that activated granulocytes destroy the tissue without apparent participation of bacterial infection.

Catecholamines Induce Ca^{2+} Influx of Granulocytes, but not Lymphocytes

A common feature underlying the conditions of high atmospheric pressure and daytime is high physical activity. Such conditions may be induced by increased activity of the sympathetic nervous system. To determine whether increased sympathetic activity activates granulocytes, in vitro stimulation with epinephrine of either human granulocytes or lymphocytes isolated from the blood was carried out (Fig. 6). The influx of Ca^{2+} was used as an indicator of their activation. Although a positive control, ionomycin (1 μM), induced an influx of Ca^{2+} for both granulocytes and lymphocytes, epinephrine (5 to 50 μg/ml) induced an influx of Ca^{2+} only for granulocytes.

A Continuous Injection of Epinephrine Induces Granulocytosis in Mice

To directly prove whether catecholamines induce granulocytosis, we conducted a mouse study in which epinephrine (0.2 mg/mouse/week) was injected by a perfusion pump (Fig. 7). Our preliminary studies determined that this dose would not kill mice but would induce a change in leukocyte counts (data not shown). It was demonstrated that a continuous injection of epinephrine eventually induced granulocytosis in all organs tested.

DISCUSSION

We investigated the mechanism underlying external environments, physical condition and the onset of disease, in patients with acute appendicitis. One important factor, namely, variation in the ratio of granulocytes and lymphocytes was hypothesized to be involved in the above mechanism. This might be a key factor connecting physical condition with the onset of disease. The simplest example for this concept is as follows: high atmospheric pressure → sympathetic nerve dominance → granulocytosis → high incidence of the onset of suppurative diseases. Although many clinicians have experienced that the incidence of the onset of some diseases is influenced by the weather (2, 3, 5–7, 32, 35, 39), a comprehensive scheme showing the relationship of the factors involved has not been proposed. If the ratio of granulocytes and lymphocytes, which may be influenced by physical conditions (i.e. the activity state of the autonomic nervous system) is involved, light is shed on the relationship between

	Control	Epinephrine
Peripheral Blood	19.0	35.2
Spleen	9.6	16.4

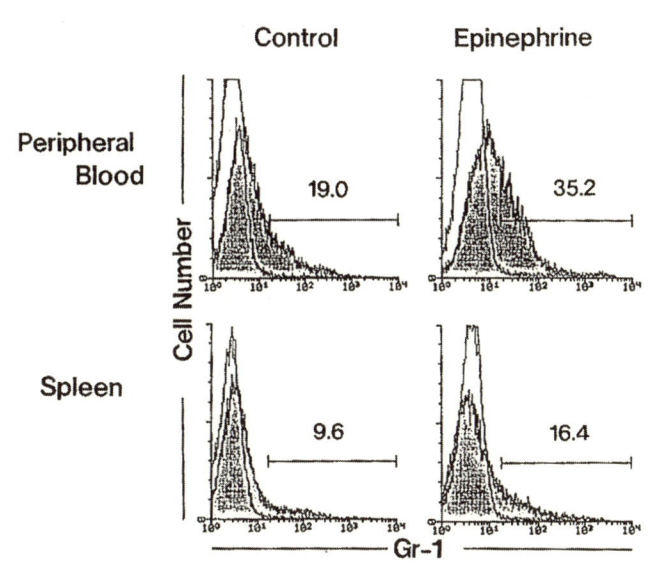

Fig. 7 A continuous injection of epinephrine by a perfusion pump into mice induced granulocytosis in various organs, including the blood and spleen. To prove whether our hypothesis (a sympathetic dominance induces granulocytosis) makes sense or not, mice were injected with epinephrine for 1 week (0.2 mg/mouse/week) and the level of granulocytes was examined in various organs. In tested organs, the levels of granulocytes increased. At this time, the absolute number of granulocytes also increased in the spleen, showing 40% splenomegaly 1 week after treatment. A thin line indicates a negative control with FITC-conjugated unrelated mAb.

the external environment and the incidence of the onset of disease.

When the appendectomized patients were divided into three groups according to levels of granulocyte infiltration into the appendix, levels of granulocytes in the blood were found to vary in parallel with those in the tissue. For example, patients with gangrenous type appendicitis showed prominent ganulocytosis and lymphocytopenia in the blood. It is presumed that the granulocytosis induced by sympathetic activity may be a generalized phenomenon in the body. The pathological determination of the type of appendicitis was confirmed by the cell analysis in this study.

Initially, to study the mechanism underlying atmospheric pressure and the onset of appendicitis, we investigated whether variation of atmospheric pressure affects the levels of granulocytes and lymphocytes in the blood of both patients and healthy individuals. One stimulus to the present study was the earlier studies by Saito (27-30), in which sympathetic nerve strain was reported to induce granulocytosis and, inversely, parasympathetic nerve strain was found to induce lymphocytosis. It is well-established that granulocytosis is prevalent in the daytime (i.e., sympathetic dominance) whereas lymphocytosis is prevalent at night (i.e., parasympathetic dominance (1, 4, 8). It is also a common observation that people feel more energetic under conditions of high atmospheric pressure accompanying fine weather, and feel more lethargic or even depressed under conditions of low atmospheric pressure (9, 17, 24, 25, 31, 35).

Granulocytosis appeared under conditions of high atmospheric pressure, while lymphocytosis under low atmospheric pressure (Fig. 2). However, the significance of these findings is limited, though not negligible (9), since many factors other than atmospheric pressure are related to the regulation of physical conditions.

A question of interest is how sympathetic nervous system dominance induces granulocytosis. In this regard, we are reminded of adrenergic receptors on granulocytes (19, 25). Although many investigators have reported the existence of such receptors, their physiological significance has remained unclear. Some studies have shown the suppressive effects of catecholamines on the exocytosis of enzymes in granulocytes and macrophages *in vitro* (12–14). In the present study, influx of Ca^{2+} into human granulocytes was found to be induced by epinephrine.

We injected epinephrine into mice by a perfusion pump and found that the injection resulted in granulocytosis in both the blood and spleen. Thymic atrophy and a subsequent cytopenia of T cells were prominent at this time (data not shown). Similar results were previously reported (11). These lines of investigation (i.e., catecholamine levels and the host defense system) appear to be important in future studies. Taken together with the present human and mouse study, sympathetic activity seems to increase the levels of granulocytes in the entire body.

The next question is how the induced granulocytosis is associated with the subsequent onset of disease. On examining the sites of granulocyte-infiltration in the appendices in several cases of gangrenous appendicitis, we found that many arterioles were dilated and that massive infiltration of granulocytes (mainly neutrophils) occurred at such sites (Fig. 5). Surprisingly, no bacteria were found around granulocytes and in the cytoplasma of granulocytes. It can be speculated that activated, apoptotic granulocytes disrupt the tissue, e.g., epithelia of the appendix. It has recently been shown that tumor necrosis factor (TNF), produced mainly in macrophages (TNFα) and lymphocytes (TNFβ), triggers a release of free radicals and superoxides from the granulocytes (36, 40). Granulocytes can damage the tissue by these free radicals and superoxides, if the activation is beyond the threshold.

In the electron micrographs of appendicitis tissue samples, we sometimes encountered adenovirus, the most common virus for the common cold, in the epithelia of the appendix (data not shown). It is presumed that some cases of appendicitis are induced by viral infection. If this is the case, the initial response may be catarrhal due to the response of lymphocytes. The response of granulocytes would occur at a final stage. Similar serial responses are seen in rhinitis of the common cold, with an initial catarrhal nasal discharge and subsequent purulent nasal discharge in a later stage. When such granulocytic response is beyond the threshold, acute appendicitis may be induced. The similarity in the distribution of lymphocyte subsets between the appendix and the tonsil is very interesting in relation to the above notion.

In the present study, our attention was focused on the relationship between atmospheric pressure and the onset of acute appendicitis. To explain the relationship of these factors, we propose the possibility that the autonomic nervous system is closely related to the changes in the ratio of granulocytes and lymphocytes in the tissue. Even to date, there are many suppurative diseases whose etiology remains unknown; these include ulcerative colitis, cholecystitis after gasterectomy (accompanying vagotomy), gastritis (and gastric ulcer) by stress, and periproctal abscess. A common feature of these suppurative diseases is granulocyte-infiltration into the tissues with or without apparent bacterial infection. Some physical conditions such as high atmospheric pressure, mental and physical stresses, vagotomy after surgery, heavy consumption of alcohol, over-exercise, etc., may induce sympathetic nerve dominance (17, 24, 31, 35, 39), and result in granulocytosis. It is likely that physiologically induced granulocytosis contributes to the incidence of suppurative diseases.

We wish to thank Mrs Masako Watanabe for her help in preparing the manuscript. This work was supported in part by a grant-in-aid for cancer research from the Ministry of Education, Science and Culture, Japan.

Receive 4 January 1996; and accepted 2 February 1996

REFERENCES

1. ABO T., KAWATE T., ITOH K. and KUMAGAI K. (1981) Studies on the bioperiodicity of immune respose I. Circadian rhythms of human T, B, and K cell traffic in the peripheral blood. *J. Immunol.* **126**, 1360–1363
2. ANDERSON T. W. and LE RICHE W. H. (1970) Cold weather and myocardial infraction. *Lancet* I, 291–296
3. BAKER-BLOCKER A. (1970) Winter weather and cardiovascular mortality in Minneapolis-St. Paul. *Amer. J. Public Health* **72**, 261–265
4. CARTER J. B., BARR G. D., LEVIN A. S., BYERS V. S., PONCE B., FUDENBERG H. H. and GERMAN D. F. (1975) Standardization of tissue culture conditions for spontaneous thymidine-2-^{14}C incorporation by unstimulated normal human peripheral lymphocytes: Circadian rhythm of DNA synthesis. *J. Allerg. Clin. Immunol.* **56**, 191–205
5. DEQUEKER J. and WUESTENREAD L. (1986) The effect of biometerological factors on Ritchie articular index and pain in rheumatoid arthritis. *Scand. J. Rheumatol.* **15**, 280–284
6. DRISCOLL D. M. (1971) The relationship between weather

and mortality in ten major metropolitan area in the United States. *Int. J. Biomet.* **15**, 23–29
7. EASTWOOD M. R. and PEACOCKE J. (1976) Seasonal patterns of suicide, depression and electroconvulsive therapy. *Brit. J. Psychiat.* **129**, 472–475
8. ELMADJIAN F. and PINCUS G. (1946) A study of the diurnal variations in circulating lymphocytes in normal and psychotic subjects. *J. Clin. Endocrinol.* **6**, 287–294
9. FECHTALI T., ABRAINI J. H., KRIEM B. and ROSTAIN J. C. (1994) Pressure increases de novo synthesized striatal dopamine release in free-moving rats. *Neuroreport* **5**, 725–728
10. GRASSI G. M., SOMERS V. K., RENK W. S., ABBOUD F. M. and MARK A. L. (1989) Effects of alcohol intake on blood pressure and sympathetic nerve activity in normotensive humans: a preliminary report. *J. Hypertention* **7**, Suppl. 6, S20–S21
11. HENSON E. C. and BRUNSON J. G. (1969) Prevention of experimental allergic encephalomyelitis by combination of eipnephrine and a phenothiazine derivative, propiomazine. *Proc. Soc. Exp. Biol. Med.* **131**, 752–755
12. HIGGINS T. J. and DAVID J. R. (1976) Effect of isoproterenol and aminophylline on cyclic AMP levels of guinea pig macrophages. *Cell. Immunol.* **27**, 1–10
13. IGNARRO L. J. and COLOMBO C. (1973) Enzyme release from polymorphonuclear leukocyte lysosomes: regulation by autonomic durgs and cyclic nucleotides. *Science* **180**, 1181–1183
14. IGNARRO L. J., LINT T. F. and GEORGE W. J. (1974) Hormonal control of lysosomal enzyme release from human neutrophils. Effects of autonomic agents on enzyme release, phagocytosis, and cyclic nucleotide levels. *J. Exp. Med.* **139**, 1395–1414
15. IIAI T., WATANABE H., IWAMOTO T., NAKASHIMA I. and ABO T. (1994) Predominant activation of extrathymic T cells during melanoma development of metallothionein/ret transgenic mice. *Cell. Immunol.* **153**, 412–427
16. IIAI T., WATANABE H., SEKI S., SUGIURA K., HIROKAWA K., UTSUYAMA M., TAKAHASHI-IWANAGA H., IWANAGA T., OHTSUKA T. and ABO T. (1992) Ontogeny and development of extrathymic T cells in mouse liver. *Immunology* **77**, 556–563
17. INOUE H., INOUE C., OKAYAMA M., SEKIZAWA K., HIDA W. and TAKISHIMA T. (1989) Breathing 30 per cent oxygen attenuates bronchial responsiveness to methacholine in asthmatic patients. *Eur. Resp. J.* **2**, 506–512
18. IRELAND M. A., VANDONGEN R., DAVIDSON L., BEILIN L. J. and ROUSE I. L. (1984) Acute effects of moderate alcohol consumption on blood pressure and plasma catecholamines. *Clin. Sci.* **66**, 643–648
19. LANDMANN R. M. A., MULLER F. B., PERINI C. H., WESP M, ERNE P. and BUHLER F. R. (1984) Changes of immunoregulatory cells induced by psychological and physical stress: relatioship to plasma catecholamines. *Clin. Exp. Immunol.* **58**, 127–135
20. MAIN J. and THOMAS T. (1990) Ethanol predominantly alters sodium influx in human leucocytes. *Clin. Sci.* **78**, 235–238
21. MYERS D. H. and DAVIES P. (1978) The seasonal incidence of mania and its relatioship to climatic variables. *Psychol. Med.* **8**, 433–440
22. OGAWA M., IIAI T., HIRAHARA H., TOMIYAMA K., KAWACHI Y., WATANABE H., SHIMOZI T. and ABO T. (1993) Immunologic state induced by starvation: Suppression of intrathymic T-cell differentiation but relative resistance of extrathymic T-cell differentiation. *Acta Med. Biol.* **41**, 177–187
23. OHTSUKA K., IIAI T., WATANABE H., TANAKA T., MIYASAKA M., SATO K., ASAKURA H. and ABO T. (1994) Similarities and differences between extrathymic T cells residing in mouse liver and intestine. *Cell. Immunol.* **153**, 52–66
24. OKABE S., HIDA W., KIKUCHI Y., KUROSAWA H., MIDORIKAWA J., CHONAN T., TAKISHIMA T. and SHIRATO K. (1993) Upper airway muscle activity during sustained hypoxia in awake humans. *J. Appl. Physiol.* **75**, 1552–1558
25. PANOSIAN J. O. and MARINETTI G. V. (1983) α_2-Adrenergic receptors in human polymorphonuclear leukocyte membranes. *Biochem. Pharmacol.* **32**, 2243–2247
26. ROTNES J. S., AAS V. and IVERSEN J. G. (1994) Interferongamma modulates cytosolic free calcium in human neutrophilic granulocytes. *Eur. J. Haematol.* **53**, 65–73
27. SAITO A. (1970) Autoadaptation mechanism of the human body. *Tohoku J. Exp. Med.* **102**, 289–312
28. SAITO A. (1971) Acute adaptational disturbances due to the imbalance of the autonomic nervous system. *Tohoku J. Exp. Med.* **103**, 71–92
29. SAITO A. (1971) Chronic adaptational disturbances due to the imbalance of the autonomic nervous system. *Tohoku J. Exp. Med.* **103**, 93–114
30. SAITO A. (1971) Relationship between acute and chronic diseases observed from the viewpoint of the autonomic nervous system. *Tohoku J. Exp. Med.* **103**, 285–302
31. SEKIZAWA K., YANAI M., SAKURAI M., KIKUCHI R., SASAKI H. and TAKISHIMA T. (1985) Effect of hypoxia on bronchial reactivity in dogs. *Bull. Eur. Physiopathol. Respir.* **21**, 485–489
32. SIBLEY J. T. (1985) Weather and arthritis symptoms. *J. Rheumatol.* **12**, 707–710
33. SOMMER F., BISCHOF S., ROLLINGHOFF M. and LOHOFF M. (1994) Demonstration of organic anion transport in T lymphocytes. L-lactate and fluo-3 are target molecules. *J. Immunol.* **153**, 3523–3532
34. SPENGLER R. N., ALLEN R. M., REMICK D. G., STRIETER R. M. and KUNKE S. L. (1990) Stimulation of α-adrenergic receptor augments the production of macrophage-derived tumor necrosis factor. *J. Immunol.* **145**, 1430–1434
35. SYMONDS R. L. and WILLIAMS P. (1976) Seasonal variation in the incidence of mania. *Brit. J. Psychiat.* **129**, 45–48
36. TAKEDA Y., WATANABE H., YONEHARA S., YAMASHITA T., SAITO S. and SENDO F. (1993) Rapid acceleration of neutrophil apoptosis by tumor necrosis factor-α. *Int. Immunol.* **5**, 691–694
37. TSUCHIDA M., HASHIMOTO M., ABO T., MIYAMURA H., HIRANO T. and EGUCHI S. (1993) CD5$^+$B cells in the thymus of patients with myasthenia gravis. *Biomedical Res.* **14**, 19–25
38. WATANABE H., OHTSUKA K., KIMURA M., IKARASHI Y., OHMORI K., KUSUMI A., OHTEKI T., SEKI S. and ABO T. (1992) Details of an isolation method for hepatic lymphocytes in mice. *J. Immunol. Method* **146**, 145–154
39. WEHR T. A., SACK D. A. and ROSENTHAL N. E. (1987) Seasonal affective disorder with summer depression and winter hypomania. *Amer. J. Psychiat.* **144**, 1602–1603
40. YUO A., KITAGAWA S., SUZUKI I., URABE A., OKABE T., SAITO M. and TAKAKU F. (1989) Tumor necrosis factor as an activator of human granulocytes. Potentiation of the metabolisms triggered by the Ca^{2+}-mobilizing agonists. *J. Immunol.* **142**, 1678–1684

C-KIT+ STEM CELLS AND THYMOCYTE PRECURSORS IN THE LIVERS OF ADULT MICE

成体マウス肝臓におけるc-kit+幹細胞と
胸腺前駆細胞

The Journal of Experimental Medicine, 184: 987-693, 1996

chapter 5

c-kit⁺ Stem Cells and Thymocyte Precursors in the Livers of Adult Mice

成体マウス肝臓におけるc-kit⁺幹細胞と胸腺前駆細胞

By Hisami Watanabe,* Chikako Miyaji,* Shuhji Seki,*[±] and Toru Abo*

【要約】

　成体マウスの肝臓にはc-kit⁺幹細胞が存在し、胸腺細胞、複数系統の細胞や骨髄（BM）幹細胞を再構築できる。BALB/cマウスの肝単核球 (MNC)(1×10^7)、あるいは肝c-kit⁺細胞（5×10^4）をCB17/-SCIDマウス（4グレイ（Gy）照射）に移植した場合、1週間以内にDP胸腺細胞が出現した。しかし、骨髄細胞または骨髄c-kit⁺細胞を移植した場合、DP胸腺細胞出現まで2週間を要した。さらに、BALB/cマウスの肝単核球移植により救済されたSCIDマウスの骨髄細胞または肝単核球（いずれもB細胞を排除）は、他の放射線照射SCIDマウスの胸腺とB細胞を再構築した。C57BL/6(B6)マウスの骨髄細胞と肝単核球における$CD3^-IL\text{-}2R\beta^-$集団は、照射したB6 SCIDマウスの胸腺の再構築前に、肝臓においてTCR^{int}細胞（胸腺外分化T細胞；大部分は$NK1.1^-$）を産生できた。さらに、B6 Ly 5.1マウスの肝c-kit⁺細胞を放射線照射B6 SCID(Ly5.2)マウスに移植すると、肝c-kit⁺細胞が骨髄および赤血球系細胞を再構築できることが明らかになった。これら結果が強く示唆するのは、肝臓は多分化能幹細胞を有し、成人においても重要な造血臓器の役目を果たすことである。

髄細胞は、c-kit⁺幹細胞を含み (1, 2) 複数の白血球系統を発生させることができる。マウス骨髄（BM）[1]のT細胞前駆細胞は胸腺へ移動し、成熟胸腺細胞に分化する；ほとんどの末梢T細胞はこのようにして生まれる。しかし、最近、T細胞が胸腺外において分化することが明らかになった。胸腺外分化の場は腸であると報告した研究グループもあるが (3-7)、著者らは肝臓でも分化が起こる可能性があることを明らかにした (8-13)。胸腺外分化した肝臓の$\alpha\beta$T細胞は、$NK1.1^+$または$NK1.1^-$T細胞（中程度のTCRを発現している）である

(13)。しかし、肝臓に造血前駆細胞が存在するか否かは不明であった。本研究では、正常マウスの肝単核球（MNC）をSCIDマウスに移植し、どのように移動し、再配置されるか検証した。そして、正常マウス（成体）の肝単核球を移植すると、非照射SCIDマウスにおいてダブル・ポジティブ（DP）胸腺細胞が出現すると同時に胸腺が一時的に再構築されることが明らかになった。SCIDマウスでは、TCR遺伝子も免疫グロブリン遺伝子も再構成は起こらない (14)。故にSCIDマウスは、放射線骨髄キメラによるある細胞集団にTとB細胞を再構築さ

---

[1] 本論文における略語；B6, C57BL/6；BM, 骨髄；DP, ダブルポジティブ；NMC, 単核球

chapter 5

せる能力があるか検証を行うのに適切なモデルである。さらに、B6-Ly5.1マウス（15）を用いて、肝c-kit$^+$細胞が骨髄や赤血球系の細胞を再構築できるか検証可能であった。本研究で明らかになったのは成体正常マウスの肝単核球にはc-kit$^+$細胞が存在すること、また、これを放射線照射SCIDマウスに移植すると胸腺細胞、複数の系統細胞および骨髄幹細胞を再構築できることである。

材料と方法

マウス

CB17/-SCIDマウス（H-2^d）、BALB/cマウス（H-2^d）およびC57BL/6マウス（H-2^b）（全て6-8週齢，雄）を（株）クレア・ジャパン（東京，日本）より購入した。C57BL/6-SCID（H-2^b）は、公益財団法人実験動物中央研究所（神奈川，日本）より購入した。C57BL/6-Ly5.1(B6-Ly5.1,H-2^b)マウスは岸原健二博士（九州大学生体防御医学研究所，福岡，日本）から寄与された。マウスは全て特定病原体未感染（SPF）環境下で飼育した。

細胞分離

マウス鎖骨下動脈および静脈より脱血を行い、肝臓と脾臓を摘出した。肝臓は200ゲージステンレススチールメッシュで濾し、一回洗浄した。細胞塊を、溶血用緩衝液（155mM NH$_4$Cl, 10mM KHCO$_3$, 1mM EDTA, 170mM Tris, PH7.3）で処理した。定法に従い肝単核球を分離した（16, 17）。略述すると、肝臓をステンレススチールメッシュで濾して、5mM Hepesおよび2% FCSを添加したEagle's MEM培養液に懸濁させた。洗浄後、細胞を100 U/mlヘパリン添加したPercoll溶液（30-35%）に再懸濁させ、室温で遠心分離を行った（2,000rpm, 15分間）。Percoll溶液の適切な濃度は、各研究室で30-35%間に設定する必要がある。細胞塊を溶血用緩衝液に再懸濁させ、培養液で二回洗浄した。骨髄細胞を、培養液で大腿骨内を洗浄して採取した。細胞懸濁液を、200-ゲージ ナイロンメッシュで濾過して組織片を除去した。胸腺を200-ゲージ スチールメッシュで濾過して胸腺細胞を採取した。溶血後の末梢血細胞を使用した。

モノクロナール抗体、フローサイトメトリー解析および細胞純化

抗CD4（RM4-5）、抗CD8（53-6.7）、抗CD3（145-2C11）、抗IL-2Rβ鎖（TM-β1）、抗NK1.1（PK136）、抗B220（RA3-6B2）、抗Mac-1（M1/70）、抗マウスIgM（R6-60.2）、抗Gr-1（RA3-8C5）、TER119（赤血球系マーカー）および抗c-kit（3C1）モノクロナール抗体は、すべてPharMingen（San Diego, CA）より購入した。マウス抗Ly5.1抗体（A20.1.7）は、喜納辰夫博士（結核胸部疾患研究所，京都大学，京都，日本）より寄与された。モノクロナール抗体はすべて、FITC、PEまたはビオチン標識されたものを使用した。ビオチン標識抗体は、FITCまたはPE標識ストレプトアビジン（Becton-Dickinson Co., Mountain View, CA）またはTRI-COLOR標識ストレプトアビジン（CALTAG Lab., San Francisco, CA）を用いて発色させた。モノクロナール抗体の非特異的な結合を防ぐため、CD32/16(24G2)抗体で前処理を行った後、標識モノクロナール抗体で染色した。細胞懸濁液（10^5 – 2×10^6）をモノクロナール抗体で染色し、FACScan（Beeton-Dickinson）を用いて解析した。死細胞は、前方散乱、側方散乱およびPIゲーティングで除外した。肝単核球と骨髄細胞におけるc-kit$^+$ Lin$^-$（CD3$^-$、B220$^-$、Mac-1$^-$、Gr-1$^-$およびTER119$^-$）をFACS$^®$Vantage (Becton-Dickinson)を用いて純化した。実験によっては、肝単核球や骨髄細胞からCD3$^+$またはB220$^+$および/またはIL-2Rβ$^+$細胞を除去した。

細胞移植

4Gy照射後（18）、BALB/cマウスの骨髄細胞、肝単核球および脾臓細胞（等量, 1×10^7）を、CB17/-SCIDマウスに静脈注射した。いくつかの実験では肝単核球または骨髄細胞より純化したc-kit$^+$ Lin-細胞（5×10^4）、CD3$^-$B220$^-$細胞（2×10^6）またはc-kit-細胞（2×10^6）をそれぞれ移入した。C57BL/6マウスの肝臓または骨髄細胞より純化したCD3$^-$IL-2Rβ^-（2×10^6）をC57BL/6-SCIDマウスに移植した実験もあった。さらに、B6-Ly5.1マウス肝臓c-kit$^+$ Lin$^-$細胞（2×10^5）を放射線照射B6 SCIDマウスに移植した。

結果

放射線照射SCIDマウスの胸腺再構築

肝単核球は、非照射SCIDマウスの胸腺細胞を一時的に再構築できた（Fig. 1）。SCIDマウスへの低線量照射が、骨髄細胞の効果的再構築に必要という報告がある（18）。そこで、BALB/cマウスの肝単核球または骨髄細胞を4Gy照射したCB17/-SCIDマウスに移植した。

結果が示すのは、骨髄細胞だけでなく肝単核球が胸腺細胞を完全に再構築できたことであった（Fig. 1, Table I）。さらに、肝単核球は、骨髄細胞より早く胸腺を再構築できた。正常マウスの肝単核球を移植すると1週以内に、SCIDマウスの胸腺にDP胸腺細胞が出現した。一方、骨髄細胞を移植した場合、DP胸腺細胞出現まで2週を要した（Fig. 1）。肝臓または骨髄単核球を移植すると4週後に、T細胞（CD3$^+$）とB細胞（B220$^+$）が脾臓に出現した。肝単核球を移植すると、IL-2Rβ^- CD3^{bright}細胞だけでなくIL-2Rβ^+CD3^{int}細胞が脾臓に出現した。一方、骨髄細胞を移植すると、少数のIL-2Rβ^+CD3^{int}細胞のみが出現した。前述のTとB細胞の中には、移植された細胞中の前駆細胞から分化した細胞だけでなく、移植された肝単核球または骨髄細胞のT細胞とB細胞が増殖した場合を含む可能性がある。BALB/cマウスの骨髄細胞または肝単核球移植の4か月後も、CB17/-SCIDマウスは生存していた。一方、脾臓細胞の移植後2週以内に、CB17/-SCIDマウスは死亡した。

Figure.1

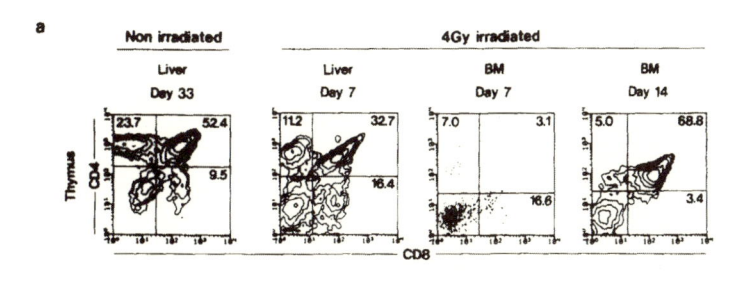

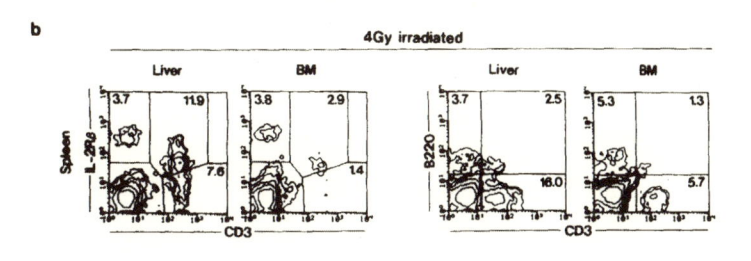

(a) 肝単核球が、SCIDマウス（非照射および照射有）のDP胸腺細胞を誘導する。BALB/C マウスの肝単核球10^7を、非照射SCIDマウスに移入した（1st panel）。SCIDマウス（4Gy照射有）（BALB/Cマウスの10^7/肝単核球移入7日後）における胸腺細胞CD4およびCD8発現（2nd panel）。SCIDマウス（照射有）（BALB/Cマウスの10^7/肝骨髄移入7日後および17日後）における胸腺細胞CD4およびCD8発現（3rdおよび4th panel）。(b) 正常マウスの肝臓および骨髄単核球を移植し、脾臓にT細胞とB細胞が出現した。移植4週後の脾臓を検証した。

Table.I		BALB/cマウスの肝単核球または骨髄細胞で再構築された放射線照射CB17/-SCIDマウスにおける細胞数			
			Number of cells in organs		
Mouse	Transferred cells	Days after transfer	Liver	Spleen	Thymus
			X10⁶ ± SD		
BALB/c	None		4.8 ± 0.8	157.9 ± 59.9	225.0 ± 61.3
SCID	None		1.1 ± 0.2	10.0 ± 3.6	5.0 ± 1.6
SCID(4Gy)	Liver MNC	7	0.8 ± 0.1	21.7 ± 5.7	0.3 ± 0.0
		14	2.1 ± 0.1	31.5 ± 4.5	33.5 ± 9.5
		21	2.7 ± 0.4	45.0 ± 5.1	220.0 ± 45.0
		82	10.4 ± 0.9	227.0 ± 55.3	121.0 ± 20.0
	BM	7	0.8 ± 0.2	15.8 ± 2.7	0.1 ± 0.0
		14	1.2 ± 0.1	18.5 ± 3.9	8.8 ± 2.9
		21	9.0 ± 1.0	17.4 ± 2.3	284.0 ± 38.2

BALB/cマウスの肝単核球と骨髄細胞（10⁷）を照射した（4Gy）SCIDマウスに移植した。肝臓、脾臓と胸腺の細胞数は移植後、各時点で検証した。平均値±1SDはマウス5匹を用いて算出した。

Figure.2

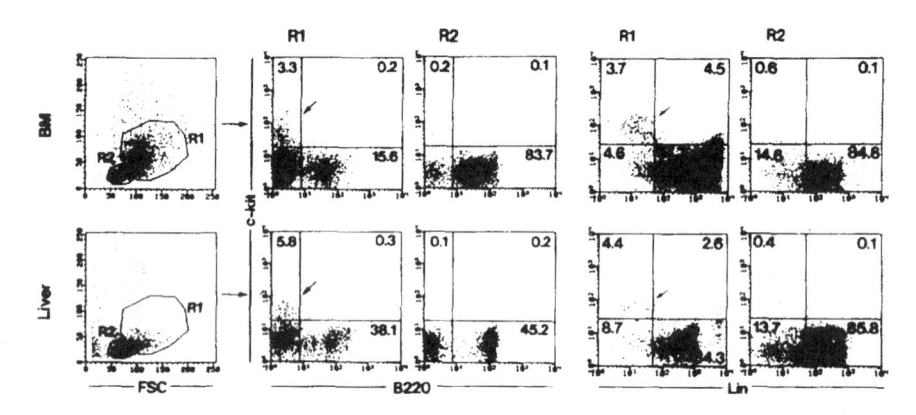

c-kit⁺細胞は、BALB/cマウスの骨髄細胞と同じく肝単核球に存在する。R1は大きい細胞集団であり、そして、R2はより小さな細胞集団をゲーティングした。これらのc-kit⁺細胞は、Lin⁻である。

c-kit⁺細胞は、骨髄細胞だけでなく肝臓にも存在する

肝単核球が胸腺を再構築できたこと、胸腺外分化T細胞分化が肝臓で起った（8-13）事実に基づき、肝臓の前駆細胞の存在を検証した。c-kit⁺が、比率は小さいが、正常マウスの肝臓（主として芽球状の大きな細胞集団）に存在することが判明した（Fig. 2）。肝臓におけるこのc-kit⁺細胞は、lineageマーカー陰性であった（CD3⁻、B220⁻、Mac-1⁻、Gr-1⁻および TER119⁻）（Fig. 2）。肝c-kit⁺細胞は、PBSでの門脈灌流の影響を受けず、同様のことが他の肝リンパ球でも見られた（16）（本研究では示さない）。

肝c-kit⁺細胞あるいはCD3⁻B220⁻分画（c-kit⁻細胞でない）移植によるDP胸腺細胞出現

肝c-kit⁺細胞およびCD3⁻B220⁻細胞を移植すると1週以内に、DP胸腺細胞が出現した、一方、骨髄c-kit⁺細胞を移植すると、DP胸腺

Figure.3

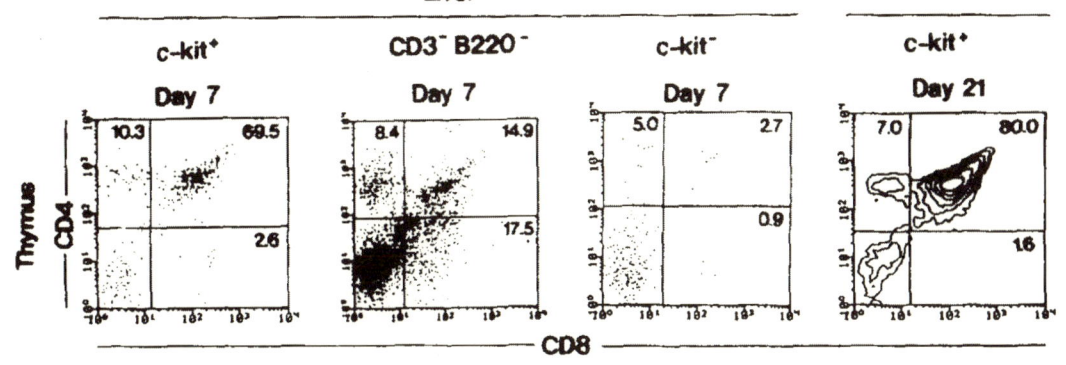

	Liver			BM
	c-kit⁺ Day 7	CD3⁻ B220⁻ Day 7	c-kit⁻ Day 7	c-kit⁺ Day 21

(Thymus: CD4 vs CD8 プロット)
- c-kit⁺ Day 7: 10.3 / 69.5 / — / 2.6
- CD3⁻B220⁻ Day 7: 8.4 / 14.9 / — / 17.5
- c-kit⁻ Day 7: 5.0 / 2.7 / — / 0.9
- c-kit⁺ Day 21: 7.0 / 80.0 / — / 1.6

BALB/cマウス肝臓のc-kit⁺細胞および非T細胞非B細胞分画（非c-kit⁻）を移植すると1週以内にDP胸腺細胞が出現した。BALB/cマウスの骨髄c-kit⁺細胞を移植すると、DP胸腺細胞出現まで2週以上必要である。BALB/cマウスの肝臓から純化したc-kit⁺Lin⁻細胞（5 x 10⁴）、CD3⁻B220⁻細胞（2 x 10⁶）、c-kit⁻Lin⁻細胞（2 x 10⁶）をSCIDマウス（4Gy照射有）に移植し、胸腺細胞のCD4とCD8染色を検証した（1st - 3rd panel）。骨髄c-kit⁺細胞（5 x 10⁴）の移植21日後の胸腺細胞も検証した（4th panel）。

Table.II

BALB/cマウスの肝臓c-kit⁺細胞で再構築されたCB17/-SCIDマウスの胸腺細胞数

Transferred cells	Days after transfer	Mean no of thymocytes ×10⁵
Liver c-kit⁺	7	1.4
	14	2
	21	9.7
Liver c-kit⁻	7	1
	10	1.9
Liver c-kit⁺+c-kit⁻	7	1.8
	14	14.5
	21	140
Liver c-kit⁺+ splenocytes	7	2
	14	1.8
	21	5.2

純化した肝c-kit⁺細胞（5 x 10⁴）およびc-kit⁺細胞（5 x 10⁴）に肝臓c-kit⁻細胞（2 x 10⁶）または脾臓細胞（2 x 10⁶）を添加して、SCIDマウス（照射有）に移植した。SCIDマウスの肝単核球、脾臓細胞と胸腺細胞の数を移植後、各時点で計測した。2週以内に肝臓c-kit⁻細胞を用いて再構築したSCIDマウスは死亡した。実験を繰り返し同様の結果を得た。

細胞産生まで2週を要した（Fig. 3）。しかし、肝c-kit⁺細胞のみを移植しても、胸腺細胞を効果的に再構築できなかったことは、注目に値する；特に再構築初期、肝臓c-kit⁻細胞は効率的に胸腺を再構築するためにも必要だった。このことは、c-kit⁻細胞が存在しないと胸腺のサイズが十分に大きくならなかったことから明らかである（Table II）。興味深いことに、肝c-kit⁻細胞には胸腺を育成する役割があるが、脾臓細胞には見られなかった（Table II）。

肝単核球移植後のSCIDマウス肝臓および骨髄におけるc-kit⁺細胞の増加

肝単核球を照射したSCIDマウスに移植した2週後、c-kit⁺細胞は肝臓でだけでなく骨髄でも著しく増加した。これは、c-kit⁺細胞が両方の場所で活発に増殖したことを示唆する（Fig. 4）。

肝単核球は、骨髄幹細胞を再構築できる

肝単核球は、TとB細胞にコミットしている（分化すると運命づけられている）骨髄幹細胞を再構築できるだろうか。また、SCIDマウス末梢中に出現したB細胞は、移植した正常マウスの肝単核球のB細胞が増殖した結果に過ぎないだけだろうか。これらのことを検証するため実験を行った。先ず、正常マウスから採取した肝単核球をSCIDマウスに移植し、このSCIDマウスの骨髄細胞を肝単核球と同様にレス

Figure.4

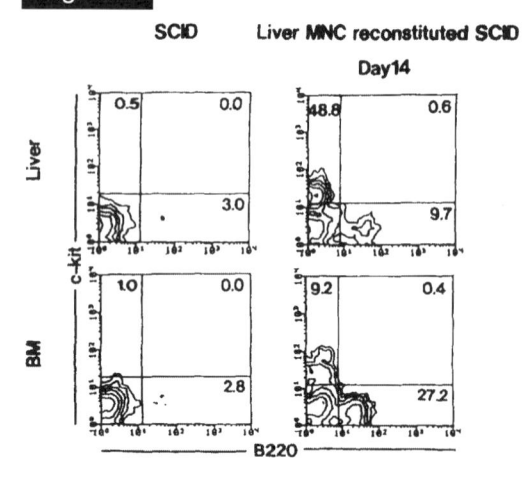

肝単核球移植後、SCIDマウス（照射有）の肝臓と骨髄にc-kit⁺細胞が大量出現した。SCIDマウス（照射有）に全肝単核球（1×10^7）移植をした2週間後、SCIDマウスの骨髄と肝単核球を検証した。

Figure.5

肝単核球でレスキューしたSCIDマウスの肝単核球または骨髄細胞を再移植すると、SCIDマウス（照射有）にDP胸腺細胞とB細胞が出現する。
BALB/cマウスの肝単核球でレスキューしたSCIDマウス（照射有）の肝単核球や骨髄細胞（いずれもB細胞を除去、10^7）を、他のSCIDマウス（照射有）に移植した。移植2週後、胸腺細胞のCD4とCD8発現を検証し（1stと2nd panel）、移植4週間後、脾臓細胞のCD3とB220もしくは細胞表面のIgM発現を検証した。

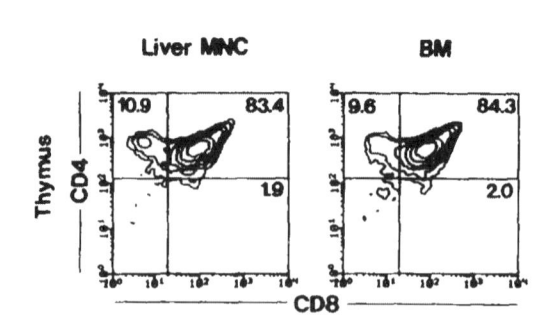

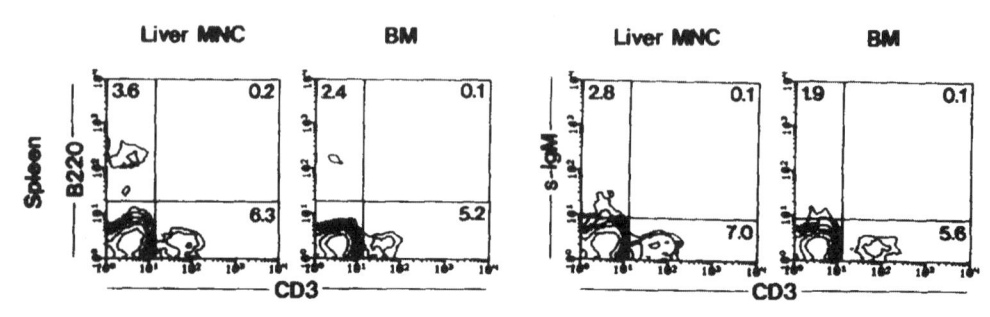

キューした。そして12週間後、このレスキューされたSCIDマウスの肝単核球、あるいは骨髄細胞（どちらもB細胞除去）を他のSCIDマウス（照射有）に移植した。その結果、胸腺は充分に再構築され、B細胞（表面IgM⁺同様B220⁺も）が4週以内に再び出現した（Fig. 5）。

肝c-kit⁺細胞は、赤血球系のみならず、骨髄系をも再構築する

肝c-kit⁺細胞が、複数の細胞系列を産生する能力があるかどうかについてB6-Ly5.1マウスの肝c-kit⁺細胞を、B6 SCID(Ly5.2)マウス（照射有）に移植した。抗Ly5.1抗体を用いて、ドナー由来の細胞（成熟赤血球以外）を、宿主のLy5.2⁺細胞と区別できる。移植後4週以内に、赤血球系細胞と同様に、骨髄系のLy5.1⁺細胞が、骨髄または末梢血に出現した（Fig. 6）。多量な骨髄のGr-1⁺細胞（顆粒球系）とTER-119⁺細胞（赤血球系）が骨髄と末梢血に出現した。Ly5.1⁺ Mac-1⁺Gr-1⁻細胞（マクロファージ系）も三重染色によるフローサイトメトリー解析を行い骨髄で同定できた。これら結果は、肝

Figure.6

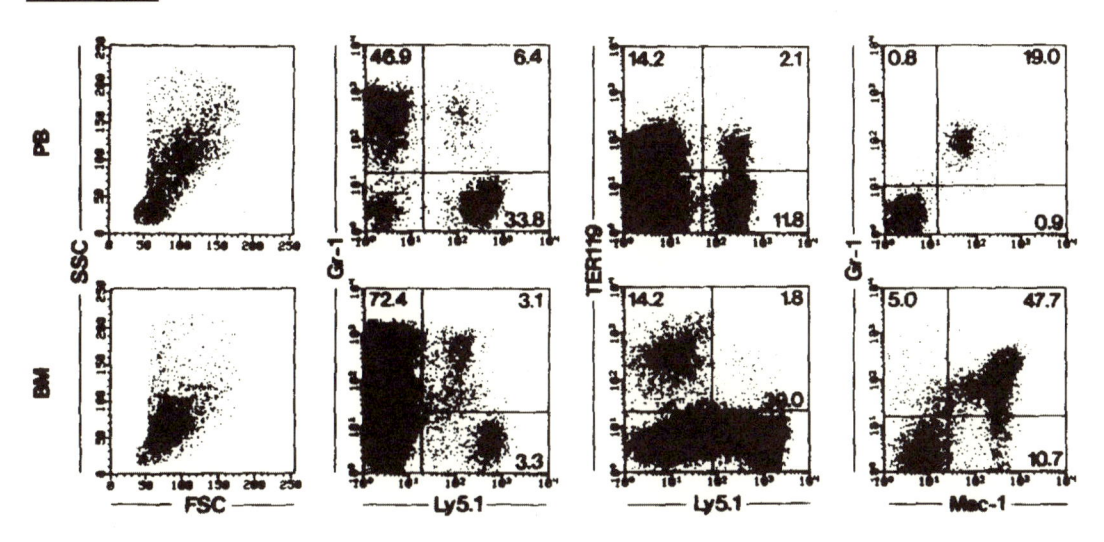

B6Ly5.1マウスの肝臓c-kit⁺細胞を移植すると、赤血球系統細胞のみならず骨髄系細胞を誘導できた。B6-Ly5.1マウスのc-kit⁺細胞（2 x 10⁵）をB6 SCIDマウス（Ly5.2）（照射有）に移植4週後、末梢血（PB）と骨髄を、モノクロナール抗体（抗Ly5.1、Gr-1、TER119とMac-1）を用いて染色した。抗Ly5.1、Mac-1とGr-1モノクロナール抗体の染色後、三重染色フローサイトメトリー解析を行った。

c-kit⁺細胞が真に多分化能幹細胞であることを強く示唆する。

肝TCR^{int}細胞は、肝臓で胸腺外分化する

次に、C57BL/6マウス肝単核球 または骨髄細胞中のCD3⁻IL-2Rβ⁻細胞を放射線照射B6 SCIDマウスに移植した。移植10日後、CD3⁺IL-2Rβ⁺細胞（大部分はNK1⁻）が数多く肝臓に出現した。この細胞の場合、胸腺由来のIL-2Rβ⁻ TCR^{bright}細胞と比較すると、TCRは中程度の発現である；既報（11-13）および本研究の結果が示すように、TCRの中程度の発現は、胸腺外分化T細胞の特徴である（Fig. 7）。つまり、通常肝T細胞は、IL-2Rβ⁺TCR^{int}細胞とIL-2Rβ⁻ TCR^{bright}細胞から構成されている。しかし、CD3⁻IL-2Rβ⁻の肝単核球または骨髄細胞で再構築されたSCIDマウスの肝T細胞は、実質的に全て、TCR^{int}細胞（主にIL-2Rβ⁺）であった（Fig. 7）。正常マウスの肝CD3⁻IL-2Rβ⁻細胞を用いて再構築した肝T細胞の数は、骨髄 CD3⁻IL-2Rβ⁻細胞を用いたものよりもずっと数が多かった（Fig. 7）。一方、骨髄 CD3⁻IL-2Rβ⁻細胞移植は、肝臓CD3⁻IL-2Rβ⁻細胞移植よりも、出現したNK細胞は、はるかに多かった（Fig. 7）。少量のTCR^{int}細胞

Figure.7

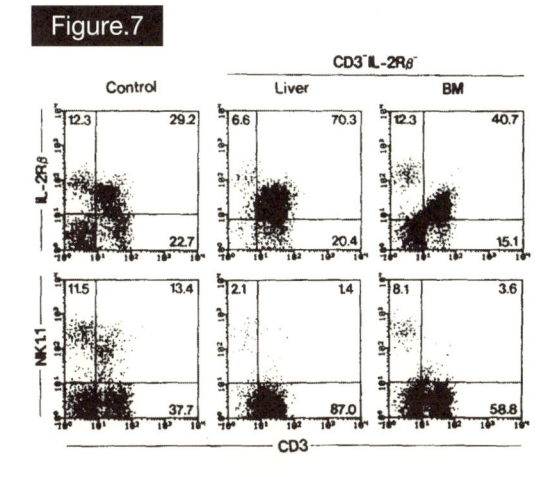

B6マウスの肝単核球または骨髄細胞のCD3⁻IL-2Rβ⁻細胞を移植すると、B6 SCIDマウス肝臓にTCR^{int}細胞とNK細胞が出現した。C57BL/6マウスの肝単核球の骨髄細胞を純化し採取したCD3⁻IL-2Rβ⁻細胞（1 x 10⁶）をB6 SCIDマウス（照射有）に移植した10日後、肝単核球のフェノタイプを検証した。対照データは正常B6マウスである。

（≠TCR^{bright}細胞）が、再構築初期に脾臓でも出現した。しかし、胸腺再構築後（肝臓または骨髄単核球移植の2週以上後）、SP（CD4$^+$あるいはCD8$^+$）T細胞（TCR^{bright}である）が出現し、TCR^{bright}細胞が、徐々に肝臓のみならず脾臓と末梢で増加した（データは示さない）。

考察

胎児の肝臓が、主要造血臓器であることはよく知られているが（19, 20）、肝造血機能はヒトの胎生後期やマウスの出生後、失われるようである。しかし、本研究では、成体マウス肝単核球は、c-kit$^+$胸腺前駆細胞だけでなくSCIDマウスの複数系統の細胞を再構築できるc-kit$^+$幹細胞も含むことが明らかになった。

肝単核球または骨髄細胞を移植すると、放射線照射したSCIDマウスの胸腺を完全に再構築できた。さらに、肝単核球またはc-kit$^+$細胞は、骨髄細胞や骨髄c-kit$^+$細胞より遥かに迅速に胸腺を再構築できた。また、正常マウスの肝単核球の移植でレスキューできたSCIDマウスの肝単核球と同様に骨髄細胞を他の放射線照射SCIDマウスへ移植すると、胸腺とB細胞を再構築することができた。この結果が示すのは、肝単核球が骨髄幹細胞を再構築できることである。

さらに、B6-Ly5.1マウスの肝c-kit$^+$細胞を放射線照射したB6 SCIDマウスに移植した。すると、Ly5.1$^+$の骨髄系と赤血球系細胞が、末梢血や骨髄に出現した。さらに、C57BL/6マウスの肝単核球または骨髄細胞のCD3$^-$IL-2Rβ$^-$細胞を放射線照射B6 SCIDマウスへ移植した。その結果、胸腺の再構築前に、肝臓で中程度のTCRを発現するCD3$^+$IL-2Rβ$^+$細胞が多数出現した。このことから、肝臓が、胸腺外分化T細胞の分化が起こる部位であることを確認した。c-kit（原がん原遺伝子の1つ）は、チロシン・キナーゼ遺伝子ファミリーの膜貫通型レセプターをエンコードし（21）骨髄造血を担う不可欠な分子であると報告されている（22, 23）。そして、骨髄の多分化能幹細胞はc-kit$^+$（1, 2）を発現している。本研究は、これらのc-kit$^+$多分化能幹細胞が、成体マウスの肝臓でも存在することを強く示唆する。

さらに、肝c-kit$^+$細胞は、骨髄c-kit$^+$細胞より迅速に、DP胸腺細胞を産生できるということ、そして、肝CD3$^-$IL-2Rβ$^-$単核球は、骨髄CD3$^-$IL-2Rβ$^-$細胞に比較して、中程度のTCRを持つ肝CD3$^+$細胞をより効率的に産生できたということである。そして、この結果が示唆するのは、肝c-kit$^+$細胞には、胸腺内分化T細胞と胸腺外分化T細胞の2系列に分化できるもう一段階分化したT細胞前駆細胞を含んでいることである。また、肝単核球を移植すると、骨髄でc-kit$^+$細胞が増加した。これら結果が示すのは、肝単核球は、多能性分化期の幹細胞を含むことである。

胸腺c-kit$^+$細胞には、もはや多能性はない。しかし、胸腺c-kit$^+$細胞も、骨髄c-kit$^+$細胞よりも迅速に胸腺細胞を再構築するという報告がある（24-26）。肝c-kit$^+$細胞集団は、胸腺に特異的に移動する可能性がある。これに対して他の細胞集団は、主に骨髄に移動し骨髄c-kit$^+$細胞を再構築している可能性がある。現在、肝臓、骨髄および胸腺におけるc-kit$^+$細胞の表面マーカーの詳細な比較を行っている。

もう一つ興味深い点がある。肝臓c-kit$^-$細胞は、胸腺を充分に再構築するのに必要である。その理由は、肝c-kit$^+$細胞のみを移植した場合、再構築された胸腺が極端に小さかったからである。しかし、肝臓c-kit$^-$細胞のこのような育成作用は、脾細胞にはない。この事実が示唆するのは、胸腺を充分に再構築するのは（特に再構築初期）、脾細胞ではなく、肝臓の細胞と胸腺

上皮細胞の相互作用に依存しているということである。宿主骨髄内のドナー肝臓由来c-kit$^+$細胞には、肝c-kit$^-$細胞は不要であることも示唆された。というのは、肝単核球でレスキューされたSCIDマウスの全骨髄細胞を用いて、他のSCIDマウス（照射有）の胸腺を充分に再構築できたからである。

　本研究の結果より、これら幹細胞が骨髄で生まれ、出生後、肝臓に移動する可能性が高くなった。もう一つは、出生後にも、胎児肝臓の幹細胞が少数残留している可能性である。現時点では、結論には至らない。肝細胞と密接に相互作用している肝単核球の中にはディッセ腔で見つかったものもあり、肝細胞損傷により肝T細胞が顕著に減少したと最近報告された（27）。肝臓の灌流により、肝臓のc-kit$^+$細胞集団は変化しない事実を考えると、肝臓の幹細胞や前駆細胞の成熟と分化は、肝臓類洞でよりは、むしろこのような実質隙（ディッセ腔）で起きている可能性が高い。

　最後に、本研究の結果は、肝移植後の宿主寛容に対する新しい見識を提供する可能性がある(28-31)。ドナー肝臓の幹細胞が、宿主に白血球をもたらす可能性がある。これは、ドナー・ホスト・キメラとして、ホストにとって、他の臓器移植拒絶率減少に役立つ可能性がある。

c-kit$^+$ Stem Cells and Thymocyte Precursors in the Livers of Adult Mice

By Hisami Watanabe,* Chikako Miyaji,* Shuhji Seki,*‡ and Toru Abo*

From the *Department of Immunology, Niigata University School of Medicine, Niigata 951, Japan; and the ‡Clinic of Shibata Base, National Defense Force, Shibata 957, Niigata, Japan

Summary

Livers of the adult mice contain c-kit$^+$ stem cells that can reconstitute thymocytes, multiple lineage cells, and bone marrow (BM) stem cells. Transfer of 1×10^7 hepatic mononuclear cells (MNC) and 5×10^4 hepatic c-kit$^+$ cells of BALB/c mice induced DP thymocytes within a week in four Gy-irradiated CB17/-SCID mice, but 2 wk were required for BM cells or BM c-kit$^+$ cells to produce DP thymocytes. Moreover, B cell–depleted BM cells or liver MNC of SCID mice that had been rescued by hepatic MNC of BALB/c mice again reconstituted thymus and B cells of other irradiated SCID mice. CD3$^-$ IL-2Rβ^- populations of both BM cells and hepatic MNC of C57BL/6 (B6) mice could generate T cells with intermediate TCR (mostly NK1.1$^-$) in the liver of irradiated B6 SCID mice before thymic reconstitution (extrathymic T cells). Furthermore, transfer of liver c-kit$^+$ cells of B6-Ly 5.1 mice into irradiated B6 SCID (Ly5.2) mice revealed that liver c-kit$^+$ cells can reconstitute myeloid and erythroid lineage cells. These results strongly suggest that the liver contains pluripotent stem cells and serves an important hematopoietic organ even into adulthood.

B M cells contain c-kit$^+$ stem cells (1, 2) which can give rise to multiple leukocyte lineages. Murine T cell precursor from bone marrow (BM)[1] migrate to the thymus and differentiate into mature thymocytes, which are the origin of most peripheral T cells. Recently, however, it has been demonstrated that T cell can differentiate in extrathymic sites. Several groups of researchers proposed that the intestine is such a site (3–7), and we demosntrated that the liver is also a candidate (8–13). Extrathymically developed αβ T cells in the liver are NK1.1$^+$ or NK1.1$^-$ T cells with intermediate TCR (13). However, it was not known whether the liver contains hematopoietic precursor cells. During an investigation as to how liver mononuclear cells (MNC) of normal mice transferred into SCID mice migrate and repopulate, we found that the liver MNC from normal adult mice could transiently reconstitute thymus accompanied by the appearance of double positive (DP) thymocytes in nonirradiated SCID mice. Since SCID mice can not rearrange either the TCR gene or the immunoglobulin gene (14), these mice are a proper model to examine whether or not a population of cells has a capacity to reconstruct T and B cells by radiation bone marrow chimera. In addition, B6-Ly5.1 mice (15) enabled us to determine whether or not myeloid and erythroid lineage cells are reconstituted by liver c-kit$^+$ cells. Here, we demonstrate that hepatic MNC of adult normal mice contain c-kit$^+$ cells which can reconstitute thymocytes, multiple lineage cells and BM stem cells of irradiated SCID mice.

Materials and Methods

Mice. Male CB17/-SCID mice (H-2^d), BALB/c mice (H-2^d) and C57BL/6 mice (H-2^b), 6-8 weeks of age, were purchased from CLEA Japan Inc. (Tokyo, Japan). C57BL/6-SCID (H-2^b) were purchased from Central Institute for Experimental Animals (Kanagawa, Japan). C57BL/6-Ly5.1 (B6-Ly5.1, H-2^b) mice were kindly provided by Dr. K. Kishihara (Medical Institute of Bioregulation, Kyushu University, Fukuoka, Japan). All mice were fed under the specific pathogen-free condition.

Cell Preparations. Mice were euthanized by exsanguination from the subclavian artery and vein, and liver and spleen were removed. The spleen was pressed on a 200-gauge stainless steel mesh and washed. The pellet was treated with RBC lysis solution (155 mM NH4Cl, 10 mM KHCO$_3$, 1 mM EDTA, 170 mM Tris, pH 7.3). Hepatic MNC were prepared as previously described (16, 17). Briefly, the liver was pressed through a stainless steel mesh and suspended in Eagle's MEM medium supplemented with 5 mM Hepes and 2% FCS. After one washing, the cells were resuspended in 30–35% Percoll solution containing 100 U/ml heparin and centrifuged at 2,000 rpm for 15 min at room temperature. An appropriate density of Percoll solution should be determined between 30 and 35% in each laboratory. The pellet was resuspended in RBC lysis solution, then washed twice with medium. BM cells were obtained by flushing femurs with medium.

---

[1] *Abbreviations used in this paper:* B6, C57BL/6; BM, bone marrow; DP, double positive; MNC, mononuclear cells.

The cell suspensions were filtrated through a 200-gauge nylon mesh to remove debris. Thymocytes were obtained by forcing thymus through a 200-gauge steel mesh. Peripheral blood cells were used after lysing red blood cells.

mAbs, Flowcytometric Analysis and Cell Sorting. Anti-CD4 (RM4-5), anti-CD8 (53-6.7), anti-CD3 (145-2C11), anti-IL-2Rβ chain (TM-β1), anti-NK1.1 (PK136), anti-B220 (RA3-6B2), anti-Mac-1 (M1/70), anti-mouse IgM (R6-60.2), anti-Gr-1 (RA3-8C5), TER119 (erythroid lineage marker), and anti-c-kit (3C1) Abs were all purchased from PharMingen (San Diego, CA). Mouse anti-Ly5.1 Ab(A20. 1.7) was kindly provided by Dr. T. Kina (Chest Disease Research Institute, Kyoto University, Kyoto, Japan). All mAbs were used with FITC-, PE-, or biotin-conjugated form. Biotinylated reagents were developed with FITC or PE-conjugated streptavidin (Becton-Dickinson Co., Mountain View, CA) or TRI-COLOR-conjugated streptavidin (CALTAG Lab., San Francisco, CA). To prevent nonspecific binding of mAbs, CD32/16 (24G2) was added before staining with labeled mAbs. Cell suspensions (10^5 to 2×10^6) were stained with mAbs and analyzed by FACScan (Becton-Dickinson). Dead cells were excluded by forward scatter, side scatter, and PI gating. c-kit$^+$ Lin$^-$ (CD3$^-$, B220$^-$, Mac-1$^-$, Gr-1$^-$, and TER119$^-$) cells of hepatic MNC and BM cells were sorted by FACS® Vantage (Becton-Dickinson). In some cases, CD3$^+$ or B220$^+$, and/or IL-2Rβ$^+$ cells were also depleted from hepatic MNC or BM cells by sorting.

Cell Transfer. After 4 Gy irradiation (18), equal number (1×10^7) of BM cells, hepatic MNC and splenocytes of BALB/c mice were injected intravenously into CB17/-SCID mice. In some experiments, 5×10^4 sorted c-kit$^+$ Lin$^-$ cells of hepatic MNC or of BM cells, sorted 2×10^6 CD3$^-$ B220$^-$ cells, or 2×10^6 c-kit$^-$ cells were injected into different mice groups. 2×10^6 sorted CD3$^-$IL-2Rβ$^-$ cells of liver or BM cells of C57BL/6 mice were also transferred into C57BL/6-SCID mice in another experiment. Further, 2×10^5 c-kit$^+$ Lin$^-$ cells of liver of B6-Ly5.1 mice were transferred into irradiated B6 SCID mice.

Results

Thymus Reconstruction in Irradiated SCID Mice. Liver MNC could transiently reconstitute thymocytes of non-irradiated SCID mice (Fig. 1). Since it was reported that low-dose irradiation of SCID mice is required for effective BM reconstitution (18), 4 Gy irradiation CB17/-SCID mice were transferred with liver MNC or BM cells of BALB/c mice. The results demonstrated that liver MNC as well as BM cells could fully reconstitute thymocytes (Fig. 1, Table 1). In addition, hepatic MNC could reconstruct thymus more rapidly than BM cells. After transfer of hepatic MNC from normal mice, DP thymocytes emerged in the thymus of SCID mice within 1 wk, whereas 2 wk were required for BM cells to induce DP thymocytes (Fig. 1). 4 wk after liver or BM MNC transfer, T cells (CD3$^+$) and B cells (B220$^+$) were detected in the spleen. In the case of liver MNC transfer, IL-2Rβ$^+$ intermediate CD3$^+$ cells as well as IL2Rβ$^-$ bright CD3$^+$ cells appeared in the spleen, while BM cells transfer induced only a small population of IL-2Rβ$^+$ intermediate CD3$^+$ cells. These T and B cells may include cells expanded from T and B cells contained in transferred liver MNC or BM cells or normal mice as well as cells from their precursors. CB17/-SCID mice that received either BM cells or hepatic MNC of BALB/c mice were still alive 4 mo later, whereas mice that received splenocytes died within 2 wk.

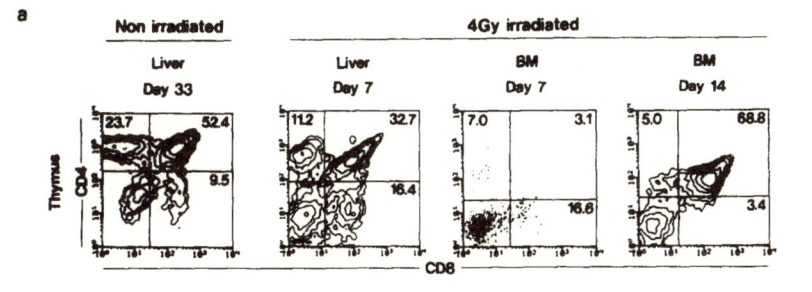

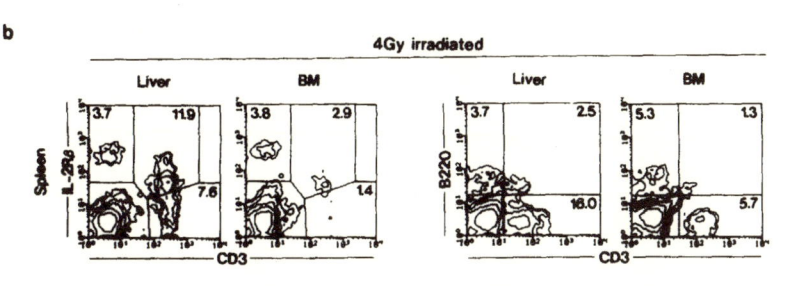

Figure 1. (*a*) Liver MNC induce DP thymocytes in non-irradiated and irradiated SCID mice. 10^7 hepatic MNC of BALB/C mice were injected into non-irradiated SCID mice (*1st panel*). CD4 and CD8 expression of thymocytes of 4 Gy irradiated SCID mice 7 d after injection of 10^7/hepatic MNC of BALB/C mice (*2nd panel*). CD4 and CD8 expression of thymocytes of irradiated SCID mice 7 and 14 d after injection of 10^7 BM cells of BALB/C mice (*3rd and 4th panels*). (*b*) Transfer of liver and BM MNC of normal mice could induce T cells and B cells in the spleen. 4 wk after transfer, spleens were examined.

Table 1. *Number of Cells Obtained from Irradiated CB17/-SCID Mice Reconstituted with Liver MNC or BM Cells of BALB/c Mice*

Mouse	Transferred cells	Days after transfer	Number of cells in organs		
			Liver	Spleen	Thymus
				$\times 10^6 \pm SD$	
BALB/c	None		4.8 ± 0.8	157.9 ± 59.9	225.0 ± 61.3
SCID	None		1.1 ± 0.2	10.0 ± 3.6	5.0 ± 1.6
SCID (4Gy)	Liver MNC	7	0.8 ± 0.1	21.7 ± 5.7	0.3 ± 0.0
		14	2.1 ± 0.1	31.5 ± 4.5	33.5 ± 9.5
		21	2.7 ± 0.4	45.0 ± 5.1	220.0 ± 45.0
		82	10.4 ± 0.9	227.0 ± 55.3	121.0 ± 20.0
	BM	7	0.8 ± 0.2	15.8 ± 2.7	0.1 ± 0.0
		14	1.2 ± 0.1	18.5 ± 3.9	8.8 ± 2.9
		21	9.0 ± 1.0	17.4 ± 2.3	284.0 ± 38.2

10^7 liver MNC and BM cells of BALB/c mice were transferred into 4 Gy irradiated SCID mice, the cell numbers in livers, spleens and thymus were examined on indicated days after transfer. Data shown are mean ± SD of five individual mice.

c-kit$^+$ Cells are Present Not Only in BM but Also in the Liver. The fact that liver MNC can reconstitute thymus and extrathymic T cell development takes place in the liver (8–13) led us to search for precursors in the liver. It was found that a small proportion of c-kit$^+$ cells are also present in the liver of normal mice, which were mainly detected in a large blastic population (Fig. 2). These c-kit$^+$ cells in the liver are lineage marker negative (CD3$^-$, B220$^-$, Mac-1$^-$, Gr-1$^-$, and TER119$^-$) (Fig. 2). The population of hepatic c-kit$^+$ cells was unaffected by perfusion of the liver with PBS from portal vein, as was previously demonstrated in the case of other lymphoid cells in the liver (16) (not shown).

Induction of DP Thymocytes by Hepatic c-kit$^+$ Cells and CD3$^-$B220$^-$ Fraction but Not c-kit$^-$ Cells. Transfer of hepatic c-kit$^+$ cells and CD3$^-$B220$^-$ cells could induce production of DP thymocytes within 1 wk, while BM c-kit$^+$ cells took 2 wk to generate DP thymocytes (Fig. 3). It is noteworthy, however, that hepatic c-kit$^+$ cells alone could not effectively reconstitute thymocytes; hepatic c-kit$^-$ cells were also needed to efficiently reconstruct the thymus, especially at early period of reconstitution, as revealed by a greatly reduced thymus size when c-kit$^-$ cells were absent (Table 2). Interestingly, splenocytes could not fulfill the supporting role played by hepatic c-kit$^-$ cells (Table 2).

Increase of c-kit$^+$ Cells in the Liver and BM of SCID Mice after Transfer of Liver MNC. 2 wk after transfer of hepatic MNC into irradiated SCID mice, c-kit$^+$ cells markedly increased not only in the liver but also in BM, which suggest that c-kit$^+$ cells were actively proliferating in both sites (Fig. 4).

Hepatic MNC Can Reconstitute BM Stem Cells. To test whether or not hepatic MNC can reconstitute BM stem cells that are committed to T and B cells, and to confirm that B cells found in the periphery of SCID mice was not merely the result of expansion of B cells contained in hepatic MNC of normal mice, BM cells as well as liver MNC from SCID mice, which had been rescued with hepatic

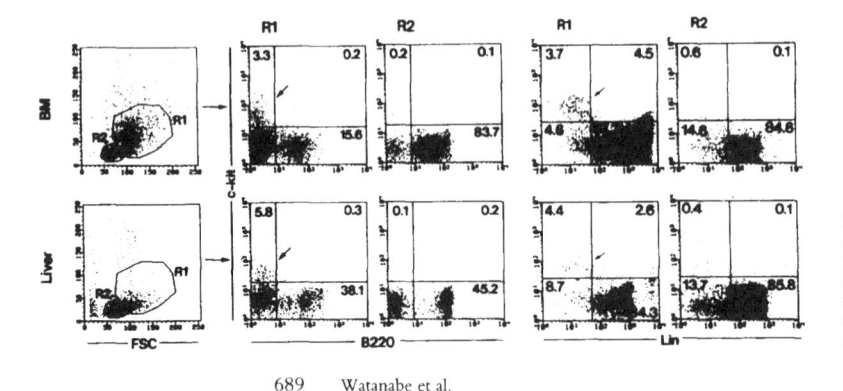

Figure 2. c-kit$^+$ cells are present in hepatic MNC as well as in BM cells of BALB/c mice. R1 gated a large blastic population and R2 gated a population of smaller cells. These c-kit$^+$ cells are Lin$^-$.

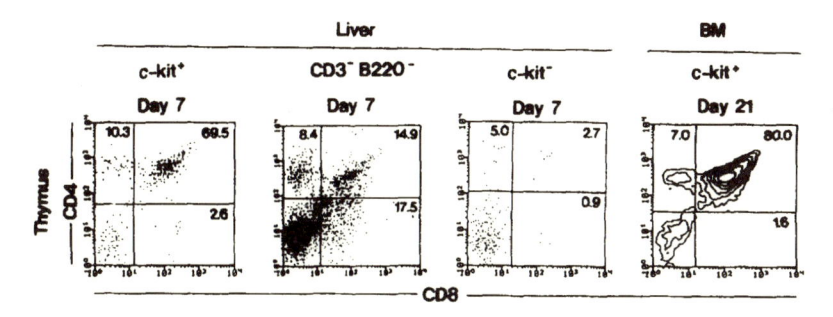

Figure 3. Transfer of c-kit⁺ cells and the fraction of non-T and non-B cells of BALB/c mice, but not c-kit⁻ cells, in the liver induced DP thymocytes within a week. Transfer of BM c-kit⁺ cells of BALB/c mice requires 2 wk or more to induce DP thymocytes. 5×10^4 sorted c-kit⁺ Lin⁻ cells, 2×10^6 CD3⁻B220⁻ cells and 2×10^6 c-kit⁻ Lin⁻ cells in the liver of BALB/c mice were transferred into 4Gy irradiated SCID mice (*1st to 3rd panels*) and CD4 and CD8 staining of thymocytes was examined at indicated day. 5×10^4 BM c-kit⁺ cells were also injected and thymocytes were examined on day 21 (*4th panel*).

MNC from normal mice 12 wk before, were further transferred into other irradiated SCID mice after depletion of B cells. The result showed that thymus was efficiently reconstituted and B cells (B220⁺ as well as surface Ig M⁺) could again emerge within 4 wk (Fig. 5).

Hepatic c-kit⁺ Cells Can Reconstitute Myeloid as Well as Erythroid Lineage Cells. To examine the capability of hepatic c-kit⁺ cells to produce multiple lineage cells, hepatic c-kit⁺ cells of B6-Ly5.1 mice were transferred into irradiated B6 SCID (Ly5.2) mice. Donor derived cells (except mature erythrocytes) can be descriminated by anti-Ly5.1 Ab from host Ly5.2⁺ cells. Within 4 wk after transfer, Ly5.1⁺ myeloid as well as erythroid lineage cells appeared in BM or peripheral blood (Fig. 6). Significant populations of BM Gr-1⁺ cells (granulocyte lineage) and TER-119⁺ cells (erythroid lineage) appeared in the BM and peripheral blood. Ly5.1⁺ Mac-1⁺ Gr-1⁻ cells (macrophage lineage) were also detected in BM by three-color flowcytometric analysis. These results strongly suggest that liver c-kit⁺ cells are indeed pluripotent stem cells.

Liver Intermediate TCR Cells Differentiate Extrathymically in the Liver. Next, CD3⁻IL-2Rβ⁻ populations of hepatic MNC or BM cells of C57BL/6 mice were transferred into irradiated B6 SCID mice. 10 d after transfer, many CD3⁺ IL-2Rβ⁺ cells (mostly NK1⁻) appeared in the liver. Here, the intensity of TCR is intermediate level, as compared to thymus derived IL-2Rβ⁻ bright TCR cells; intermediate

Table 2. *Number of thymocytes in CB17/-SCID Mice Reconstituted with Liver c-kit⁺ Cells of BALB/c Mice*

Transferred cells	Days after transfer	Mean no. of thymocytes
		$\times 10^5$
Liver c-kit⁺	7	1.4
	14	2.0
	21	9.7
Liver c-kit⁻	7	1.0
	10	1.9
Liver c-kit⁺ + c-kit⁻	7	1.8
	14	14.5
	21	140.0
Liver c-kit⁺ + splenocytes	7	2.0
	14	1.8
	21	5.2

5×10^4 sorted hepatic c-kit⁺ cells, and 5×10^4 c-kit⁺ cells with either 2×10^6 hepatic c-kit⁻ cells or 2×10^6 splenocytes were transferred into irradiated SCID mice. The number of liver MNC, splenocytes and thymocytes were counted on indicated days after transfer. SCID mice reconstituted by liver c-kit⁻ cells died within 2 wk. Repeated experiments showed similar results.

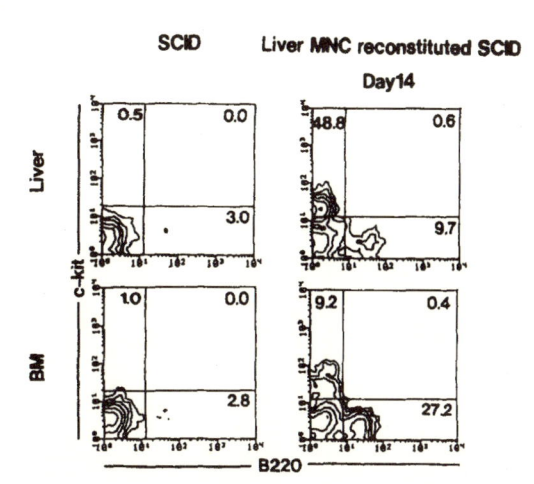

Figure 4. Appearance of a large number of c-kit⁺ cells in the liver and BM of irradiated SCID mice after transfer of hepatic MNC. 2 wk after transfer of 1×10^7 of total hepatic MNC into irradaited SCID mice, BM and liver MNC were examined.

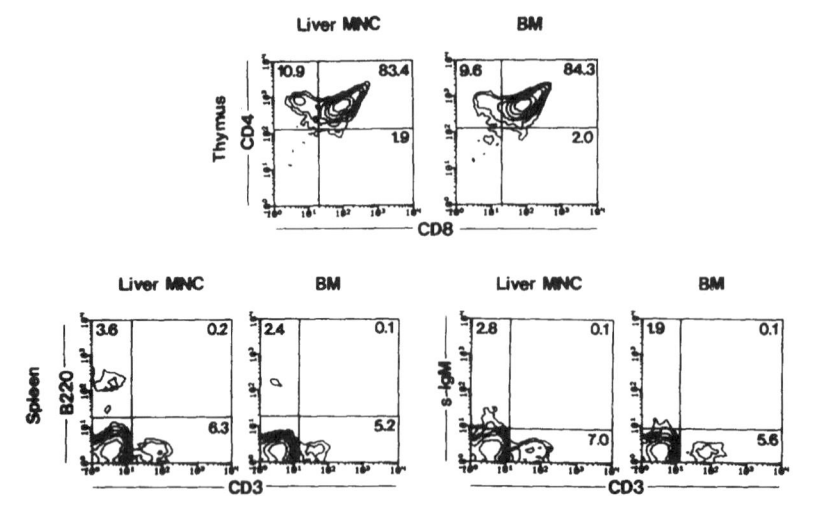

Figure 5. Induction of DP thymocytes and B cells in the irradiated SCID mice by hepatic MNC or BM cells of SCID mice, which had been rescued by hepatic MNC. B cell depleted 10^7 hepatic MNC or BM cells of SCID mice that had been irradiated and rescued by hepatic MNC of BALB/c mice were further transferred into other irradiated SCID mice. 2 wk after transfer, thymocytes were examined for their CD4 and CD8 expression (*1st and 2nd panels*), and splenocytes were examined for their CD3 and B220 or surface IgM expression 4 wk after transfer.

TCR is characteristic of extrathymic T cells, as shown previously (11–13) and demonstrated here (Fig. 7). Namely, although control liver T cells consist of IL-2Rβ^+ intermediate TCR cells and IL-2Rβ^- bright TCR cells, virtually all liver T cells of SCID mice reconstituted with CD3$^-$IL-2Rβ^- liver or BM cells were intermediate TCR cells (mainly IL-2Rβ^+) (Fig. 7). The number of these T cells in the liver reconstituted by hepatic CD3$^-$IL-2Rβ^- cells of normal mice was much greater than that induced by BM CD3$^-$IL-2Rβ^- cells (Fig. 7), while a larger population of NK cells were induced by the transfer of BM CD3$^-$IL-2Rβ^- cells than the transfer of hepatic CD3$^-$IL-2Rβ^- cells (Fig. 7). A smaller population of intermediate TCR cells (but not bright TCR cells) was also found in the spleen at an early stage of reconstruction, but after thymic reconstitution (beyond 2 wk after liver or BM MNC transfer) accompanied by the appearance of single positive T cells with bright TCR, bright TCR cells gradually increased in the spleen and periphery as well as in the liver (data not shown).

Discussion

It is well known that the fetal liver is a major hematopoietic organ (19, 20), whereas the hematopoietic function of the liver seems to be abrogated at later stage of the fetus in humans and after birth in mice. In this report, however, we demonstrate that the adult mouse liver MNC contain not only c-kit$^+$ thymocyte precursors but also c-kit$^+$ stem cells that can reconstitute multiple lineage cells in SCID mice.

The thymus of irradiated SCID mice could be fully reconstructed by the transfer of hepatic MNC or BM cells. In addition, hepatic MNC or c-kit$^+$ cells could reconstitute thymus more rapidly than BM cells or BM c-kit$^+$ cells. BM cells as well as liver MNC from SCID mice which had been rescued with hepatic MNC from normal mice could further reconstitute thymus and B cells of other irradiated SCID mice, suggesting that liver MNC can reconstitute BM stem cells. Moreover, when liver c-kit$^+$ cells of B6-Ly5.1 mice were transferred into irradiated B6 SCID mice, Ly5.1$^+$ myeloid and erythroid lineage cells were detected in peripheral blood or BM. Further, transfer of CD3$^-$IL-2Rβ^-

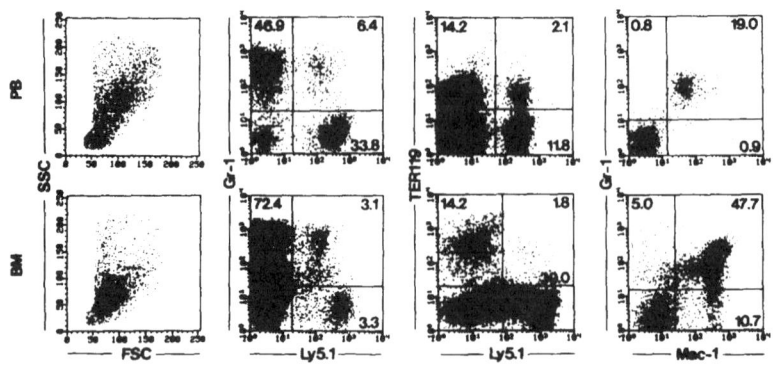

Figure 6. Liver c-kit$^+$ cells of B6–Ly5.1 mice could induce myeloid as well as erythroid lineage cells. 4 wk after transfer of 2×10^5 c-kit$^+$ cells of B6-Ly5.1 mice into irradiated B6 SCID mice (*Ly5.2*), peripheral blood cells (*PB*) and BM were stained by anti-Ly5.1, Gr-1, TER119, and Mac-1 mAbs. For Mac-1 and Gr-1 staining, three-color flowcytometric analysis of cells was carried out after staining with anti-Ly5.1, Mac-1 and Gr-1 mAbs.

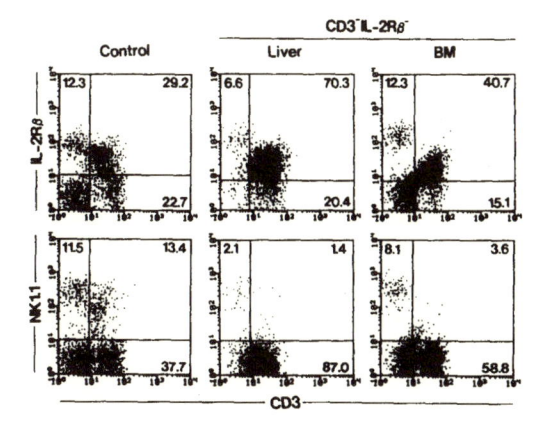

Figure 7. Induction of T cells with intermediate TCR and NK cells in the liver of B6 SCID mice from CD3$^-$IL-2Rβ^- cells of hepatic MNC or BM cells of B6 mice. 1×10^6 sorted CD3$^-$IL-2Rβ^- cells of hepatic MNC or BM cells of C57BL/6 mice were transferred into irradiated B6 SCID mice. 10 d after transfer, phenotype of liver MNC were examined. Control data is from a normal B6 mouse.

populations of hepatic MNC or BM cells of C57BL/6 mice into irradiated B6 SCID mice resulted in the appearance of many CD3$^+$IL-2Rβ^+ cells with intermediate TCR in the liver before thymic reconstitution, confirming that liver is the site where extrathymic T cell differentiation occurs.

The proto-oncogene, c-kit, encodes a transmembrane receptor of the tyrosine kinase gene family (21) and is reported to be an essential molecule for constitutive hematopoiesis in BM (22, 23), and pluripotent stem cells in BM are surface c-kit$^+$ (1, 2). This study strongly suggests that these c-kit$^+$ pluripotent stem cells are also present in the liver of adult mice. In addition, the fact that the hepatic c-kit$^+$ cells can generate DP thymocytes faster than BM c-kit$^+$ cells and that hepatic CD3$^-$IL-2Rβ^- MNC could more efficiently produce hepatic CD3$^+$ cells with intermediate TCR than BM CD3$^-$IL-2Rβ^- cells indicates that the hepatic c-kit$^+$ cells contain more differentiated T cell progenitors of both intrathymic and extrathymic T cell lineages. Further, hepatic MNC transfer could increase c-kit$^+$ cells in BM. These findings suggest that hepatic MNC contain stem cell populations at heterogeneous stages of differentiation. It was reported that c-kit$^+$ cells in the thymus also can reconstitute thymocytes faster than BM c-kit$^+$ cells, although they were not already pluripotential (24–26). It is possible that a population of liver c-kit$^+$ cells preferentially migrate into thymus, while another population mainly migrates into BM to reconstitute BM c-kit$^+$ cells. A detailed comparison of surface markers of c-kit$^+$ cells in the liver, BM and thymus is now underway.

Another interesting point is that hepatic c-kit$^-$ cells are needed to efficiently reconstruct thymus, because hepatic c-kit$^+$ cells alone could only reconstruct a thymus of much smaller size. However, the fact that this supporting effect of c-kit$^-$ cells of the liver could not be assumed by splenocytes indicates that effective thymic reconstruction, especially in early period of reconstitution, depends upon the interaction of thymic epithelial cells with certain cells in the liver different from splenocytes. It is also suggested that donor liver derived c-kit$^+$ cells in host BM do not need liver c-kit$^-$ cells any more, because whole BM cells of SCID mice rescued by liver MNC could effectively reconstitute thymus of other irradiated SCID mice.

The present results raise the possibility that these stem cells may originate in bone marrow and migrate to the liver after birth. Another possibility is that a small number of stem cells in fetal liver remain in the liver even after birth. At present, it can not be decided which is the case. According to a recent report (27) some hepatic MNC which firmly interact with hepatocytes have been detected in Disse's space and hepatocyte damage markedly decreased liver T cells. Considering the fact that the perfusion of the liver do not change the population of c-kit$^+$ cells in the liver, the possibility is raised that the maturation and differentiation of stem cells or precursor cells in the liver could occur in such parenchymal spaces rather than in the liver sinusoids.

Finally, the present results may offer a new insight into the host tolerance after liver transplantation (28–31). Stem cells in the liver of the donor may provide leukocytes to the host and create a donor host chimera that may contribute for decreasing the rate of rejection of other organ transplantations in the host.

Address correspondence to H. Watanabe, Department of Immunology, Niigata University School of Medicine, Niigata 951 Japan.

Received for publication 15 January 1996 and in revised form 20 May 1996.

References

1. Ogawa, M., Y. Matsuzaki, S. Nishikawa, S. Hayashi, T. Kunisada, T. Sudo, T. Kina, H. Nakauchi, and S.-I. Nishikawa. 1991. Expression and function of c-kit in hematopoietic progenitor cells. *J. Exp. Med.* 174:63–71.
2. Okada, S., H. Nakauchi, K. Nagayoshi, S. Nishikawa, S.-I. Nishikawa, Y. Miura, and T. Suda. 1991. Enrichment and characterization of murine hematopoietic stem cells that express c-kit molecule. *Blood.* 78:1706–1712.
3. Ferguson, A., and D.M. Parrott. 1972. The effect of antigen deprivation on thymus-dependent and thymus-independent lymphocytes in the small intestine of the mouse. *Clin. Exp. Immunol.* 12:477–488.
4. Mosley, R.L., D. Styre, and J.R. Klein. 1990. Differentiation and functional maturation of bone marrow-derived intestinal

epitherial T cells expressing membrane T cell receptor in athymic radiation chimeras. *J. Immunol.* 145:1369–1375.
5. Mosley, R.L., D. Styre, and J.R. Klein. 1990. CD4+CD8+ murine intestinal intraepithelial lymphocytes. *Int. Immunol.* 2: 361–365.
6. Bandeira, A., S. Itohara, M. Bonneville, O. Burlen-Defranoux, T. Mota-Santos, A. Coutinho, and S. Tonegawa. 1991. Extrathymic origin of intestinal intraepithelial lymphocytes bearing T-cell antigen receptor gamma delta. *Proc. Natl. Acad. Sci. USA.* 88:43–47.
7. Rocha, B., P. Vassalli, and D. Guy-Grand. 1991. The Vβ repertoire of mouse gut homodimeric α CD8+ intraepithelial T cell receptor α/β+ lymphocytes reveals a major extrathymic pathway of T cell differentiation. *J. Exp. Med.* 173: 483–486.
8. Ohteki, T., S. Seki, T. Abo, and K. Kumagai. 1990. Liver is a possible site for proliferation of abnormal CD3+4−8− double-negative lymphocytes in autoimmune MRL-lpr/lpr mice. *J. Exp. Med.* 172:7–12.
9. Seki, S., T. Abo, T. Masuda, T. Ohteki, A. Kanno, K. Takeda, H. Rikiishi, H. Nagura, and K. Kumagai. 1990. Identification of activated T cell receptor γδ lymphocytes in the liver of tumor-bearing hosts. *J. Clin. Invest.* 86:409–415.
10. Ohteki, T., T. Abo, S. Seki, T. Kobata, H. Yagita, K. Okumura, and K. Kumagai. 1991. Predominant appearance of γδ T lymphocytes of mice after birth. *Eur. J. Immunol.* 21:1733–1740.
11. Seki, S., T. Abo, T. Ohteki, K. Sugiura, and K. Kumagai. 1991. Unusual α β-T cells expanded in autoimmune lpr mice are probably a counterpart of normal T cells in the liver. *J. Immunol.* 147:1214–1221.
12. Abo, T., H. Watanabe, T. Iiai, M. Kimura, K. Ohtsuka, K. Sato, M. Ogawa, H. Hirahara, S. Hashimoto, H. Sekikawa, and S. Seki. 1994. Extrathymic pathways of T-cell differentiation in the liver and other organs. *Inter. Rev. Immunol.* 11: 61–102.
13. Sato, K., K. Ohtsuka, K. Hasegawa, S. Yamagiwa, H. Watanabe, H. Asakura, and T. Abo. 1995. Evidence for extrathymic generation of intermediate T cell receptor cells in the liver revealed in thymectomized, irradiated mice subjected to bone marrow transplantation. *J. Exp. Med.* 182: 759–767.
14. Bosma, G.C., R.P. Custer, and M.J. Bosma. 1983. A severe combined immunodeficiency mutation in the mouse. *Nature (Lond.).* 301:527–530.
15. Scheid, M.P., and D. Triglia. 1979. Further description of the Ly-5 system. *Immunogenetics.* 9:423–433.
16. Fulop, G.M., and R.A. Phillips. 1986. Full reconstitution of the immune deficiency in scid mice with normal stem cells requires low-dose irradiation of the recipients. *J. Immunol.* 136:4438–4443.
17. Watanabe, H., K. Ohtsuka, M. Kimura, Y. Ikarashi, K. Ohmori, A. Kusumi, T. Ohteki, S. Seki, and T. Abo. 1992. Details of an isolation method for hepatic lymphocytes in mice. *J. Immunol. Methods.* 146:145–154.
18. Goossens, P.L., H. Jouin, G. Marchal, and G. Milon. 1990. Isolation and flow cytometric analysis of the free lympho-myeloid cells present in murine liver. *J. Immunol. Methods.* 132:137–144.
19. Abramson, S., R.G. Miller, and R.A. Phillips. 1977. The identification in adult bone marrow of pluripotent and restricted stem cells of myeloid and lymphoid systems. *J. Exp. Med.* 145:1567–1579.
20. Owen, J.J., and M.A. Ritter. 1969. Tissue interaction in the development of thymus lymphocytes. *J. Exp. Med.* 129: 431–442.
21. Qiu, F.H., P. Ray, K. Brown, P.E. Barker, S. Jhanwar, F.H. Ruddle, and P. Besmer. 1988. Primary structure of c-kit: relationship with the CSF-1/PDGF receptor kinase family-oncogenic activation of v-kit involves deletion of extracellular domain and C terminus. *EMBO (Eur. Mol. Biol. Organ.) J.* 7:1003–1011.
22. Geissler, E.N., M.A. Ryan, and D.E. Housman. 1988. The dominant-white spotting (W) locus of the mouse encodes the c-kit proto-oncogene. *Cell.* 55:185–192.
23. Chabot, B., D.A. Stephenson, V.M. Chapman, P. Besmer, and A. Bernstein. 1988l The proto-oncogene c-kit encoding a transmembrane tyrosine kinase receptor maps to the mouse W locus. *Nature (Lond.).* 335:88–89.
24. Godfrey, D.I., A. Zlotnik, and T. Suda. 1992. Phenotypic and functional characterization of c-kit expression during intrathymic T cell development. *J. Immunol.* 149:2281–2285.
25. Wu, L., M. Antica, G.R. Johnson, R. Scollay, and K. Shortman. 1991. Developmental potential of the earliest precursor cells in the adult mouse thymus. *J. Exp. Med.* 174:1617–1627.
26. Matsuzaki, Y., J. Gyotoku, M. Ogawa, S.-I. Nishkawa, Y. Katsura, G. Gachelin, and H. Nakauchi. 1993. Characterization of c-kit positive intrathymic stem cells that are restricted to lymphoid differentiation. *J. Exp. Med.* 178:1283–1292.
27. Kawachi, Y., K. Arai, T. Moroda, T. Kawamura, H. Umezu, M. Naito, K. Ohtsuka, K. Hasegawa, H. Takahashi-Iwanaga, T. Iwanaga, et al. 1995. Supportive elements for hepatic T cell differentiation: T cell expressing intermediate levels of the T cell receptor are cytotoxic against syngeneic hepatoma, and are lost after hepatocyte damage. *Eur. J. Immunol.* 25: 3452–3459.
28. Kamada, N., H.S. Davies, and B. Koser. 1981. Reversal of transplantation immunity by liver grafting. *Nature (Lond.).* 292:840–842.
29. Starzl, T.E., A.J. Demetris, N. Murase, A.W. Thomson, M. Trucco, and C. Ricordi. Donor cell chimerism permitted by immunosuppressive drugs: a new view of organ transplantation. 1993. *Immunol. Today.* 14:326–332.
30. Calne, R., and H. Davies, 1994. Organ graft tolerance; the liver effect. *Lancet.* 343:67–68.
31. Lu, L., J. Woo, A.S. Rao, Y. Li, S.C. Watkins, S. Qian, T.E. Starzl, A.J. Demetris, and A.W. Thomson. 1994. Propagation of dendritic cell progenitors from normal mouse liver using granulocyte/macrophage colony-stimulating factor and their maturational development in the presence of type-1 collagen. *J. Exp. Med.* 179:1823–1834.

IDENTIFICATION OF NICOTINIC ACETYLCHOLINE RECEPTORS ON LYMPHOCYTES IN THE PERIPHERY AS WELL AS THYMUS IN MICE

マウスの胸腺および末梢リンパ球の
ニコチン性アセチルコリン受容体の同定

Immunology, 92: 201-205, 1997

chapter **6**

Identification of nicotinic acetylcholine receptors on lymphocytes in the periphery as well as thymus in mice

マウスの胸腺および末梢リンパ球のニコチン性アセチルコリン受容体の同定

S. TOYABE,*† T. IIAI,* M. FUKUDA,‡ T. KAWAMURA,* S. SUZUKI,* M. UCHIYAMA‡ & T. ABO*

*Department of Immunology and ‡Department of Paediatrics, Niigata University School of Medicine, Niigata, and †Sakamachi Hospital, Sakamachi, Niigata, Japan

【要約】

　リンパ球のニコチン性アセチルコリン受容体 (nAChR) の存在が議論されているが、本研究の目的は、マウスのリンパ球上のnAChRの存在を示すことである。ニコチン腹腔内投与3日後、脾臓においてリンパ球が増加した。採取した新鮮リンパ球は、フルオレッセインイソチオシアネート (FITC) 標識したαブンガロトキシン (αBuTx) に少量しか結合できなかった。しかし、培養液で培養すると、αBuTxと結合し始めた。顆粒球と対照的に、各リンパ臓器から採取した各リンパ球サブセットは、αBuTxを結合できることが明らかになった。αBuTxが結合した蛋白の親和性純化を行ったところ、リンパ球には筋肉と同じnAChR分子が存在することが明らかになった。逆転写ポリメラーゼ連鎖反応 (RT-PCR) 分析法で、リンパ球にnAChRのαサブユニットmRNAが発現していることが示された。この結果が示唆するのは、リンパ球表面には、nAChRが存在し、副交感神経刺激により、リンパ球はnAChRを介して直接刺激を受けることである。

はじめに

　リンパ球のニコチン性アセチルコリン受容体 (nAChR) の存在が議論されている。結合実験と細胞増殖実験を行った結果、リンパ球上のnAChRの存在を示す複数の報告がある[1-3]。これら報告の目的は、重症筋無力症 (MG) の病因の探究であり、胸腺構成要素のnAChR発現は重視されなかった[4,5]。これらの実験の中には、胸腺や末梢血リンパ球のnAChR発現が示された実験もあったが、胸腺上皮や胸腺筋様細胞のみnAChR発現が示された実験もあった[6-8]。それ故、結果を巡り賛否両論があり、リンパ球上のnAChRの確実な同定法は現在のところ定まっていない。

　本研究の目的は、マウスのリンパ球表面にnAChRが存在することを明らかにすることである。リンパ球表面には、nAChRが存在し、副交感神経が刺激されると、リンパ球はnAChRにより直接刺激を受けることが示唆される。

Received 3 September 1996; revised and accepted 18 May 1997.
略語：Abbreviations: αBuTx, αブンガロトキシン；ACh, acetylcholine; AChR, アセチルコリン受容体；n, ニコチン性；m, ムスカリン性；MGN, 筋原性；myogenin; MG, 重症筋無力症
Correspondence: Dr T. Abo, Department of Immunology, University School of Medicine, Asahimachi 1, Niigata 951, Japan.

材料と方法

マウスとニコチン投与

C3H/Heマウス（6-8週齢）を使用した。マウスは全て、新潟大学（新潟，日本）動物飼育施設内にて、特定病原体未感染（SPF）環境下で飼育した。マウスに、ニコチン（Sigma, St Louis, MO）（20μg／匹）を腹腔内投与した。

細胞分離

脾臓単核球（MNC）を、Ficoll-Isopaque勾配（1.090）遠心分離を行い、純化した。胸腺および鼠径リンパ節をステンレススチールメッシュで濾して、胸腺細胞およびリンパ節細胞を採取した。肝臓リンパ球を100U/mlヘパリンを添加した35%Percoll溶液で比重遠心分離を行い採取した[9]。末梢血細胞は、2%デキストラン沈降（40分間）を行い、バッフィーコートより採取した。混入した赤血球は、塩化アンモニウム（0.83%塩化アンモニウム-Tris緩衝液、PH 7.6）で溶血させた。脾臓単核球は、マクロファージを、プラスチックに接着させることにより純化した[9]。

フローサイトメトリー解析

リンパ球、顆粒球とマクロファージは、ヘマトキシリン・エオシン染色後、塗抹標本の組織学的検証を行った。顆粒球とマクロファージは、モノクローナル抗体（mAb）を用いフローサイトメトリー解析も行い同定した。顆粒球はGr-1$^+$、マクロファージはMac-1$^+$であった。リンパ球サブセットも、フローサイトメトリー解析により同定した。T細胞はCD3$^+$、ナチュナル・キラー（NK）細胞はインターロイキン-2受容体（IL-2R）β^+、ヘルパーT細胞はCD4$^+$、細胞傷害性T細胞はCD8$^+$、そして、B細胞はB220$^+$であった。これらマーカーのモノクロナール抗体は、全てPharMingen Co.（San Diego, CA）製である。蛍光陽性細胞を、FACScan（Becton Dickinson, Mountain View, CA）を用いて解析した。ゲーティングを行い、ヨウ化プロピジウム陽性の死細胞を除外した。

細胞へのαBuTx結合

C3H/Heマウスの脾臓単核球を採取し、10%牛胎仔血清を添加したRPMI-1640培養液中で培養した。各時点において細胞を採取、洗浄して、フルオレッセインイソチオシアネート（FITC）標識α-ブンガロトキシン（αBuTx）（Sigma; 1x10^{-7}M）を細胞塊に加えた（4℃, 30分間）。洗浄後蛍光陽性細胞をFACScanを用い解析した。陰性対照は、FITC標識αBuTx染色前、標識していないαBuTxを過剰処理（1x10^{-4}M）した（4℃, 30分間）リンパ球である。

nAChR親和性純化

ポリフッ化ビニリデン樹脂（PDVF）膜にαBuTxを結合させるために、膜をαBuTx（1x10^{-4}M）を添加したリン酸緩衝食塩水（PBS）中で培養した（4℃, 12時間）。そしてこの膜を10%ウシ血清アルブミン（BSA）を添加したPBSでブロッキングした（4℃, 12時間）。脾臓単核球を培養した（37℃, 12時間）。そして、採取した細胞を洗浄し、細胞表面の蛋白質を標識するため、1.0mg/dlビオチン-N-ヒドロキシ-スクシンイミド（Sigma）を添加したPBS中で培養した（4℃, 1時間）。そして、放射性免疫沈降分析緩衝液で溶解した。緩衝液の内容は以下の通り：0.5%ノニデット P-40（NP-40）, 0.02%アジ化ナトリウム, 1%アプロチニン, 1mMフルオロ燐酸ジイソプロピル, 5mMヨードアセトアミドおよび1mM PMSF。細胞溶解物を、αBuTxリガンドを純化するためαBuTxが結合したPDVF膜を用い培養した（4℃, 2時間）。そして、膜を5% 2-メルカプトエタノールを添加したドデシル硫酸ナトリウム（SDS）試料緩衝液の中で加熱した（95℃, 5分間）。沈殿物の

SDS電気泳動（8%ポリアクリルアミド）を行い、他のPDVF膜上にブロットし（写し取り）、ストレプト-アビディン標識ホースラディッシュペルオキシダーゼ（Sigma）染色後、増強化学発光（ECL）（Amersham Int., Amersham, UK）を用いて検証した。

AChRのαサブユニットおよびMGN mRNAのRT-PCR

総RNAを、酸性グアニジン・フェノール・クロロホルム法により、細胞（5×10^6）または組織（50mg）から抽出した。RNAをcDNAに、モロニーマウス白血病ウイルス逆転写酵素（RT）（Gibco BRL, Grand Island, NY）とオリゴ（dT）プライマー（宝酒造（株）, 京都, 日本）を用いて変換した（37℃）。cDNAをnAChRのα-サブユニットのプライマーセット（5'-TGGGCTCCGAACATGAGACGと3'-TGGACGCAAITGACAAAGACC）とミオゲニン（MGN）プライマー（5'-TCACCTCCATCGTGGACAGCと3'-AAACCACTGGAAGGTTCCC）とを混和した[10]。β-アクチンのプライマーは、RNA調整の整合性の評価にも用いた。ポリメラーゼ連鎖反応（PCR）を、Perkin-Elmer/Cetus thermocycler（Norwalk, CT）で、30サイクル（94℃, 55秒間；55℃, 30秒間；72℃, 2分間）、200μM dNTPおよび2.5U Taq DNAポリメラーゼ（東洋紡績（株）, 大阪, 日本）を用いて行った。PCR産物を2%アガロースゲルで泳動し、エチジウムブロマイドで染色した。

統計分析

実験群間の有意差検定には、ANOVA検定を用いた。

結果

マウスにニコチンの腹膜内投与すると、リンパ球増加症が出現した

ニコチンの腹腔内投与3日後、C3H/Heマウスの脾臓にはリンパ球増加が見られた（Fig. 1）。しかし、顆粒球にはほとんど影響が見られなかった。（胸腺由来）CD3$^+$T細胞の数は倍増したが、IL-2Rβ$^+$NK細胞の数の変化は少なかっ

Figure.1

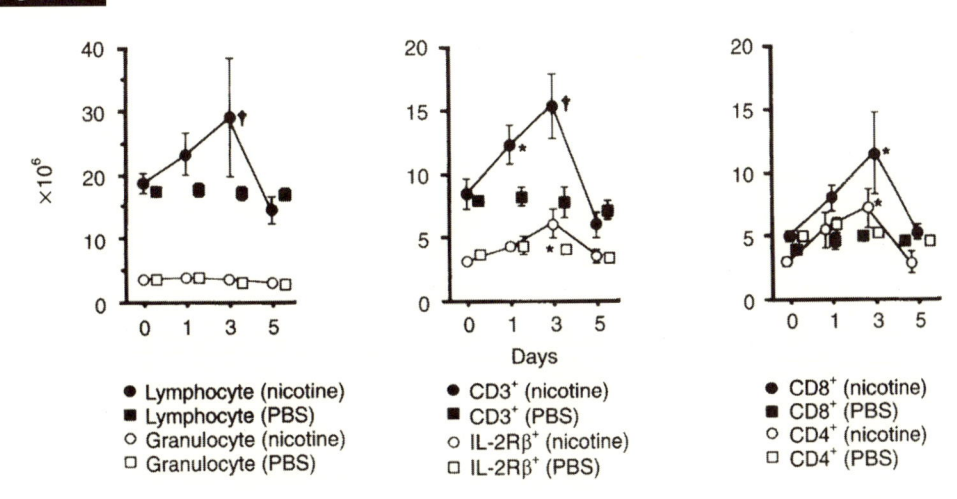

マウスにニコチンを腹腔内投与すると脾臓でリンパ球が増加した。8週齢のC3H/Heマウスに腹腔内投与し（20μgニコチン/匹）、リンパ球、顆粒球と各リンパ球サブセットの数を各時点で測定した。投与3日後にリンパ球増加が見られた。平均±1 SDは3匹のマウスを用いて算出した。*$P<0.05$, †$P<001$

Figure.2

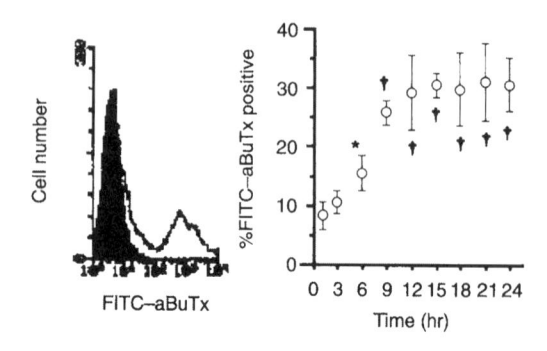

リンパ球表面上のαBuTx結合。培養液中で培養後、結合の経時的変化（右）。データは、3回の実験の平均±SDである。*P<0.05, †P<001 染色データの代表例を示す（左）。陰性対照は、染色前、未標識αBuTx過剰処理を行ったリンパ球である。

Figure.3

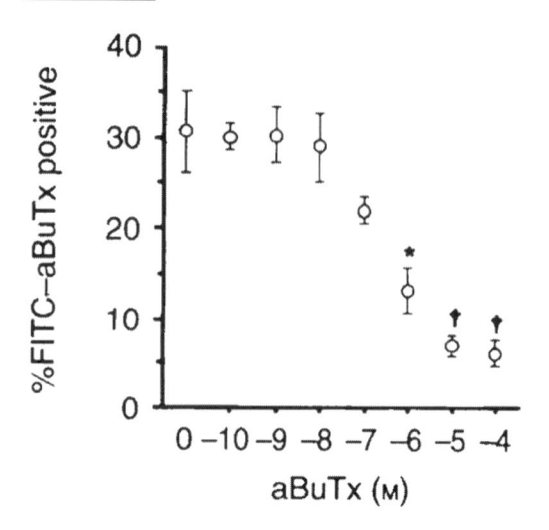

FITC標識αBuTxの結合は、未標識αBuTxとのプレ培養で抑制された。脾臓リンパ球を培養した（37℃，12時間）。洗浄後、染色前、細胞を各濃度のαBuTx（標識なし）を添加して培養した（4℃，30分間）。平均±1 SDは実験を三度行い算出した。*P<0.05, †P<001

た。CD4$^+$T細胞およびCD8$^+$T細胞両サブセットは増加した。

リンパ球を予め培養すると、αBuTx結合が促進する

マウスからすぐ採取した脾臓リンパ球は、nAChR αサブユニットに特異的に結合するFITC標識αBuTxの結合はわずかであったが[11]、10%牛胎仔血清を添加した培養液中で培養すると（37℃）αBuTxが結合し始めた（Fig. 2）。結合が最大に達したのは（陽性細胞＝約30%）は、培養12時間であった。12時間染色のデータを示す（Fig. 2）。

FITC-αBuTx結合の特異性を標識を確認するため、標識していないαBuTxを用いて遮断（ブロッキング）実験を行った（Fig. 3）。FITC標識αBuTx染色前、細胞にαBuTx（標識なし）を各濃度（1 x 10^{-10} to 10^{-4} M）を添加し培養した（4℃，30分間）。FITC-αBuTxの結合80%以上は、濃度10^{-5}Mでブロックできた。

各白血球およびリンパ球サブセットにおけるnAChRの局在

そして、白血球およびリンパ球サブセット（T細胞、B細胞、顆粒球やマクロファージなど）のどの種類にnAChRが発現するのか検証した。FITC標識αBuTx、フィコエリトリン（PE）標識抗白血球抗原およびヨウ化プロピジウムで三重染色を行った。ヨウ化プロピジウム陽性の死細胞を除外した。ゲーティング解析を行い、CD3$^+$ T細胞とB220$^+$ B細胞においては、陽性細胞は22-25%であることが明らかになった。対照的に、Gr-1$^+$顆粒球にはほとんど発現が見られなかったが、Mac-1$^+$マクロファージはかなりの比率の陽性細胞が見られた（Fig. 4a）。リンパ球を各リンパ臓器から採取したが、未熟T細胞を含む胸腺においてさえ、すべてにnAChR$^+$細胞が含まれていた（Fig. 4b）。胸腺細胞を構成する細胞には、CD3$^-$、CD3^{dull}とCD3^{high}細胞があるが、さらに各サブセットのnAChRの発現程度を検証した（Fig. 4c）。成熟したCD3^{high}細胞のみならず、未熟なCD3$^-$およ

Figure.4

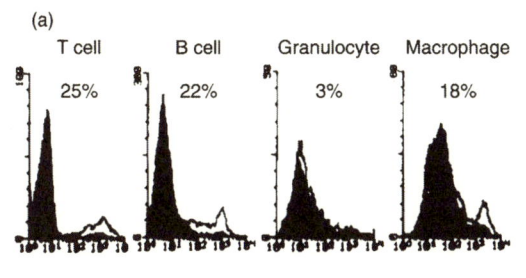

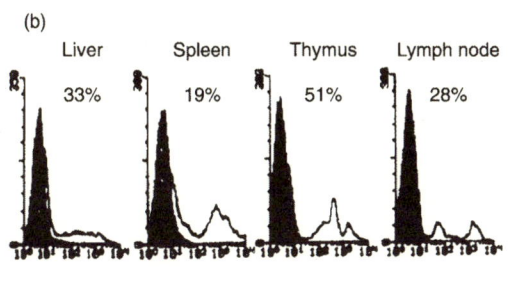

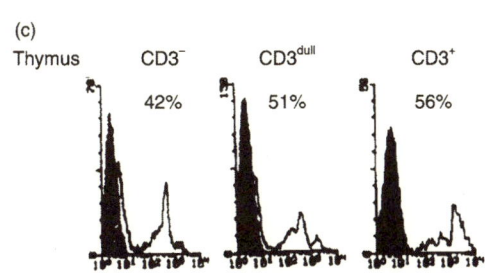

(a) T cell 25% / B cell 22% / Granulocyte 3% / Macrophage 18%

(b) Liver 33% / Spleen 19% / Thymus 51% / Lymph node 28%

(c) Thymus / CD3⁻ 42% / CD3^dull 51% / CD3⁺ 56%

各細胞分画におけるnAChR陽性細胞の比率の比較。(a) 脾臓の各細胞分画におけるnAChR⁺細胞；(b) 各リンパ臓器のリンパ球におけるnAChR⁺細胞；(c) 胸腺の未熟および成熟細胞サブセットにおけるnAChR⁺細胞。FITC標識αBuTx、PE標識モノクロナール抗体およびヨウ化プロピジウムで三重染色を行った。ゲーティング解析を行い、PE標識モノクロナール陽性でヨウ化プロピジウム陰性の細胞を表した。陰性対照（黒塗部分）は、染色前、未標識αBuTx過剰処理を行ったリンパ球である。

Figure.5

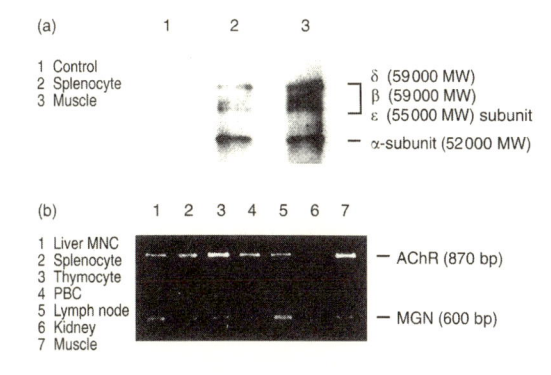

(a)
1 Control
2 Splenocyte
3 Muscle

δ (59000 MW)
β (59000 MW)
ε (55000 MW) subunit
α-subunit (52000 MW)

(b)
1 Liver MNC
2 Splenocyte
3 Thymocyte
4 PBC
5 Lymph node
6 Kidney
7 Muscle

AChR (870 bp)
MGN (600 bp)

リンパ球上のnAChRの直接同定。(a) マウス脾臓細胞からのnAChRの親和性純化。脾臓リンパ球の細胞表面蛋白（2）筋肉抽出物．（3）αBuTxとの反応を示す。(b) 各細胞と各組織のnAChRαサブユニットおよびMGNののmRNAを表示する。nAChRαサブユニット（870bp）およびMGN（600bp）mRNAのPCR産物は、各リンパ臓器のリンパ球で検出した。

びCD3^dull細胞にも相当数のnAChR⁺細胞が存在することが判明した。

リンパ球からのnAChRの分離と同定

次に、リンパ球表面からnAChR分子の分離を試みた（Fig. 5a）。分子の親和性純化を、αBuTx標識PDVF膜を用いて行った。陽性対照は筋肉抽出物（lane 3）で、一方、陰性対照はBSAのみを標識した膜を使用して沈降させた。12時間プレ培養した脾臓リンパ球から、分子量55000 - 59000（β、δおよびε-サブユニット）と52000（α-サブユニット）の蛋白質を抽出した[12]。その結果は、筋肉抽出物と同一であった。マウスからすぐに分離した脾臓リンパ球は、分子量52000バンドを僅かに示すのみだった（未発表データ）。

そして、RT-PCR法を用い、リンパ球がnAChRαサブユニットmRNAおよびMGN mRNA（nAChR産生に必要）を発現するか検証した（Fig. 5b）。腎臓（陰性対照）と筋肉（陽性対照）の結果を同時に示す。筋肉だけでなくリンパ球もnAChR（α-サブユニット）およびMGNのmRNAを発現することが明らかになった。PCR産物は、DNA配列により正しいnAChR mRNAであった（未発表データ）。

考察

本研究では、各リンパ臓器におけるリンパ球表面のnAChRの存在を示し、実際にnAChR分子を分離した。nAChRの発現は、数が多い顆

粒球上ではなく、成熟および未熟T細胞とB細胞上に見られた。ニコチンを投与すると、脾臓においてリンパ球が増加した。従って、リンパ球表面にはnAChRが存在し、副交感神経を刺激するとnAChRを介してリンパ球は直接刺激を受けることが示唆される。一方、顆粒球はαおよびβアドレナリン受容体を発現することが知られている[13-15]。それ故、免疫系は、自律神経系機能の直接支配を受ける可能性がある。

FITC標識αBuTxとの結合がリンパ球を培養すると増加したか、その理由の全てはわからない。しかし、αBuTxとの結合には受容体特異的である。理由は、FITC標識αBuTxとの結合がリンパ球を未標識αBuTxとプレ培養すると用量依存的に遮断（ブロック）されるからであった。nAChRは、培養中、リンパ球表面に出現するのではないかと推測された。

細胞の中には、刺激がなくとも培養中、nAChRを発現するという報告がある[16,17]。この現象は、リンパ球表面のnAChRにも当てはまる可能性がある。

リンパ球表面（特に胸腺細胞表面）にnAChRが存在することは、重症筋無力症の病因を理解するのに重要である。この分野の研究者は、患者の血清に抗nAChR抗体が含まれることをこれまで証明した[8]。これらの抗体は、筋肉のnAChRでだけでなく胸腺細胞のものにも反応するようである。胸腺摘出が重症筋無力症患者に効果があるという報告がある[18]。これは、胸腺が重症筋無力症において抗nAChR抗体に反応する抗原を供給する主要器官の1つであり[19]、そして、胸腺細胞は、筋nAChRに対する自己免疫反応を誘発する主要な抗原である可能性があるかもしれないという仮説を裏打ちするものである。一方、他の胸腺の細胞（例、胸腺上皮および筋様細胞）がnAChRを発現するという報告もある[6-8]。抗nAChR抗体の標的細胞について更なる研究を行うことは、重症筋無力症患者における自己免疫機構を理解するのに有益である。

謝辞

本研究は、日本国文部科学省癌研究助成金による。原稿浄書について木村京奈氏に感謝する。

Identification of nicotinic acetylcholine receptors on lymphocytes in the periphery as well as thymus in mice

S. TOYABE,*† T. IIAI,* M. FUKUDA,‡ T. KAWAMURA,* S. SUZUKI,* M. UCHIYAMA† & T. ABO*
*Department of Immunology and †Department of Paediatrics, Niigata University School of Medicine, Niigata, and ‡Sakamachi Hospital, Sakamachi, Niigata, Japan

SUMMARY

The existence of nicotinic acetylcholine receptors (nAChR) on lymphocytes remains controversial. We attempted to show the existence of nAChR on murine lymphocytes. The intraperitoneal injection of nicotine induced the lymphocytosis in the spleen on day 3. Although freshly isolated lymphocytes bound small quantities of fluorescein isothiocyanate (FITC)-conjugated α-bungarotoxin (αBuTx), they began to bind αBuTx after incubation in medium. In contrast to granulocytes, various lymphocyte subsets obtained from various lymphoid organs were found to bind αBuTx. Affinity purification of αBuTx-binding protein revealed that lymphocytes expressed the same nAChR molecules as those of muscle. Reverse transcriptase-polymerase chain reaction (RT-PCR) analysis showed that lymphocytes expressed the α-subunit mRNA of nAChR. These results suggest that lymphocytes carry nAChR on the surface and are stimulated directly via their nAChR by parasympathetic nerve stimuli.

INTRODUCTION

The existence of nicotinic acetylcholine receptor (nAChR) on lymphocytes remains controversial. In some reports, lymphocytes have been shown by binding assays and cell-proliferation assays to bear nAChR.[1-3] Whether thymic components express nAChR, in connection with the search for the aetiology of myasthenia gravis (MG), has also been examined.[4,5] Some of these experiments showed that thymic or peripheral lymphocytes express nAChR but others showed that only thymic epithelial or myoid cells express nAChR.[6-8] The results are therefore controversial and a more definite identification of nAChR on lymphocytes remains to be achieved.

In this study, we attempted to show the existence of nAChR on murine lymphocytes. We show that lymphocytes carried nAChR on the surface and it is suggested that they are stimulated directly via their nAChR by parasympathetic nerve stimuli.

MATERIALS AND METHODS

Mice and nicotine administration
C3H/He mice (aged 6-8 weeks) were used. All mice were fed

Received 3 September 1996; revised and accepted 18 May 1997.

Abbreviations: αBuTx, α-bungarotoxin; ACh, acetylcholine; AChR, acetylcholine receptor; n, nicotinic; m, muscarinic; MGN, myogenin; MG, myasthenia gravis.

Correspondence: Dr T. Abo, Department of Immunology, University School of Medicine, Asahimachi 1, Niigata 951, Japan.

© 1997 Blackwell Science Ltd

under specific pathogen-free conditions in the animal facility of Niigata University (Niigata, Japan). Mice were injected intraperitoneally with 20 μg nicotine (Sigma, St Louis, MO)/mouse.

Cell preparation
Splenic mononuclear cells (MNC) were purified by Ficoll–Isopaque gradient (1·090) centrifugation. Thymocytes and lymph node cells were obtained by teasing the thymus and inguinal lymph nodes, respectively, and passing through a stainless steel mesh. Liver lymphocytes were obtained by Percoll gradient centrifugation (35% Percoll containing 100 U/ml heparin).[9] Peripheral blood cells were obtained from the buffy coat (2% dextran sedimentation for 40 min). The contaminating erythrocytes were lysed by ammonium chloride buffer (0·83% NH$_4$Cl–Tris buffer, pH 7·6). Macrophages were purified from splenic MNC by the plastic adherence method.[9]

Immunofluorescence test
Lymphocytes, granulocytes and macrophages were morphologically identified in cell smears after staining with haematoxylin and eosin. Granulocytes and macrophages were also identified by immunofluorescence tests using monoclonal antibodies (mAb). Granulocytes were Gr-1$^+$ and macrophages were Mac-1$^+$. Lymphocyte subsets were also identified by immunofluorescence tests. T cells were CD3$^+$, natural killer (NK) cells were interleukin-2 receptor (IL-2R) β$^+$, helper T cells were CD4$^+$, cytotoxic T cells were CD8$^+$, and B cells were B220$^+$. All mAb against these markers were obtained from PharMingen Co. (San Diego, CA). The fluorescence-positive cells were analysed by FACScan (Becton Dickinson,

Mountain View, CA). The dead cells positive for propidium iodide were excluded by gating.

Binding of αBuTx onto cells

Splenic MNC isolated from C3H/He mice were incubated in RPMI-1640 medium supplemented with 10% fetal calf serum. At the identified times, cells were harvested and washed. Fluorescein isothiocyanate (FITC)-conjugated α-bungarotoxin (αBuTx) (Sigma; 1×10^{-7} M) was then added to the cell pellet for 30 min at 4°C. After washing, the fluorescence-positive cells were analysed by FACScan. As a negative control, cells were treated with an excess of unlabelled αBuTx (1×10^{-4} M) for 30 min at 4° before staining with FITC-conjugated αBuTx.

Affinity purification of nAChR

To bind αBuTx to polyvinylidene difluoride (PDVF) membrane, the membranes were incubated with phosphate-buffered saline (PBS) with 1×10^{-4} M αBuTx for 12 hr at 4°. The membranes were then blocked by PBS containing 10% bovine serum albumin (BSA) for 12 hr at 4°. Splenic MNC were cultured at 37° for 12 hr. The cells were harvested, washed and incubated in PBS containing 1·0 mg/dl biotin-N-hydroxy-succimide (Sigma) for 1 hr at 4° to label cell-surface proteins. The cells were then lysed in radioimmunoprecipitation assay buffer containing 0·5% nonidet P-40 (NP-40), 0·02% azide, 1% aprotinin, 1 mM diisopropyl fluorophosphate, 5 mM iodoacetamide, and 1 mM PMSF. The cell lysates were incubated for 2 hr at 4° with the αBuTx-binding PDVF membrane to purify the ligands for αBuTx. The membranes were then heated at 95° for 5 min in sodium dodecyl sulphate (SDS) sample buffer with 5%, 2-mercaptoethanol. The precipitates were electrophoresed through 8% polyacrylamide in the presence of SDS, blotted onto another PDVF membrane, and detected using the enhanced chemiluminescence (ECL) system (Amersham Int., Amersham, UK) after staining with strepto-avidin-conjugated horseradish peroxidase (Sigma).

RT-PCR of α-subunit of AChR and MGN mRNA

Total RNA was isolated from 5×10^6 cells or 50 mg tissue by the acid-guanidium-phenol-chloroform method. RNA was converted to cDNA using Molony murine leukaemia virus reverse transcriptase (RT) (Gibco BRL, Grand Island, NY) and an oligo(dT) primer (Takara Shuzo Co., Kyoto, Japan) at 37°. The cDNA was mixed with the α-subunit of nAChR primer set (5'-TGGGCTCCGAACATGAGACG and 3'-TGGACGCAATGACAAAGACC), and the myogenin (MGN) primer (5'-TCACCTCCATCGTGGACAGC and 3'-AAACCACTGGAAGGTTCCC).[10] Primers for β-actin were also used to assess the integrity of the RNA preparation. Polymerase chain reaction (PCR) was performed with 200 μM dNTP and 2·5 U Taq DNA polymerase (Toyobo Co., Osaka, Japan) for 30 cycles (94° for 55 seconds, 55° for 30 seconds, and 72° for 2 min) in a Perkin-Elmer/Cetus thermocycler (Norwalk, CT). Part of the reaction mixture was separated on 2% agarose gel and stained with ethidium bromide.

Statistical analysis

The differences were analysed statistically by the ANOVA method.

RESULTS

Lymphocytosis induced by an intraperitoneal administration of nicotine into mice

We found that an intraperitoneal injection of nicotine induced lymphocytosis in the spleen of C3H/He mice on day 3 (Fig. 1). However, the effect on granulocytes was minimal. A twofold increase was seen in the number of conventional CD3$^+$ T cells, but the change in the number of IL-2Rβ$^+$ NK cells was smaller. Both CD4$^+$ and CD8$^+$ T-cell subsets increased.

Preincubation of lymphocytes facilitates the binding of αBuTx

Although freshly isolated splenic lymphocytes bound small quantities of FITC-conjugated αBuTx, which was specifically bound to the α-subunit of nAChR,[11] they began to bind αBuTx after incubation in medium supplemented with 10% fetal calf serum at 37° (Fig. 2). The maximum binding (about 30% positive cells) was achieved by a 12-hr incubation. The staining profile at 12 hr is shown in Fig. 2.

To examine whether the binding of FITC-αBuTx occurred specifically, a blocking experiment with unlabelled αBuTx was conducted (Fig. 3). Before staining cells with FITC-conjugated αBuTx, cells were incubated with unlabelled αBuTx at the indicated concentration (1×10^{-10} to 10^{-4} M) at 4° for 30 min. More than 80% binding of FITC-αBuTx was blocked at a concentration of 10^{-5} M.

Distribution of nAChR in various leucocytes and lymphocyte subsets

We then examined what cell types of lymphocyte subsets or leucocytes express nAChR, including T cells, B cells, granulocytes and macrophages. Three-colour staining for FITC-conjugated αBuTx, phycoerythrin (PE)-conjugated anti-leucocyte antigens, and propidium iodide was carried out. The dead cells positive for propidium iodide were excluded. The gated analysis revealed 22–25% positive cells in CD3$^+$ T cells and B220$^+$ B cells. In contrast, Gr-1$^+$ granulocytes almost lacked expression, whereas Mac-1$^+$ macrophages contained a considerable proportion of positive cells (Fig. 4a).

When lymphocytes were obtained from various lymphoid organs, they all included nAChR$^+$ cells, even in the thymus which contains immature T cells (Fig. 4b). Since thymocytes consist of CD3$^-$, CD3^{dull} and CD3^{high} cells, the expression levels of nAChR on each subset were examined further (Fig. 4c). It was found that immature CD3$^-$ and CD3^{dull} cells as well as mature CD3^{high} cells contained nAChR$^+$ cells at comparable levels.

Isolation and identification of nAChR from lymphocytes

We then attempted to isolate nAChR molecules from the surface of lymphocytes (Fig. 5a). Affinity purification of the molecules was performed by using an αBuTx-conjugated PDVF membrane. The positive control was muscle extract (lane 3), whereas the negative control was the precipitates using membrane conjugated only with BSA. Proteins of 55 000–59 000 MW (β, δ and ε-subunits) and 52 000 MW (α-subunit) were extracted from splenic lymphocytes preincubated for 12 hr.[12] This result was identical to muscle extract.

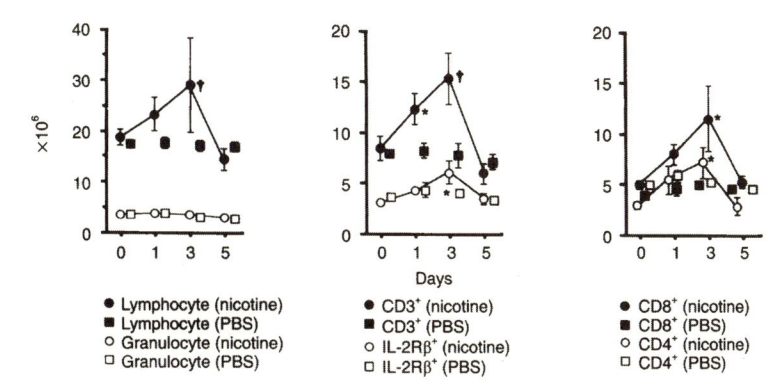

Figure 1. Induction of lymphocytosis in the spleen by an intraperitoneal injection of nicotine in mice. C3H/He mice at the age of 8 weeks were intraperitoneally injected with 20 μg nicotine/mouse and the numbers of lymphocytes, granulocytes and various lymphocyte subsets were enumerated at the indicated days. Lymphocytosis was seen at 3 days after injection. The mean+1 SD from three mice is represented. $*P<0·05$, $\dagger P<0·01$ versus 0 day by ANOVA.

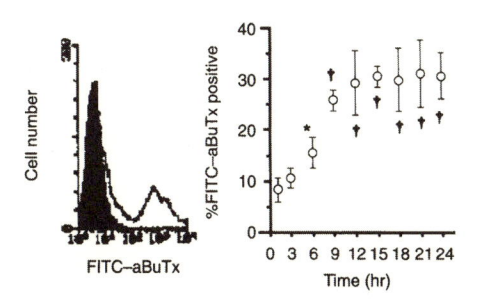

Figure 2. Binding of αBuTx onto lymphocytes. Time kinetics of the binding after incubation in medium (right). Data represented are the mean±SD of three investigations. $*P<0·05$, $\dagger P<0·01$ versus 0 hr by ANOVA. The staining profile is also represented (left). The negative control is lymphocytes treated with an excess of unlabelled αBuTx before staining.

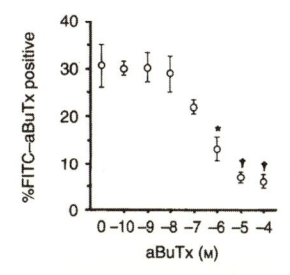

Figure 3. The binding of FITC-conjugated αBuTx was inhibited by the preincubation with unlabelled αBuTx. Splenic lymphocytes were cultured at 37° for 12 hr. After washing, cells were incubated at 4° for 30 min with unlabelled αBuTx at the indicated concentrations before staining. Data represented are mean±SD of three investigations. $*P<0·05$, $\dagger P<0·01$ versus 0 M αBuTx by ANOVA.

© 1997 Blackwell Science Ltd, *Immunology*, **92**, 201–205

The freshly isolated splenic lymphocytes showed only a faint 52 000 MW band (data not shown).

We then examined whether lymphocytes produced the α-subunit mRNA of nAChR and MGN mRNA (which is required for the production of nAChR), by using an RT-PCR method (Fig. 5b). The results from the kidney (negative control) and muscle (positive control) are presented in parallel. It was demonstrated that lymphocytes as well as muscle produced mRNA of nAChR (α-subunit) and MGN. It was confirmed that the PCR product was truly mRNA of known nAChR by DNA sequencing (data not shown).

DISCUSSION

In the present study, we have demonstrated the existence of nAChR on lymphocytes in various lymphoid organs and isolated the actual molecules of nAChR. The expression of nAChR was seen in both mature and immature T cells and B cells, but not on the majority of granulocytes. The administration of nicotine induced the lymphocytosis in the spleen. Therefore, it is suggested that lymphocytes carry nAChR on their surface and are directly stimulated via their nAChR by parasympathetic nerve stimuli. On the other hand, granulocytes are known to express α- and β-adrenergic receptors.[13–15] So the immune system might be regulated directly under the function of the autonomic nervous system.

We cannot fully understand why the binding of FITC-conjugated αBuTx increased with the incubation of lymphocytes. But the binding of αBuTx is specific for the receptors, since the binding of FITC-conjugated αBuTx was blocked with preincubation of lymphocytes with unlabelled αBuTx in a dose-dependent manner. We speculated that the nAChR was induced on lymphocytes during the incubation. Several kinds of cells have been reported to express nAChR during incubation without any stimuli.[16,17] This phenomenon might be also true for nAChR on lymphocytes.

The existence of nAChR on lymphocytes, especially on thymocytes, is also important for understanding the aetiology of MG. Investigators in this field have already demonstrated that sera from patients contain anti-nAChR antibodies.[8] These

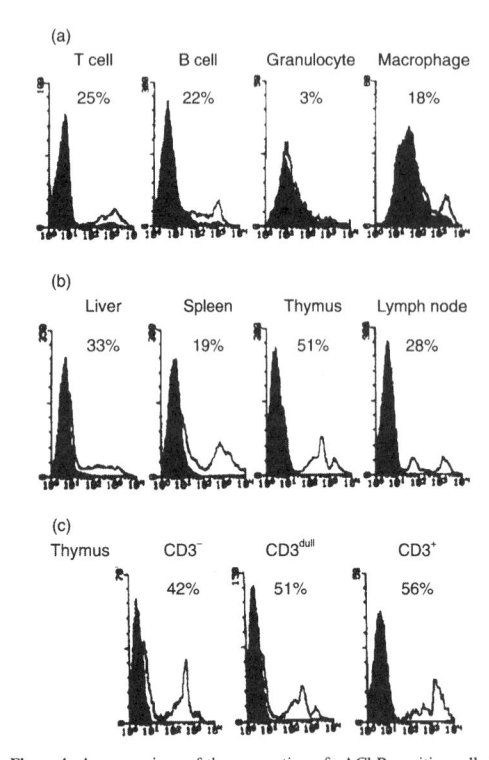

Figure 4. A comparison of the proportion of nAChR-positive cells in various cell fractions. (a) nAChR$^+$ cells among various cell fractions in the spleen; (b) nAChR$^+$ cells among lymphocytes in various lymphoid organs; (c) nAChR$^+$ cells on immature and mature T-cell subsets in thymus. Three-colour staining of FITC-conjugated αBuTx, PE-conjugated mAb and propidium iodide was performed. By gated analysis, PE-conjugated mAb-positive and propidium iodide-negative cell fractions are represented. The negative control (filled areas) was lymphocytes treated with an excess of unlabelled αBuTx before staining.

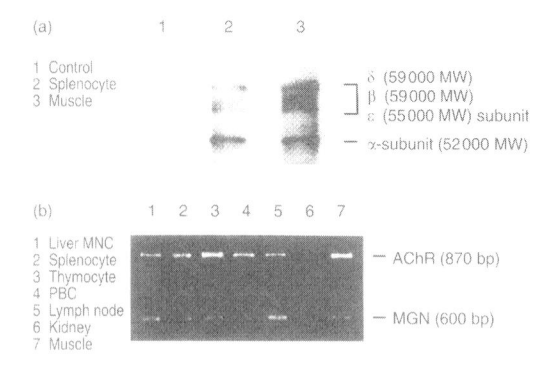

Figure 5. Direct identification of nAChR on lymphocytes. (a) Affinity purification of nAChR from murine splenocytes. Cell-surface proteins from splenic lymphocytes (2) and muscle extract (3) reactive to αBuTx were precipitated as indicated. (b) Demonstration of mRNA of the α-subunit of nAChR and MGN in various cells and tissues. The PCR product of the α-subunit of nAChR (870 bp) and MGN (600 bp) mRNA was detected in lymphocytes from various lymphoid organs.

antibodies seem to be reactive not only with nAChR on muscle but also with that on thymocytes. It has been reported that thymectomy is effective for patients with MG.[18] This supports the hypothesis that thymus is one of the major organs providing antigens reactive with anti-nAChR antibody in MG,[19] and thymocytes might be the primary antigen that induces autoimmune responses to muscle nAChR. On the other hand, it is also reported that other thymic cells, such as thymic epithelial and myoid cells, express nAChR.[6–8] Further investigations about target cells of anti-nAChR antibody will be useful in understanding the autoimmune mechanism in MG patients.

ACKNOWLEDGMENTS

This work was supported in part by a grant-in-aid for cancer research from the Ministry of Education, Science, and Culture, Japan. We wish to thank Mrs Kyona Kimura for preparation of the manuscript.

REFERENCES

1. Fuchs S., Schmidt-Hopfeld I., Tridente G. & Tarrab-Hazdai R. (1980) Thymic lymphocytes bear a surface antigen which cross-reacts with acetylcholine receptor. *Nature* **287**, 162.
2. Richman D.P. & Arnason B.G. (1979) Nicotinic acetylcholine receptor: evidence for a functionally distinct receptor on human lymphocytes. *Proc Nat Acad Sci USA* **76**, 4632.
3. Richman D.P., Antel J.P., Burns J.B. & Arnason B.G. (1981) Nicotinic acetylcholine receptor on human lymphocytes. *Ann NY Acad Sci* **377**, 427.
4. Kaminski H.J., Fenstermaker R.A., Abdul-Karim F.W., Clayman J. & Ruff R.L. (1993) Acetylcholine receptor subunit gene expression in thymic tissue. *Muscle Nerve* **16**, 1332.
5. Kornstein M.J., Asher O. & Fuchs S. (1995) Acetylcholine receptor alpha-subunit and myogenin mRNAs in thymus and thymomas. *Am J Pathol* **146**, 1320.
6. Hara Y., Ueno S., Uemichi T., Takahashi N., Yorifuji S., Fujii Y. & Tarui S. (1991) Neoplastic epithelial cells express alpha-subunit of muscle nicotinic acetylcholine receptor in thymomas from patients with myasthenia gravis. *FEBS Lett* **279**, 137.
7. Schluep M., Willcox N., Vincent A., Dhoot G.K. & Newsom-Davis J. (1987) Acetylcholine receptors in human thymic myoid cells *in situ*: an immunohistological study. *Ann Neurol* **22**, 212.
8. Toyka K.V., Drachman D.B., Griffin D.E. *et al.* (1977) Myasthenia gravis. Study of humoral immune mechanisms by passive transfer to mice. *New Engl J Med* **296**, 125.
9. Iiai T., Watanabe H., Seki S. *et al.* (1992) Ontogeny and development of extrathymic T cells in mouse liver. *Immunology* **77**, 556.
10. Asher O., Kues W.A., Witzemann V., Tzartos S.J., Fuchs S. & Souroujon M.C. (1993) Increased gene expression of acetylcholine receptor and myogenic factors in passively transferred experimental autoimmune myasthenia gravis. *J Immunol* **151**, 6442.
11. Ralston S., Sarin V., Thanh H.L., Rivier J., Fox J.L. & Lindstrom J. (1987) Synthetic peptides used to locate the alpha-bungarotoxin binding site and immunogenic regions on alpha subunits of the nicotinic acetylcholine receptor. *Biochemistry* **26**, 3261.
12. Gotti C., Conti-Tronconi B.M. & Raftery M.A. (1982) Mammalian muscle acetylcholine receptor purification and characterization. *Biochemistry* **21**, 3148.

13. IGNARRO L.J. & COLOMBO C. (1973) Enzyme release from polymorphonuclear leukocyte lysosomes: regulation by autonomic drugs and cyclic nucleotides. *Science* **180,** 1181.
14. LANDMANN R.M., MULLER F.B., PERINI C., WESP M., ERNE P. & BUHLER F.R. (1984) Changes of immunoregulatory cells induced by psychological and physical stress: relationship to plasma catecholamines. *Clin Exp Immunol* **58,** 127.
15. PANOSIAN J.O. & MARINETTI G.V. (1983) Alpha 2-adrenergic receptors in human polymorphonuclear leukocyte membranes. *Biochem Pharmacol* **32,** 2243.
16. DE KONINCK P. & COOPER E. (1995) Differential regulation of neuronal nicotinic ACh receptor subunit genes in cultured neonatal rat sympathetic neurons: specific induction of alpha 7 by membrane depolarization through a Ca^{2+}/calmodulin-dependent kinase pathway. *J Neurosci* **15,** 7966.
17. JENSEN J.J., WINZER-SERHAN U.H. & LESLIE F.M. (1997) Glial regulation of alpha 7-type nicotinic acetylcholine receptor expression in cultured rat cortical neurons. *J Neurochem* **68,** 112.
18. BLOSSOM G.B., ERNSTOFF R.M., HOWELLS G.A., BENDICK P.J. & GLOVER J.L. (1993) Thymectomy for myasthenia gravis. *Arch Surgery,* **128,** 855.
19. HARA H., HAYASHI K., OHTA K., ITOH N. & OHTA M. (1993) Nicotinic acetylcholine receptor mRNAs in myasthenic thymuses: association with intrathymic pathogenesis of myasthenia gravis. *Biochem Biophys Res Comm* **194,** 1269.

CIRCADIAN RHYTHM OF LEUCOCYTES AND LYMPHOCYTE SUBSETS AND ITS POSSIBLE CORRELATION WITH THE FUNCTION OF THE AUTONOMIC NERVOUS SYSTEM

白血球とリンパ球サブセットの日内変動及び
自律神経機能との間の相関関係の可能性

Clinical Experimental Medicine, 110: 500-508, 1997

chapter 7

Circadian rhythm of leucocytes and lymphocyte subsets and its possible correlation with the function of the autonomic nervous system

白血球とリンパ球サブセットの日内変動及び自律神経機能との間の相関関係の可能性

S. SUZUKI*†, S. TOYABE, T. MORODA†, TUKADA†, A. TSUKAHARA†, T. IIAI†, M. MINAGAWA†,
S. MARUYAMA†, K. HATAKEYAMA†, K. ENDOH‡ & T. ABO*

*Departmen Immnology, †First Departmenl of Surgery,. and ‡Department of
Hygienics, Niigata University, School of Medicine, Niigata, Japan
(Accepted for publication 28 August 1997)

【キーワード】

日内変動、白血球、リンパ球サブセット、顆粒球、自律神経系

【要約】

　白血球値には生理的変化があるが、その中でも、日内変動は、変化が大きいので非常に重要である。近年、新たなリンパ球サブセット（胸腺外分化T細胞）が同定された。そこで幅広く日内変動の研究を行った。すると、白血球はすべて、日内変動により数や比率が変化することが明らかになり、白血球を2群に分類した。第1のグループ（昼型リズム群）では、昼間、増加を示した；顆粒球、マクロファージ、ナチュラル・キラー（NK）細胞、胸腺外分化T細胞、$\gamma\delta$ T細胞とCD8$^+$ サブセット。第2のグループ（夜型リズム群）では、夜間、増加を示した；T細胞、B細胞、$\alpha\beta$ T細胞とCD4$^+$ サブセット。ヒトは、昼間、活動的であり、交感神経緊張を示す。興味深いことに、昼型リズムを持つ顆粒球とリンパ球サブセットは、アドレナリン受容体を数多く有することが明らかになった。一方、夜型リズムを持つリンパ球サブセットには、コリン受容体を数多く有する。このことを反映し、運動をすると、昼型リズムを持つ細胞の数が顕著に増加した。これらの結果が示すのは、自律神経系が白血球の値を支配する可能性である。

はじめに

　生体の生理的状態により、各種免疫パラメータの数と機能が変化することはよく知られている[1, 2]。ヒトと動物における白血球とリンパ球サブセットの数の日内変動は、この現象の一つである[3-5]。これまで、このリンパ球リズムの評価には、形態学もしくは他の指標を用いられた。その後の研究では、モノクロナール抗体を用いてリンパ球サブセットの評価が行われ、独特のパターンを持つ日内変動が報告された[6-8]。本研究の実験の目的を以下示す；(i) 最近の研究により、ヒトの新しいリンパ球サブセット（すなわち胸腺外起源 [9, 10]のCD56$^+$ T細胞とCD57$^+$ T細胞）の存在を明らかになったが、白血球とリンパ球サブセットの日内変動の全体的な構図を得ることが必要である。(ii) 白血球とリンパ球サブセットの日内変動が起きる要因は何であるのかを説明する必要もある。ヒトを対象にした本研究の結果より、白血球には二つのグループがあり、日内変動のピーク時間が異なることが明らかになった。第1のグループは、昼型リズム（昼間、数や比率が増加する）を持つ細胞である。このグループは、単

球、顆粒球、ナチュラル・キラー（NK）細胞、胸腺外分化T細胞、CD8$^+$細胞およびγδT細胞を含む。第2のグループは、夜型リズム（夜間、比率が増加する）を持つ細胞である。このグループは、T細胞（αβT細胞を含む）、B細胞およびCD4$^+$細胞である。

全てではないにしても、昼型リズムを持つ細胞には、細胞表面にアドレナリン受容体が存在するものが多い傾向にある。対照的に、夜型リズムを持つ細胞の表面には、コリン受容体が存在することが明らかになった。このことから身体活動（カテコラミン高産生や、その逆にアセチルコリン（ACh）の高産生を伴う）により、白血球変動が決定される可能性が高い。この考察を裏付けるように、昼型リズムを持つ全細胞において、運動後、数が増加することが判明した。白血球表面上にアドレナリンおよびコリン受容体が存在すると相次ぎ報告され、身体活動（自律神経系の機能）が白血球やリンパ球サブセットの日内変動の原因であると結論される [11, 12]。

材料と方法

被験者

本研究の被験者は健康人男性であった（年齢；26 – 48歳）。うち被験者2名は運動後も検査を行い、AM8:00より4時間毎に日内変動を測定した。（被験者1；48歳，被験者2；28歳）。被験者は全員、通常通り活動し、睡眠を取った。

免疫学的指標測定

末梢血（5ml）をヘパリン化したシリンジで採血した。血液（2ml）を用いて白血球（顆粒球、リンパ球など）の数と比率、および血清アドレナリンとノルアドレナリン値の測定を新潟大学中央臨床検査室に委託した。通常、採血後数時間内に白血球を測定するが、数時間内に白血球は影響を受けないと確認されている。

残りの血液（3ml）を用いて、各リンパ球サブセットを解析した。単核球（MNC）を、Ficall-Isopaque比重分離液（1.077g/ml）を用い遠心分離を行い採取した [5]。

二重免疫蛍光染色を行い、リンパ球サブセット、NK細胞、胸腺外分化T細胞と従来型TおよびB細胞を同定した [10]。CD3とCD16（またはCD56またはCD57）の二重染色を行い、CD3$^-$CD16$^+$ NK細胞（またはCD3$^-$CD56$^+$またはCD3$^-$CD57$^+$ NK細胞）、CD3$^+$CD16$^+$胸腺外分化T細胞（またはCD3$^+$CD56$^+$またはCD3$^+$CD57$^+$胸腺外分化T細胞）およびCD3$^+$CD16$^-$通常型T細胞（またはCD3$^+$CD56$^-$またはCD3$^+$CD57$^-$通常型T細胞）を同定した。CD3とT細胞レセプター（TCR）αβ（またはTCR γδ）、そしてCD3とCD4（またはCD8）の二重染色を行い、αβT細胞（またはγδT細胞）もしくはCD4$^+$ T細胞（またはCD8$^+$ T細胞）を同定した。CD20とCD5の二重染色を行いCD20$^+$CD5-B細胞を同定した。使用したモノクローナル抗体は全てBecton Dickinson（Mountain View、CA）製である。蛍光陽性細胞をFACScan（Becton Dickinson）を用いて解析した。

細胞純化

さまざまな分画においてアドレナリンやコリン受容体の存在を測定するため各細胞分画の純化を行った。単球は単核球をプラスチックに付着させることにより純化した [13]。顆粒球は、6%デキストラン硫酸沈殿を行った末梢血のバッフィーコートをFicall-Isopaque勾配遠心分離を行い純化した。このように、モノクローナル抗体を様々に組合せ、二重染色後、細胞選別機を用いすべてのリンパ球サブセットを分離した。純度は>98%であった。

血清中カテコラミン値

定法に従い、各時点における血清中アドレナ

リンとノルアドレナリン値を、高速液体クロマトグラフィー（HPLC）システムを用いて測定した [14]。事前実験において各サンプルの一定分量を測定し、実験間における変動はアドレナリン <2pg/ml、ノルアドレナリン <10pg/ml であった。

βアドレナリン受容体測定

先ず、細胞（2×10^5）を1mMプロプラノロールを加えたEagle MEM培養液（6mM HEPES日水製薬（株），東京，日本）と2%非働化（30℃ 90分）仔牛血清添加で培養した [11, 12]。その後、細胞を^{125}I-シアノピンドロール（^{125}I-CYP; Amersham Corp., Arlington Heights, IL）各濃度培養液（10 – 200 pM）（総量600μl）で培養した。培養液で3度洗浄した後、採取した細胞塊をガンマカウンターにより同位元素結合を測定した。特異的^{125}I-CYP結合は、プロプラノロール（なし）の値からプロプラノロール（1mM）の値を減算して算出した。

細胞表面におけるコリン受容体の同定

先ず、純化した細胞分画（細胞数，2×10^5）にアセチルコリン・エステラーゼ（AChE）（1.0U/ml）を添加した培養液中で培養した。この培養（37℃，5時間）は、白血球表面上に飽和したアセチルコリンを除去するため重要である [15]。細胞を回収し、培養液で2回洗浄した。そして、各濃度のFITC標識型α-ブンガロトキシン（α-BT; Sigma Chemical Co., St Louis, MO）を細胞塊に添加した（4℃，30分）。洗浄後、蛍光陽性細胞をFACScanにより解析した。こうして、コリン受容体（ニコチン・アセチルコリン受容体：nAChR）を有する細胞の比率を得た。

運動

被験者1と2は、午後2:00より1時間走った。3時点の（運動前、運動直後、4時間後）免疫パラメータを計測した。

統計分析

日内変動評価にロジャース法を [16]、パラメータの有意差検定にスチューデントt検定を用いた。

結果

血液中の顆粒球、リンパ球および単球の日内変動

本研究では、最初に1日24時間にわたる末梢血の白血球数の変動パターンを確認した。健康被験者5名のデータを示す（Fig. 1）。白血球総数は相対的に安定しているが、顆粒球、リンパ球および単球の数と比率に日内変動が見られた。顆粒球と単球の数と比率は昼間に増加した、一方、リンパ球の数と比率は夜に増加した（統計結果はTable II最上部）。顆粒球と単球は白血球全体の60％超であるため、白血球総数の変動に若干似ている。他の研究者もこの傾向を以前報告している [3-8]。これらのうち日差変動や年内変動の報告は既報であるので繰り返さない [16]。

実験値の安定性

本研究では、多様な免疫パラメータ（各リンパ球サブセットの比率）を算出した。

実験間における値の変動を確認するため、3分割したサンプルを個別に測定した結果、変動はごく僅かであることが確認できた（Table I）。

リンパ球サブセットの日内変動は2群に分類できる

多様な組合せで二重染色を行い、末梢血（NK細胞、胸腺外分化T細胞や従来型T・B細胞）のリンパ球サブセットを特定した。健康被験者5名のデータを示す（Fig. 2）。リズムの変動を統計学的に分析した（Table II）。

CD3とCD16（またはCD56またはCD57）の二重染色を行い、$CD3^-CD16^+$（または$CD56^+$または$CD57^+$）NK細胞、$CD3^+CD16^+$（また

Figure.1

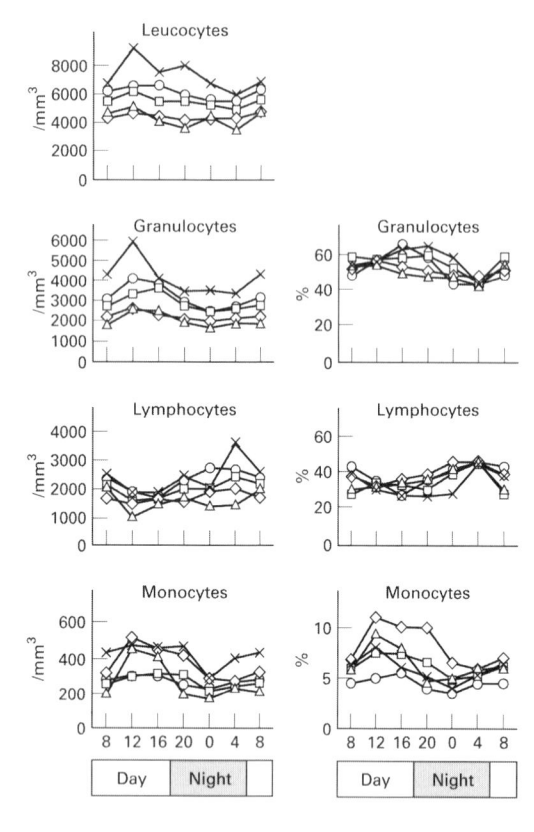

Leucocytes / Granulocytes / Granulocytes (%) / Lymphocytes / Lymphocytes (%) / Monocytes / Monocytes (%)

8:00から1日（24時間）、4時間毎に、多種の免疫パラメータを測定した。顆粒球と単球の数と比率には昼型リズムがあるのに対し、リンパ球の数と比率には、夜型リズムがあることが明らかになった。Fig1-3において、各個人のデータを記号別に示す。

Table.I

実験値の安定性

Subpopulation		Mean ± s.d. (%)
$CD3^-CD16^+$	NK	19.4 ± 0.4
$CD3^-CD56^+$	NK	19.0 ± 0.6
$CD3^-CD57^+$	NK	8.2 ± 0.8
$CD3^+CD16^+$	extrathymic T	0.4 ± 0.2
$CD3^+CD56^+$	extrathymic T	4.6 ± 0.5
$CD3^+CD57^+$	extrathymic T	5.8 ± 0.8
$CD3^+CD16^-$	T	61.5 ± 0.9
$CD3^+CD56^-$	T	58.3 ± 2.5
$CD3^+CD57^-$	T	56.4 ± 2.7
$\alpha\beta$ T	(% of $CD3^+$T)	86.7 ± 0.9
$\gamma\delta$ T	(% of $CD3^+$T)	13.3 ± 0.9
$CD4^+$ Th		33.0 ± 0.5
$CD8^+$ Te		32.0 ± 1.2
$CD20^+$ B		9.7 ± 0.9

平均値±SDは、3度個別に行った実験のデータを用いて算出した。

はCD56$^+$またはCD57$^+$）胸腺外分化T細胞、およびCD3$^+$CD16$^-$（またはCD56$^-$はCD57$^-$）従来型T細胞を同定した。

NK細胞と胸腺外分化T細胞（CD3$^+$CD16$^+$細胞以外）は、日内変動すると考えられ、昼間に比率の増加を示した。一方、通常型T細胞も日内変動し、夜間に比率の増加を示した；昼間、γδT細胞の比率が増加したが、夜間、αβT細胞の比率が増加した。CD4$^+$ T細胞は、夜間、増加した。一方、CD8$^+$ T細胞は、昼間、増加した。CD20とCD5の二重染色を行い、T細胞と同様にB細胞を同定した。CD20$^+$CD5$^-$B細胞およびCD20$^-$CD5$^+$T細胞には日内変動があり、夜間、増加を示した。

血清カテコラミン値の日内変動

身体活動は、最大の日内変化の一つであるが、これはカテコラミン産生量に影響する可能性がある。本実験では、健康被験者（5名）の血清カテコラミン値の変動を先ず確認した（Fig. 3）。以前、日内変動を検証したのと同時刻に血清を採取した。アドレナリンとノルアドレナリン値は日内変動を示し、昼間に増加した（P < 0.001 Roger法）。

昼型リズムを持つ細胞にはアドレナリン受容体が多い

白血球表面にはアドレナリン受容体が存在することは知られている。この点について、白血球各タイプにおいてアドレナリン受容体の発現量が日内変動のパターンと関連しているか検証した（Fig. 4a）。プロプラノロール（1μM）前

Figure.2

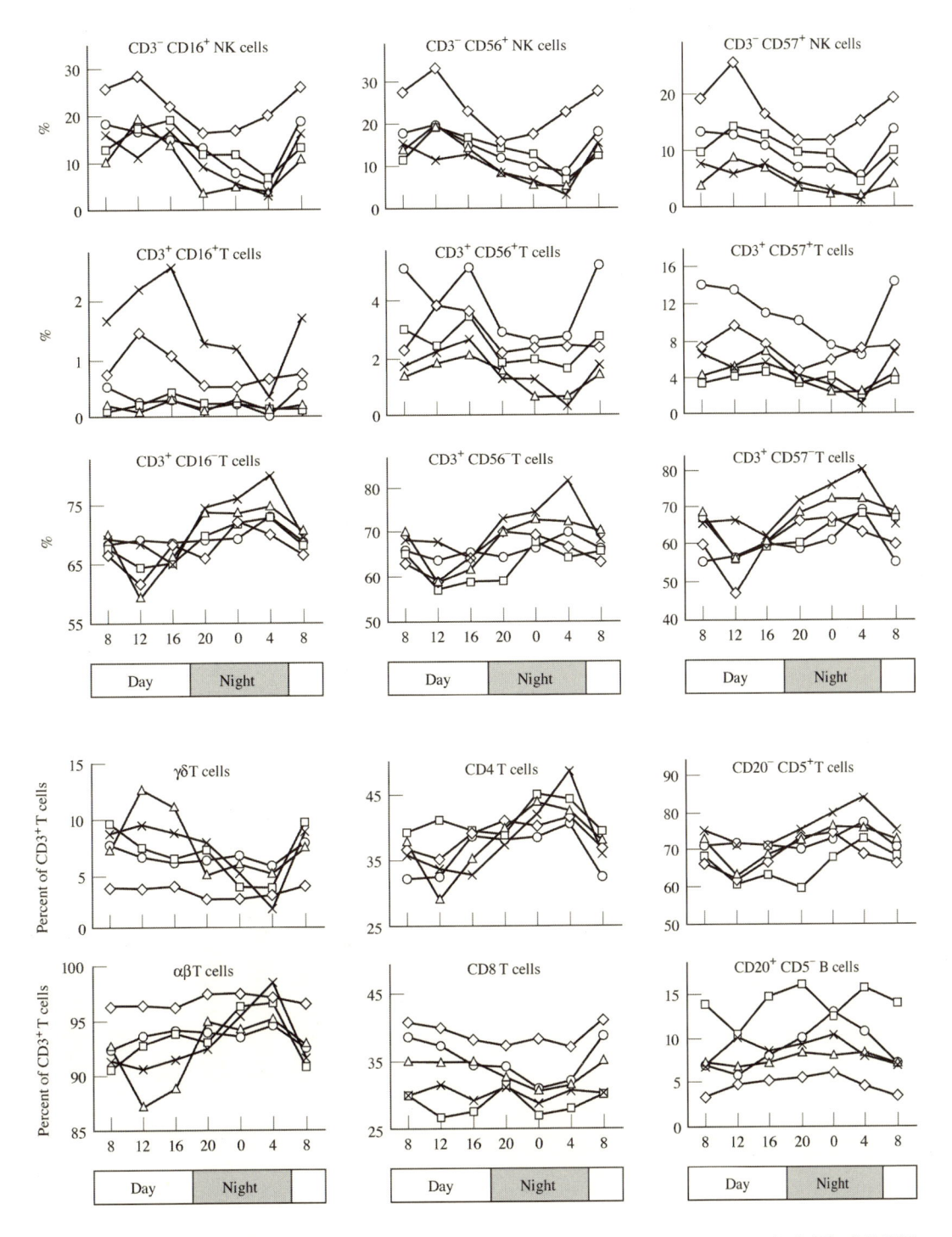

リンパ球サブセットの日内変動。被験者は、健常人5名である。他のリンパ球サブセット同様、ナチュラル・キラー（NK）細胞、胸腺外分化T細胞および従来型T細胞を、モノクローナル抗体の様々な組合で二重染色を行い同定した。リンパ球サブセットを、2群に分類した；昼型リズム群（例、NK細胞や胸腺外分化T細胞）および夜間リズム群（例、通常型TやB細胞）。

Table.II

免疫パラメータの統計解析

Subpopulation		Increase	γ	P
Leucocytes		Daytime	27903	<0.001*
Granulocytes		Daytime	281.4	<0.001*
Lymphocytes		Night	163.5	<0.001*
Monocytes		Daytime	34.3	<0.001*
CD3⁻CD16⁺	NK	Daytime	77.0	<0.001*
CD3⁻CD56⁺	NK	Daytime	79.5	<0.001*
CD3⁻CD57⁺	NK	Daytime	51.8	<0.001*
CD3⁺CD16⁺	extrathymic T		3.8	=0.15
CD3⁺CD56⁺	extrathymic T	Daytime	12.8	=0.002*
CD3⁺CD57⁺	extrathymic T	Daytime	30.4	<0.001*
CD3⁺CD16⁻	T	Night	336.7	<0.001*
CD3⁺CD56⁻	T	Night	325.9	<0.001*
CD3⁺CD57⁻	T	Night	314.4	<0.001*
αβ T		Night	466.4	<0.001*
γδ T		Daytime	33.8	<0.001*
CD4⁺ Th		Night	190.2	<0.001*
CD8⁺ Tc		Daytime	163.8	<0.001*
CD20⁺ B		Night	45.8	<0.001*

データは、図1-3に示す以外に、被験者5名を加えた被験者10名の結果である。*有意差有り

Figure.3

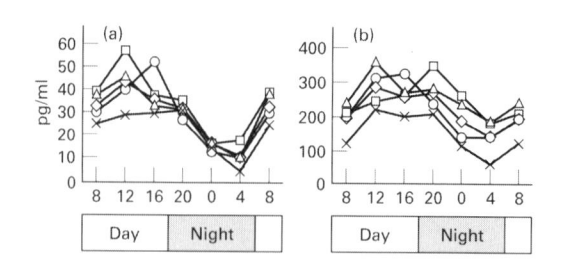

血清中アドレナリン（a）とノルアドレナリン（b）値における日内変動。身体活動により交感神経系の機能が変化するかどうか確認するために、5名の健康な被験者における血中カテコラミン値を測定した。

Figure.4

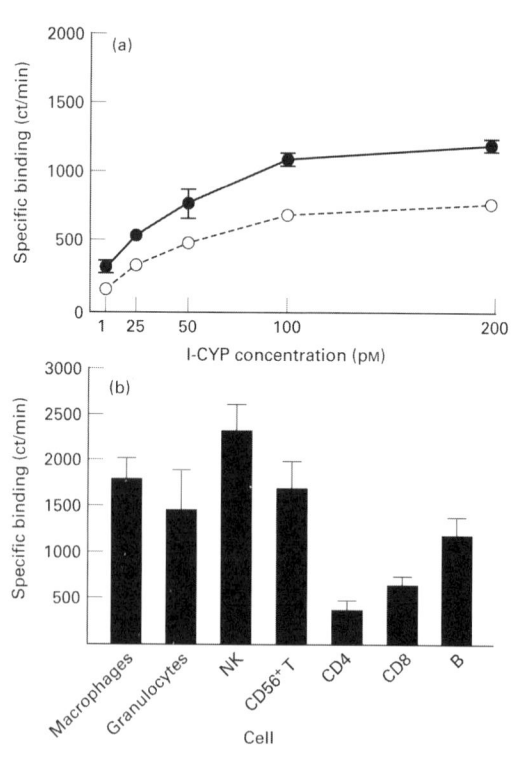

白血球におけるアドレナリン受容体の発現。（a）顆粒球（●）およびリンパ球（○）における¹²⁵I-シアノ・ピンドロール（¹²⁵I-CYP）の特異的結合。（b）白血球と各リンパ球サブセットにおけるアドレナリン受容体の発現の比較。実験（Figs 4および5）では、朝10:00に検体採取を行った。昼型リズムを持つ単球、顆粒球、NK細胞と（胸腺外起源である）CD56⁺ T細胞の表面にはアドレナリン受容体は高値を示した。平均値±SDは、被験者3名のデータを用いて算出した。

処理の有無にかかわらずβアドレナリン受容体の特異的結合の確認には、¹²⁵I-CYP（βアドレナリン作動薬）を用いた。そして、アドレナリン受容体は、リンパ球表面よりも、顆粒球表面に断然多いことが明らかになった。同様に、アドレナリン受容体との特異的結合を、セルソーターで純化を行い各分画間で比較した（Fig. 4b）。単球、顆粒球、NK細胞とCD56⁺ T細胞（胸腺外分化）には、アドレナリン受容体がより多く存在し、一方、リンパ球サブセットCD4⁺、CD8⁺およびB細胞では発現量は低かった。はっきりした昼型リズムを持つ細胞（貪食細胞やNK細胞）には、アドレナリン受容体の密度が高い傾向があった。

夜型リズムを持つ細胞にはコリン受容体が多い

最近、リンパ球表面上のnAChRの直接同定

Figure.5

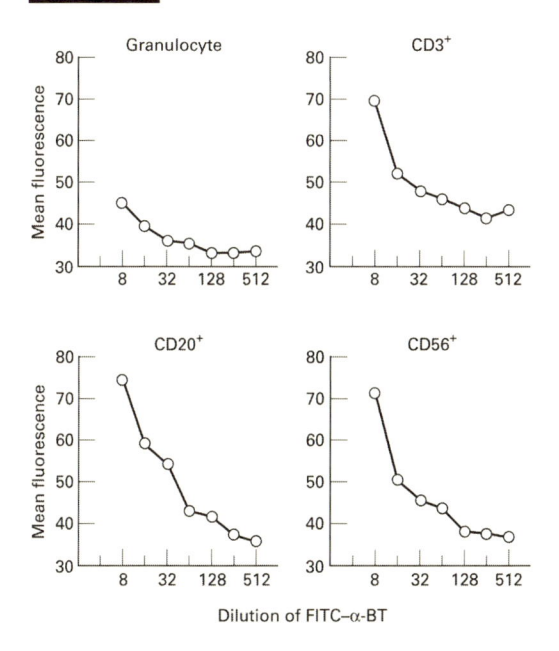

Figure.6

白血球とリンパ球サブセットにおけるコリン受容体の発現の比較。全細胞を、1.0U/mlアセチルコリン・エステラーゼ（AChE）で前培養（5時間）して、FITC標識α-ブンガロトキシ（α-BT）染色を行った。ニコチン・アセチルコリン受容体（nAChR）の発現レベルには、以下の差が見られた；CD20$^+$ B細胞＞CD3$^+$ T細胞＞CD56$^+$ NK細胞＞顆粒球。3度実験を行った典型例を示す。

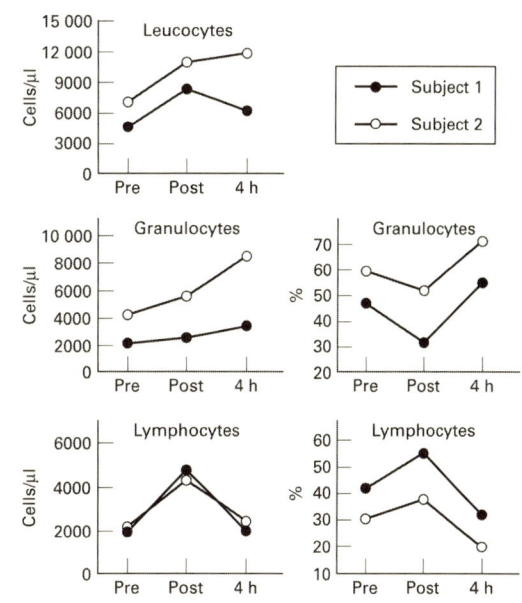

運動後における顆粒球およびリンパ球の数や比率の変化。健康被験者（2名）は1時間走った。末梢血における免疫パラメータを示した時間において測定した。運動直後に、リンパ球数は増加した、そして、顆粒球数は、その後徐々に増加した。次の実験（Fig. 7）において、リンパ球数増加は、NK細胞数増加が原因であることが明らかになった。Fig. 6の実験開始時刻は、午後2:00pmであった。

法を確立した［15］。

リンパ球表面のnAChRは、通常Achで飽和しているため、リンパ球をAChEで5時間前処理して、FITC-α-BTを特異的に結合させる必要がある。この方法を用いて、純化したリンパ球分画のコリン受容体の量を検証した（Fig. 5）。顆粒球と比較してCD3$^+$ T細胞、CD20$^+$ B細胞およびCD56$^+$ NK細胞におけるnAChR$^+$細胞の比率が大きいことが明らかになった。本研究では、各サブセット間におけるコリン受容体量の相対的な違いのみを示した。

運動により昼型リズムを持つ細胞の数と比率が増加した

昼型リズムを持つ細胞のグループには、アドレナリン受容体の量がより多い傾向があった。

この発見が本当であれば、運動（カテコラミン高産生を伴う激しい身体活動）により、特異的な変動パターンが出現する可能性がある。この可能性を、健康被験者（2名）が1時間走り検証した。白血球とリンパ球サブセットの数と比率を、運動前後の3時点で計測した（Fig. 6）。両被験者とも、運動後、白血球総数と顆粒球数は、大幅に増加した（運動直後および4時間後）。顆粒球の比率は、運動直後に減少したが、顆粒球数は僅かに増加を示した。リンパ球の数と比率は、運動直後、一時的に増加したものの、運動4時間後、通常もしくは通常より低値に戻った。後述するように、リンパ球の数と比率の増加は、NK細胞と胸腺外分化T細胞の数と比率によるものであった。

運動後に見られた比率が増加した全リンパ球サブセットは昼型リズムを持つ細胞であった

運動後、リンパ球サブセットの比率の変化を検証した (Fig. 7)。運動直後、両被験者とも、NK細胞と胸腺外分化T細胞の全比率が増加した。全く対照的に、従来型T細胞の比率は、顕著に減少した。同様に日内変動と関連して、$\gamma\delta$T細胞の比率は増加したが、$\alpha\beta$T細胞とCD4$^+$T細胞の比率は減少した。このように、運動により、昼型リズムを持つサブセットの比率が増加した。CD8$^+$T細胞とCD20$^+$CD5$^-$B細胞は、運動による変化は比較的小さかった。

考察

本研究の第一の目的は、顆粒球と単球の数と比率の日内変動の検証であるが、その日内変動のピークは昼間であった（昼型リズム）。一方、リンパ球総数のピークは夜間であった（夜型リズム）。既報を参考に [3-8] 実験を行い、胸腺外分化T細胞（CD56$^+$T細胞およびCD57$^+$T細胞）[9, 10] を含む各リンパ球サブセットのリズムの特徴を検証した [9, 10]。その結果、白血球には2つのグループがあることが明らかになった：一つのグループは、昼型リズムを有し、それは、単球、顆粒球、ナチュラル・キラー（NK）細胞、胸腺外分化T細胞、CD8$^+$細胞および$\gamma\delta$T細胞である。もう一つのグループは、夜型リズムを有し、それは、従来型T細胞、B細胞、$\alpha\beta$T細胞およびCD4$^+$細胞である。NK細胞、胸腺外分化T細胞と$\gamma\delta$T細胞は、自然免疫を担当し、系統発生の進化上、通常型T（$\alpha\beta$T）細胞、B細胞よりも原始的であると広く知られている。故に、昼型リズムを持つ白血球集団は、原始的な白血球の系列に属する可能性がある。

CD8$^+$細胞は、従来型T細胞と胸腺外分化T細胞で構成されている通常健常者では、CD8$^+$胸腺外分化T細胞は、CD8$^+$通常型T細胞よりも高値である。故に、CD8$^+$細胞全体としては、昼型リズムを持つ細胞の変化が見られる可能性がある。

本研究の第二の目的は、生体内で白血球の日内変動が起きる原因の特定である。以前、マウス（夜行性）では、検証した全器官においてリンパ球には日内変動が見られることが明らかになったが、マウスの日内変動はヒトの反対である [17]。ヒトとマウスにおいて、糖質コルチコイドの大量分泌が、身体活動開始直前（ヒトにおける糖質コルチコイドの早朝分泌）に見られる [5]。換言すると、糖質コルチコイドの早朝分泌の刺激で、覚醒し、昼間型活動のリズムが始まる。この時、血清カテコラミン値も上昇する。そこで、副腎摘出マウスを使用し、日内変動に対して起こりうる影響を検証した [17]。副腎摘出マウスでは、この日内変動が消失したことから、ホルモン関与が示唆された。しかし、このマウスには、運動に障害があるため、24時間の身体活動の変化も消失した。自律神経系の活動が変動すると、アドレナリンやコリン受容体を持つ白血球サブセットが影響を受ける可能性がある [11, 12]。運動後、末梢血中の白血球が変化すると多数報告されている [2, 12, 18-20]。

そこで、本研究では、白血球と各リンパ球サブセットにおけるアドレナリンもしくはコリン受容体を比較した。昼型リズムを持つ細胞の表面には、アドレナリン受容体が高密度で存在する一方、夜型リズムを持つ細胞には、高密度のコリン受容体が存在する傾向があった。このことから、二種類の受容体のバランスにより、日内変動が出現する可能性が高まった。例えば、B細胞は夜のリズムを有するにもかかわらず例

Figure.7

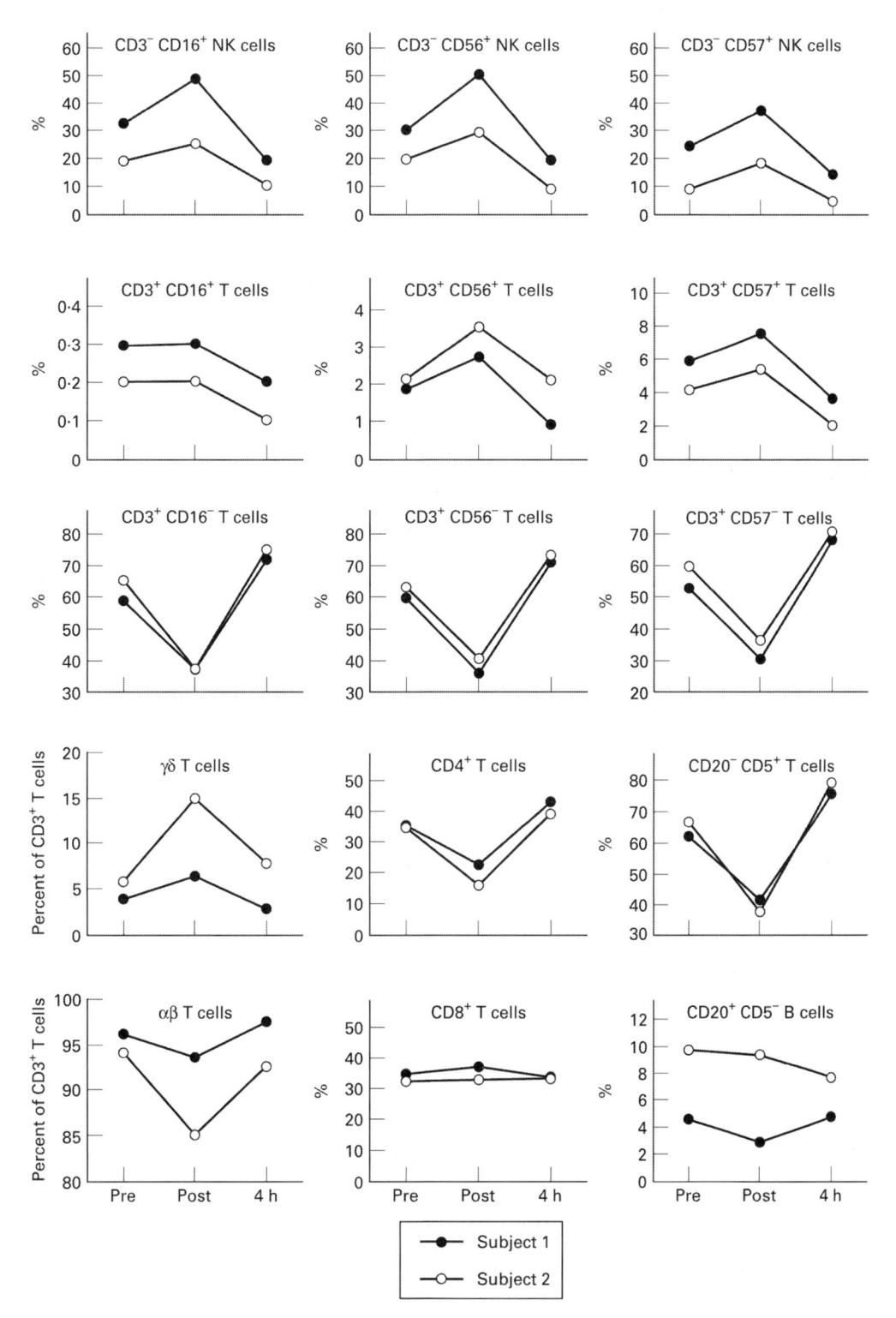

運動後におけるリンパ球サブセットにおける比率の変化。健康被験者（2名）は1時間走った。末梢血における免疫パラメータを示した時間において測定した。運動により、昼型リズムを持つ細胞（アドレナリン受容体をより多く持つ細胞）の比率の増加が出現した。但し、反応には時間差も見られた（例、顆粒球）。

chapter 7 147

外的に多数のアドレナリン受容体をあるが、B細胞には、多数のコリン受容体も存在するのである。

身体活動や自律神経系活動の結果起こる変動が、本当に、白血球の日内変動を引き起こす原因であれば、運動により昼型リズムを持つサブセットの数の増加が出現するはずである。この予測は、本実験の結果により、顆粒球、NK細胞、胸腺外分化T細胞など昼型リズムを持つ細胞の数または比率が、顕著に増加していたことから確認できた。血中のカテコラミン値は、昼間や運動後産生が増加を示していた。身体活動や交感神経緊張が、白血球変動が出現する直接的な要因である可能性がある。従って、夜型リズムを持つサブセットは、ほとんど運動後減少する傾向が見られた。白血球循環（例、血液からリンパ節まで）の中には、この現象と関連するものもある可能性がある [16]。

NK細胞のみならず顆粒球でも、急速な変化が見られた。他にも類似した現象の報告がある：カテコラミンを投与すると末梢血中NK細胞が増加したのである [21]。NK細胞や顆粒球の急速な反応には、どこかにこの細胞集団の貯留場所があり利用していると仮定する研究者は多い。上述の研究では、カテコラミン投与しても脾臓を摘出した患者ではNK細胞の反応に変化がないことを明らかにした。このことから、脾臓はNK細胞や顆粒球の貯留場所（境界顆粒球プール）ではなさそうである。マウスを用いた予備研究において、骨髄自体がそのような貯留場所（特に顆粒球）である可能性を示した [22]。顆粒球の寿命は、非常に短命であることが知られている（2, 3日）。それ故、顆粒球の代謝回転自体は、非常に速い。従って、交感神経が刺激を受け、骨髄内の顆粒球分化や末梢への顆粒球運搬を促進する可能性がある。骨髄には、その可能性が大いにある。単球のみならず、顆粒球、NK細胞と胸腺外分化T細胞は、通常型TとB細胞よりもより原始的である（系統学的に初期に進化した）[23]。白血球の原始的系統では、コリン受容体よりもこのアドレナリン受容体が白血球表面に多く存在すると考えられる。従って、本実験の結果より、以下の推察ができる：原始白血球は、交感神経の刺激を受けてより効率的に活性化し、一方、CD4$^+$ $\alpha\beta$T細胞とB細胞は、副交感神経の刺激を受け活性化する。換言すると、昼間、活動中には、自然免疫系への転換が起こるのである。その反対に、微生物や外来抗原など白血球が貪食するには小さすぎる抗原に対する特異的反応には夜間が有利である可能性がある。

謝辞

本研究は、文部科学省科学研究費補助金による。渡辺正子氏の原稿浄書と橋本哲夫氏の動物飼育に感謝する。

Circadian rhythm of leucocytes and lymphocyte subsets and its possible correlation with the function of the autonomic nervous system

S. SUZUKI*†, S. TOYABE*, T. MORODA†, T. TADA†, A. TSUKAHARA†, T. IIAI†, M. MINAGAWA†, S. MARUYAMA†, K. HATAKEYAMA†, K. ENDOH‡ & T. ABO* *Department of Immunology, †First Department of Surgery, and ‡Department of Hygienics, Niigata University School of Medicine, Niigta, Japan

(Accepted for publication 28 August 1997)

SUMMARY

There are physiological variations in the levels of leucocytes. Among these, the circadian rhythm is very important in terms of the magnitude. Since newly identified lymphocyte subsets (i.e. extrathymic T cells) have recently been detected, a comprehensive study of the circadian rhythm was conducted. All leucocytes were found to vary in number or proportion with a circadian rhythm and were classified into two groups. One group — granulocytes, macrophages, natural killer (NK) cells, extrathymic T cells, $\gamma\delta$ T cells, and $CD8^+$ subset — showed an increase in the daytime (i.e. daytime rhythm). The other group — T cells, B cells, $\alpha\beta$ T cells, and $CD4^+$ subset — showed an increase at night. Humans are active and show sympathetic nerve dominance in the daytime. Interestingly, granulocytes and lymphocyte subsets with the daytime rhythm were found to carry a high density of adrenergic receptors. On the other hand, lymphocyte subsets with the night rhythm carried a high proportion of cholinergic receptors. Reflecting this situation, exercise prominently increased the number of cells with the daytime rhythm. These results suggest that the levels of leucocytes may be under the regulation of the autonomic nervous system.

Keywords circadian rhythm leucocytes lymphocyte subset granulocytes autonomic nervous system

INTRODUCTION

It is well known that various immunoparameters vary in number and function, depending on physical conditions in the host [1,2]. One such phenomenon is circadian variation in the number of leucocytes and lymphocyte subsets in humans and animals [3–5]. In earlier studies, such rhythms of lymphocytes were estimated by morphological and other criteria. In a subsequent study, lymphocyte subsets were estimated by MoAbs, and a unique pattern of the circadian rhythm was reported [6–8]. In this study, experiments were further conducted for the following purposes: (i) since recent studies have revealed the existence of new lymphocyte subsets in humans, i.e. $CD56^+$ T cells and $CD57^+$ T cells of extrathymic origin [9,10], it is desirable that an overall picture of circadian variation of leucocytes and lymphocyte subsets should be obtained; (ii) it should also be elucidated what is the major factor causing the circadian rhythm of leucocytes and lymphocyte subsets.

The results obtained in the present study in humans demonstrate that there are two groups of leucocytes with different peak times of the circadian rhythm. One group consists of cells with a daytime rhythm, namely, cells which increase in number or proportion in the daytime. This group includes monocytes, granulocytes, natural killer (NK) cells, extrathymic T cells, $CD8^+$ cells, and $\gamma\delta$ T cells. The other group comprises cells with a night rhythm, namely, cells which increase in number or proportion at night. This group includes T cells (including $\alpha\beta$ T cells), B cells, and $CD4^+$ cells.

Many, if not all, of the cells with the daytime rhythm tend to express a higher level of adrenergic receptors on the surface. In contrast, cells with the night rhythm were found to carry a large proportion of cholinergic receptors on the surface. This raises the possibility that physical activity, which accompanies the high production of catecholamines or inversely the high production of acetylcholine (ACh), determines the rhythm of leucocytes. Supporting this speculation, it was found that all cells with the daytime rhythm increased in number after exercise. In conjunction with accumulating evidence for adrenergic and cholinergic receptors on leucocytes [11,12], it is concluded that physical activity, a function of the autonomic nervous system, causes the circadian rhythm of leucocytes and lymphocyte subsets.

Correspondence: Toru Abo, Department of Immunology, Niigata University School of Medicine, Asahimachi 1, Niigata 951, Japan.

SUBJECTS AND METHODS

Subjects
The subjects in this study were 10 healthy men, their ages ranging from 26 to 48 years. Two of them, subject 1 being 48 years old and subject 2 being 28 years old, were also tested after exercise. The samples for a circadian rhythm were taken every 4 h from the beginning at 8.00 am. All donors worked and slept in bed, in a regular way.

Immunoparameters examined
Peripheral blood (5 ml) was aspirated into a heparinized syringe. Two millilitres of the blood were sent to the Central Laboratory Unit of Niigata University to examine the numbers and proportions of leucocytes, including granulocytes and lymphocytes, and to measure the serum levels of adrenaline and noradrenaline. The enumeration of leucocyte count was usually done within several hours after sampling. During this time, we confirmed that the result was not affected.

The remaining 3 ml of the blood was used to determine the levels of various lymphocyte subsets. Mononuclear cells (MNC) were isolated by Ficoll–Isopaque gradient (1·077 g/ml) centrifugation [5].

Two-colour immunofluorescence tests were applied to identify lymphocytes subsets, NK cells, extrathymic T cells, and conventional T and B cells [10]. Two-colour staining for CD3 and CD16 (or CD56 or CD57) identified $CD3^-CD16^+$ NK cells (or $CD3^-CD56^+$ or $CD3^-CD57^+$ NK cells), $CD3^+CD16^+$ extrathymic T cells (or $CD3^+CD56^+$ or $CD3^+CD57^+$ extrathymic T cells), and $CD3^+CD16^-$ conventional T cells (or $CD3^+CD56^-$ or $CD3^+CD57^-$ conventional T cells). Two-colour staining for CD3 and T cell receptor (TCR) $\alpha\beta$ (or TCR $\gamma\delta$) or for CD3 and CD4 (or CD8) was also performed to identify $\alpha\beta$ T cells (or $\gamma\delta$ T cells) and $CD4^+$ T cells (or $CD8^+$ T cells). $CD20^+CD5^-$ B cells were identified by two-colour staining for CD20 and CD5. All MoAbs used were obtained from Becton Dickinson (Mountain View, CA). The fluorescence-positive cells were analysed by FACScan (Becton Dickinson).

Cell purification
To determine the presence of adrenergic or cholinergic receptors on various cell fractions, cell purification was performed. Monocytes were purified from whole MNC by adherence to a plastic surface [13]. Granulocytes were isolated from the buffy coat of the blood (sedimented by 6% dextran sulphate) by Ficoll–Isopaque gradient centrifugation. All lymphocyte subsets were isolated by the cell sorter after two-colour staining in various combinations of MoAbs as shown above. Purity was >98%.

Serum level of catecholamines
Plasma at the indicated time was used to measure the concentration of adrenaline and noradrenaline. Its concentrations were analysed by the high performance liquid chromatography (HPLC) system, as described elsewhere [14]. Preliminary experiments of separated aliquots in one sample showed us that experiment-to-experiment variation was <2 pg/ml for adrenaline and <10 pg/ml for noradrenaline.

Measurement of β-adrenergic receptors
Pre-incubation of 2×10^5 cells with 1 μM propranolol was first performed in Eagle's MEM medium supplemented with 6 mM HEPES (Nissui Pharmaceutical Co., Tokyo, Japan) and 2% heat-inactivated newborn calf serum for 90 min at 30°C. Cells were then incubated with different concentrations (10–200 pM) of ^{125}I-cyanopindolol (^{125}I-CYP; Amersham Corp., Arlington Heights, IL) in a total volume of 600 μl medium [11,12]. After being washed three times with medium, cell pellets were obtained to measure isotope-binding levels in a gamma counter. Specific ^{125}I-CYP binding was determined by subtracting the value in the presence of 1 μM propranolol from the total counts in its absence.

Identification of cholinergic receptors on the cell surface
Purified cell fractions (2×10^5 cells) were first incubated with a medium containing ACh esterase (AChE) (1·0 U/ml). This incubation at 37°C for 5 h is critical to eliminate saturated ACh on the cell surface of leucocytes [15]. Cells were harvested and washed twice with medium. FITC-conjugated α-bungarotoxin (α-BT; Sigma Chemical Co., St Louis, MO) was then added at various concentrations to the cell pellet for 30 min at 4°C. After washing, fluorescence-positive cells were analysed by FACScan. This method identified the proportion of cells carrying cholinergic receptors (i.e. nicotinic acetylcholine receptors; nAChR).

Exercise
Subjects 1 and 2 ran for 1 h, starting at 2.00 pm. Immunoparameters were examined at three points of time, i.e. before, just after, and 4 h after the exercise.

Statistical analysis
Rogers' method was applied to estimate the rhythmicity [16]. Student's *t*-test was also used to estimate the difference of some parameters.

RESULTS

Circadian rhythm of granulocytes, lymphocytes and monocytes in the blood
In this study, we first confirmed the pattern of variation in the number of leucocytes in the peripheral blood over the 24-h period of a day. Data from five healthy donors are represented (Fig. 1). Although the number of total leucocytes was seen to be relatively constant, the number (as well as the proportion) of granulocytes, lymphocytes and monocytes varied, showing a circadian rhythm. The number and proportion of granulocytes and monocytes increased in the daytime, whereas the number and proportion of lymphocytes increased at night (statistical analysis of these parameters is included at the top of Table 2). Since granulocytes and monocytes comprise >60% of the total leucocytes, the variation in the number of total leucocytes slightly resembled this variation. This tendency was previously reported by us as well as by other investigators [3–8]. Since we have already reported the day-to-day variation and annual variation in some of these factors [16], we did not repeat it.

Stability of the value in experiments
In the present study, we enumerated many immunoparameters, namely the proportion of various lymphocyte subsets. To determine the variation of such values between experiments, one sample was separated into three aliquots and the values were enumerated independently (Table 1). It was confirmed that the variaton was very small.

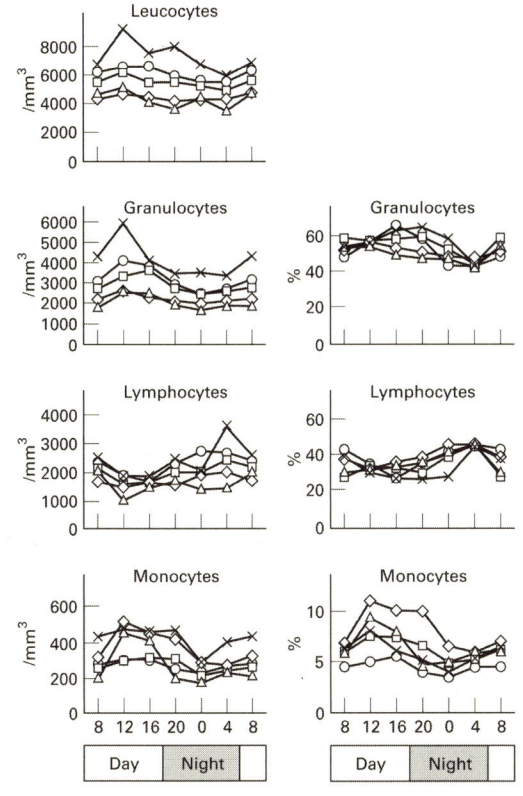

Fig. 1. Circadian rhythm in the number and proportion of total leucocytes, granulocytes, lymphocytes, and monocytes. Five healthy donors were examined on various immunoparameters every 4 h from the beginning at 8.00 am during the 24-h period of a day. It was confirmed that the number and proportion of granulocytes and monocytes had daytime rhythm, while those of lymphocytes had night rhythm. The same symbols in Figs 1–3 indicate data from the same individual.

Table 1. Stability of the value in experiments

Subpopulation		Mean ± s.d. (%)
$CD3^-CD16^+$	NK	19.4 ± 0.4
$CD3^-CD56^+$	NK	19.0 ± 0.6
$CD3^-CD57^+$	NK	8.2 ± 0.8
$CD3^+CD16^+$	extrathymic T	0.4 ± 0.2
$CD3^+CD56^+$	extrathymic T	4.6 ± 0.5
$CD3^+CD57^+$	extrathymic T	5.8 ± 0.8
$CD3^+CD16^-$	T	61.5 ± 0.9
$CD3^+CD56^-$	T	58.3 ± 2.5
$CD3^+CD57^-$	T	56.4 ± 2.7
$\alpha\beta$ T	(% of $CD3^+$T)	86.7 ± 0.9
$\gamma\delta$ T	(% of $CD3^+$T)	13.3 ± 0.9
$CD4^+$ Th		33.0 ± 0.5
$CD8^+$ Tc		32.0 ± 1.2
$CD20^+$ B		9.7 ± 0.9

Mean and s.d. were obtained from three independent experiments.

Circadian rhythm of lymphocyte subsets was classified into two groups

Two-colour staining in various combinations was conducted to identify lymphocyte subsets in the peripheral blood, e.g. NK cells, extrathymic T cells, and conventional T and B cells. Data from five healthy subjects are represented (Fig. 2). The significance of the rhythms is statistically analysed in Table 2. By two-colour staining for CD3 and CD16 (or CD56 or CD57), $CD3^-CD16^+$ (or $CD56^+$ or $CD57^+$) NK cells, $CD3^+CD16^+$ (or $CD56^+$ or $CD57^+$) extrathymic T cells, and $CD3^+CD16^-$ (or $CD56^-$ or $CD57^-$) conventional T cells were determined. NK cells and extrathymic T cells (except $CD3^+CD16^+$ cells) were estimated to vary with a circadian rhythm, showing an increase in the proportion in the daytime. In contrast, conventional T cells varied with a circadian rhythm, showing an increase in the proportion at night. $\gamma\delta$ T cells increased in the daytime, whereas $\alpha\beta$ T cells increased at night. $CD4^+$ T cells increased at night, whereas $CD8^+$ T cells increased in the daytime. B cells as well as T cells were also identified by two-colour staining for CD20 and CD5. Both $CD20^+CD5^-$ B cells and $CD20^-CD5^+$ T cells were evaluated to vary with a circadian rhythm, showing an increase in proportion at night.

Circadian rhythm in the serum level of catecholamines

One of the greatest circadian variables is physical activity. It may influence the production level of catecholamines. In these experiments, the variation in serum level of catecholamines was first confirmed in five healthy donors (Fig. 3). Sera were obtained at the same times as their circadian rhythms had been examined previously. The levels of both adrenaline and noradrenaline varied with a circadian rhythm, showing an increase in the daytime ($P < 0.001$ in Roger's method).

Cells with daytime rhythm expressed a higher level of adrenergic receptors

Leucocytes are known to express adrenergic receptors on their surface. In this regard, it was examined whether the expression level of adrenergic receptors on various types of leucocytes was related to the pattern of their circadian variation (Fig. 4a). ^{125}I-CYP (β-adrenergic agonist) was used to identify the specific binding for β-adrenergic receptors with or without pretreatment with propranolol (1 μM). It was found to be greater on granulocytes than on lymphocytes.

Similarly, specific binding for adrenergic receptors was compared among various cell fractions purified by the cell sorter (Fig. 4b). Monocytes, granulocytes, NK cells and $CD56^+$ T cells (of extrathymic origin) showed a greater density of adrenergic receptors, whereas lymphocyte subsets, i.e. $CD4^+$, $CD8^+$ and B cells, showed a lower density. Cells which had a clear daytime rhythm (i.e. phagocytic cells and NK cells) tended to express a higher level of adrenergic receptors.

Cells with night rhythm expressed a higher level of cholinergic receptors

We recently established a method of directly identifying nAChR on lymphocytes [15]. Since nAChR on lymphocytes is usually saturated by ACh itself, pretreatment of lymphocytes with AChE for 5 h is required to induce the specific binding of FITC–α-BT.

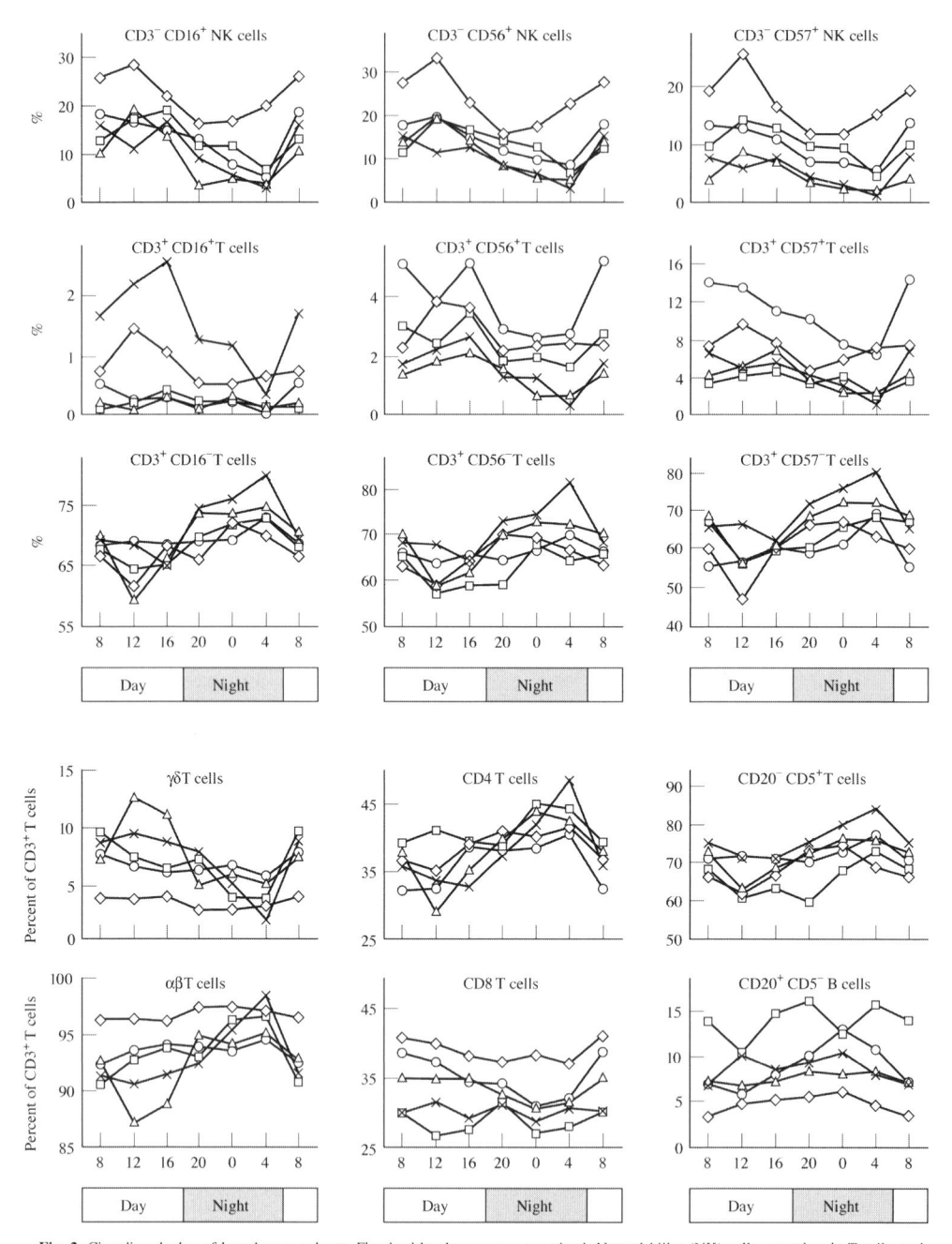

Fig. 2. Circadian rhythm of lymphocyte subsets. Five healthy donors were examined. Natural killer (NK) cells, extrathymic T cells, and conventional T cells, as well as other lymphocyte subsets, were identified by two-colour staining in various combinations of MoAbs. Lymphocyte subsets were classified into two groups, namely, a daytime rhythm group (e.g. NK cells and extrathymic T cells) and a night rhythm group (e.g. conventional T and B cells).

Table 2. Statistical analysis of immunoparameters

Subpopulation		Increase	r	P
Leucocytes		Daytime	2790·3	<0·001*
Granulocytes		Daytime	281·4	<0·001*
Lymphocytes		Night	163·5	<0·001*
Monocytes		Daytime	34·3	<0·001*
CD3$^-$CD16$^+$	NK	Daytime	77·0	<0·001*
CD3$^-$CD56$^+$	NK	Daytime	79·5	<0·001*
CD3$^-$CD57$^+$	NK	Daytime	51·8	<0·001*
CD3$^+$CD16$^+$	extrathymic T		3·8	=0·15
CD3$^+$CD56$^+$	extrathymic T	Daytime	12·8	=0·002*
CD3$^+$CD57$^+$	extrathymic T	Daytime	30·4	<0·001*
CD3$^+$CD16$^-$	T	Night	336·7	<0·001*
CD3$^+$CD56$^-$	T	Night	325·9	<0·001*
CD3$^+$CD57$^-$	T	Night	314·4	<0·001*
$\alpha\beta$ T		Night	466·4	<0·001*
$\gamma\delta$ T		Daytime	33·8	<0·001*
CD4$^+$ Th		Night	190·2	<0·001*
CD8$^+$ Tc		Daytime	163·8	<0·001*
CD20$^+$ B		Night	45·8	<0·001*

Data are results from 10 donors, including five donors indicated in Figs 1–3 and an additional five donors.
*Significant.

Using this method, the level of cholinergic receptors on purified fractions of lymphocytes was examined (Fig. 5). CD3$^+$ T cells, CD20$^+$ B cells and CD56$^+$ NK cells were found to contain a greater proportion of nAChR$^+$ cells than the proportion contained by granulocytes. In this study, we showed only a relative difference in the expression of cholinergic receptors among various subsets.

Exercise induced an increase in the number and proportion of cells with daytime rhythm

There was a tendency for the group of cells with the daytime rhythm to have a higher level of adrenergic receptors. If this finding is valid, exercise (i.e. high physical activity accompanied by a high production of catecholamines) may induce some specific variation patterns. This possibility was examined in two healthy subjects who ran for 1 h. The number and proportion of leucocytes and lymphocyte subsets were enumerated at three points of time

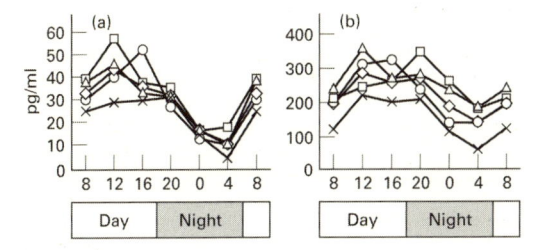

Fig. 3. Circadian variation in the serum levels of adrenaline (a) and noradrenaline (b). To confirm whether physical activity changes the function of the sympathetic nervous system, catecholamine levels in the blood were examined in five healthy donors.

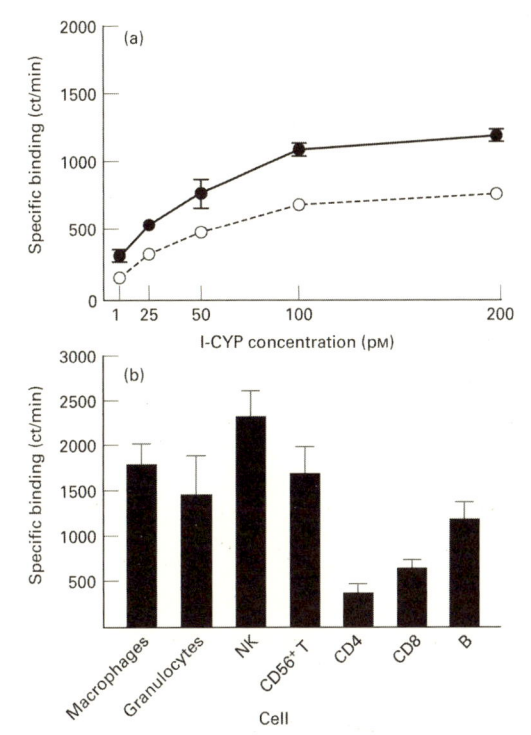

Fig. 4. Expression of adrenergic receptors on leucocytes. (a) Specific binding of ^{125}I-cyanopindolol (^{125}I-CYP) on granulocytes (●) and lymphocytes (○). (b) A comparison of the expression of adrenergic receptors among leucocytes and various lymphocyte subsets. The sampling time was 10.00 am for the experiments of Figs 4 and 5. Monocytes, granulocytes, NK cells, and CD56$^+$ T cells (of extrathymic origin) with the daytime rhythm expressed a higher level of adrenergic receptors on the surface. The mean and 1 s.d. of the data from three donors are represented.

before and after exercise (Fig. 6). In both subjects, the number of total leucocytes and granulocytes increased substantially at the post-exercise time (i.e. just and 4 h after exercise). Although the proportion of granulocytes decreased just after exercise, their absolute number increased slightly. In the case of lymphocytes, the absolute number and proportion transiently increased (just after exercise), but these retured to normal or even lower levels 4 h after exercise. As shown later, this increase in the number and proportion of lymphocytes was due to the increase in the number and proportion of NK cells and extrathymic T cells.

All proportional increases of lymphocyte subsets seen after exercise were for cells with daytime rhythm

The variation in the proportion of lymphocyte subsets was then examined after exercise (Fig. 7). The proportion of NK cells and extrathymic T cells increased just after exercise, without exception, in both subjects. In sharp contrast, the proportion of conventional T cells decreased prominently. Similarly with regard to the circadian rhythm, the proportion of $\gamma\delta$ T cells increased, whereas that of $\alpha\beta$ T cells and CD4$^+$ T cells decreased. Thus, exercise induced an increase in the proportion of the subsets

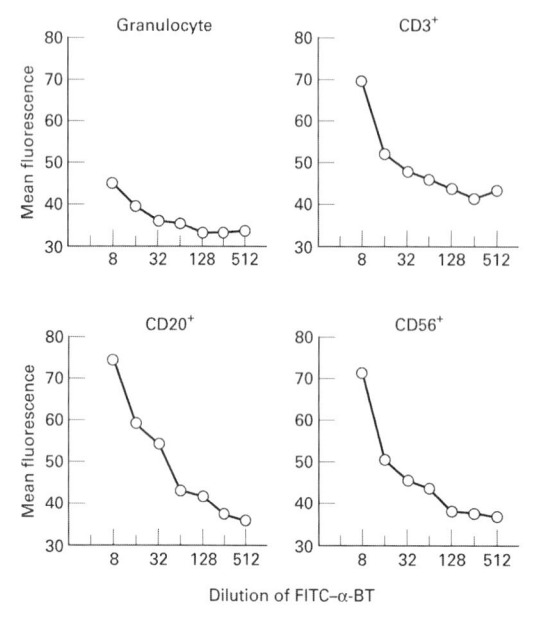

Fig. 5. A comparison of the expression of cholinergic receptors among leucocytes and lymphocyte subsets. All cells were pre-incubated with 1·0 U/ml acetylcholine esterase (AChE) for 5 h and then stained with FITC-conjugated α-bungarotoxin (α-BT). There was an order in the expression level of nicotinic acetylcholine receptor (nAChR), i.e. CD20$^+$ B cells > CD3$^+$ T cells > CD56$^+$ NK cells > granulocytes. Representative results from three experiments are depicted.

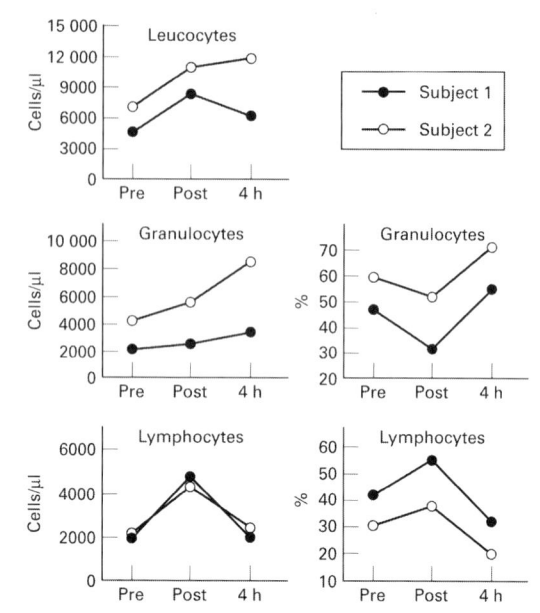

Fig. 6. Variation in the number or proportion of granulocytes and lymphocytes after exercise. Two healthy subjects ran for 1 h and various immunoparameters in the peripheral blood were examined at the indicated points of time. Just after exercise, the number of lymphocytes increased and that of granulocytes gradually increased thereafter. Subsequent experiments (see Fig. 7) revealed that the increase of lymphocytes was due to that of NK cells. The sampling for the experiments of Fig. 6 was started at 2.00 pm.

with the daytime rhythm. The levels of T cells estimated by CD8 and CD20$^+$CD5$^-$ B cells were relatively stationary after exercise.

DISCUSSION

In this study, we first confirmed that granulocytes and monocytes varied in number and proportion, showing a circadian rhythm with a peak in the daytime (i.e. daytime rhythm), whereas total lymphocytes showed a peak at night (i.e. night rhythm). Based on this earlier evidence [3–8], experiments were then conducted to characterize the rhythm of various lymphocyte subsets, including possible extrathymic T cells (i.e. CD56$^+$ T cells and CD57$^+$ T cells) [9,10]. It was found that cell populations could be classified into two groups: one group with daytime rhythm includes granulocytes, monocytes, NK cells, extrathymic T cells, γδ T cells, and CD8$^+$ cells. The other, with night rhythm, includes conventional T and B cells, αβ T cells, and CD4$^+$ cells. It is well known that NK cells, extrathymic T cells and γδ T cells are involved in natural immunity and are more primitive than conventional T (and αβ T) and B cells in phylogenetic development. Therefore, cell populations with daytime rhythm might belong to a primitive lineage of leucocytes.

CD8$^+$ cells consist of both conventional T cells and extrathymic T cells. In usually healthy pearsons, CD8$^+$ extrathymic T cells are much more dominant than CD8$^+$ conventional T cells. In this situation, total CD8$^+$ cells may behave as the cells with daytime rhythm.

The next objective of this study was to determine what causes the circadian rhythm of leucocytes in the body. Previously, we found that mice (which are nocturnal) have a circadian rhythm of lymphocytes in all tested organs, which is opposite to that of humans [17]. A secretion burst of glucocorticoids is seen in both humans and mice just before the start of physical activity (e.g. an early morning secretion of glucocorticoids in humans) [5]. In other words, the early morning secretion of glucocorticoids stimulates and awakes us, and results in the subsequent daily rhythm of our activity, accompanying the serum elevation of catecholamines. Therefore, we used adrenalectomized mice in an attempt to identify possible influences on the circadian rhythm [17]. These mice lost such circadian rhythms, implying some hormonal regulation. However, because of impaired mobility, they also lost the variation of their physical activity round the clock. Changes in the activity of the autonomic nervous system might affect leucocyte subsets, some of them carrying adrenergic or cholinergic receptors [11,12]. There are many reports on changes in blood leucocytes after exercise [2,12,18–20].

We therefore compared adrenergic or cholinergic receptors among leucocytes and various lymphocyte subsets in this study. There was a tendency for cells with daytime rhythm to express a higher density of adrenergic receptors on the surface, while cells with night rhythm were found to express a

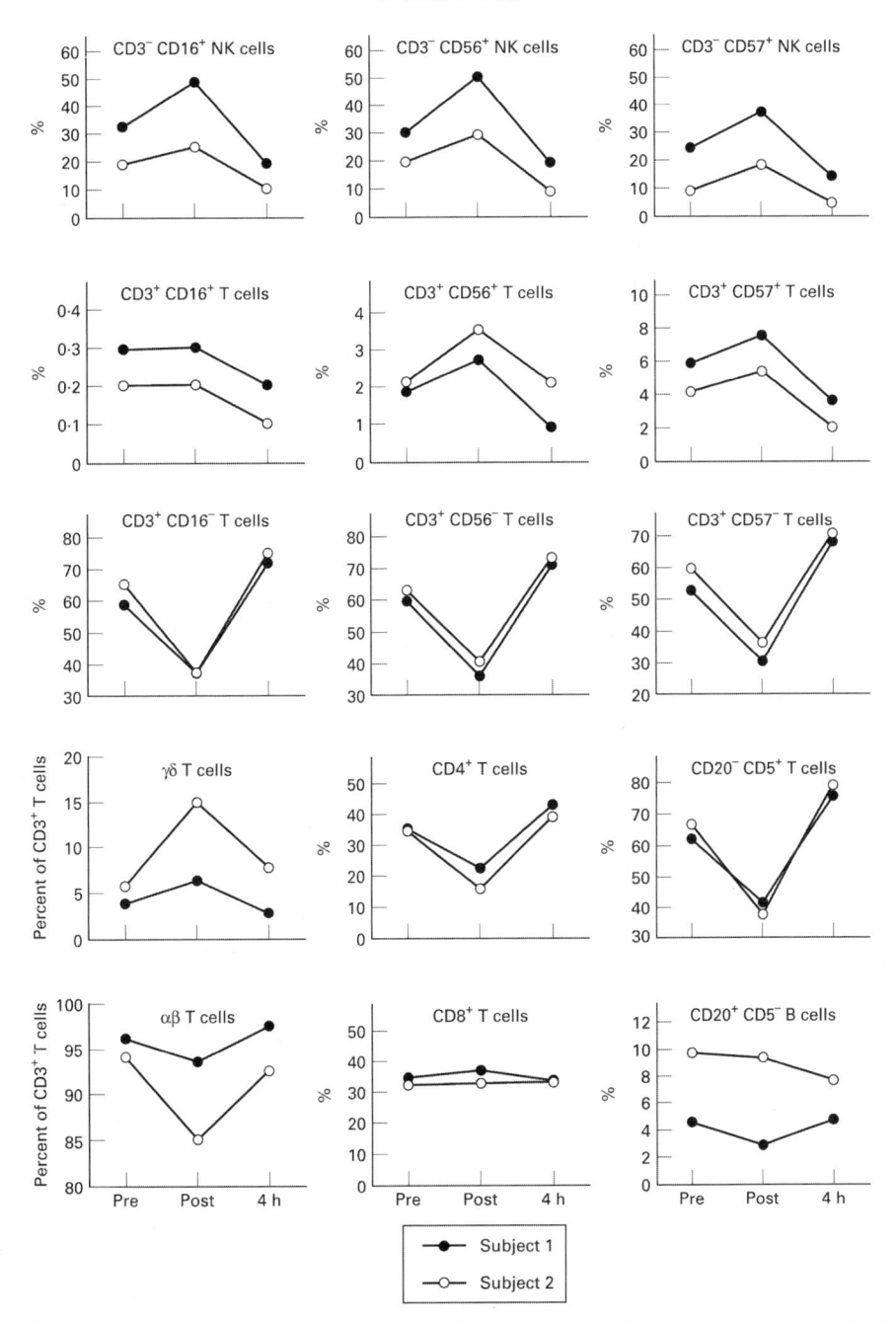

Fig. 7. Variation in the proportion of lymphocyte subsets after exercise. Two healthy subjects ran for 1 h and various immunoparameters in the peripheral blood were exmained at the indicated points of time. Exercies induced an increase in the proportion of cells with the daytim rhythm (i.e. cells carrying a higher level of adrenergic receptors), although there was a time lag (e.g. granulocytes).

high proportion of cholinergic receptors. This raises the possibility that the rhythm is determined by a combination of the expression of both receptors. For example, B cells which had night rhythm exceptionally expressed a high density of adrenergic receptors, but also expressed a high proportion of cholinergic receptors.

If physical activity and the resultant changes in the activity of the autonomic nervous system do indeed produce a circadian rhythm of leucocytes, exercise should induce an increase in the number of those subsets with daytime rhythm. This predicton was confirmed by our present finding of a prominent increase in number or proportion of cells with daytime rhythm, including granulocytes, NK cells, extrathymic T cells, etc. In conjunction with the data on the production of catecholamines in the blood, in which the production increased in the daytime or after exercise, the physical activity and resultant sympathetic nerve strain might be a direct factor causing the variation of leucocytes. Consequently, most subsets with night rhythm tended to decrease after exercise. Some effects on the leucocyte circulation (e.g. from the blood to the lymph nodes) might also be associated with this phenomenon [16].

The most rapid changes were seen in granulocytes as well as NK cells. A similar phenomenon was observed by other investigators, namely, the administration of catecholamine was found to increase NK cells in the peripheral blood [21]. Given a quick response of NK cells or granulocytes, many investigators postulate the existence of an accessible reservoir of these populations somewhere. In the above cited study, the authors revealed that the response of NK cells to an administration of catecholamine did not change in patients who underwent splenectomy. In this regard, the spleen may not be the site of a reservoir (or marginal pool) of these cells. In a preliminary study using mice, we demonstrated that the bone marrow itself might be the site of such a reservoir, especially of granulocytes [22]. As is well known, the life span of granulocytes is very short (i.e. 2 or 3 days). In this respect, the turnover itself of granulocytes is very quick. Therefore, the differentiation of granulocytes in the bone marrow and their export to the periphery might be accelerated by sympathetic nerve stimulation. The bone marrow possibly has such a great potential.

It is obvious that granulocytes, NK cells, and extrathymic T cells, as well as monocytes, are more primitive (i.e. developed phylogenetically earlier) than conventional T and B cells [23]. The primitive lineage of leucocytes is considered to carry dominantly such adrenergic receptors, rather than cholinergic receptors on the surface. The present results, therefore, lead us to speculate that primitive leucocytes are more efficiently activated by sympathetic nerve stimulation, while both $CD4^+$ $\alpha\beta$ T cells and B cells are activated by parasympathetic nerve stimulation. In other words, there is a shift towards the innate immune system during exercise in the daytime. Conversely, specific responses to small fragments of microbial and foreign antigens, which are too small to be phagocytosed by leucocytes, might be favoured at night.

ACKNOWLEDGMENTS

This paper was supported by a Grant-in-Aid for Scientific Research from the Ministry of Education, Science and Culture, Japan. The authors wish to thank Mrs Masako Watanabe for manuscript preparation and Mr Tetsuo Hashimoto for animal maintenance.

REFERENCES

1 Abo T, Kumagai K. Studies of surface immunoglobulins on human B lymphocytes. III. Physiological variations of SIg^+ cells in peripheral blood. Clin Exp Immunol 1978; **33**:441–52.

2 Edwards AJ, Bacon TH, Elms CA, Verardi R, Felder M, Knight SC. Changes in the populations of lymphoid cells in human peripheral blood following physical exercise. Clin Exp Immunol 1984; **58**:420–7.

3 Elmadjian F, Pincus G. A study of the diurnal variations in circulating lymphocytes in normal and psychotic subjects. J Clin Endocrinol 1946; **6**:287–4.

4 Carter JB, Barr GD, Levin AS, Byers VS, Ponce B, Fudenberg HH, German DF. Standardization of tissue culture conditions for spontaneous thymidine-2-^{14}C incorporation by unstimulated normal human peripheral lymphocytes: circadian rhythm of DNA synthesis. J Allergy Cin Immunol 1975; **56**:191–205.

5 Abo T, Kawate T, Itoh K, Kumagai K. Studies on the bioperiodicity of the immune response. I. Circadian rhythms of human T, B, and K cell traffic in the peripheral blood. J Immunol 1981; **126**:1360–3.

6 Ritchie AWS, Oswald I, Micklem HS, Boyd JE, Elton RA, Jazwinska E, James K. Circadian variation of lymphocyte subpopulations: a study with monoclonal antibodies. Brit Med J 1983; **286**:1773–5.

7 Bertouch JV, Roberts-Thomson PJ, Bradley J. Diurnal variation of lymphocyte subsets identified by monoclonal antibodies. Brit Med J 1983; **286**:1171–2.

8 Levi FA, Canon C, Blum J-P, Mechkouri M, Reinberg A, Mathe G. Circadian and/or circahemidian rhythms in nine lymphocyte-related variables from peripheral blood of healthy subjects. J Immunol 1985; **134**:217–22.

9 Takii Y, Hashimoto S, Iiai T, Watanabe H, Hatakeyama K, Abo T. Increase in the proportion of granulated $CD56^+$ T cells in patients with malignancy. Clin Exp Immunol 1994; **97**:522–7.

10 Okada T, Iiai T, Kawachi Y, Moroda T, Takii Y, Hatakeyama K, Abo T. Origin of $CD57^+$ T cells which increase at tumor sites in patients with colorectal cancer. Clin Exp Immunol 1995; **102**:159–66.

11 Khan MM, Sansoni P, Silverman ED, Engleman EG, Melmon KL. Beta-adrenergic receptors on human suppressor, helper, and cytolytic lymphocytes. Biochem Pharmacol 1986; **35**:1137–42.

12 Ratge D, Wiedemann A, Kohse KP, Wisser H. Alterations of β-adrenoceptors on human leukocyte subsets induced by dynamic exercise: effect of prednisone. Clin Exp Pharm Phys 1988; **15**:43–53.

13 Abo T, Sugawara S, Amenomori A, Itoh H, Rikiishi H, Moro, I, Kumagai K. Selective phagocytosis of Gram-positive bacteria and interleukin 1-like factor production by a subpopulation of large granular lymphocytes. J Immunol 1986; **136**:3189–97.

14 Yazawa K, Wang CH, Maruoka Y, Nakajima T, Saito H, Nishiyama N. Determination of catecholamines and their metabolites in adrenals of stress-loaded and wild suncrus (*Suncus murinus*). Jap J Pharmacol 1989; **51**:443–5.

15 Toyabe S, Iiai T, Fukuda M, Kawamura T, Suzuki S, Uchiyama M, Abo T. Identification of nicotinic acetylocholine receptors of lymphocytes in the periphery as well as thymus in mice. Immunology, in press.

16 Kawate T, Abo T, Hinuma S, Kumagai K. Studies on the bioperiodicity of the immune response. II. Co-variations of murine T and B cells and a role of corticosteroid. J Immunol 1981; **126**:1364–7.

17 Maisel AS, Harris T, Rearden CA, Michel MC. β-adrenergic receptors in lymphocyte subsets after exercise. Alterations in normal individuals and patients with congestive heart failure. Circulation 1990; **82**:2003–10.

18 Maisel AS, Knowlton KU, Fowler P, Rearden A, Ziegler MG, Motulsky HJ, Insel PA, Michel MC. Adrenergic control of circulating lymphocyte subpopulations. Effects of congestive heart failure, dynamic exercise, and terbutaline treatment. J Clin Invest 1990; **85**:462–7.

19 Murray DR, Irwin M, Rearden CA, Ziegler M, Motulsky H, Maisel AS. Sympathetic and immune interactions during dynamic exercise. Mediation via a β_2-adrenergic-dependent mechanism. Circulation 1992; **86**:203–13.

© 1997 Blackwell Science Ltd, *Clinical and Experimental Immunology*, **110**:500–508

20 Iversen PO, Arvesen BL, Benestad HB. No mandatory role for the spleen in the exercise-induced leucocytosis in man. Clin Sci 1994; **86**:505–10.

21 Schedlowski M, Hosch W, Oberbeck R, Benschop RJ, Jacobs R, Raab H-R, Schmidt RE. Catecholamines modulate human NK cell circulation and function via spleen-independent β_2-adrenergic mechanisms. J Immunol 1996; **156**:93–99.

22 Tsukahara A, Tada T, Suzuki S et al. Adrenergic stimulation simultaneously induces the expansion of granulocytes and extrathymic T cells in mice. Biomed Res 1997; **18**:237–46.

23 Abo T, Watanabe H, Iiai T et al. Extrathymic pathways of T-cell differentiation in the liver and other organs. Int Rev Immunol 1994; **11**:61–102.

Neonatal Granulocytosis Is a Postpartum Event Which Is Seen in the Liver as well as in the Blood

分娩後、末梢血のみならず肝臓においても新生児顆粒球増多が出現する

Hepatology, 26: 161-172, 1997

chapter **8**

Neonatal Granulocytosis Is a Postpartum Event Which Is Seen in the Liver as well as in the Blood

分娩後、末梢血のみならず肝臓においても新生児顆粒球増多が出現する

TOSHIHIKO KAWAMURA,[1] SHINICHI TOYABE,[2] TETSUYA MORODA,[1] TSUNEO IIAI,[1]
HIROMI TAKAHASHI-IWANAGA,[3]
MINORU FUKUDA,[1] HISAMI WATANABE,[1] HIROHO SEKIKAWA,[1] SHUJI SEKI,[1] AND TORU ABO[1]

From the [1] Department of Immunology, [2] Department of Pediatrics, and [3] Third Department of Anatomy, Niigata University School of Medicine, Niigata, Japan.

【要約】

　最近の一連の研究において、顆粒球表面にはアドレナリン受容体が存在するため、ヒトと動物にストレスを与えると交感神経緊張が出現し、顕著な顆粒球増多が出現することを証明した。活性化した顆粒球がフリーラジカルと超酸化物を産生するので、ストレスが強すぎたり長期化したりする場合、顆粒球が組織を破壊することもある。ヒト新生児の末梢血において顆粒球高値が見られることも知られている。本研究では、この新生児顆粒球増症は、出生時のストレス関連反応であるかを検証した。対象は、出生前後のヒトとマウスで行った。血清を用いた各項目検査および血中白血球総数の計測を行なった。顆粒球値はヒト胎児およびマウス胎仔で低値を示したが、出生後、急激に増加した。この出生後顆粒球増多症と共に、血清中トランスアミナーゼ値が一過性に増加した。マウス出生時にカテコラミン値が一過性に上昇するという結果からも、これらすべての現象は、ストレス関連反応に類似している。実際、マウスとヒトにおいて、肝臓において脂肪肝や造血破壊が見られた。この時、肝臓では、顆粒球による一酸化窒素シンターゼ（iNOS）産生が起こることが明らかになった。これらの結果が示唆するのは、新生児顆粒球増多症は、出生時にさまざまなストレス（例、酸素ストレス）が原因で分娩後生ずる現象である。この現象は、新生児にみられる胎児の肝造血の消失や新生児黄疸と知られている現象の原因である可能性である。

　篤であるが一過性である顆粒球増多（15-20 x 10^3/mm^3）が、決まって新生児に出現するが、生後3日以内に顆粒球値は正常に回復する[1-3]。しかし、顆粒球増多が出生前に存在しているかは不明である。本研究室におけるマウスを用いた実験より、新生児に見られる顆粒球増多は、ストレスにより肝臓に激しい組織破壊が出現した結果ではないかと考えた。この説の裏付けとして、出生後、顆粒球増多と共に特に肝臓で組織破壊の徴候が数多く見られることが判明した。組織破壊の原因は、出生時、主として顆粒球が産生するフリーラジカルと超酸化物である可能性がある[4-7]。ヒトとマウスに見られるこのような徴候には、トランスアミナーゼ値の上昇、肝造血の消失や脂肪肝の形成がある。

略語：iNOS, 一酸化窒素シンターゼ；mRNA, メッセンジャー RNA.
Received April 14, 1997; accepted July 29, 1997.
Supported in part by a grant-in-aid for scientific research from the Ministry of Education, Science, and Culture, Japan.
Address reprint requests to: Toru Abo, M.D., Department of Immunology, Niigata University School of Medicine, Asahimachi 1, Niigata 951, Japan. Fax: 81-25-228-0868.
Copyright © 1997 by the American Association for the Study of Liver Diseases.
0270-9139/97/2606-0027$3.00/0

新生児顆粒球増多症は出生後の一過性の現象であり、出生前には見られないと仮定した。本研究の目的は、上記の仮説を検証することである；実際、共通して見られる顆粒球増多が、出生過程と関連するのかどうか。そして、関連するのであれば、出生と関連する顆粒球増多症として考えられる基本的メカニズムを明らかにすることである。本研究のデータは全て、新生児顆粒球増多症は、ストレス関連の反応と非常に似ていることを示す。例えば、マウスの出生時における血清中カテコールアミン値の一時的な上昇が原因でアドレナリン受容体を持つ顆粒球の増多が見られる可能性がある。この仮説が実証されるのであれば、この結果は、出生後、胎児の肝造血が突然消失する理由と必ず新生児黄疸が出現する理由を説明できるかもしれない。

材料と方法

ヒト検体

健康な新生児の白血球を、出生時の臍帯血、または、出生1,3および7日後の末梢血より採取した。白血球総数を先ず計測し、その後、顆粒球とリンパ球の比率はメイグリュンワルド・ギムザ法により白血球染色を行い検証した。新生児の両親よりインフォームド・コンセントを得た。

マウス検体

新生仔または胎仔BALB/cマウスに、エーテル麻酔を行い、白血球は、胎生期で（妊娠19日目）、新生仔期で（1日齢）、成体期の（8週齢）における白血球を各臓器より採取した。肝臓の非実質細胞（主に造血細胞）を、パーコール（100U/mLヘパリンを加えた35%パーコール）勾配遠心分離で採取した[8]。略述すると、胎仔の肝臓を200-ゲージ・ステンレススチールメッシュで漉し、2%仔牛血清を添加した培養液（RPMI1640, 30mL）に懸濁させたたものを、一度洗浄した後、パーコール溶液に縦走した。こうして分離した細胞塊には非実質細胞を含む。

肺単核球は、肺を細切し、RPMI1640培養液で培養した；0.05%コラゲナーゼ（和光純薬工業（株），大阪，日本）と0.01%トリプシン阻害剤（Sigma, St. Louis, MO）を加えた後、撹拌した（37℃ 30分間）。上清とともに200-ゲージ・ステンレス・スチール・メッシュで漉した後、細胞を培養液で洗浄し、パーコール法を用いて分離した。

ヘパリン化した血液からファイコール-イソパーク勾配法（1.090）により、白血球を分離した[8]。骨髄細胞はシリンジ（注射器）に培養液を入れ大腿骨の洗浄を行い採取した。分離した細胞塊のペレットを、溶血用緩衝液（0.83%塩化アンモニウム/TRIS-HCl緩衝液）[pH7.65]）に再懸濁して溶血した後、培養液で二度洗浄した。

マウスに対する身体的ストレスの影響を検証するため、成年マウス（8週齢-）をステンレス・スチール・メッシュ筒で18時間拘束した。そして、エーテル麻酔下のマウスより臓器を摘出した。

フローサイトメトリー解析

マウスの顆粒球（$Gr-1^+Mac-1^+$）の同定は、抗顆粒球（Gr-1）と抗骨髄系細胞（Mac-1）モノクロナール抗体（PharMingen Co., San Diego, CA）による二重染色を行いフローサイトメトリー FACScan（Becton Dickinson Co., Mountain View, CA）を用いて染色パターンを解析した[8]。

血清中カテコラミン値測定

アドレナリン、ノルアドレナリンおよびドーパミン値を、HPLC（標準高性能液体クロマトグラフィー）を用いて測定した。

電顕標本

透過電子顕微鏡検査のため、肝臓を2.5%グ

ルタルアルデヒドを添加したリン酸塩緩衝液（0.1mol/L）（pH 7.4）で固定した。固定剤に浸漬後（2時間）、1%OsO$_4$添加したリン酸塩緩衝液に組織塊を再固定した（1.5時間）。その後、複数回、段階的にエタノール脱水を行い、酸化プロピレンを添加したアラルダイトに包埋した[9]。超薄切片をウラニル・アセテートおよびクエン酸鉛により着色した後、日立H-7000透過型電子顕微鏡（(株)日立製作所,日立,日本）を用い検証した。

逆転写酵素-ポリメラーゼ連鎖反応（RT-PCR法）

胎児や成年期における様々な週齢のBALB/cマウスからパーコール法により非実質細胞を採取した。iNOSメッセンジャーRNA（mRNA）を検証するため、特異的なプライマーを用いて逆転写酵素-ポリメラーゼ連鎖反応を用いた[10,11]。

成年マウスに高圧酸素を与える

高圧酸素はストレスであるか、また、顆粒球増多症の原因となるかを検証するため、成年BALB/cマウス（n=4）を新潟大学高圧酸素室内で3時間 60%酸素下においた。3時間後に（実験開始6時間後）、マウスにエーテル麻酔を施した後、各臓器の細胞のフェノタイプを解析した。

超音波検査

脂肪肝出現の検証するため、分娩2-6日後における新生児の肝臓と脾臓の超音波画像を記録した。当該臓器における脂質濃度が上昇すると、必然的にエコー輝度も上昇するので確認可能である。超音波画像エコー輝度の比率（肝臓／脾臓）（n=14）を算出し、出生後の日数と比較した。

統計分析

スチューデントのt検定とピアソンの積率相関係数を用いた。

結果

ヒトにおける顆粒球増多

健康なヒト新生児臍静脈血および末梢静脈血（出生1、3そして7日後）を検証した。出生時（臍帯血）、白血球と顆粒球の数も、トランスアミナーゼ値（アスパラギン酸トランスアミナーゼおよびアラニン・トランスアミナーゼ）も上昇しなかった（Fig. 1）。予想通り、これらの値は出生1日後、顕著な上昇を示したが、出生3または7日後までには正常値に回復した。

マウス新生仔における顆粒球増多

胎仔（妊娠19日後）新生仔マウス（分娩1日後）マウスの各臓器より白血球を採取した。顆粒球（Gr-1$^+$Mac-1$^+$）を抗顆粒球（Gr-1）と抗骨髄系細胞（Mac-1）モノクロナール抗体を用いて同定したところ、顆粒球は、胎仔の血液には見られなかったが、分娩後の血液では数多く見られた（Fig. 2A）。分娩後における顆粒球増

Figure.1

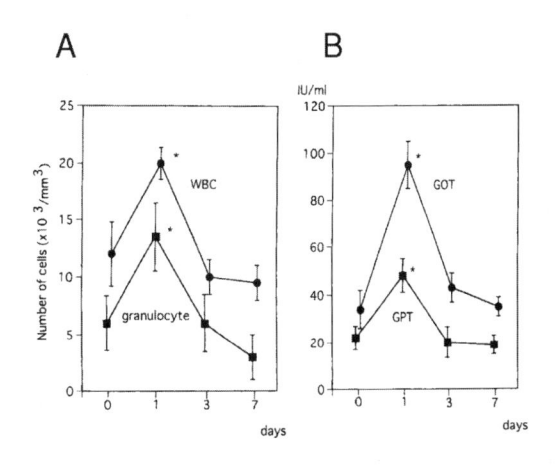

(A) WBCおよび顆粒球数の経時的変化。(B) 出生から新生児7日目までの血清中トランスアミナーゼ値の経時的変化。ポイントとバーで、平均値±1SD（n=8）を示す。*P＜0.05スチューデントのt検定。

Figure.2

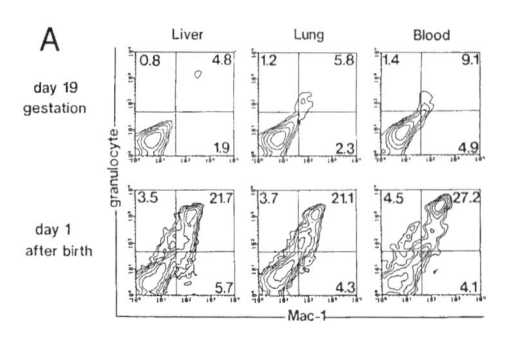

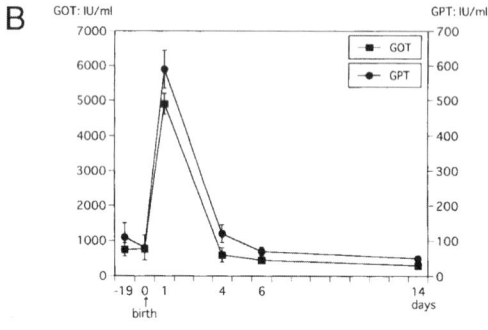

マウスにおける出生時顆粒球増多。(A) 胎仔マウスの組織では顆粒球増多は見られなかったが（上）、分娩後のマウスの組織にでは顆粒球増多が出現した（下）。(B) 新生仔マウスの血清中のトランスアミナーゼ値の一過性上昇。(A) 3実験を行った典型例を示す。各分画内の数値は蛍光陽性細胞の比率を示す。顆粒球増多は、出生後のみ新生仔の全臓器に出現した。(B) 出生後のBALB/cマウス (n=4) より血清を採取した。

Figure.3

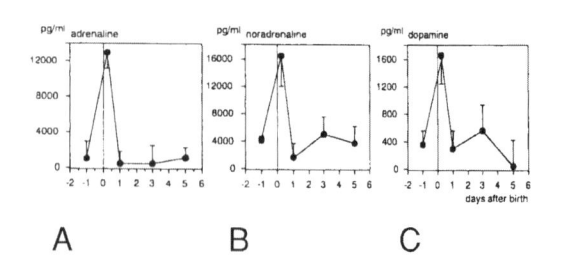

出生後のマウスにおける血清中カテコールアミン値が、ストレス関連反応が出生時に、一過性に上昇するかを検証するため、各時点における血清中カテコールアミン値（(A) アドレナリン (B) ノルアドレナリンおよび (C) ドーパミン）を測定した (n=6)。おそらく重篤なストレスを反映して、血清中カテコールアミン値が出生直後に急激に上昇した。

多は、実際、出生3-6時間後に観察された（未発表データ）。ヒトに見られたトランスアミナーゼ高値は、出生1日後に見られた (Fig. 2B)。

マウス出生時における血清中カテコールアミン値の一時的な上昇

新生仔顆粒球増多症とそれに伴う組織破壊の原因が出生時のストレス関連反応ならば、必然的に、交感神経は緊張しているはずである。そこで、その可能性を検証した (Fig. 3)。血清中カテコールアミン値測定を (n=6) を、出生の前後における4つの時点で行なった。全カテコラミン（アドレナリン，ノルアドレナリンおよびドーパミン）値の顕著な上昇が、出生直後に見られた。

出生前後のマウス肝臓電子顕微鏡検査

出生前後のマウス肝臓を、電子顕微鏡を用いて検証した (Fig. 4)。肝細胞は、出生前は正常であったが（妊娠19日後；Fig. 4A）、出生後、肝細胞の細胞質中に脂肪滴が大量に出現した（分娩1日後；Fig. 4B）。この変化を反映して、肉眼的に肝臓の色が赤から白に変化した。対照群の成年マウスの肝臓（8週齢）(Fig. 4C) と拘束ストレスマウス（16時間）(Fig. 4D) の間にも、全く同様のことが観察された。

ヒト新生児における一過性の脂肪肝の出現

ヒト新生児 (n=14) における肝臓と脾臓の超音波画像（分娩2-6日後）を使用して、エコー輝度における肝臓/脾臓比率を算出した。この比率は、分娩2日後に最高値を示した後、減少を続け、正常値に回復したのは分娩6日後であった (Fig. 5)；生後の日数と肝臓／脾臓の比率の間に相関関係が認められた (r=-0.711, p<0.05)。これらの結果が示唆するのは、ヒト新生児においてさえ、出生時に脂肪肝が出現したことであった。

Figure.4

出生時における肝細胞内の脂肪滴の出現。(A) 胎仔（妊娠19日目）の肝臓；(B) 新生仔（出生後1日目）の肝臓；(C) 成年マウス（8週齢）の肝臓；および (D) 成年マウス（8週齢）拘束ストレス（16時間）後の肝臓（倍率×2000）。肝細胞の細胞質において脂質滴が大量に見られた。おそらくマウスの出生ストレスや拘束ストレスが原因であろう。

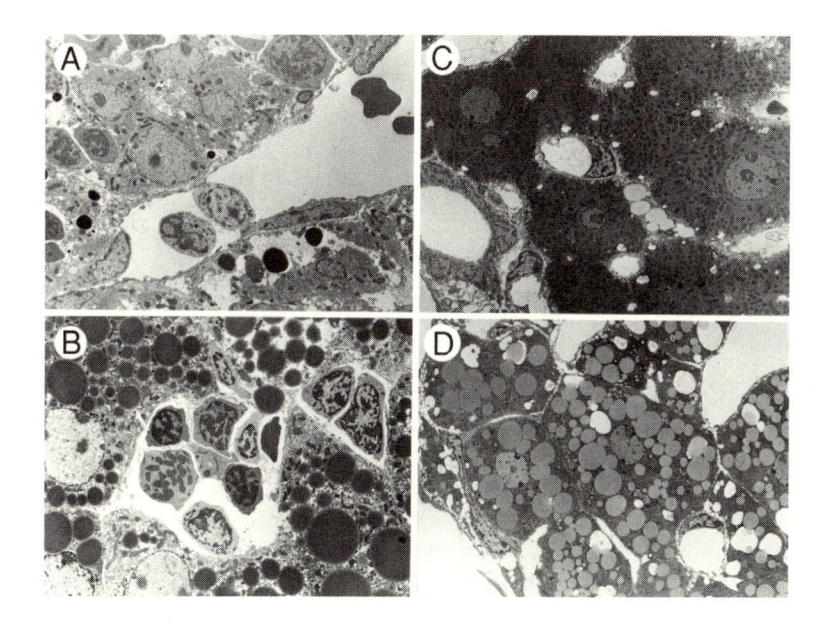

Figure.5

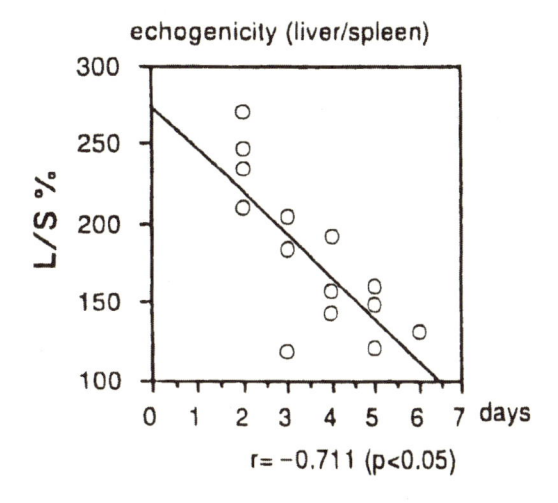

ヒト新生児の肝臓および脾臓の超音波画像。分娩2-6日後の超音波画像を使用した（n=14）。
出生後の日数（X軸）および肝臓／脾臓の比率（Y軸）を示す。出生後の日数と肝臓／脾臓の比率の間に相関関係が認められた（r=-0.711[n=14],p<0.05)。

出生時に造血細胞が破壊される

マウス肝臓における造血細胞数の経時的変化を検証した（n=4）。造血細胞（非実質細胞）の数は、胎齢に相関して安定して増加したが、出生後、急速な減少を示した（Fig. 6A）。BALB/cマウス新生仔（分娩3, 6, 24および48時間後）の白血球におけるiNOS mRNA発現を検証した。出生3時間後の肝臓における白血球でiNOS mRNAの発現が見られたが、この発現は、6時間以内に減弱し、分娩後24および48時間後には完全に消失した（Fig. 6B）。

酸素ストレスと顆粒球増多

BALB/Cマウス（n=3）を3時間 60%酸素下においた。その3時間後に、マウスの各臓器おける顆粒球値を計測した。測定を行なった全臓器（特に肺と末梢血）において、Gr-1$^+$Mac-1$^+$顆粒球の比率が増加した（Fig. 7）。肺では単核細胞数は二倍になったが、他臓器ではそれほどの増加を示さなかった（最高30%）。

考察

本研究以前には、ヒト新生児における顆粒球数の顕著に高い理由も、胎児の肝造血の組織破壊（新生児黄疸や新生児肝炎が起きる）が、出生の直後に始まる理由も不明であった。本研究の結果は、これらの現象の原因は、ヒトとマウスが出生する際のストレスであることを示唆する。

Figure.6

A (グラフ: Number of hematopoietic cells in the liver (×10^6) vs days 11, 13, 14, 15, 17, 19, ↑birth, 1, 7, 14)

B (電気泳動像: size marker, before birth, after birth 3hr, 6hr, 24hr, 48hr)
- iNOS (479bp) — 450bp, 250bp マーカー
- β-actin (373bp) — 350bp, 250bp マーカー

出生後、造血細胞が破壊される（活性化した顆粒球が産生する遊離基が原因の可能性がある）と思われる。(A) マウス肝臓における造血細胞数の経時的変化。(B) 新生仔（BALB/cマウス）の白血球による出生後 iNOS mRNAの発現。造血細胞（非実質細胞）の数は、胎齢に相関して安定して増加したが、出生後、急速な減少を示した。細胞数は、分娩後7-14日前後に安定した。実験（A）では、4匹のマウスを用いて検査標本を採取した。出生3時間後の肝臓における白血球はではiNOS mRNAの発現を示した。しかし、この発現は、6時間以内に減弱し、分娩後24および48時間後には完全に消失した。

Figure.7

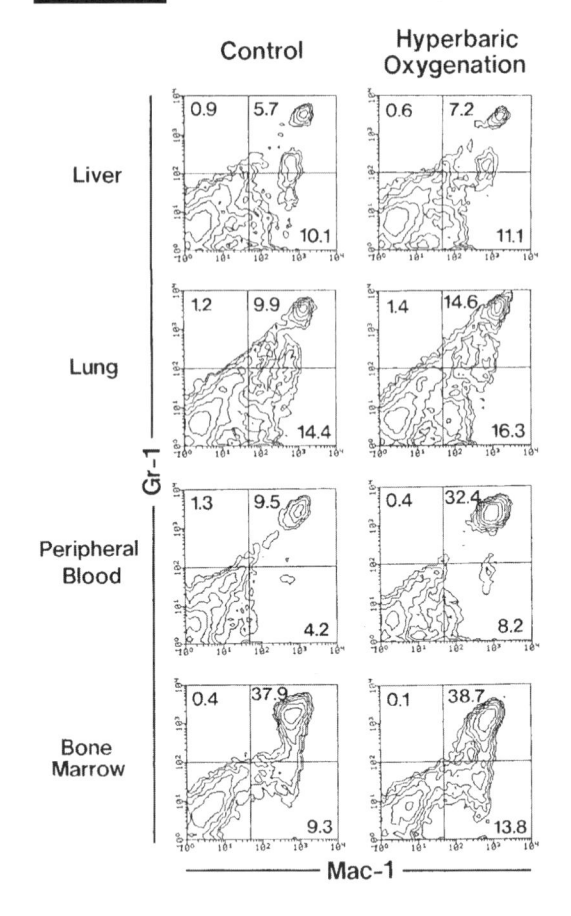

(フローサイトメトリー像: Control / Hyperbaric Oxygenation、Liver, Lung, Peripheral Blood, Bone Marrow、縦軸 Gr-1、横軸 Mac-1)

臓器	Control (左上/右上/右下)	Hyperbaric Oxygenation (左上/右上/右下)
Liver	0.9 / 5.7 / 10.1	0.6 / 7.2 / 11.1
Lung	1.2 / 9.9 / 14.4	1.4 / 14.6 / 16.3
Peripheral Blood	1.3 / 9.5 / 4.2	0.4 / 32.4 / 8.2
Bone Marrow	0.4 / 37.9 / 9.3	0.1 / 38.7 / 13.8

マウス各臓器における酸素ストレスにより顆粒球増多の出現。8週齢のBALB/Cマウスを3時間60％酸素下（1 atom）においた。その3時間後に、マウスの顆粒球値を計測した。Gr-1とMac-1の二重染色を行なった。高酸素ストレスの結果、肺と末梢血における顆粒球比率が顕著に増加した（実験群，右：対照群，左）。3度実験を行った典型例を示す。

なぜ、ストレスにより顆粒球増多が出現するのか？

この点について、顆粒球表面にαおよびβアドレナリン受容体が存在することを忘れてはならない[12-14]；故に、いろいろなストレッサーにより交感神経系緊張となり、顆粒球が増多する[15]。マウスで出生時には、血清中カテコールアミン値の一時的な上昇が見られた。顆粒球はフリーラジカルと超酸化物を産生する主な細胞であるので、後に出現する組織破壊に密接に関与している可能性がある[16,17]。一酸化窒素（NO）の過剰産生が出現し、低値ではない場合、DNA損傷や組織破壊が出現することが知られている[10,11]。あるいは、出生時の一酸化窒素産生は、反対に、組織保護と関係している可能性もある。いずれにせよ、肝臓の白血球における

iNOS mRNA発現は、ストレスの指標としてすぐれているようである。

研究者と臨床医の多くは、胎児期に、胎児型肝造血から成人型骨髄造血に徐々に移行すると思っている。本研究では出生前と出生直後における肝造血細胞の経時的変化を検証し徐々に移行するわけではないことを明らかにした。出生後、肝造血細胞の数が突然減少する。

何度も大量の酸素にさらされると、特定の副作用（例えば組織破壊、肺線維症または白内障）が出現することが知られている[4,5]。さらに、脂肪肝は過度のアルコール摂取結果として有名である[18,19]。換言すると、生体にいろいろなストレッサーを与えると、肝細胞に脂肪滴が数多く見られるのは共通した特徴である。本研究では、成年マウスへ多量の酸素を暴露すると顆粒球増多症が誘導された。このような副作用は顆粒球や他の細胞が産生するフリーラジカルと超酸化物が原因であると仮定される[16,17]。

空気呼吸する新生児も、初めて酸素を吸い込むことがストレスになる。ヒト胎児では、動脈血PO_2値28 ± 8mmHg前後であるが、出生4時間後、62 ± 14mmHgまで急激に上昇する[20]。末梢血中の酸素濃度がこのように上昇することが、激しいストレッサーになると容易に想像できる。この時、主として組織破壊が起こる臓器の1つが肝臓であるようだ。出生後、トランスアミナーゼ値が高いことからもこの概念は裏打ちされる。本研究では、脂肪滴が大量にある肝細胞（脂肪肝）の状況を、マウスでは直接的に、そしてヒトでは間接的に（超音波検査）検証を行った。出生でも拘束ストレスでも、ストレッサーから解放されると生体は回復を示した。

その後の研究において（未発表データ）、呼吸開始後および孵化前のニワトリにも脂肪肝を発見されたことからも、新生児顆粒球増多症に対する酸素ストレスの関与は、出産ストレスのものよりも密であると仮定できる。もっとも、身体的または精神的ストレスが顆粒球増多症の原因となることが知られている[21-23]。帝王切開で生まれた新生児にも出生後顆粒球増多と新生児黄疸が見られることから（未発表データ）この仮説は有効と考えられる。

本研究が示唆するのは、肺呼吸する生物はすべてこの現象を経験し、進化の歴史において上陸しようとしたすべての生命体が類似した現象に直面したことである。生物や生命体の上陸作戦の多くは、酸素ストレスが原因で挫折した可能性もありそうだ。造血器官が肝臓から骨髄（成人型造血）へと上手く移動出来た時のみ上陸に成功できたのである。出生時は、肺呼吸する生体の新生児は、上陸への歴史現象を繰返す可能性がある。

いずれにせよ、出生前後のヒトとマウスの各臓器における顆粒球値の詳細な観察により、新生児顆粒球増多症は分娩後の現象であること、そして、それはストレス関連の反応に似ていることが明らかになった。出生時のストレスについて更なる研究が必要である。

謝辞

木村京菜氏と金子裕子氏の浄書に感謝する。

Neonatal Granulocytosis Is a Postpartum Event Which Is Seen in the Liver as Well as in the Blood

Toshihiko Kawamura,[1] Shinichi Toyabe,[2] Tetsuya Moroda,[1] Tsuneo Iiai,[1] Hiromi Takahashi-Iwanaga,[3] Minoru Fukada,[1] Hisami Watanabe,[1] Hiroho Sekikawa,[1] Shuhji Seki,[1] and Toru Abo[1]

In a recent series of studies, we demonstrated that stress in humans and animals, with resultant sympathetic nerve strain, induces severe granulocytosis, because granulocytes carry adrenergic receptors on the surface. Because activated granulocytes produce free radicals and superoxides, they sometimes induce tissue damage if the stress is too strong or continuous. Human neonates are also known to show high levels of granulocytes in the peripheral blood. In this study, we investigated whether such neonatal granulocytosis are a stress-associated response at birth. Both human and mouse materials, before and after birth, were used. The number of leukocytes in the blood, as well as some other factors in the serum, were measured. Although levels of granulocytes were found to be low in fetal humans and mice, they increased sharply after birth. In parallel with this postpartal granulocytosis, transaminases in sera increased transiently. In reference to results of a transient elevation in the levels of catecholamines at birth in mice, all these phenomena resemble stress-associated responses. Indeed, fatty liver and hematopoietic destruction in the liver were also observed in mice and humans. At this time, the production of inducible nitric oxide synthase (iNOS) by granulocytes in the liver was evident. These results suggest that neonatal granulocytosis is a postpartum event which results from various stresses (e.g., oxygen stress) at birth. This event may be responsible for such well-known neonatal phenomena as the termination of fetal hematopoiesis in the liver and as neonatal jaundice. (HEPATOLOGY 1997;26:1567-1572.)

Severe but transient granulocytosis (15 to 20 × $10^3/mm^3$) is always seen in neonates, and a return to normal granulocyte levels occurs within 3 days.[1-3] However, it is not known whether or not this condition exists before birth. In our laboratory, incidental observations in mice led us to suspect that the granulocytosis seen in neonates may result from some stresses, with the liver suffering the greatest tissue destruction. In support of this idea, it was found that many signs of tissue destruction, especially in the liver, are seen in parallel with granulocytosis after birth. It is speculated that tissue damages are induced by free radicals and superoxides, which are mainly produced by granulocytes at that time.[4-7] Such signs in humans and mice include the elevation of transaminases, termination of hematopoiesis in the liver, and the formation of fatty liver.

We postulated that neonatal granulocytosis is a transient phenomenon following birth and does not appear before birth. The present study was designed to test our hypothesis, i.e., to determine whether or not the commonly observed granulocytosis is, in fact, related to the birth process, and if so, to elucidate possible mechanisms underlying birth-related granulocytosis. All data from the present study suggest that neonatal granulocytosis is quite similar to stress-associated responses. For example, a transient elevation in serum levels of catecholamines at birth in mice may induce granulocytosis, which carries adrenergic receptors on the surface. If our hypothesis is validated, the results may explain why fetal hematopoiesis suddenly ceases in the liver after birth and why neonates consistently experience jaundice.

MATERIALS AND METHODS

Human Materials. Leukocytes of healthy neonates were obtained from the cord blood at birth or from the peripheral blood on postpartum days 1, 3, and 7. The number of total leukocytes was first enumerated, after which the proportion of granulocytes and lymphocytes was determined from cell smears stained by the May-Grüwald-Giemsa method. Informed consent was obtained from the parents of the babies.

Mouse Materials. Neonatal or fetal BALB/c mice were euthanized by ether anesthesia. Leukocytes were obtained from various organs at fetal (day 19 of gestation), neonatal (postpartum day 1), and adult (8 week) ages. Non-parenchymal cells in the liver, mainly hematopoietic cells, were obtained by Percoll (35% Percoll containing 100 U/mL of heparin) gradient centrifugation.[8] Briefly, fetal liver was pressed through 200-gauge stainless steel mesh and suspended in 30 mL of RPMI1640 medium supplemented with 2% newborn calf serum. After being washed once, the suspension was overlapped onto the Percoll cushion. The resulting cell pellets contained non-parenchymal cells.

Lung leukocytes were obtained by cutting the lung into small pieces and by incubating them in RPMI1640 medium; 0.05% collagenase (WAKO, Osaka, Japan) and 0.01% trypsin inhibitor (Sigma, St. Louis, MO) was added to the mixture, which was then stirred for 30 minutes at 37°C. The pieces and supernatant were pressed through 200-gauge stainless steel mesh. The cells were then washed with the medium and fractionated by the Percoll method.

Blood leukocytes were isolated from heparinized blood by the Ficoll-Isopaque gradient (1.090) method.[8] Bone marrow cells were obtained by flushing the femurs with a syringe containing the medium. The pellet was resuspended in the lysing buffer solution

---

Abbreviations: iNOS, inducible nitric oxide synthase; mRNA, messenger RNA.
From the [1]Department of Immunology, [2]Department of Pediatrics, and [3]Third Department of Anatomy, Niigata University School of Medicine, Niigata, Japan.
Received April 14, 1997; accepted July 29, 1997.
Supported in part by a grant-in-aid for scientific research from the Ministry of Education, Science, and Culture, Japan.
Address reprint requests to: Toru Abo, M.D., Department of Immunology, Niigata University School of Medicine, Asahimachi 1, Niigata 951, Japan. Fax: 81-25-228-0868.
Copyright © 1997 by the American Association for the Study of Liver Diseases.
0270-9139/97/2606-0027$3.00/0

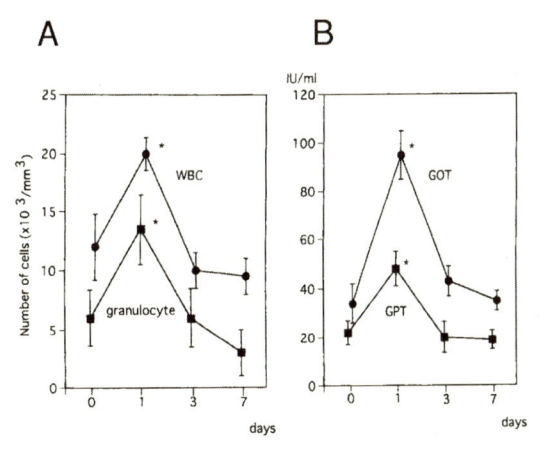

FIG. 1. (A) Time-kinetics of the numbers of WBC and granulocytes, and (B) time-kinetics of the levels of serum transaminase from birth through day 7 in human neonates. The *point* and *bar* represent ± 1 SD (n = 8). *$P < .05$ by Student's t test.

(0.83% ammonium chloride/TRIS-HCl buffer [pH 7.65]) to deplete erythrocytes and was then washed twice in the medium.

To examine the effects of physical stress on mice, adult mice (8-weeks old) were physically restrained in a stainless steel mesh sleeve for 18 hours. The mice were then euthanized by ether anesthesia and their organs were harvested.

Immunofluorescence Test. Identification of mouse granulocytes (Gr-1$^+$Mac-1$^+$) was performed using anti-granulocyte (Gr-1) and anti-myeloid cell (Mac-1) mAbs (PharMingen Co., San Diego, CA) in conjunction with a two-color immunofluorescence test.[8] The staining pattern was produced by a FACScan (Becton Dickinson Co., Mountain View, CA).

Measurement of Catecholamines in Sera. Levels of adrenaline, noradrenaline, and dopamine were measured by a regular high-performance liquid chromatography method.

Electron Microscopy. For transmission electron microscopy, the livers were fixed with 2.5% glutaraldehyde in 0.1 mol/L phosphate buffer (pH 7.4). After being immersed in the fixative for 2 hours, the tissue blocks were postfixed for 1.5 hours in 1% OsO$_4$ dissolved in the phosphate buffer, were dehydrated through a series of graded ethanol, and were embedded in Araldite with propylene oxide.[9] The ultra-thin sections were stained with uranyl acetate and lead citrate and were then examined under a Hitachi H-7000 transmission electron microscope (Hitachi Seisakusho, Hitachi, Japan).

Reverse Transcriptase-Polymerase Chain Reaction. BALB/c mice at various fetal and adult ages were used to obtain non-parenchymal cells by the Percoll method. To detect iNOS messenger RNA (mRNA), reverse transcriptase–polymerase chain reaction was applied. Specific primers were used in conjunction with reverse transcriptase–polymerase chain reactions.[10,11]

Exposure of Adult Mice to a High Concentration of Oxygen. To determine if hyperbaric oxygenation is stressful and if it induces granulocytosis, adult BALB/c mice (n = 4) were exposed to 60% oxygen at 1 Atm for 3 hours in the hyperbaric chamber of Niigata University. Three hours later (6 hours after initiation), the mice were killed by deep ether anesthesia to analyze the phenotype of cells in various organs.

Ultrasonography. Ultrasonograms of the liver and spleen of human neonates were recorded on postpartum days 2 through 6 to detect the presence of fatty livers. It followed that if lipid levels increased in the corresponding tissues, the echogenicity should be elevated.

Ratios (liver/spleen) of echogenicity of 14 ultrasonograms were calculated and compared with days since birth.

Statistical Analysis. Differences were analyzed by the Student's t test. The correlation coefficient was determined by Pearson's method.

RESULTS

Granulocytosis in Humans. Blood from healthy human neonate umbilical vein and from peripheral veins on postpartum days 1, 3, and 7 were examined. At birth (i.e., in umbilical cord blood), the numbers of white blood cells and granulocytes were not elevated, nor were the levels of transaminases (i.e., aspartate transaminase and alanine transaminase) (Fig. 1). As expected, these levels were significantly higher on postpartum day 1 and recovered to normal levels postpartum by days 3 or 7.

Neonatal Granulocytosis in Mice. Leukocytes were isolated from various organs in fetal (day 19 after gestation) and in neonatal mice (postpartum day 1) mice. Granulocytes (Gr-1$^+$Mac-1$^+$), identified by anti-granulocyte (Gr-1) and anti-myeloid cell (Mac-1) monoclonal antibodies, were absent in the fetal blood but abundant in the postpartal blood (Fig. 2A). Postpartum granulocytosis was actually observed 3 to 6 hours after birth (data not shown). As in humans, elevated levels of transaminases were seen on day 1 after birth (Fig. 2B).

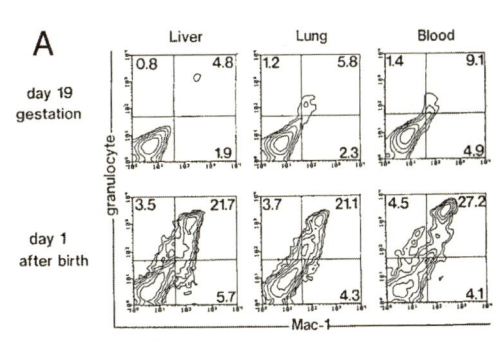

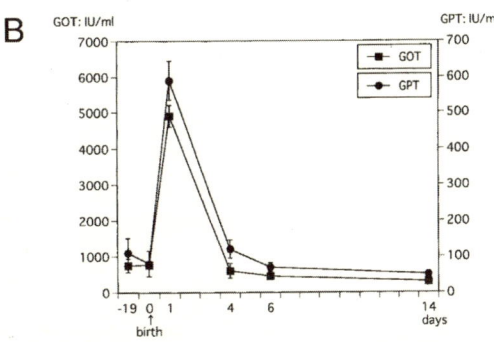

FIG. 2. Postpartal granulocytosis in mice. (A) Absence of granulocytosis in tissues of fetal mice (*upper panels*) and appearance of granulocytosis in tissues of postpartum mice (*lower panels*). (B) Transient elevation of transaminases in sera of neonatal mice. (A) Representative data of three experiments are depicted. Numbers in the figure represent the percentages of fluorescence-positive cells in corresponding areas. Granulocytosis was observed in all organs of neonates only after birth. (B) Sera were obtained from BALB/c mice (n = 4) after birth.

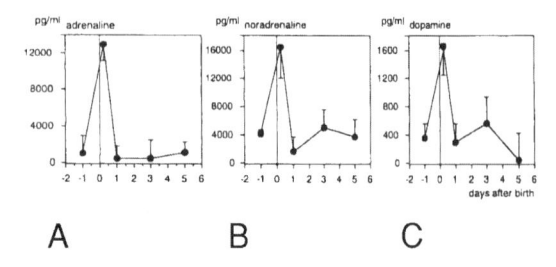

FIG. 3. A transient increase in serum levels of catecholamines after birth in mice. To examine whether some stress-associated responses were induced at birth, serum levels of catecholamines, including (A) adrenaline, (B) noradrenaline, and (C) dopamine, were measured at the indicated time points (n = 6). Possibly reflecting severe stress, serum levels of catecholamines were sharply elevated just after birth.

A Transient Elevation in Serum Levels of Catecholamines at Birth in Mice. Logically, if neonatal granulocytosis and subsequent tissue destruction result from a stress-associated response at birth, the sympathetic nerve strain should be present. This possibility was then investigated (Fig. 3). Serum levels of catecholamines (n = 6) were measured at four time points before and after birth. It was shown that a sharp elevation in the levels of all catecholamines, including adrenaline, noradrenaline, and dopamine, occurred just after birth.

Pre- and Postpartum Electron Microscopical Examination of Mouse Liver. Mouse livers before and after birth were examined by electron microscopy (Fig. 4). Hepatocytes seemed normal before birth (day 19 of gestation; Fig. 4A), but after birth (postpartum day 1; Fig. 4B), many lipid droplets appeared in the hepatocyte cytoplasm. Reflecting this change, the color of the liver changed from red to white macroscopically. This appearance was quite similar to that observed in the liver of normal adult (8 weeks old; Fig. 4C) mice and adult mice 16 hours after exposure to restriction stress (Fig. 4D).

Transient Appearance of Fatty Liver in Human Neonates. Ultrasonograms of livers and spleens of human neonates (n = 14) were obtained from postpartum days 2 to 6 and the liver/spleen ratios of echogenicity were calculated. The ratios were highest at postpartum day 2 and steadily decreased until normal levels were achieved at postpartum day 6 (Fig. 5); the correlation between ratio and days was significant ($r = -.711$; $P < .05$). These results suggested that steatosis in the liver occurred at birth, even in human neonates.

Hematopoietic Destruction Occurs at Birth. The time-kinetics of hematopoietic cell numbers was examined in mouse livers (n = 4). The number of hematopoietic cells (i.e., non-parenchymal cells) increased steadily as a function of fetal age but dropped precipitously after birth (Fig. 6A).

iNOS mRNA expression by leukocytes of neonatal BALB/c mice at 3, 6, 24, and 48 hours postpartum was determined. Leukocytes isolated from the liver 3 hours after birth expressed iNOS mRNA, but the expression was diminished within 6 hours and was completely absent at 24 and 48 hours postpartum (Fig. 6B).

Oxygen Stress and Granulocytosis. Granulocyte levels were determined in various organs of adult mice (n = 3) 3 hours after the mice had been exposed to hyperbaric oxygenation (60% oxygen) for 3 hours. In all of the organs examined, the proportion of Gr-1$^+$Mac-1$^+$ granulocytes increased, especially in the lung and blood (Fig. 7). The number of mononuclear cells in the lung doubled, whereas the increase in other organs was moderate (up to 30%).

DISCUSSION

Until the present study, it has neither been clear why the number of granulocytes is extremely high in human neonates

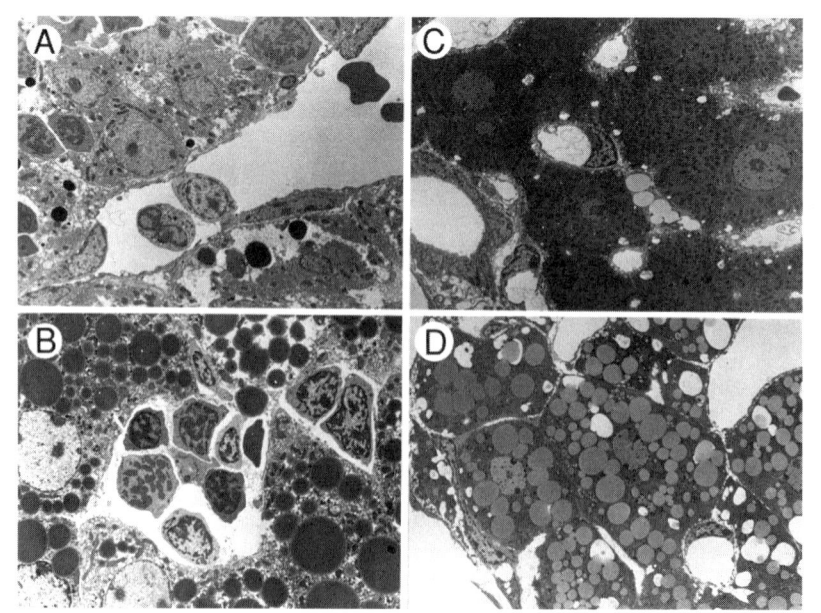

FIG. 4. Appearance of hepatocytes with lipid droplets at birth. (A) The liver of a fetus, day 19 after gestation; (B) the liver of a neonate, day 1 after birth; (C) the liver of a normal 8-week-old adult mouse; and (D) the liver of an 8-week-old adult mouse after 16 hours of restriction stress. (Original magnification ×2,000.) Many lipid droplets appeared in the cytoplasm of hepatocytes, possibly caused by the stress of birth and by restriction stress in mice.

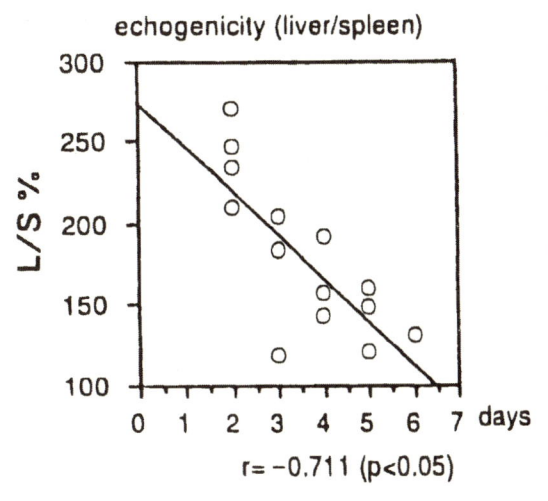

FIG. 5. Ultrasonograms of livers and spleens of human neonates. Samples were obtained from postpartum days 2 to 6 (n = 14). The liver/spleen ratios were calculated and plotted against days after birth. The correlation between ratio and days was significant ($r = -.711$ [n = 14], $P < .05$).

nor why the destruction of fetal hepatic hematopoietic tissue, accompanied by newborn jaundice and neonatal hepatitis, commences immediately after birth. Results of the present study suggest that these events are caused by stress at birth in humans and mice.

Why Does Stress Induce Granulocytosis? In this regard, it should be remembered that granulocytes bear α- and β-adrenergic receptors on the cell surface[12-14]; therefore, various stressors stimulate the sympathetic nervous system and result in granulocytosis.[15] A transient elevation in serum levels of catecholamines was demonstrated at birth in mice. Because granulocytes are the main cells that produce free radicals and superoxides, they may be intimately involved in subsequent tissue destruction.[16,17] In the case of nitic oxide, over-production and not low-level production, is known to induce DNA damage or tissue damage.[10,11] Alternatively, there is a possibility that nitric oxide production at birth may, instead, be associated with tissue protection. In any case, the expression of iNOS mRNA by leukocytes in the liver seems to be a good marker of stress.

Many investigators and clinicians believe that fetal hematopoiesis in the liver is gradually switched to an adult type of hematopoiesis in the bone marrow during the fetal stage. In the present study, the time-kinetic study of hematopoietic cells in the liver before and immediately after birth revealed that this is not the case. The decrease in the number of hepatic hematopoietic cells following birth is abrupt.

Repeated hyperbaric oxygenation is known to have certain side effects, such as tissue destruction, pulmonary fibrosis, or cataracts.[4,5] Furthermore, fatty liver is a well-known consequence of excessive alcohol consumption.[18,19] In other words, hepatocytes with many lipid droplets are a common feature when animals are exposed to various stressors. In the present study, granulocytosis was induced by hyperbaric oxygenation in adult mice. It is postulated that such side effects are induced by the free radicals and superoxides produced by granulocytes and other cells.[16,17]

Air breathing neonates also undergo stress induced by their initial exposure to inspired O_2. In the case of the human fetus, the level of PO_2 in the arteries is around 28 ± 8 mm Hg; it increases sharply to 62 ± 14 mm Hg within 4 hours after birth.[20] It can be easily imagined that this elevation of oxygen concentration in the blood is a severe stressor. One of the prime target organs of tissue destruction at this time seems to be the liver. Elevated levels of transaminases after birth support this notion. In this study, the appearance of hepatocytes with many lipid droplets (i.e., fatty liver) was observed directly in mice and indirectly (by ultrasonography) in humans. In both the cases of birth and restriction stress,

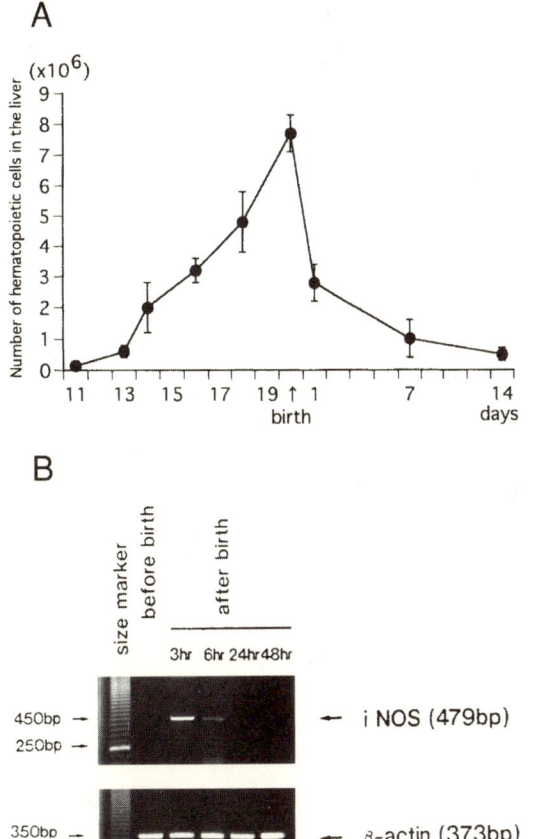

FIG. 6. Destruction of hematopoietic cells after birth, possibly caused by the production of free radicals by activated granulocytes. (A) Time-kinetics of hematopoietic cell numbers in mouse livers. (B) Postpartal iNOS mRNA expression by leukocytes of neonatal BALB/c mice. The numbers of hematopoietic cells (i.e., non-parenchymal cells) increased steadily as a function of fetal age but dropped precipitously after birth. The number of cells stabilized around partum days 7 to 14. In these experiments (A), materials were obtained from 4 mice. Leukocytes isolated from the liver 3 hours after birth expressed iNOS mRNA, but the expression was diminished within 6 hours and was completely absent at 24 and 48 hours postpartum.

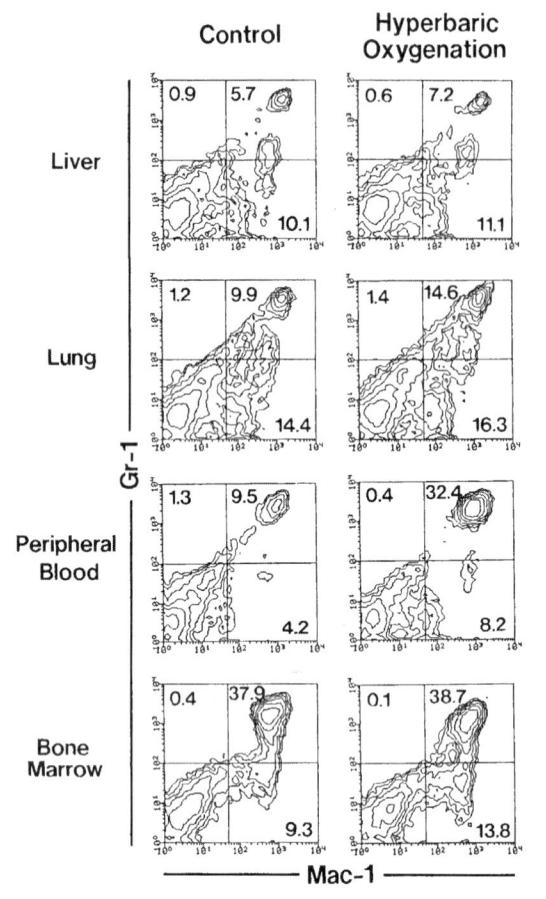

FIG. 7. Oxygen stress induced granulocytosis in various organs of mice. BALB/C mice at 8 weeks of age were exposed to 60% oxygen at 1 Atm for 3 hours. After another 3 hours, mice were killed to determine the levels of granulocytes. Two-color staining for Gr-1 and Mac-1 was performed. A prominent increase in the proportion of granulocytes, as a result of the hyperbaric stress, was seen in lungs and blood (exposed animals, *right panels*; control animals, *left panels*). Representative data of three experiments are depicted.

this phenomenon is reversible when the stressors are removed.

In a subsequent study (Kawamura et al., Unpublished observation, March 1997), the detection of fatty livers in chickens after the initiation of respiration and before hatching also prompts us to speculate that neonatal granulocytosis is more intimately related to oxygen stress at birth than to the stress of delivery, although physical or mental stress is also known to induce granulocytosis.[21-23] This speculation seems to be valid, as neonates that are delivered by Cesarean Section also show granulocytosis after birth and experience neonatal jaundice (Kawamura et al., unpublished observations, April 1996).

We suggest that all these events are experienced by living beings with lungs and that it is evolutionarily possible that a similar phenomenon confronted all organisms that attempted to emerge onto land. It is likely that many of these attempts resulted in failure because of oxygen stress. Only when the hematopoietic organ was successfully moved from the liver to the bone marrow (i.e., adult type of hematopoiesis), could emergence onto land be successful. At birth, neonates of animals with lungs may repeat the historical event of emergence onto land.

In any case, detailed observations on the levels of granulocytes in various organs of humans and mice before and after birth has revealed that neonatal granulocytosis is a postpartum event and that it resembles stress-associated responses. Details of stresses at birth should be investigated further.

Acknowledgment: We wish to thank Mrs. Kyona Kimura and Mrs. Yuko Kaneko for preparation of the manuscript.

REFERENCES

1. Robinson WA, Mangalik A. The kinetics and regulations of granulopoiesis. Semin Hematol 1975;12:7-25.
2. Boxer LA. Diseases of the blood. In: Behrman RE, ed. Nelson Textbook of Pediatrics. 14 Ed. Chap. 16. Philadelphia: WB Saunders, 1992:1264.
3. Lim FT, van Winsen L, Willemze R, Kanhai HH, Falkenburg JH. Influence of delivery on numbers of leukocytes, leukocyte subpopulations, and hematopoietic progenitor cells in human umbilical cord blood. Blood Cells 1994;20:547-559.
4. Lee AK, Hester RB, Coggin JH, Gottlieb SF. Increased oxygen tensions influence subset composition of the cellular immune system in aged mice. Cancer Biother 1994;9:39-54.
5. Fechtali T, Abraini JH, Kriem B, Rostain JC. Pressure increases de novo synthesized striatal dopamine release in free-moving rats. Neuroreport 1994;5:725-728.
6. Yuo A, Kitagawa S, Suzuki I, Urabe A, Okabe T, Saito M, Takaku F. Tumor necrosis factor as an activator of human granulocytes. Potentiation of the metabolisms triggered by the Ca^{2+}-mobilizing agonists. J Immunol 1989;142:1678-1684.
7. Takeda Y, Watanabe H, Yonehara S, Yamashita T, Saito S, Sendo F. Rapid acceleration of neutrophil apoptosis by tumor necrosis factor-α. Int Immunol 1993;5:691-694.
8. Iiai T, Watanabe H, Seki S, Sugiura K, Hirokawa K, Utsuyama M, Takahashi-Iwanaga H, et al. Ontogeny and development of extrathymic T cells in mouse liver. Immunology 1992;77:556-563.
9. Watanabe H, Miyaji C, Kawachi Y, Iiai T, Ohtsuka K, Iwanaga T, Takahashi-Iwanaga H, et al. Relationships between intermediate TCR cells and NK1.1$^+$ T cells in various immune organs. NK1.1$^+$ T cells are present within a population of intermediate TCR cells. J Immunol 1995; 155:2972-2983.
10. Yim C-Y, McGregor JR, Kwon O-D, Bastian NR, Rees M, Mori M, Hibbs JB Jr., et al. Nitric oxide synthesis contributes to IL-2-induced antitumor responses against intraperitoneal Meth A tumor. J Immunol 1995;155: 4382-4390.
11. Yang J, Kawamura I, Zhu H, Mitsuyama M. Involvement of natural killer cells in nitric oxide production by spleen cells after stimulation with *Mycobacterium bovis* BCG. J Immunol 1995;155:5728-5735.
12. Aarons RD, Nies AS, Gal J, Hegstrand LR, Molinoff PB. Elevation of β-adrenergic receptor density in human lymphocytes after propranolol administration. J Clin Invest 1980;65:949-957.
13. Panosian JO, Marinetti GV. α_2-adrenergic receptors in human polymorphonuclear leukocyte membranes. Biochem Pharmacol 1983;32:2243-2247.
14. Ratge D, Wiedemann A, Kohse KP, Wisser H. Alterations of β-adrenoceptors on human leukocyte subsets induced by dynamic exercise; effect of prednisone. Clin Exp Pharmac Physiol 1988;15:43-53.
15. Fukuda M, Moroda T, Toyabe S, Iiai T, Kawachi Y, Takahashi-Iwanaga H, Iwanaga T, et al. Granulocytosis induced by increasing sympathetic nerve activity contributes to the incidence of acute appendicitis. Biomed Res 1996;17:171-181.
16. Nguyen T, Brunson D, Crespi CL, Penman BW, Wishnok JS, Tannenbaum SR. DNA damage and mutation in human cells exposed to nitric oxide *in vitro*. Proc Natl Acad Sci U S A 1992;89:3030-3034.
17. Huang F-P, Feng G-J, Lindop G, Stott DI, Liew FY. The role of interleukin 12 and nitric oxide in the development of spontaneous autoimmune disease in MRL/MP-*lpr/lpr* mice. J Exp Med 1996;183:1447-1459.

18. Guido MG, Virend KS, William SR, Francois MA, Mark AL. Effects of alcohol intake on blood pressure and sympathetic nerve activity in normotensive humans: a preliminary report. J Hypertension 1989;7:20-21.
19. Gao W, Connor HD, Lamesters JJ, Mason RP, Thurman RG. Primary nonfunction of fatty livers produced by alcohol is associated with a new, antioxidant-insensitive free radical species. Transplantation 1995; 59:674-679.
20. Klaus M. Respiratory function and pulmonary disease in the newborn. in Barnett H, ed. Pediatrics. New York: Appleton-Century-Crofts, 1972:1255.
21. Iversen PO, Arvesen BL, Benestad HB. No mandatory role for the spleen in the exercise-induced leucocytosis in man. Clin Sci 1994;86:505-510.
22. Murray DR, Irwin M, Rearden CA, Ziegler M, Motulsky H, Maisel AS. Sympathetic and immune interactions during dynamic exercise. Circulation 1992;86:203-213.
23. Landmann RMA, Müller FB, Perini C, Wesp M, Erne P, Bühler FR. Changes of immunoregulatory cells induced by psychological and physical stress: relationship to plasma catecholamines. Clin Exp Immunol 1984;58:127-135.

ASSOCIATION OF GRANULOCYTES WITH ULCER FORMATION IN THE STOMACH OF RODENTS EXPOSED TO RESTRAINT STRESS

拘束ストレスを与えた齧歯類の胃における
潰瘍形成への顆粒球の関与

Biomedical Research, 18: 423-437, 1997

chapter 9

ASSOCIATION OF GRANULOCYTES WITH ULCER FORMATION IN THE STOMACH OF RODENTS EXPOSED TO RESTRAINT STRESS

拘束ストレスを与えた齧歯類の胃における潰瘍形成への顆粒球の関与

TETSUYA MORODA[1,2], TSUKAHARA[2], AKIHIRO TSUKAHARA[2], MINORU FUKUDA[1], SUSUMU SUZUKI[2], TAKASH1 TADA[2], KATSUYOSHI HATAKEYAMA[2] and TORU ABO[1,3]

[1]Department of Immunology, and [2]First Department of Surgery, Niigata University School of Medicine, Niigata 951, Japan

【要約】

　先ず、胃潰瘍患者の血液中において顆粒球値が上昇すると考えた。そこで、齧歯類（マウスやラット）を用いた実験を行なった。拘束ストレスを与えるため齧歯類をステンレススチールメッシュで固定した。マウス各臓器への顆粒球などの細胞の浸潤を、モノクロナール抗体を用いてフローサイトメトリーにて解析を行った。拘束ストレス24時間後に各臓器（胃、末梢血および肝臓）において顕著に顆粒球が増多していた。興味深いことに、胸腺外分化T細胞（増殖が速い自己細胞を傷害する能力があると知られている）も同時に増加した。更に重要なことは、抗顆粒球抗体を用いて前もって顆粒球の除去を行なったところ、ラットでは潰瘍形成は出現しなかった。一方、G-CSFを用いて前もって顆粒球を活性化させると潰瘍形成が促進された。本研究の結果は、生体の背景または基礎状態が胃潰瘍形成と他の臓器傷害出現に非常に重要である可能性を示唆する。

胃　潰瘍形成の原因は、胃の中のpHは酸性下において、ペプシンの分泌過剰が原因で胃粘膜が消化されることだとこれまで長い間信じられてきた（「胃潰瘍の酸説」）(21)。しかし、近年、Helicbacter pylori（胃の常在菌）が、胃潰瘍形成と密接に関連していると報告された (3, 4, 16, 22, 24)。実際に、抗生物質でH pyloriを除去すると、胃潰瘍再発防止に効果がある (7, 31, 32)。つまり、胃潰瘍の原因はまだ議論の余地がありそうである。そこで、大規模に胃潰瘍患者の臨床データ検証を行ったところ、末梢血中の顆粒球値が対照群（本研究のデータ）よりも顕著に高値であることが判明した。さらに、多くの胃潰瘍患者における胃切片の組織を検証したところ、顆粒球による胃粘膜侵襲が数多く見られた。従って、顆粒球が常在菌とともに胃潰瘍形成に関連している可能性が高まった。この可能性を実験により検証したところ、活性化した顆粒球が細菌を傷害するためフリーラジカルと超酸化物を産生するが、このような物質の過剰産生が組織破壊の原因であることが判明した。このことより「胃潰瘍の顆粒球説」が確認できた (6, 34, 36, 40)。

　本研究では、胃潰瘍モデルとしてマウスとラットモデルを使用した。そして、実験動物に拘束ストレスを与えた（8時間と24時間）。拘束ストレスを与えると、標的臓器（胃）のみならずいろいろな臓器で、顕著な顆粒球増多が出

略語：NSAID，非ステロイド性抗炎症薬；TCR[int] cells，TCR[int] 細胞；MNC，単核球；DN，ダブル・ネガティブ
[3]Correspondence to: T. Abo at the above address. Fax: (81) 25-228-0868

現した（>95% 好中球）。顆粒球表面には、アドレナリン受容体（αおよびβタイプ）が高密度で存在すると知られているので (5, 17, 20, 28, 39)、ストレスとそれに続く交感神経緊張に誘導される顆粒球増多が胃潰瘍形成の要因の一つである可能性が考えられる。胸腺外分化T細胞（自己応答性がある）も顆粒球とともに潰瘍形成および組織損傷に関与している可能性を提案する。

材料と方法

被験者

胃潰瘍患者（n=30：年齢，32-54歳；平均年齢，44.3）の末梢血における顆粒球およびリンパ球値を測定した。被験者は新潟県坂町病院（日本）の外来患者であった。対照群は同年齢の健康成人であった。(n=33：年齢，30-53歳；平均年齢，43.8)。

実験動物

6-8週齢のBALB/cマウスとDDラットを使用した。実験動物は、日本チャールズ・リバー（株式会社）（神奈川）より購入し、新潟大学動物飼育施設においてSPF（特定病原体未感染）環境下にて飼育した。

拘束ストレス

実験動物をケージ内にてステンレススチールメッシュで固定した（8時間と24時間）。

細胞分離

エーテル麻酔したマウスの、腋窩動脈と静脈より完全に脱血した。摘出した肝臓、脾臓と胸腺は、細胞分離作業中は氷上のリン酸緩衝液（PBS）（pH7.2）中で保存した。

肝臓の単核球採取のため、摘出した肝臓をハサミで細断し、200-ゲージステンレススチールメッシュで濾し、5mM HEPES（日水製薬，東京，日本）と2%非働化仔牛血清を添加した40ml Eagle MEM培養液中に懸濁させた。培養液で一度洗浄した後、この細胞に15mlの100IU/mlのヘパリンを加えた35%パーコール溶液中に再浮遊させ、遠心分離比重分離を行なった（2,000rpm，15分間）(8)。分離した細胞塊を培養液で再懸濁して洗浄し、赤血球を除去するために溶血用試薬（17mM Tris-HCl緩衝液（pH7.65）155mmM NH_4Cl, 10mM $KHCO_3$ および10mM Na_2EDTA）で分離した細胞塊に混ぜ、氷上に5分間静置した。培養液で二回洗浄後、肝臓単核球（単核球）を1mlの培養液に懸濁し、細胞数を測定した。

脾臓と胸腺を細切し200-ゲージステンレススチールメッシュで濾し、脾臓細胞と胸腺細胞を採取した。定法に従い赤血球を塩化アンモニウム/Tris-HCl緩衝液で溶血した後、培養液で二度洗浄した。6%デキストラン硫酸比重法により、白血球をバッフィーコートから末梢血白血球を分離した。

胃と関節からも細胞を採取した。組織を、それぞれ胃と関節から切除して、ハサミで細切した後、切片をコラゲナーゼで（0.1mg/ml in PBS）(Sigma Chemical, St. Louis, MO) 処理した。この切片を200-ゲージステンレスメッシュで濾し、培養液に懸濁した。この細胞浮遊液をFicoll-Isopaque勾配緩衝液（1.077）に縦走して比重遠心し分離した（12）。

フローサイトメトリー解析

細胞表面のフェノタイプを、モノクロナール抗体を用いた二重染色を行い解析した（12）。使用したモノクロナール抗体を以下に示す：フルオレセイン・イソチオシアネート(FITC)-、フィコエリスリン(PE)-、またはビオチン標識した抗CD3(145-2C11)(PharMingen, San Diego, CA)および抗IL-2Rβ⁻鎖(IL-2Rβ)(TM-β1)モノクロナール抗体 (21)。FITCまたはPE標識した抗CD4（L3T4）および抗CD8（Lyt-2）モノクロナール抗体をBecton Dickinson（Mountain

View, CA）から購入した。モノクローナル抗体の非特異的結合を防ぐためCD32/16（2.4G2）(PharMingen) モノクローナル抗体にて細胞に必ず前処理を行なった（Fc受容体ブロッキング）。ビオチン標識抗体は、PE標識ストレプトアビジン（Becton Dickinson）で発色させた。蛍光陽性細胞をLYSIS IIソフトウェア（Becton Dickinson）を用いFACScanにより解析した。

生体における顆粒球除去

RP-3（マウス抗ラット顆粒球モノクローナル抗体）（山形大学（山形，日本）仙道富士郎博士提供）を腹腔内投与すれば、ラット生体内の顆粒球を除去できることは確立されており(15, 30)、本研究ではこの手法を用いた。RP-3を週2度接種した（1mg/回/匹）。ラット体内の顆粒球値測定にRP-3も用いた。二次抗体は、PE標識抗マウスIgGモノクローナル抗体（Biomeda, Faster City, CA）を用いた。

G-CSFによる顆粒球増多

ヒト組換型G-CSF（麒麟麦酒（株），東京，日本）を用いマウスの顆粒球を増多させた。G-CSFを週3度皮下投与した（10^4 U/回/匹）。

統計分析

有意差検定には、スチューデントt検定を用いた。

結果

胃潰瘍患者の末梢血における顆粒球増多

大多数の胃潰瘍患者は、精神的もしくは身体的ストレスに苦しむようである。これまでの研究において、このストレスが交感神経緊張とそれによっておこる顆粒球増多の原因であると報告した（顆粒球表面にはαおよびβアドレナリン受容体がある）(6)。この点について、先ず、健常者群と患者群において顆粒球とリンパ球の絶対数の比較を行なった（Fig. 1）。末梢血中における顆粒球値は、健常者群よりも患者群において高値であると判明した；絶対数（$P< 0.01$），比率（$P< 0.01$）。リンパ球の絶対数は、患者群も健常者群も有意差は得られなかったが（$P>0.05$）、リンパ球比率は、患者群は健常者群に比較して低値であった（$P< 0.05$）。

Figure.1

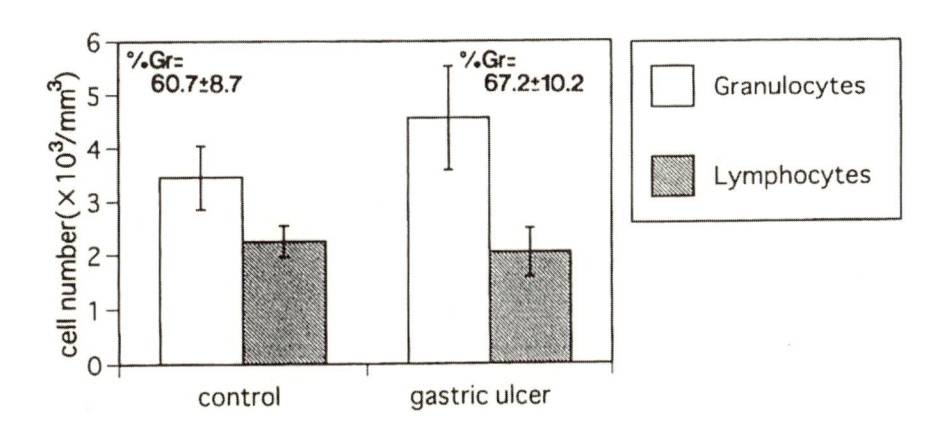

顆粒球増多症が胃潰瘍患者との関連。胃潰瘍の患者群において顆粒球およびリンパ球値を測定した（n=30）。同年齢の健常者群の値も測定した(n=33)。患者群の顆粒球の数と比率（$4.3 ± 1.2 × 10^3/mm^3$）($67.2 ± 10.2\%$)は、健常者群の顆粒球の数と比率（$3.6 ± 0.6 × 10^3/mm^3$）($60.7 ± 8.7\%$）よりも高値であった（$P <0.01$）。患者群のリンパ球数（$2.1 ± 0.3 × 10^3/mm^3$）と健常者群のリンパ球数（$2.2 ± 0.3 × 10^3/mm$）との間に有意差は見られなかった（$P>0.05$）。しかし、患者のリンパ比率（$30.6 ± 5.8\%$）は、健常者群のもの（$35.1 ± 6.1\%$）よりも低値であった（$P< 0.05$）。

Figure.2

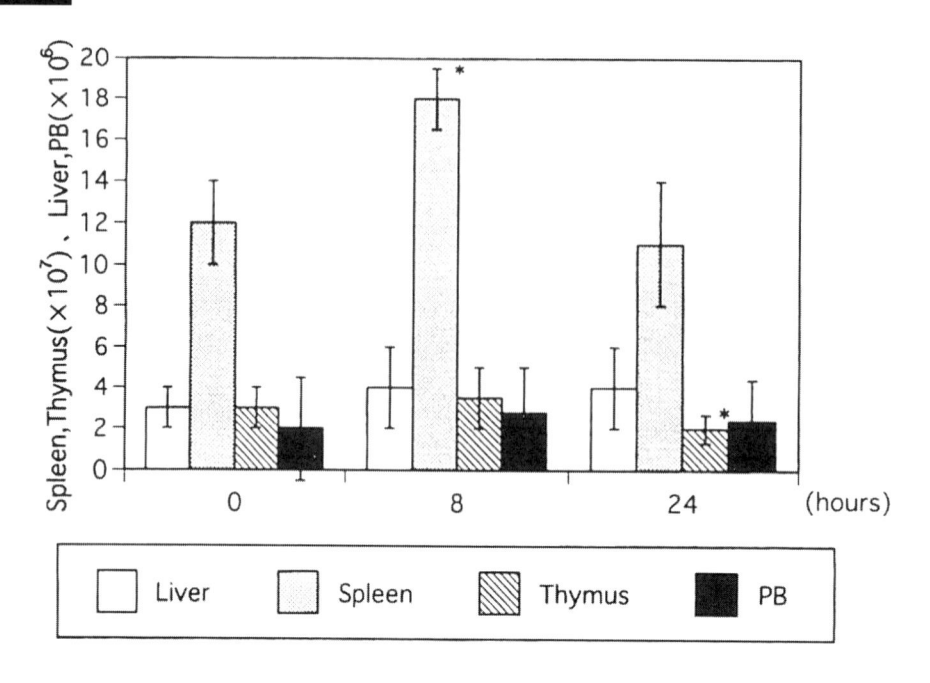

拘束ストレスによるマウス各臓器の単核球数の変化。マウスにストレスを与えた後（8,24時間後）、各臓器の単核球数を計測した。平均値±1SDは、4匹のマウスを用いて算出した。脾臓単核球は8時間後に増加した。一方、胸腺細胞の単核球は24時間後に減少した（P<0.05）。その他の値には変化は見られなかった。*P < 0.05。

拘束ストレスを与えたマウスの各免疫臓器における単核球数の経時的変化

細胞のフェノタイプを解析する前に、拘束ストレスを受けたマウスの各臓器における単核球の絶対数を計測した（Fig. 2）。マウスに拘束ストレスを与え、計測を行なった（8および24時間）。脾臓では、単核球の数がストレス8時間後に増加した一方、胸腺細胞では24時間後に減少した。肝臓、末梢血では変化は見られなかった。

拘束ストレス後の各臓器における顆粒球および胸腺外分化T細胞の数と比率の増加

顆粒球（Gr-1$^+$ Mac-1$^+$）の確認するためGr-1とMac-1の二重染色を行なった（Fig. 3A）。基本的に、マウスの顆粒球値は、どの臓器でも（末梢血中でさえも）高くない（Figの0h参照）。しかし、マウスにストレスを与えると、顆粒球増多は、先ず、末梢血（39.2%）（8時間後）に出現し、その後肝臓と脾臓を含む他の臓器が続いた（24時間後）。胸腺萎縮がストレス24時間後に誘導されたが、顆粒球浸潤は認められなかった。そこで、ストレスによるリンパ球サブセットの分布の変化を検証した。CD3とIL-2Rβの二重染色を行なった（Fig. 3B）。この染色により、同時に以下の細胞を同定できる：CD3$^-$IL-2Rβ$^+$：NK細胞（12）、CD3^{int}IL-2Rβ$^+$：胸腺外分化T細胞およびCD3^{high}IL-2Rβ$^-$従来型T細胞である。ストレス8時間以降、各臓器（特に肝臓）において胸腺外分化T細胞の比率が顕著に増加した。胸腺萎縮により未熟T細胞（CD3$^-$ or CD3^{dull}）がアポトーシスで死滅したため、成熟T細胞（CD3^{high}IL-2Rβ$^-$）の比率は反対に増加した（24時間後）。CD3$^-$IL-2Rβ$^+$ NK細胞の比率は、ストレスマウスの各

Figure.3A

A

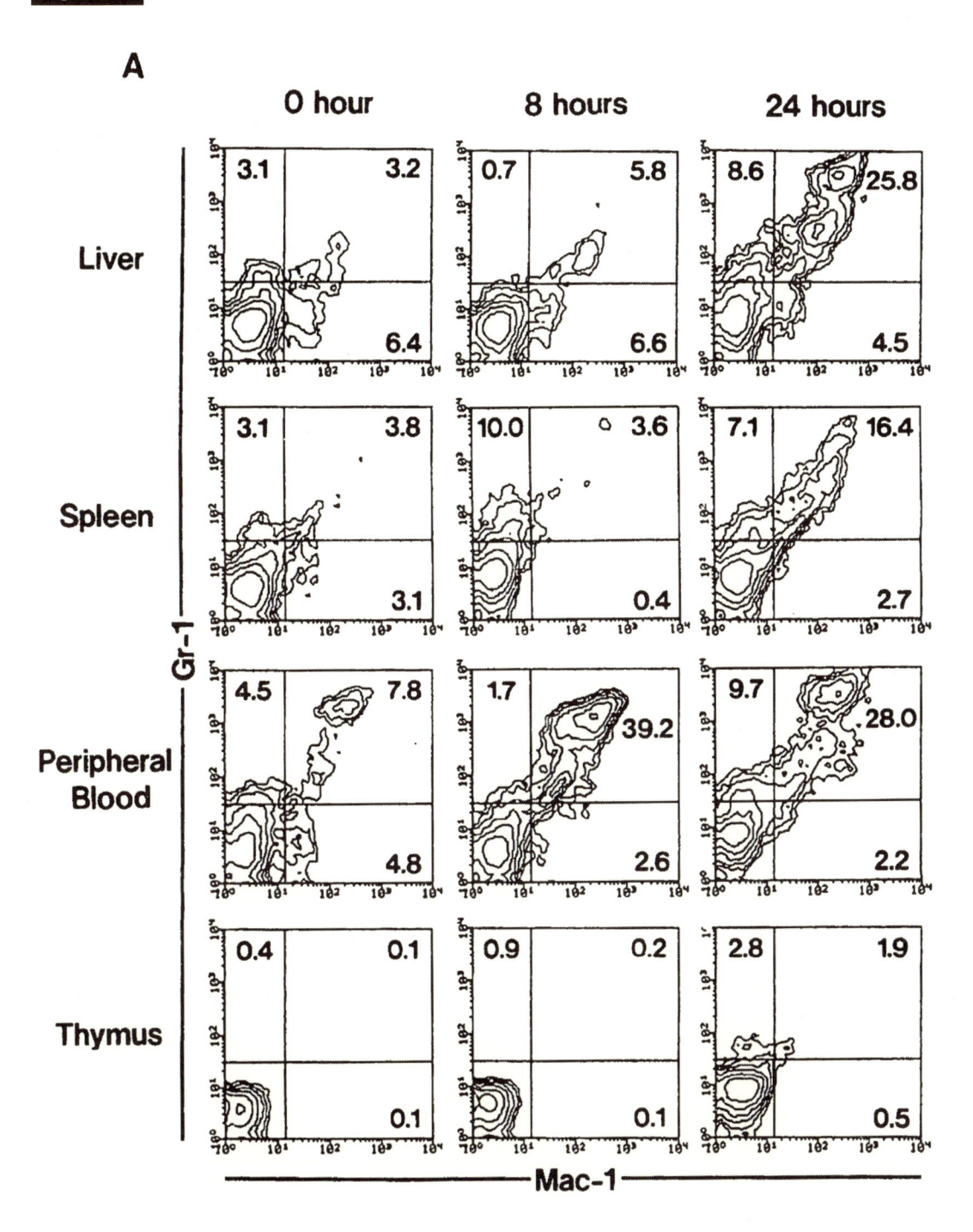

<!-- Figure: Flow cytometry contour plots, Gr-1 (y-axis) vs Mac-1 (x-axis), for Liver, Spleen, Peripheral Blood, and Thymus at 0 hour, 8 hours, and 24 hours. -->

	0 hour	8 hours	24 hours
Liver	UL 3.1, UR 3.2, LR 6.4	UL 0.7, UR 5.8, LR 6.6	UL 8.6, UR 25.8, LR 4.5
Spleen	UL 3.1, UR 3.8, LR 3.1	UL 10.0, UR 3.6, LR 0.4	UL 7.1, UR 16.4, LR 2.7
Peripheral Blood	UL 4.5, UR 7.8, LR 4.8	UL 1.7, UR 39.2, LR 2.6	UL 9.7, UR 28.0, LR 2.2
Thymus	UL 0.4, UR 0.1, LR 0.1	UL 0.9, UR 0.2, LR 0.1	UL 2.8, UR 1.9, LR 0.5

拘束ストレスを与えたマウスの各臓器における単核球のフェノタイプの特徴。A：Gr-1とMac-1の二重染色。B：CD3とIL-2Rβの二重染色。ストレスを与えたマウス（8, 24時間）を使用した。各分画内の数字は、数値は蛍光陽性細胞の比率を示す。拘束ストレスを与えると顆粒球（Gr-1$^+$Mac-1$^+$）と胸腺外分化T細胞（CD3^{int}IL-2Rβ$^+$）が各臓器に誘導された。

Figure.3B

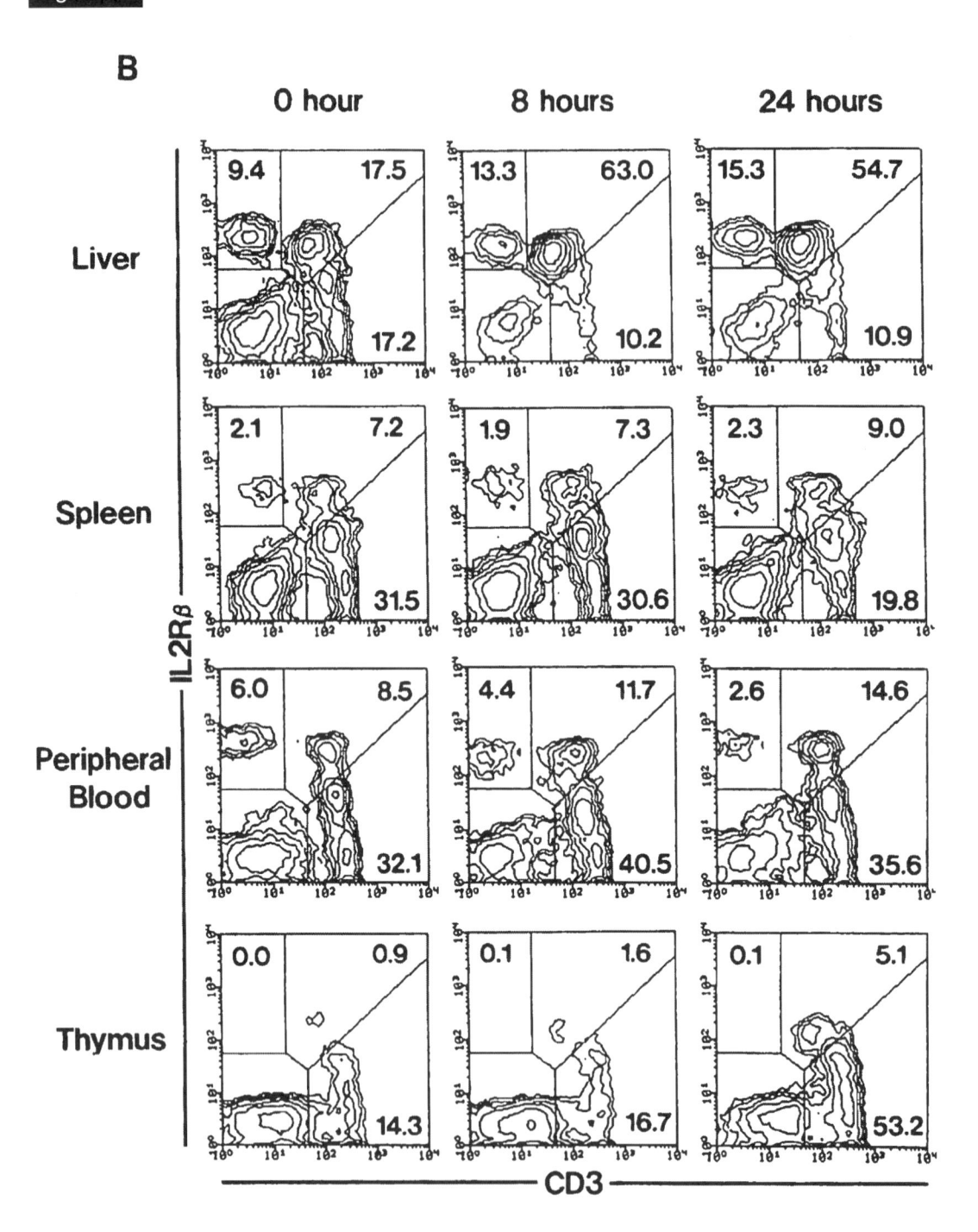

B

	0 hour	8 hours	24 hours
Liver	9.4 / 17.5 / 17.2	13.3 / 63.0 / 10.2	15.3 / 54.7 / 10.9
Spleen	2.1 / 7.2 / 31.5	1.9 / 7.3 / 30.6	2.3 / 9.0 / 19.8
Peripheral Blood	6.0 / 8.5 / 32.1	4.4 / 11.7 / 40.5	2.6 / 14.6 / 35.6
Thymus	0.0 / 0.9 / 14.3	0.1 / 1.6 / 16.7	0.1 / 5.1 / 53.2

Y-axis: IL2Rβ
X-axis: CD3

Figure.4A

A

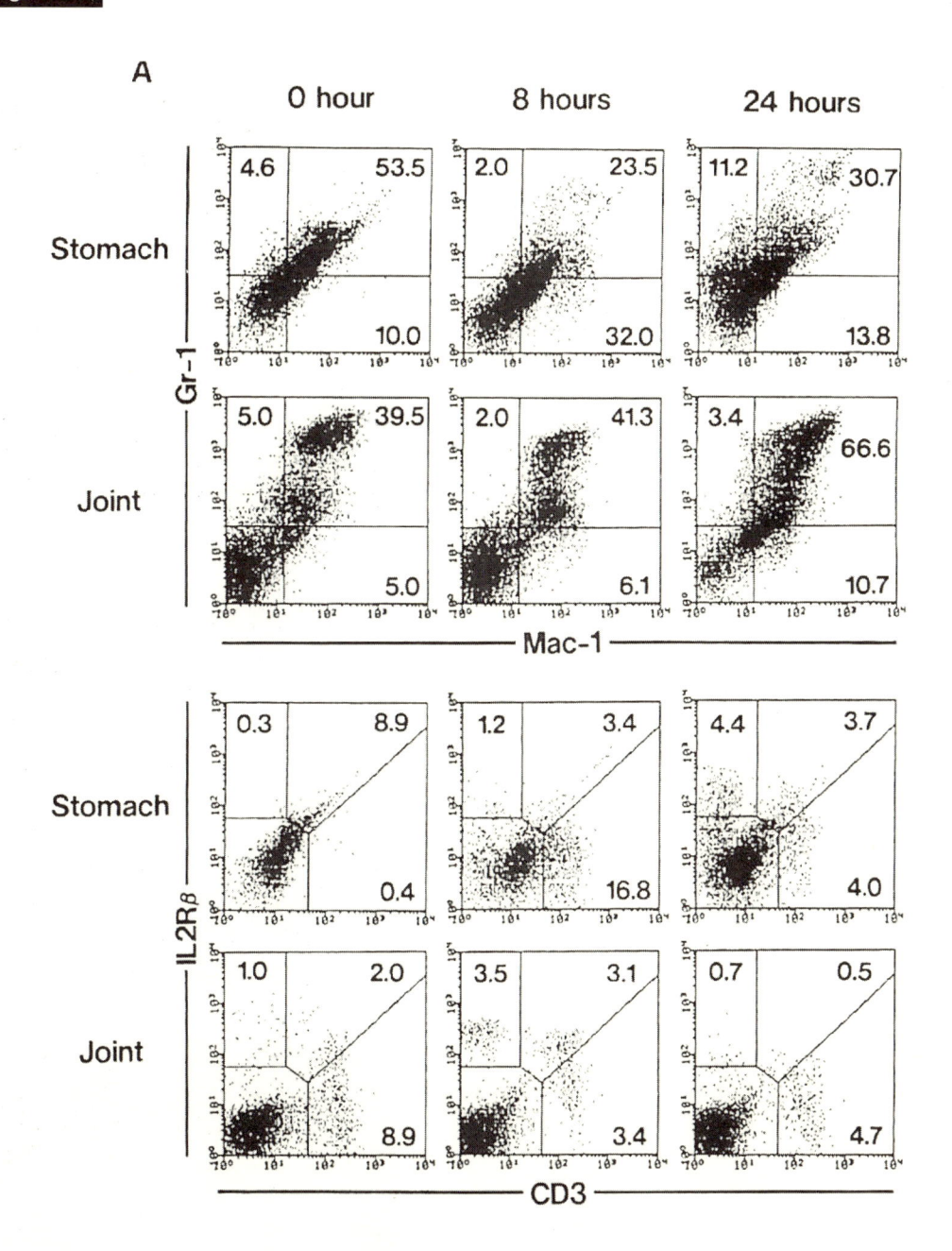

	0 hour	8 hours	24 hours
Stomach (Gr-1 / Mac-1)	4.6 / 53.5 / 10.0	2.0 / 23.5 / 32.0	11.2 / 30.7 / 13.8
Joint (Gr-1 / Mac-1)	5.0 / 39.5 / 5.0	2.0 / 41.3 / 6.1	3.4 / 66.6 / 10.7
Stomach (IL2Rβ / CD3)	0.3 / 8.9 / 0.4	1.2 / 3.4 / 16.8	4.4 / 3.7 / 4.0
Joint (IL2Rβ / CD3)	1.0 / 2.0 / 8.9	3.5 / 3.1 / 3.4	0.7 / 0.5 / 4.7

顆粒球と胸腺外分化T細胞が拘束ストレスを与えたマウスの胃に浸潤する。A：Gr-1とMac-1の二重染色およびCD3とIL-2Rβの二重染色。B：胃における単核球の光散乱分析。ストレスを与えたマウス（8,24時間）を使用した。胃と関節より白血球を採取した。ストレス24時間後のマウスの胃において顆粒球（Gr-1$^+$Mac-1$^+$）と胸腺外分化T細胞（CD3^{int}IL-2Rβ$^+$）が出現した。このマウスの関節では、顆粒球増多が見られた。

臓器で比較的変化しなかった。ところが、従来型T細胞の比率は、ストレスマウスの肝臓と脾臓で減少した（24時間後）。

ストレスマウスにおける胃への顆粒球浸潤

実験を胃と膝関節にまで拡大した（Fig. 4A）。リンパ組織と異なり、胃と膝関節の組織破片の

Figure.4B

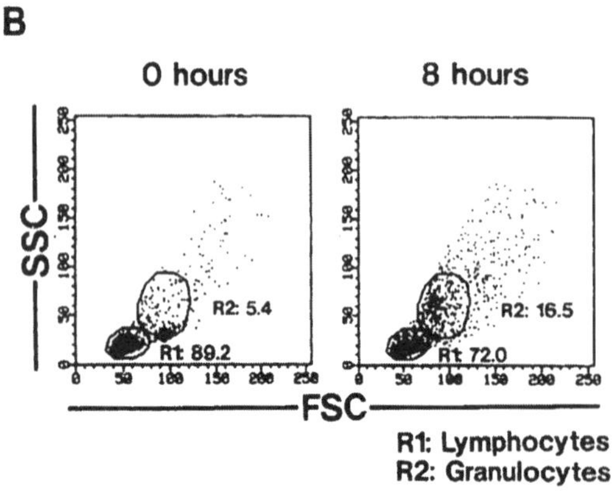

B

0 hours / 8 hours

R2: 5.4 R2: 16.5
R1 89.2 R1 72.0

SSC / FSC

R1: Lymphocytes
R2: Granulocytes

Figure.5A

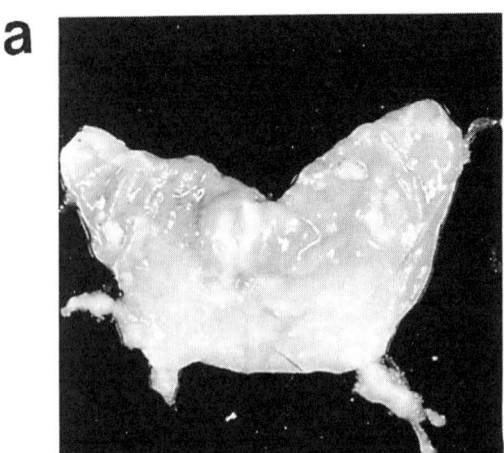

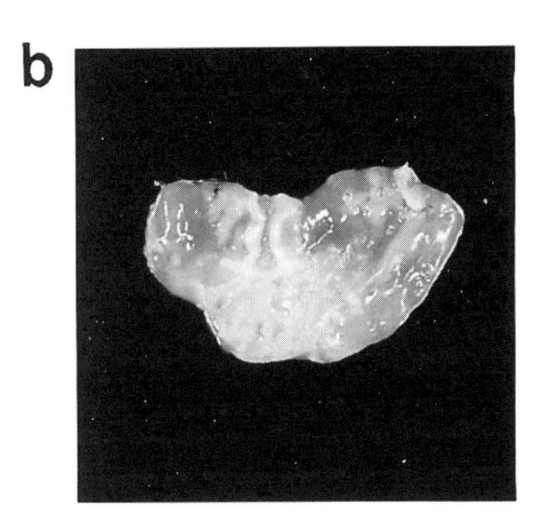

A

a

b

c

染色（Gr-1$^+$Mac-1$^+$）は（特にリンパ球でなく顆粒球に対応する光散乱領域では）偽陽性であった。しかし、ストレス有無に関係なく、関節にGr-1^{2+}Mac-1$^+$型（Gr-1の傾向強度が通常の顆粒球より高い）の顆粒球も存在した。興味深いことに、このGr-1^{2+}Mac-1$^+$細胞の小集団は、ストレスマウスの胃に新しく出現した（8および24時間）。この時、若干のリンパ球（NK細胞、胸腺外分化T細胞と従来型T細胞の混在）も、胃に出現した（Fig. 4A,下）。これらの結果より、拘束ストレスにより顆粒球とリンパ球の浸潤が見られることが明らかになった。胃の単核球のフローサイトメトリー解析を行なったが染色の結果が偽陽性であったので、胃の単核球の光散乱分析を行なった（Fig. 4B）。本図において、FSC（前方散乱）とSSC（側方散乱）の弱い光散乱部分（R1）はリンパ球群を示し、これに対して、FSCとSSCの強い光散乱部分（R2）は顆粒球群を示す。胃への顆粒球浸潤を反映して、光散乱が大きな細胞（R2）（顆粒球）が、ストレス8時間後に増加した（5.4→16.5%）。

ストレスマウスの胃の肉眼的観察

そこで、本実験プロトコルによる拘束ストレスが原因で胃潰瘍が発症したのか否か確認した（Fig. 5A）。ストレス8時間後には、はっきり

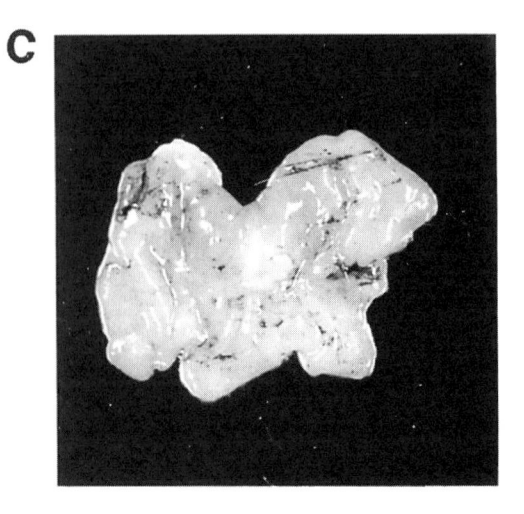

Figure.5B

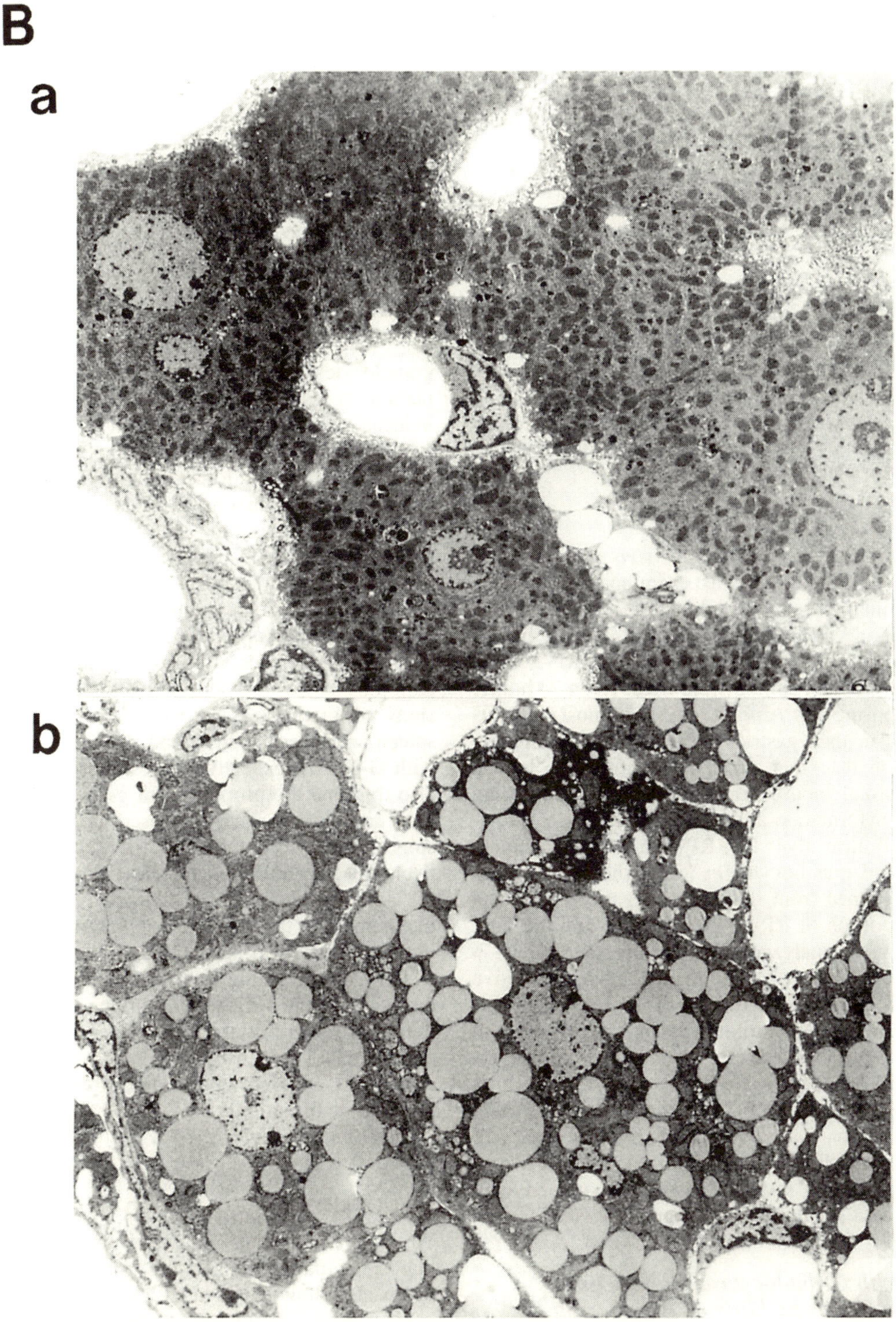

形態学的研究。A:胃の肉眼観察. a.対照群;b.ストレス群（8時間後）;c.ストレス群（24時間後）。B:ストレスによる脂肪肝形成。a.対照群の肝臓;b.ストレス群（24時間後）の肝臓。出血と潰瘍発症の顕著な徴候がストレス24時間後に観察された。この時、肝細胞の細胞質に脂肪滴が多数見られる脂肪肝が見られた。

Figure.6

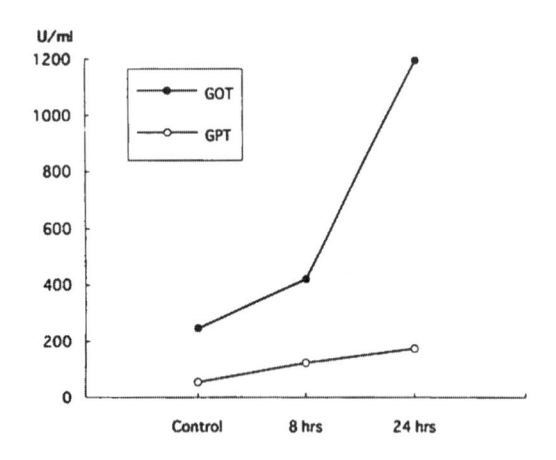

拘束ストレスによる血清トランスアミナーゼ値の上昇。血清トランスアミナーゼ値（特にGOT）がストレス24時間後に顕著に上昇した。血清3匹分を用いた平均値を示す。

Table.I

抗顆粒球抗体（RP-3）又はG-CSFの前投与に胃出血又は潰瘍形成への影響

Subject	Restriction	
	8h	24h
Control rat	0/8*	6/6
RP-3-treated rat	0/5	1/6
Control mouse	0/5	6/6
G-CSF-treated mouse	4/5	4/4

胃出血が見られた匹数/実験に使用した総匹数

とした胃粘膜損傷はまだ見られなかった（Fig. 5Ab）。出血や潰瘍形成のはっきりとした徴候は、24時間後に見られた（Fig. 5Ac）。ストレスマウスの肝臓において顕著な顆粒球増多が見られた。そこで、ストレスマウスの肝臓に顕微鏡的変化が見られるか否か検証した（Fig. 5B）。対照群マウスの肝細胞には、脂肪滴は見られなかった（Fig. 5Ba）。ストレスマウスにおいて脂肪肝（肝細胞の細胞質には脂肪滴が多い）が出現することが判明した（Fig. 5Bb）。

ストレスマウスにおける肝臓組織の損傷

このように本実験では、拘束ストレスにより肝臓に顆粒球増多が出現し、肝臓に組織学的変化（脂肪肝）が起こることが明らかになった。そこで、その時、実際に肝細胞が損傷された検証するため、血清中トランスアミナーゼ値（GOTとGPT）を測定した（Fig. 6）。ストレス8時間後に早くも、血清中GOTおよびGPT値は上昇し始めた。GOT値の顕著な上昇は、注目に値した。

顆粒球は、胃潰瘍形成に直接関与する

RP-3（ラット顆粒球に対するマウスモノクローナル抗体）をラットに投与すると顆粒球の除去ができるという報告がある（15, 30）。この点について、ラットにおいてあらかじめ顆粒球の除去を行うと、潰瘍形成に変化が起こるかどうか検証した（Table I）。本実験では、ストレスを与える3日前にラットにRP-3を事前に投与した。ストレス24時間後でも、大部分のラットにおいて胃潰瘍による出血は見られなかった（1/6）。一方、正常マウスの血清を投与した対照群の全てのラットには胃出血と潰瘍形成が見られた（6/6）。

実際に、RP-3を接種すると生体内の顆粒球を除去できるのかを確認するため、いろいろなラットの血液から白血球を採取し、RP-3$^+$顆粒球比率と光散乱を解析した（Fig.7）。対照群ラットにおいて、RP-3を投与すると顆粒球陽性の顕著なピークが消失した（22.0% → 13.1%）。このような変化はラットにストレスを与えると更に顕著なものとなった。つまり、ストレスが原因の顆粒球値の増加は（36.2%）、RP-3を事前に投与したラットにおいては顕著ではなかった（13.8%）。このことは、光散乱の結果にも示されている（Fig. 7, 右）。拘束ストレスの有無と

Figure.7

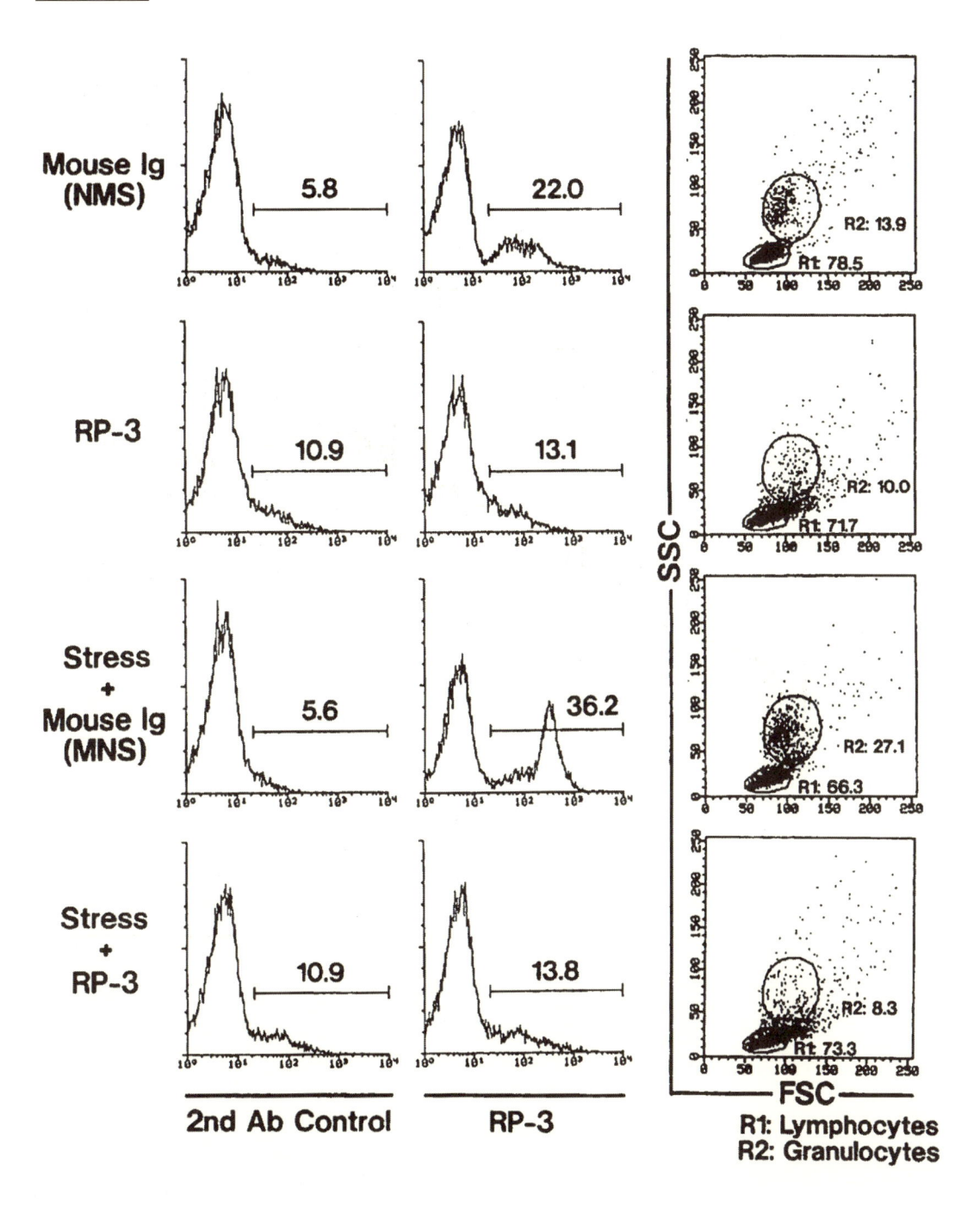

Mouse Ig (NMS) | 2nd Ab Control: 5.8 | RP-3: 22.0 | R2: 13.9 / R1: 78.5

RP-3 | 2nd Ab Control: 10.9 | RP-3: 13.1 | R2: 10.0 / R1: 71.7

Stress + Mouse Ig (MNS) | 2nd Ab Control: 5.6 | RP-3: 36.2 | R2: 27.1 / R1: 66.3

Stress + RP-3 | 2nd Ab Control: 10.9 | RP-3: 13.8 | R2: 8.3 / R1: 73.3

R1: Lymphocytes
R2: Granulocytes

抗ラット顆粒球(RP-3)モノクロナール抗体によるラットの顆粒球の除去。RP-3を週2度腹腔内投与した(1mg/回/匹)。対照群および拘束ストレス群の両群において顆粒球値が減少した。光散乱の結果も、リンパ球よりも光散乱が大きな顆粒球の減少を示した。

Figure.8A

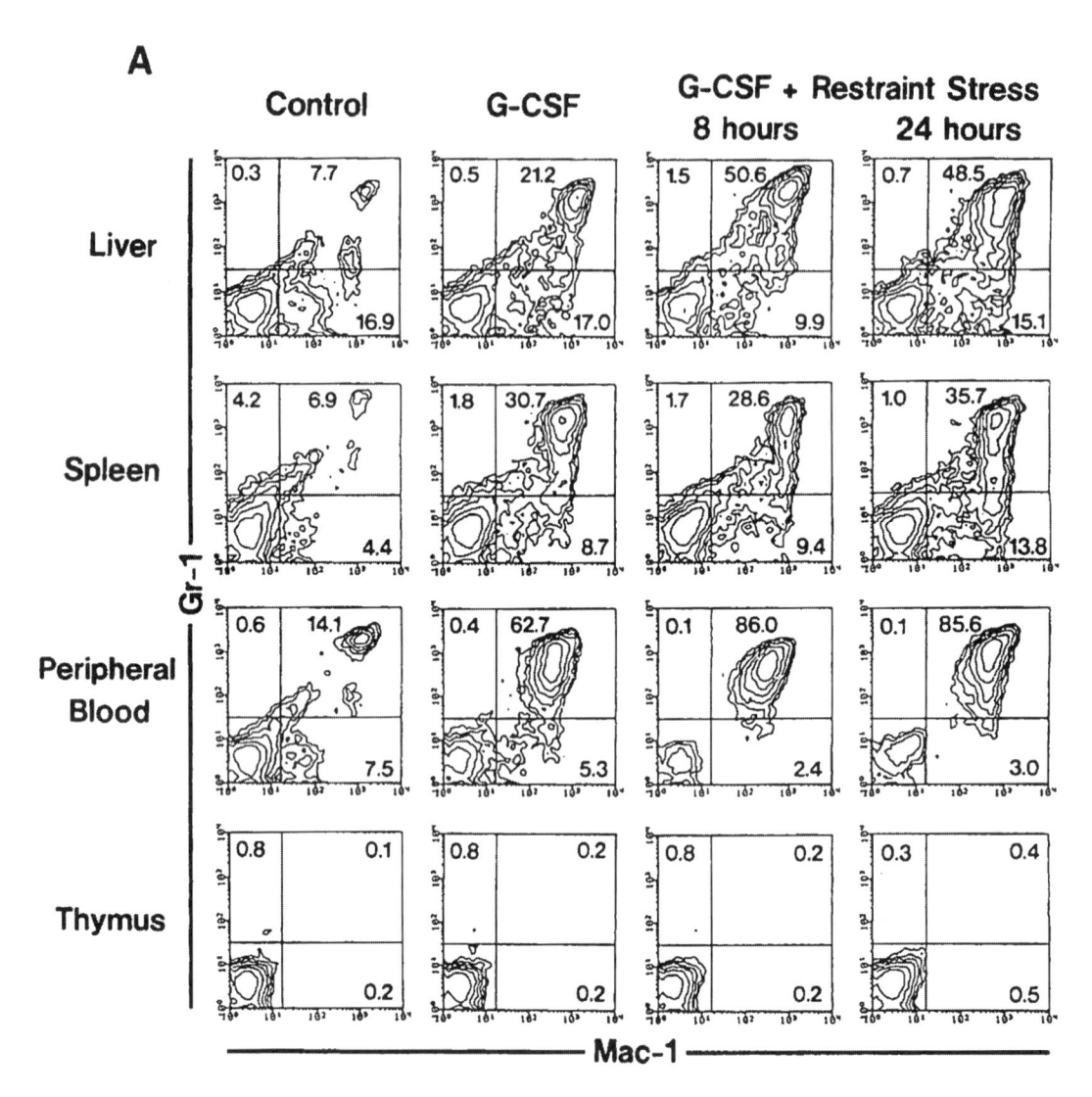

	Control	G-CSF	G-CSF + Restraint Stress 8 hours	G-CSF + Restraint Stress 24 hours
Liver	0.3 / 7.7 / 16.9	0.5 / 21.2 / 17.0	1.5 / 50.6 / 9.9	0.7 / 48.5 / 15.1
Spleen	4.2 / 6.9 / 4.4	1.8 / 30.7 / 8.7	1.7 / 28.6 / 9.4	1.0 / 35.7 / 13.8
Peripheral Blood	0.6 / 14.1 / 7.5	0.4 / 62.7 / 5.3	0.1 / 86.0 / 2.4	0.1 / 85.6 / 3.0
Thymus	0.8 / 0.1 / 0.2	0.8 / 0.2 / 0.2	0.8 / 0.2 / 0.2	0.3 / 0.4 / 0.5

(縦軸: Gr-1、横軸: Mac-1)

G-CSF投与は顆粒球を誘導し潰瘍形成を促進する。A：Gr-1とMac-1の二重染色。B：CD3とIL-2βの二重染色。各分画内の数字は、数値は蛍光陽性細胞の比率を示す。G-CSF前投与した後、拘束ストレス（24時間）を与えたマウスの肝臓と各臓器において顆粒球（Gr-1$^+$Mac-1$^+$）と胸腺外分化T細胞（CD3^{int}IL-2Rβ$^+$）の比率が顕著に増加した。

は関係なく、RP-3を投与したラットにおいて顆粒球は少なくなった。

顆粒球増多のマウスは、ストレス8時間後に早くも胃潰瘍が発症する

組換型ヒトG-CSFが、現在利用可能であり、これは、マウスにも効果的がある。顆粒球が胃潰瘍形成に直接関与しているという仮説が妥当であるならば、G-CSFを事前に投与して顆粒球を増多させることにより、潰瘍形成が早まるに違いない。この可能性を検証した（Table，下）。G-CSFを週3回腹腔注射した後、マウスに拘束ストレスを与えた。G-CSF接種をした5匹のマウスのうち4匹にストレス8時間後にすでに胃出血が見られた。

Figure.8B

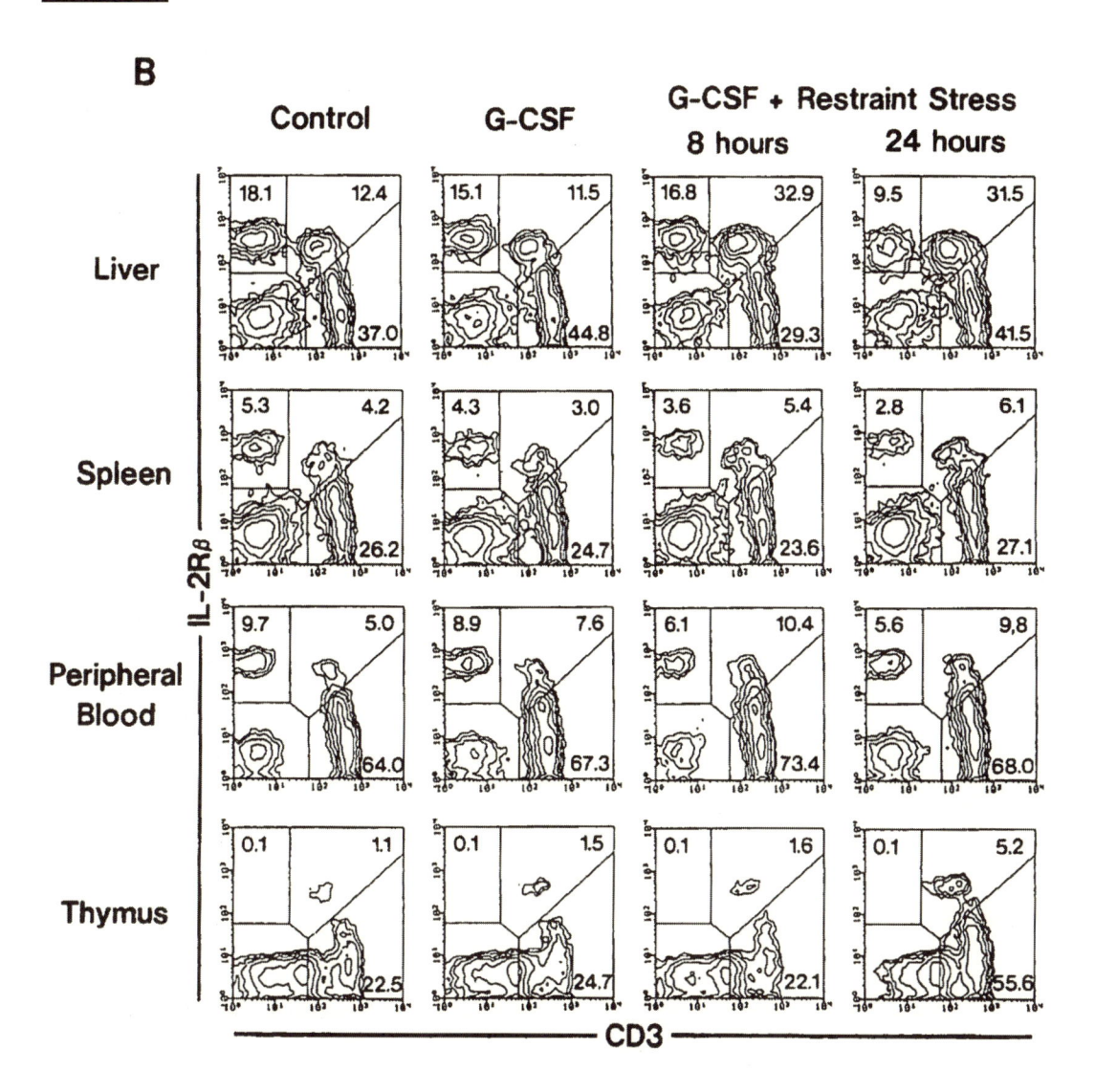

B

	Control	G-CSF	G-CSF + Restraint Stress 8 hours	G-CSF + Restraint Stress 24 hours
Liver	18.1 / 12.4 / 37.0	15.1 / 11.5 / 44.8	16.8 / 32.9 / 29.3	9.5 / 31.5 / 41.5
Spleen	5.3 / 4.2 / 26.2	4.3 / 3.0 / 24.7	3.6 / 5.4 / 23.6	2.8 / 6.1 / 27.1
Peripheral Blood	9.7 / 5.0 / 64.0	8.9 / 7.6 / 67.3	6.1 / 10.4 / 73.4	5.6 / 9.8 / 68.0
Thymus	0.1 / 1.1 / 22.5	0.1 / 1.5 / 24.7	0.1 / 1.6 / 22.1	0.1 / 5.2 / 55.6

Y軸: IL-2Rβ　X軸: CD3

　本実験のプロトコルに従いG-CSF投与により、マウスの各臓器において顆粒球増多が出現したことを確認するため、Gr-1とMac-1の二重染色を行なった (Fig. 8)。ストレスの有無に関係なくG-CSFを投与した全てのマウスの肝臓、脾臓および末梢血において、顕著な顆粒球増多徴候が見られた。ストレスを与えると肝臓と末梢血における顆粒球の比率は、さらに増大した。

G-CSF投与と拘束ストレスにより肝臓、脾臓と末梢血中の単核球数は、50％も上昇し、これらの臓器において顆粒球の絶対数の相当量増加した。CD3とIL-2Rβの二重染色を行なった (Fig 8B)。G-CSF単独投与では、各臓器においてCD3^{int}IL-2Rβ$^+$細胞の比率は上昇しなかったが、拘束ストレスを与えたマウスでは、特に肝臓において、CD3^{int}IL-2Rβ$^+$細胞の比率が増加した。

考察

臨床において、重篤な胃潰瘍の患者において肝機能不全によるトランスアミナーゼ高値が見られることがある（未発表データ）。本研究における患者の検査データが示唆するのは、胃や肝臓における組織破壊は、全身の顆粒球の活性化が原因である可能性である。この点において、マウスとラットの胃のみならずリンパ臓器における顆粒球値にも注目した。拘束ストレスにおける胃潰瘍形成に顆粒球が深く関与していることが判明した。拘束ストレスを与えると、検証を行なった胸腺以外のすべての臓器において顆粒球が増多した。形態学的に顆粒球の大部分は好中球であった（>95%）（未発表データ）。換言すると、これが、重篤な胃潰瘍患者の中には肝臓などの複数の臓器に機能障害が何故現れるかという理由である。これらの結果が示すのは、激しいストレッサーには顆粒球増多の原因となる可能性があること、そして、増多した顆粒球が過剰な活性化すると、次に複数の組織（粘膜）損傷が出現することである。拘束ストレスによりどのようにして各臓器の顆粒球増多が出現したかという疑問について顆粒球に存在するアドレナリン受容体（αとβタイプ）が鍵となる要因だと考える（5, 17, 20, 28, 39）。すなわち、ストレッサーにより、先ず、交感神経緊張が出現し、そして、この交感神経緊張が刺激となって、骨髄そして末梢血の顆粒球が活性化する可能性がある。ストレスのみならず、運動、働き過ぎやアドレナリン投与など他の交感神経刺激により顆粒球増多が誘導されることが知られている（9, 13, 18, 19, 23, 25, 29）。胸腺外分化T細胞は、細胞表面に高密度のアドレナリン受容体が存在するリンパ球であるので（未発表データ）、この考察は理にかなっている。本研究において、拘束ストレスによりCD3^{int}IL-2Rβ^+胸腺外分化T細胞の数と比率も同様に高率で増加することが判明した。

拘束ストレスを30時間以上継続すると、多臓器不全で死亡するマウスも存在した。過剰活性化した顆粒球が原因で、組織損傷が起こり、フリーラジカル、超酸化物および他の細胞質酵素の過剰産生も関与すると考えられる。胃潰瘍、肝機能不全と多臓器不全における基本的な相違は、ストレス、交感神経緊張、とそれに伴う顆粒球増多の程度によるものだという可能性がある。

拘束ストレスによる顆粒球増多と同時にCD3^{int}IL-2Rβ^+胸腺外分化T細胞が出現するのは、注目に値する。Mlsシステムと抗Vβモノクロナール抗体を用いた実験より推察できるように、これまで胸腺外分化T細胞は自己応答禁止クローンを含むが、同系の腫瘍細胞のみならず、急速に増殖する自己細胞（例、胸腺細胞、肝細胞と腸細胞）を傷害することが明らかになった（1, 4, 27, 35）。この結果は、関節リウマチ患者の関節に浸潤している細胞は、顆粒球（80%）とCD57$^+$T細胞（15%）（ヒトにおける胸腺外分化T細胞）なことと関連するかもしれない（11, 26, 37）。顆粒球が破壊した組織が、自己反応性を持つ胸腺外分化T細胞の標的となることが考えられる。

顆粒球の反応（末梢における顆粒球増多）は非常に速いので境界顆粒球プールを有する臓器もあると仮定する研究者も多い（6）。本研究において、末梢血の顆粒球増多は拘束ストレス開始8時間後という早い時点で出現した。しかし、他の研究者も我々もそのような臓器を発見できなかった、しかし、我々は骨髄自体が境界顆粒球プールであることを最近明らかにした。肝臓と脾臓が境界顆粒球プールではないことは、明らかである（Fig. 3A）。顆粒球は、非常に短命である（2-3日）。例えば、定常の状態でも、顆

粒球の30-50%が、新しい集団と入れ替えられている。この点について、骨髄自体に短時間で大量の顆粒球を産生する大きな能力がある。

　組織学的検査では、拘束ストレスマウスの胃において大量の顆粒球は見られなかった（未発表データ）。しかし、フローサイトメトリー解析では、胃に若干顆粒球が見られた。顆粒球は血管内で作用している可能性がある、従って、ストレスを受けると、一番先に、血管拡張や出血が出現している可能性がある（2, 33）。一方、胃潰瘍患者の胃切片が示すように、ストレスによる慢性刺激が胃の粘膜組織に顆粒球浸潤を誘導するようである。拘束ストレスマウスにおける脂肪肝の組織所見も、非常に興味深かった。最近、脂肪肝出現は重篤なストレスの重要な徴候である可能性を提案した（論文投稿中）。

　大量の抗顆粒球モノクロナール抗体をラットに利用できるので（15,3 0）、ラットに使用して顆粒球を除去する実験を行なった。顆粒球を除去した後、胃潰瘍形成を抑圧する効果は顕著であった。G-CSFを事前に投与した実験の結果とととともに、顆粒球が潰瘍形成に直接関与していることが明らかになった。一般に細菌感染すると局所および全身において顆粒球値が上昇すること、また、細菌とその構成成分が顆粒球の機能を効率的に活性化することが知られている（10, 34, 36, 40）。総合的に考察すると、H.pyloriがこの刺激の主因であることは十分に考察できる。しかし、本研究の結果は、ヒトと動物において交感神経緊張が、胃潰瘍形成と組織傷害の主因であるという背景または基礎状況を示すものである。

ASSOCIATION OF GRANULOCYTES WITH ULCER FORMATION IN THE STOMACH OF RODENTS EXPOSED TO RESTRAINT STRESS

TETSUYA MORODA[1,2], TSUNEO IIAI[2], AKIHIRO TSUKAHARA[2], MINORU FUKUDA[1], SUSUMU SUZUKI[2], TAKASHI TADA[2], KATSUYOSHI HATAKEYAMA[2] and TORU ABO[1,3]

[1]Department of Immunology, and [2]First Department of Surgery, Niigata University School of Medicine, Niigata 951, Japan

ABSTRACT

Increased levels of granulocytes in the blood were first estimated in patients with gastric ulcer. Then, experiments were extended to rodents, including mice and rats. Restraint stress was induced by fixing rodents in stainless steel mesh. Infiltration of granulocytes and other cells was determined in various organs of mice by using mAbs in conjunction with immunofluorescence tests. Severe granulocytosis was induced in various organs, including the stomach, blood, and liver 24 h after the exposure. Interestingly, extrathymic T cells, which are known to have the ability to kill rapidly proliferating autologous self-cells, increased in parallel. More importantly, the pre-elimination of granulocytes by anti-granulocyte mAb abrogated the formation of ulcers in rats, whereas the preactivation of granulocytes by G-CSF accelerated formation. The present results suggest that the background or basal conditions in hosts may be very critical for the formation of gastric ulcers and the occurrence of other damage to organs.

It has long been believed that gastric ulcers are formed due to the digestion on the gastric mucosa by excess levels of pepsin under conditions of acidic pH in the stomach (and termed peptic ulcer) (21). However, recent evidence shows that *Helicobactor (H.) pylori*, resident bacteria in the stomach, are intimately associated with the formation of gastric ulcers (3, 4, 16, 22, 24). Indeed, the elimination of *H. pylori* by antibiotics effectively prevents the recurrence of gastric ulcers (7, 31, 32). Taken together, the etiology of gastric ulcer seems to be still controversial.

Based on these findings, we have examined clinical data in many patients with gastric ulcers and noticed that the levels of granulocytes in blood were significantly higher than those of a control group (data shown in this study). Moreover, in many such patients, histological study of resected stomach revealed that granulocytes often invaded the gastric mucosa. The possibility is therefore raised that granulocytes may be associated with the formation of gastric ulcers in conjunction with resident bacteria. This possibility is supported by findings that activated granulocytes produce free radicals and superoxides to kill bacteria and that the excessive production of such substances induces tissue destruction (6, 34, 36, 40).

In the present study, we used mouse and rat models of gastric ulcers, the experimental animals being exposed to restraint stress for 8 and 24 h. This stress induced prominent granulocytosis (> 95% neutrophils) in various organs, including the target organ, the stomach. Since granulocytes are known to carry a high density of adrenergic receptors (α and β types) on their surface (5, 17, 20, 28, 39), it is speculated that granulocytosis induced by stress and subsequent sympathetic nerve strain might be an important factor in the formation of gastric ulcers. We also propose the possibility that extrathymic T cells, which have autoreactivity,

Abbreviations: NSAID, nonsteroidal anti-inflammatory drug; TCR[int] cells, intermediate TCR cells; MNC, mononuclear cells; DN, double-negative
[3]Correspondence to: T. Abo at the above address. Fax: (81)25-228-0868

might also be involved in ulcer formation and tissue damage in conjunction with granulocytes.

MATERIALS AND METHODS

Subjects

Patients with gastric ulcers (n = 30; age, 32 to 54 years old; mean age, 44.3) were examined as to the levels of granulocytes and lymphocytes in the peripheral blood. They were outpatients at Sakamachi Hospital, Niigata, Japan. Age-matched controls were healthy volunteers (n = 33; age, 30 to 53 years old; mean age, 43.8).

Animals

BALB/c mice and DD rats at the ages of 6 to 8 weeks were used. They were obtained from Charles River Japan, Kanagawa, Japan and were maintained in animal facilities of the Niigata University under specific pathogen-free conditions.

Restrain Stress

Animals were fixed in stainless steel mesh and kept for 8 and 24 h in a cage.

Cell Preparations

Mice anesthetized with ether were killed after complete exsanguination through incised axillary arteries and veins. Specimens from the liver, spleen, and thymus were removed and kept in phosphate-buffered saline (PBS) (pH 7.2) on ice until cell preparation.

To obtain liver non-parenchymal cells, the liver obtained from one mouse was cut into small pieces with scissors, pressed through 200-gauge stainless steel mesh, and then suspended in 40 ml Eagle's MEM supplemented with 5 mM HEPES (Nissui Pharmaceutical, Tokyo, Japan) and 2% heat-inactivated newborn calf serum. After being washed once with medium, the cells were fractionated by centrifugation in 15 ml of 35% Percoll solution containing 100 IU/ml heparin for 15 min at 2,000 rpm (8). The resultant pellet of cells containing red blood cells (RBC) was resuspended and washed with medium. To deplete RBC, 170 mM Tris-HCl buffer (pH 7.65) containing 155 mM NH_4Cl, 10 mM $KHCO_3$, and 1 mM Na_2EDTA was added (12), and the resulting mixture was kept on ice for 5 min. After being washed twice with medium, liver mononuclear cells (MNC) were suspended in 1 ml medium and the number of cells was enumerated.

Spleen cells and thymocytes were obtained by forcing each organ through 200-gauge stainless steel mesh. RBC were lysed with the ammonium chloride/Tris-HCl buffer as described for liver non-parenchymal cells and then washed twice with medium. Blood leukocytes were isolated from the buffy coat by the 6% dextran-sulphate sedimentation method.

Cell preparation was also conducted for the stomach and joints. Tissue was resected from the stomach and the joints, respectively, and cut into small pieces with scissors. Fragments were then treated with collagenase (0.1 mg/ml in PBS) (Sigma Chemical, St. Louis, MO). The treated samples were pressed through 200-gauge stainless mesh and suspended in the medium. The cell pellet was loaded onto a Ficoll-Isopaque gradient (1.077) cushion to separate leukocytes from the debris (12).

Immunofluorescence Tests

The surface phenotype of cells was analyzed using mAbs in conjunction with a two-color immunofluorescence test (12). The mAbs used here included fluorescein isothiocyanate (FITC)-, phycoerythrin (PE)-, or biotin-conjugated anti-CD3 (145-2C11) (PharMingen, San Diego, CA), and anti-IL-2R β-chain (IL-2Rβ) (TM-β1) mAb (21). FITC- or PE-conjugated anti-CD4 (L3T4), and anti-CD8 (Lyt-2) mAb were obtained from Becton Dickinson (Mountain View, CA). To prevent nonspecific binding of mAbs, the pretreatment of cells with mAb against CD32/16 (2.4G2) (PharMingen) was always performed (i.e., the blocking of Fc receptors). Biotin-conjugated reagents were developed with PE-conjugated streptavidin (Becton Dickinson). The fluorescence-positive cells were analyzed with a FACScan using LYSIS II software (Becton Dickinson).

In vivo Elimination of Granulocytes

It was established that mouse anti-rat granulocyte mAb, RP-3 (kindly provided by Dr F. Sendo, Yamagata University School of Medicine, Yamagata, Japan), was able to eliminate granulocytes in vivo in rats when it was i.p. injected (15, 30). We applied this method in this study. RP-3 was injected twice in one week (1 mg/one time/mouse). To determine the level of granulocytes in rats, RP-3 was also used. The second antibody was PE-conjugated

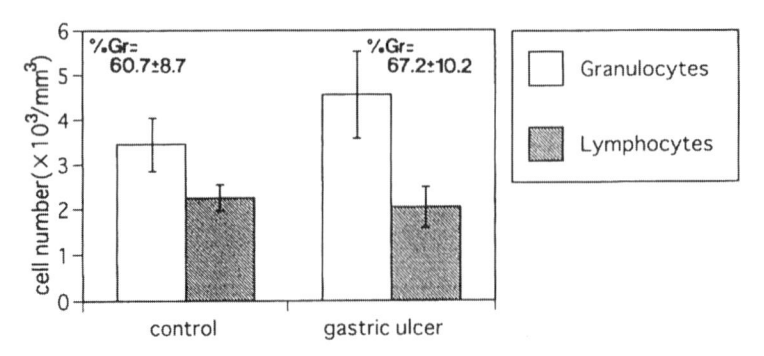

Fig. 1 Granulocytosis is associated with patients with gastric ulcers. Thirty patients with gastric ulcers were examined as to the levels of granulocytes and lymphocytes. Age-matched controls (n = 33) were also examined. The number ($4.3 \pm 1.2 \times 10^3/mm^3$) and proportion ($67.2 \pm 10.2\%$) of granulocytes in the patients were higher than the number ($3.6 \pm 0.6 \times 10^3/mm^3$) and proportion ($60.7 \pm 8.7\%$) of granulocytes in controls ($P < 0.01$). The number ($2.1 \pm 0.3 \times 10^3/mm^3$) of lymphocytes in the patients was almost comparable to that ($2.2 \pm 0.3 \times 10^3/mm^3$) in controls ($P > 0.05$). However, the proportion ($30.6 \pm 5.8\%$) of lymphocytes in the patients was lower than that ($35.1 \pm 6.1\%$) in controls ($P < 0.05$).

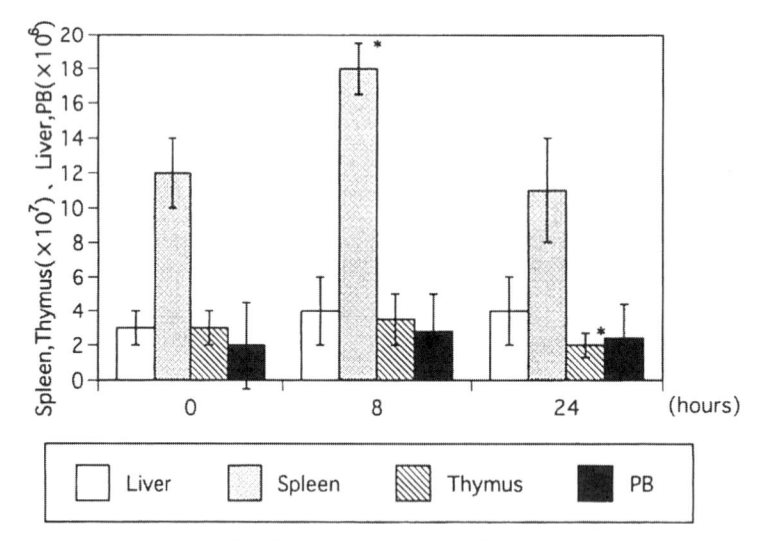

Fig. 2 Variation in the numbers of MNC yielded by various organs in mice after exposure to restraint stress. Mice were sacrificed 8 and 24 h after the exposure and the number of MNC in each organ was enumerated. To produce the mean and one SD, 4 mice were used at each time point. The number of splenic MNC increased at 8 h while that of thymocytes decreased at 24 h ($P < 0.05$). The other values remained unchanged. *$P < 0.05$

anti-mouse IgG mAb (Biomeda, Faster City, CA).

Granulocytosis Induced by G-CSF

Human recombinant G-CSF (Kirin Beer, Tokyo, Japan) was used to induce granulocytosis in mice. G-CSF was subcutaneously injected three times in one week (10^4 U/one time/mouse).

Statistical Analysis

Significance was statistically determined by Stu-

A

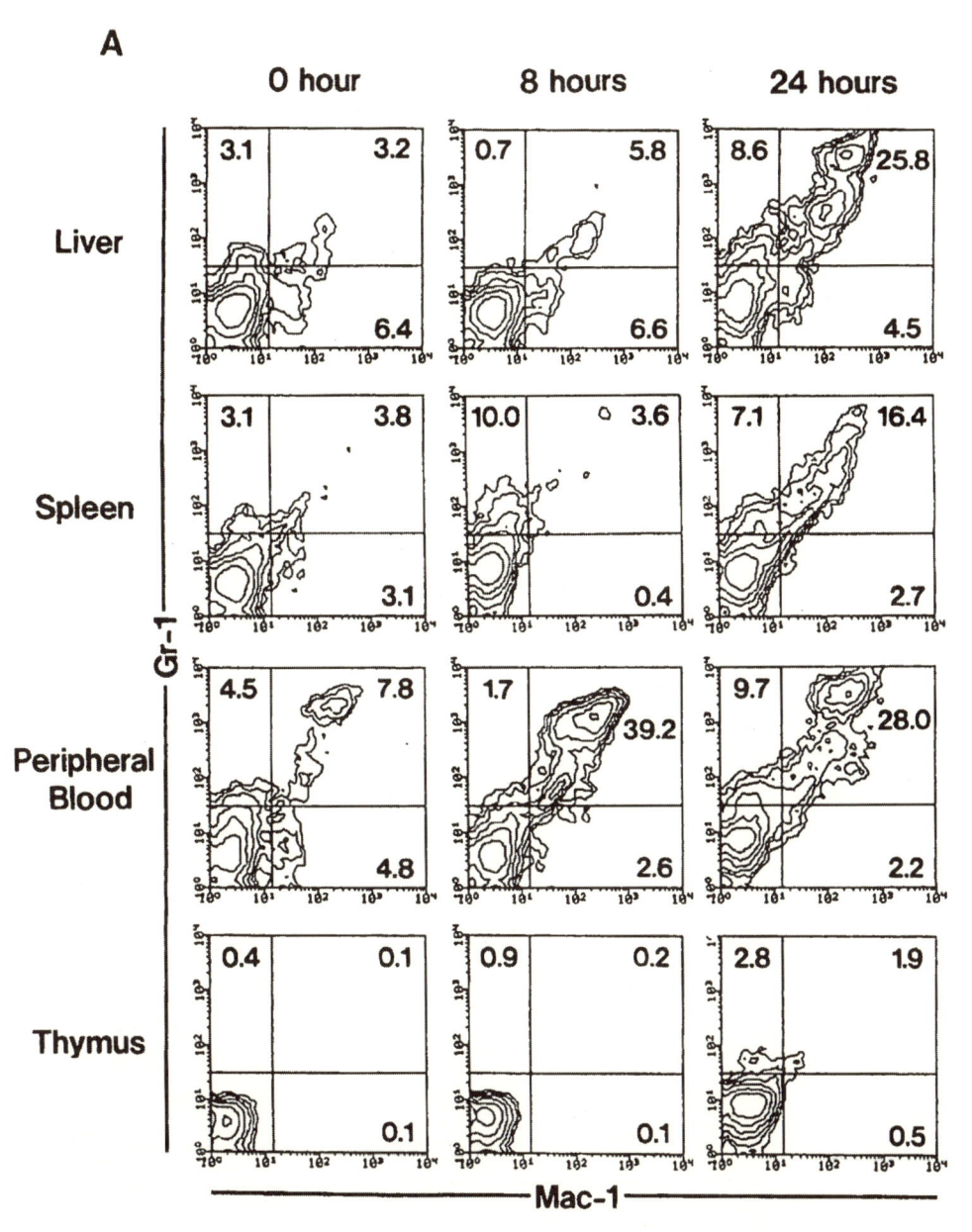

	0 hour	8 hours	24 hours
Liver	3.1 / 3.2 / 6.4	0.7 / 5.8 / 6.6	8.6 / 25.8 / 4.5
Spleen	3.1 / 3.8 / 3.1	10.0 / 3.6 / 0.4	7.1 / 16.4 / 2.7
Peripheral Blood	4.5 / 7.8 / 4.8	1.7 / 39.2 / 2.6	9.7 / 28.0 / 2.2
Thymus	0.4 / 0.1 / 0.1	0.9 / 0.2 / 0.1	2.8 / 1.9 / 0.5

Gr-1 (vertical axis) — Mac-1 (horizontal axis)

Fig. 3 Phenotypic characterization of MNC in various organs of mice exposed to restraint stress. A: Two-color staining for Gr-1 and Mac-1. B: Two-color staining for CD3 and IL-2Rβ. Mice were used 8 and 24 h after the exposure. Numbers in the figure represent the percentage of fluorescence-positive cells in corresponding areas. Granulocytes (Gr-1$^+$ Mac-1$^+$) and extrathymic T cells (CD3^{int} IL-2Rβ^+) were induced in various organs by restraint stress.

B

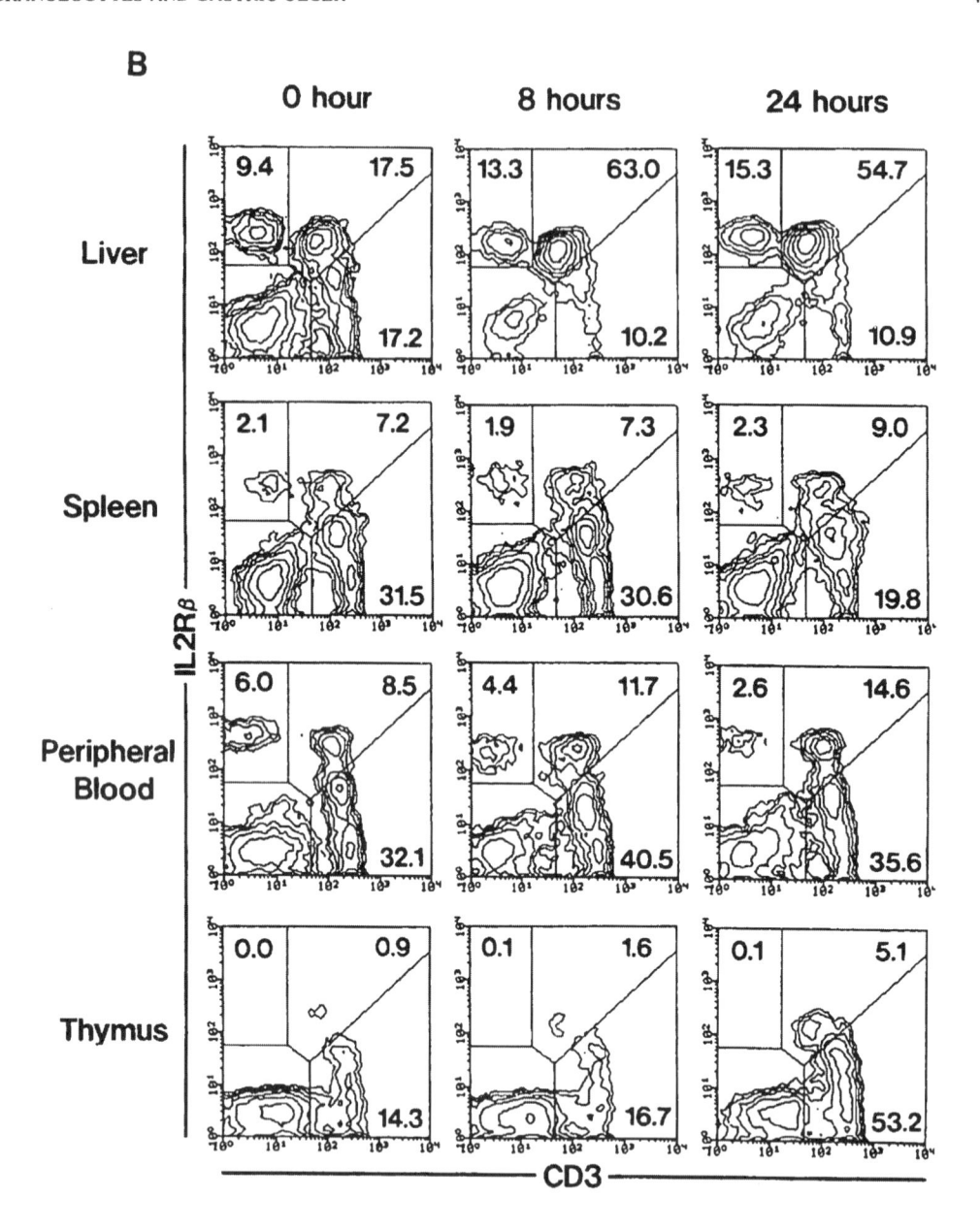

	0 hour	8 hours	24 hours
Liver	9.4 / 17.5 / 17.2	13.3 / 63.0 / 10.2	15.3 / 54.7 / 10.9
Spleen	2.1 / 7.2 / 31.5	1.9 / 7.3 / 30.6	2.3 / 9.0 / 19.8
Peripheral Blood	6.0 / 8.5 / 32.1	4.4 / 11.7 / 40.5	2.6 / 14.6 / 35.6
Thymus	0.0 / 0.9 / 14.3	0.1 / 1.6 / 16.7	0.1 / 5.1 / 53.2

Y-axis: IL2Rβ
X-axis: CD3

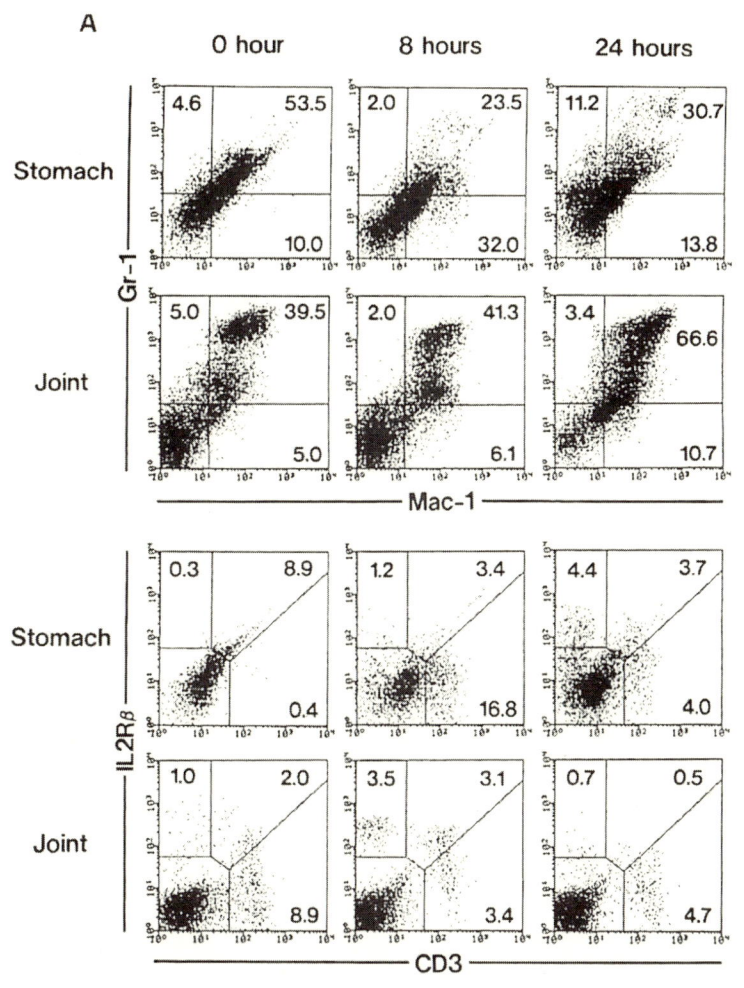

Fig. 4 Infiltration of granulocytes and extrathymic T cells into the stomach in mice exposed to restraint stress. A: Two-color staining for Gr-1 and Mac-1, and two-color staining for CD3 and IL-2Rβ. B: Light scatter analysis for MNC in the stomach. Mice were sacrificed after 8 and 24 h of exposure to the stress. Leukocytes were isolated from the stomach and joints. Gr-1$^+$Mac-1$^+$ granulocytes and CD3^{int}IL-2Rβ^+ extrathymic T cells were found in the stomach when mice were exposed to stress for 24 h. Granulocytosis was also seen in the joints in these mice.

dent's t-test.

RESULTS

Increase in the Level of Granulocytes in the Peripheral Blood of Patients with Gastric Ulcers

Almost all patients with gastric ulcers seem to suffer from mental or physical stress. We previously reported that such stress induces sympathetic nerve strain and subsequent granulocytosis (i.e., granulocytes carry α- and β-adrenegic receptors on their surface) (6). In this regard, the absolute numbers of granulocytes and lymphocytes were first compared between healthy volunteers and the patients (Fig. 1). It was found that the level of granulocytes in the blood was higher in the patients than in the healthy subjects. This was true in number ($P < 0.01$) and in proportion ($P < 0.01$). The absolute number of lymphocytes was comparable to that in the controls ($P > 0.05$), but the proportion of lymphocytes was

B

0 hours   8 hours

R2: 5.4   R2: 16.5
R1: 89.2   R1: 72.0

R1: Lymphocytes
R2: Granulocytes

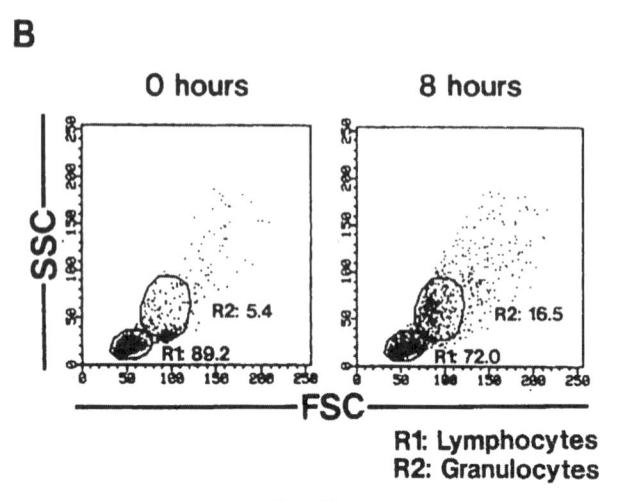

Fig. 4B

lower than that in the controls ($P < 0.05$).

Time-Kinetics in the Numbers of MNC Yielded by Various Immune Organs in Mice after Exposure to Restraint Stress

Before the analysis of the phenotype of cells, the absolute numbers of MNC yielded by various organs were examined in mice exposed to restraint stress (Fig. 2). Mice were exposed to restraint stress and sacrificed 8 and 24 h after initiation. The number of splenic MNC had increased at 8 h after the exposure, whereas that of thymocytes had decreased at 24 h after the exposure. The other numbers remained unchanged.

Increase in the Proportion and Number of Granulocytes and Extrathymic T Cells in Various Organs after Exposure to Restraint Stress

To identify granulocytes (Gr-1$^+$ Mac-1$^+$), two-color staining for Gr-1 and Mac-1 was carried out (Fig. 3A). Fundamentally, mice did not have a high level of granulocytes in various organs, even in the blood (see the data at zero h). However, when mice were exposed to stress, granulocytosis was seen first in the blood (39.2%) (8 h) and thereafter in other organs, including the liver and spleen (24 h). Although thymic atrophy was induced at 24 h after the exposure, granulocytes did not invade this organ.

It was then examined how the distribution of lymphocyte subsets varied with stress. Two-color staining for CD3 and IL-2Rβ was conducted (Fig. 3B). This staining simultaneously identifies CD3$^-$IL-2Rβ^+ NK cells (12), CD3^{int}IL-2Rβ^+ extrathymic T cells, and CD3^{high}IL-2Rβ^- conventional T cells. From 8 h after the exposure, a prominent increase in the proportion of extrathymic T cells was seen in various organs, especially in the liver. Since immature T cells (i.e., CD3$^-$ or CD3^{dull}) died of apoptosis in the atrophic thymus, the proportion of mature T cells (i.e., CD3^{high}IL-2Rβ^-) inversely increased (24 h). The proportion of CD3$^-$IL-2Rβ^+ NK cells was relatively constant in various organs of treated mice, whereas that of conventional T cells decreased in the liver and spleen of treated mice (24 h).

Infiltration of Granulocytes into the Stomach in Treated Mice

The experiments were extended to the stomach and knee joint (Fig. 4A). In contrast to the lymphoid tissues, tissue debris resulted in false-positive staining (Gr-1$^+$Mac-1$^+$) in these organs (especially in the area of light scatter corresponding to granulocytes but not lymphocytes). However, some granulocytes were identified as Gr-1^{2+}Mac-1$^+$ in the joint, irrespective of the exposure to stress. Interestingly, a small cluster of such Gr-1^{2+}Mac-1$^+$ cells newly appeared in the stomach of treated mice (at both 8 and 24 h). In parallel with this, some lymphocytes (a mixture of NK cells, extrathymic T cells, and conventional T cells) also appeared in the stomach (Fig. 4A, lower columns). These results revealed that restraint stress resulted in infiltration of granulocytes and lymphocytes into the stomach.

Since an immunofluorescence test for MNC in the stomach produced false-positive staining, light scatter analysis of MNC in the stomach is represented (Fig. 4B). In this figure, low light scatters of ESC (forward scatter) and SSC (side scatter) showed a cluster of lymphocytes, whereas high light scatters of FSC and SSC showed a cluster of granulocytes. Reflecting the invasion of granulocytes into the stomach, cells (R_2) with larger light scatter (i.e., granulocytes) increased (5.4 → 16.5%) 8 h after the exposure.

Macroscopic Observation of the Stomach in Mice Exposed to Stress

It was then confirmed whether the present protocol of restraint stress eventually induced the formation of ulcers in the stomach (Fig. 5A). At 8 h after the exposure, mucosal damage was not yet apparent in the stomach (Fig. 5Ab). However, prominent signs of bleeding and ulcer formation were seen at 24 h (Fig. 5Ac).

Since severe granulocytosis was also seen in the liver of treated mice, it was examined whether microscopic changes of the liver were induced in treated mice (Fig. 5B). In control mice, no lipid droplets were seen in hepatocytes (Fig. 5Ba). It was demonstrated that fatty liver (i.e., hepatocytes contained many lipid droplets in the cytoplasma) was induced in treated mice (Fig. 5Bb).

Tissue Damage in the Liver of Mice Exposed to Stress

The experiments thus far showed that restraint stress induced granulocytosis in the liver and changed its morphology (i.e., fatty liver). Then, to examine whether actual hepatocyte damage was induced at that time, the serum levels of transaminases (GOT and GPT) were measured (Fig. 6). As early as 8 h after the exposure, the serum levels of GOT and GPT began to increase. A great increase in the level of GOT was noteworthy.

Granulocytes Are Directly Associated with the Formation of Gastric Ulcers

It has been reported that RP-3, a mouse mAb against rat granulocytes, was able to eliminate

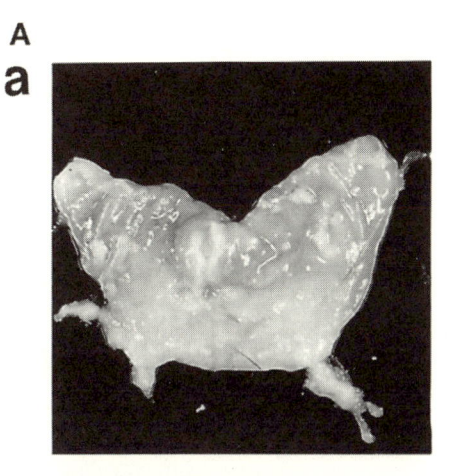

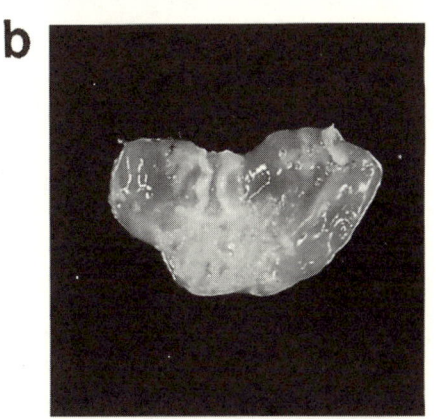

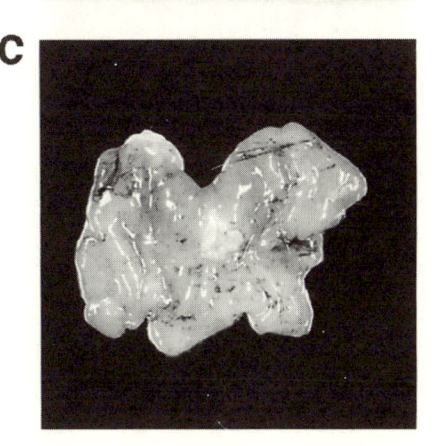

Fig. 5A

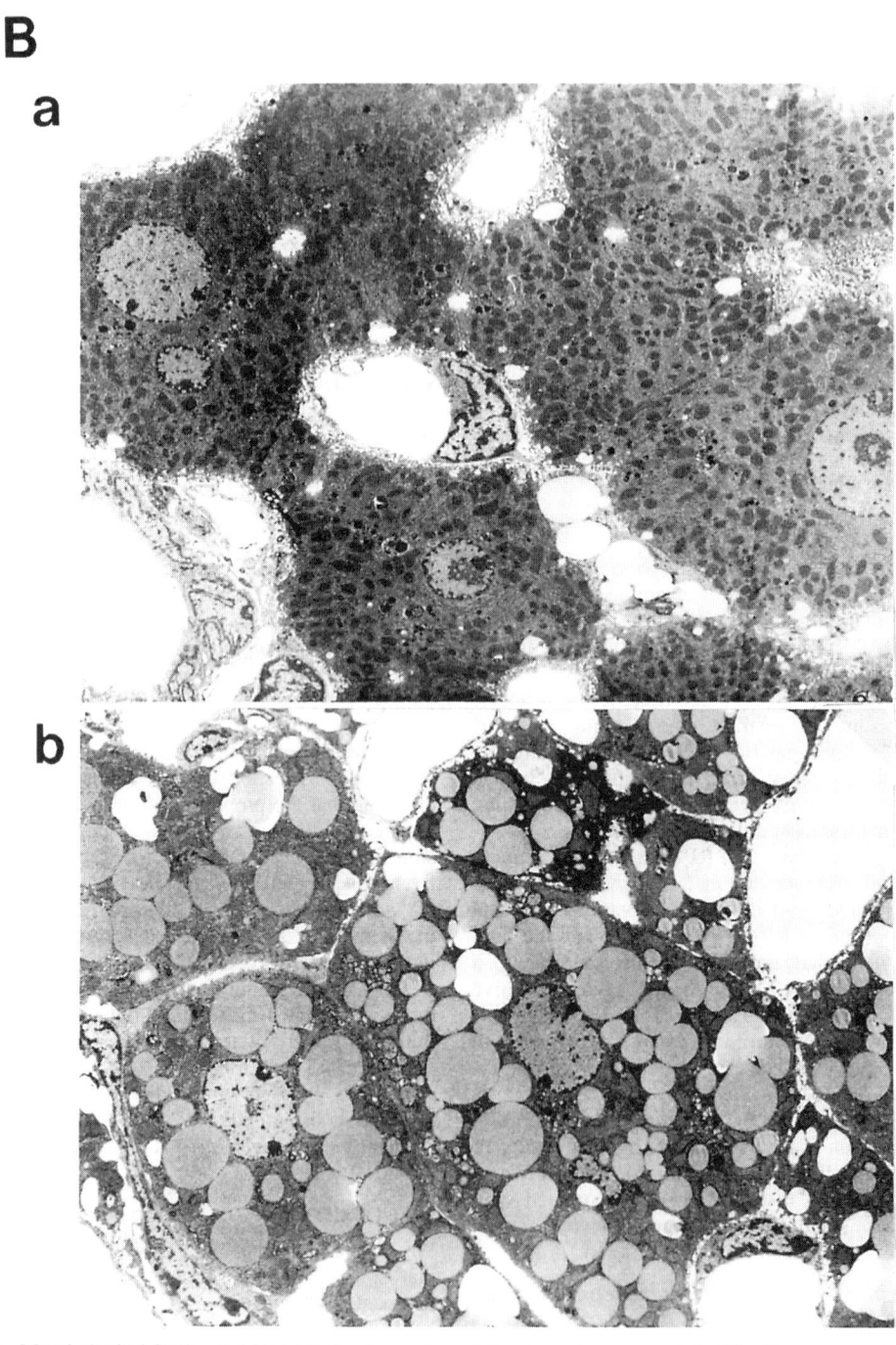

Fig. 5 Morphological Study. A: Macroscopic observation of the stomach. a, control; b, 8 h after exposure to stress; c, 24 h. B: Formation of fatty liver due to stress. a, control liver; b, liver at 24 h after the exposure. Prominent signs of bleeding and ulcer formation were observed 24 h after the exposure. At the same time, fatty liver developed in which hepatocytes contained many lipid droplets in the cytoplasm.

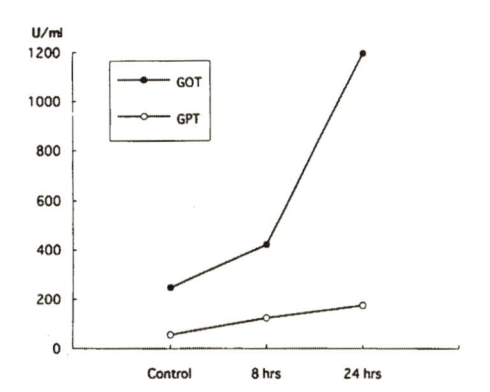

Fig. 6 Elevation in serum levels of transaminases due to restraint stress. A prominent elevation in serum levels of transaminases, especially GOT, was seen 24 h after the exposure to stress. Mean values of pooled materials (n = 3) are represented.

Table 1 *Modulation of Gastric Bleeding or Ulcer Formation by Pretreatment with Anti-Granulocyte Antibody (RP-3) or G-CSF*

Subject	Restriction	
	8 h	24 h
Control rat	0/8*	6/6
RP-3-treated rat	0/5	1/6
Control mouse	0/5	6/6
G-CSF-treated mouse	4/5	4/4

*Numbers of animals with gastric bleeding/total number of tested animals

granulocytes when injected *in vivo* into rats (15, 30). In this regard, it was examined whether the pre-elimination of granulocytes modulated the onset of ulcer formation in rats (Table 1). In this experiment, the rats pretreated with RP-3 three days before the restraint were used. Even 24 h after the exposure to restrain stress, almost all rats showed neither gastric bleeding ulcer formation (1/6). On the other hand, all control rats treated with normal mouse sera showed gastric bleeding and ulcer formation at that time (6/6).

To confirm that the RP-3 treatment actually eliminated granulocytes *in vivo*, whole leukocytes were obtained from the blood in various rats, and the proportion of RP-3$^+$ granulocytes and the light scatter were analyzed (Fig. 7). In control rats, it was found that RP-3 eliminated a clear positive peak of granulocytes (22.0% → 13.1%). This difference was more striking when rats exposed to stress were observed. Namely, the increase in the level of granulocytes caused by stress (36.2%) was not prominent in RP-3 pretreated rats (13.8%). This situation was also shown by the results of light scatter (Fig. 7, right column). Irrespective of the exposure to restraint stress, rats treated with RP-3 had a smaller cluster of granulocytes.

Mice with Granulocytosis Fall Victim to Gastric Ulcers as Early as 8 h after Stress

Recombinant human G-CSF is now available and is also effective in mice. If our hypothesis that granulocytes are directly associated with the formation of gastric ulcers is valid, granulocytosis induced by pre-treatment with G-CSF should accelerate ulcer formation. This possibility was examined (Table 1, lower lines). G-CSF was i.p. injected 3 times in one week and the mice were then exposed to restraint stress. Four of the 5 mice treated with G-CSF already showed gastric bleeding at 8 h after the exposure.

To confirm that the administration of G-CSF in the present protocol induced granulocytosis in various organs of mice, two-color staining for Gr-1 and Mac-1 was carried out (Fig. 8). Prominent signs of granulocytosis were seen in the liver, spleen, and peripheral blood of all mice treated with G-CSF, irrespective of restraint stress. It was also true that the proportion of granulocytes in the liver and blood further increased as a result of the stress. Since the numbers of MNC yielded by the liver, spleen, and blood increased up to 50% with the administration of G-CSF and restraint stress, the increase in the absolute number of granulocytes in these organs was substantial.

Two-color staining for CD3 and IL-2Rβ was then carried out (Fig. 8B). Although the administration of G-CSF by itself did not increase the proportion of CD3^{int}IL-2Rβ^+ cells in various organs, such mice exposed to restraint stress showed an increase in the proportion of CD3^{int}IL-2Rβ^+ cells, especially in the liver.

DISCUSSION

We, as well as other clinicians, have experienced that some patients suffering from severe gastric ulcers also show an elevated level of transaminases or liver dysfunction (our unpublished observation). The data from the patients examined in this study suggest that such tissue destruction of the stomach

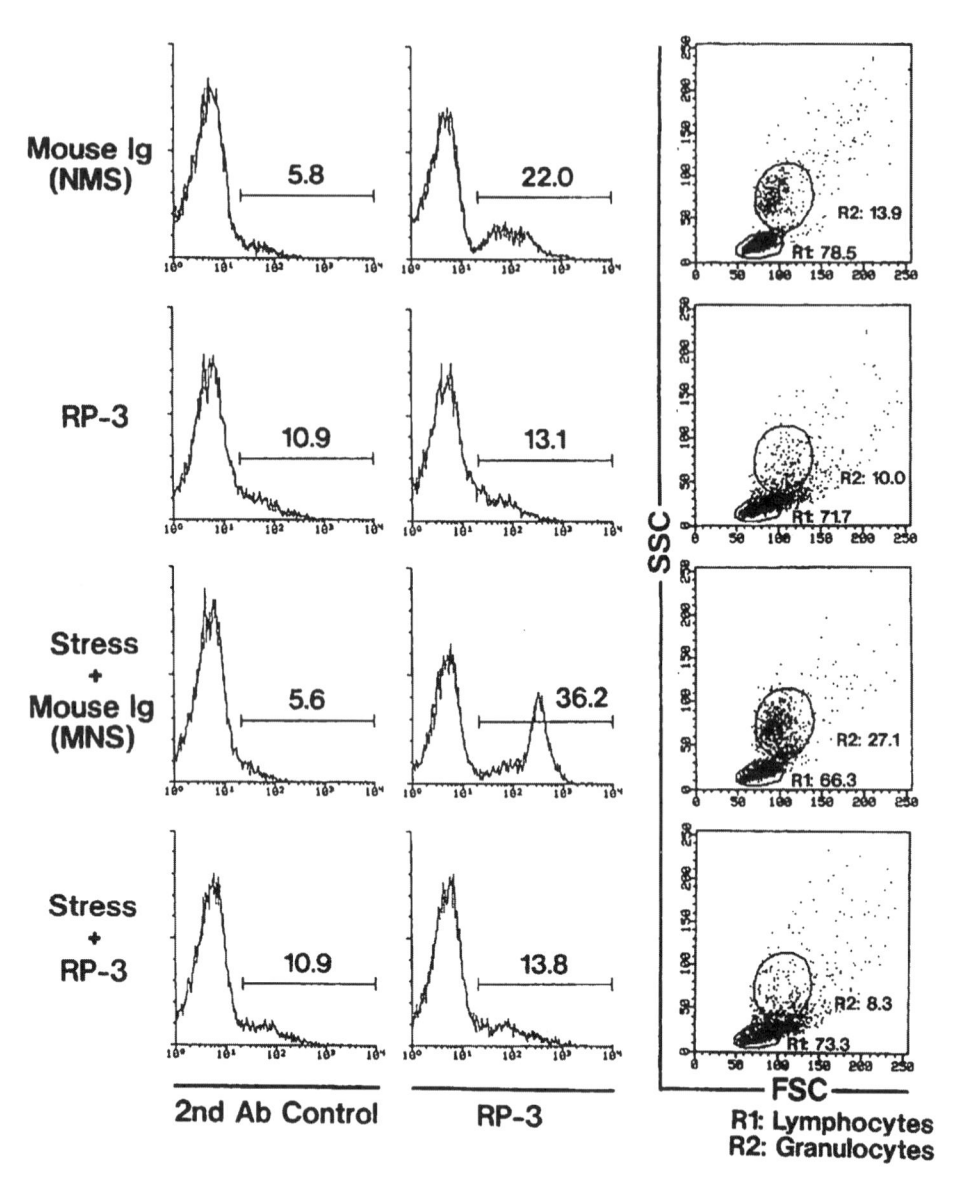

Fig. 7 Elimination of granulocytes in rats by treatment with anti-rat granulocyte (RP-3) mAb. RP-3 mAb was i.p. injected twice in one week (1 mg RP-3/one time/mouse). The levels of granulocytes decreased in both control rats and rats exposed to restraint stress. The result of light scatter also indicated the decrease of granulocytes which had larger light scatter than did lymphocytes.

and liver may be due to activated granulocytes which increase in general in the body. In this respect, attention was herein focused on the levels of granulocytes not only in the stomach but also in lymphoid organs in mice and rats. It was demonstrated that granulocytes are intimately associated with the formation of gastric ulcers in mice exposed to restraint stress. The restraint stress

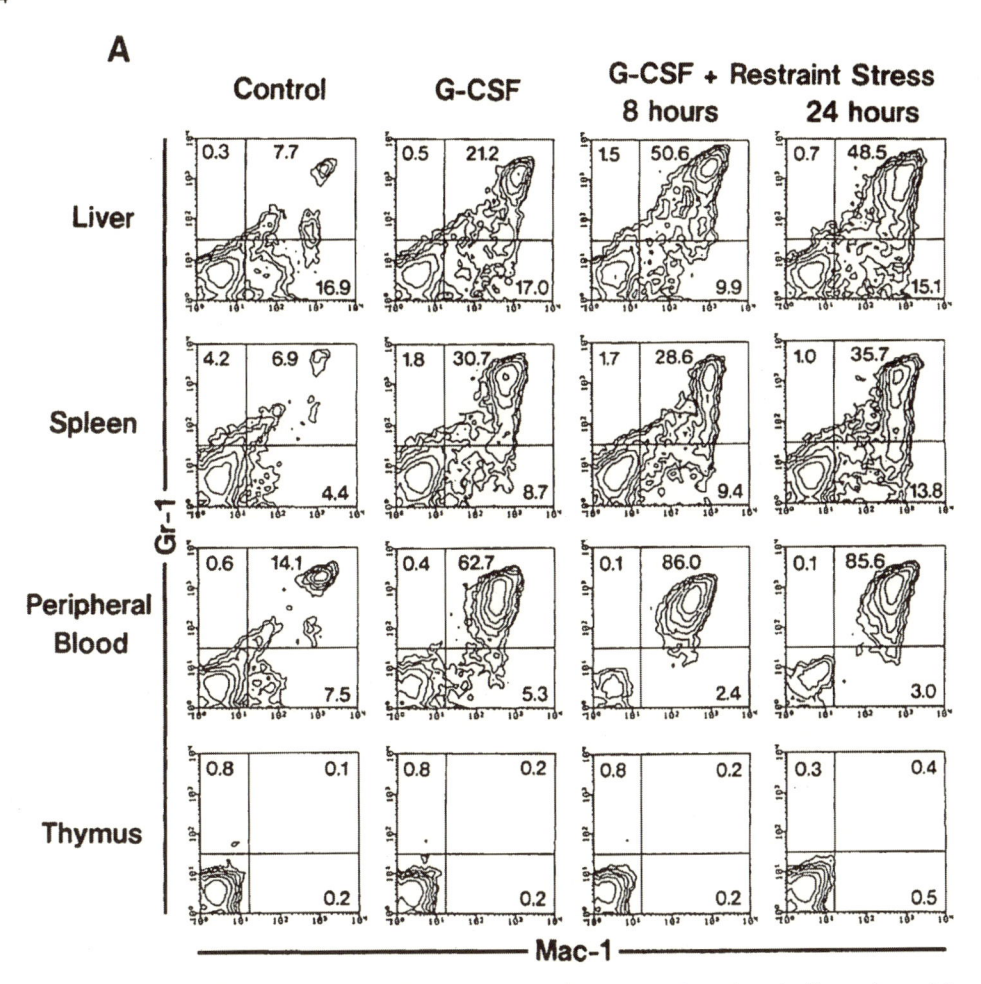

Fig. 8 Administration of G-CSF induces granulocytes and accelerates ulcer formation. A: Two-color staining for Gr-1 and Mac-1. B: Two-color staining for CD3 and IL-2Rβ. Numbers in the figure represent the percentages of fluorescence-positive cells in the corresponding areas. Gr-1$^+$ Mac-1$^+$ granulocytes and CD3^{int} IL-2Rβ$^+$ extrathymic T cells greatly increased in proportion in the liver and other organs of mice pre-treated with G-CSF and exposed to restraint (24 h) stress. The number of liver MNC increased up to 50% in treated mice (24 h).

induced granulocytosis in all organs tested except the thymus. Morphologically, almost all granulocytes (>95%) were neutrophils (data not shown). In other words, this is the reason why some patients with severe gastric ulcers suffer from dysfunction of several organs, including the liver. These results suggest that severe stressors have the potential to induce granulocytosis and that such granulocytes may subsequently induce multiple tissue (mucosal) damage if over-activated.

As to the question of how the restraint stress induces granulocytosis in various organs, we consider that adrenergic receptors (α and β types) of granulocytes (5, 17, 20, 28, 39) are key factors. Namely, stressors first induce sympathetic nerve strain and then such sympathetic nerve stimuli may activate granulocytes in the bone marrow and thereafter in the periphery. In addition to the stress, other sympathetic nerve stimuli such as exercise, overwork, and administration of adrenaline itself are known to induce granulocytosis (9, 13, 18, 19, 23, 25, 29). This speculation also seems to be rea-

B

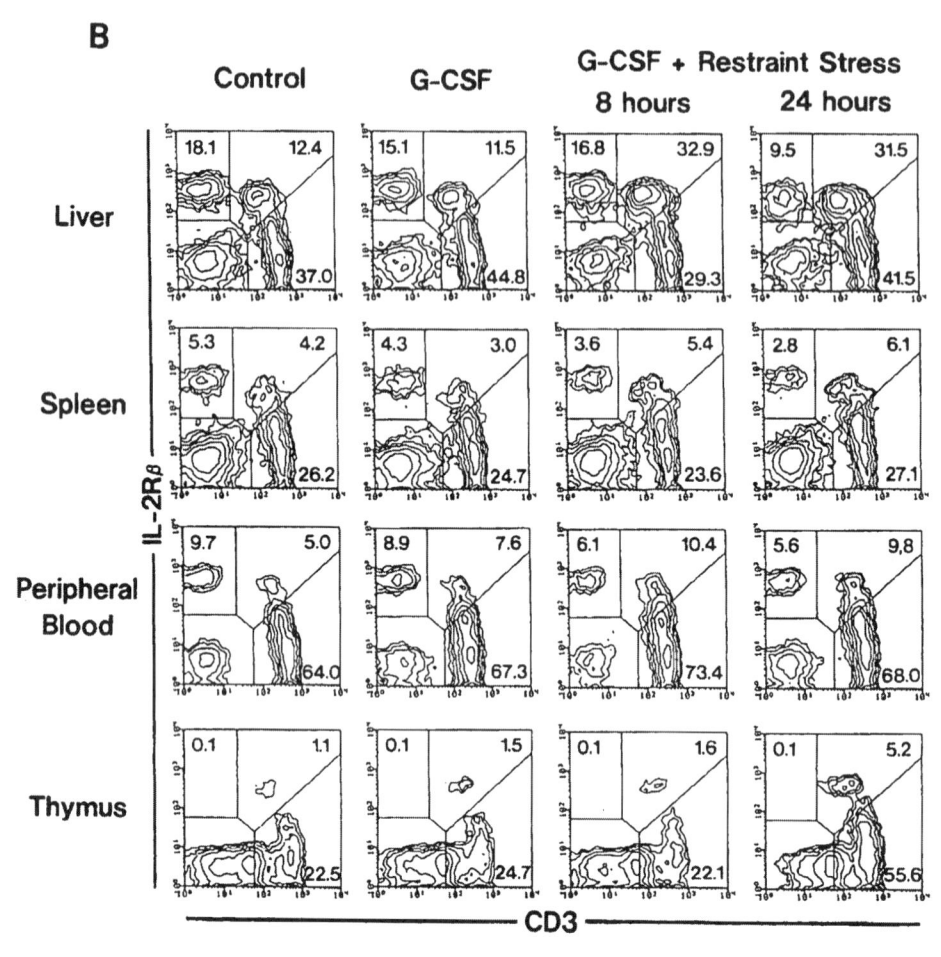

Fig. 8B

sonable, because extrathymic T cells are lymphocytes which carry a high density of adrenergic receptors on the surface (our unpublished observation). In this study, it was found that CD3^{int}IL-2Rβ^+ extrathymic T cells were efficiently augmented in number and proportion by restraint stress as well.

When restraint stress continued for more than 30 h, some mice died of multi-organ failure. It is speculated that over-activated granulocytes exerted tissue damage, mediated by the over-production of free radicals, superoxides, and other cytoplasmic enzymes. There is a possibility that the underlying differences between gastric ulcers, liver dysfunction, and multi-organ failure are due to the magnitudes of the stress, sympathetic nerve strain, and subsequent granulocytosis.

The induction of CD3^{int}IL-2Rβ^+ extrathymic T cells which parallels that of granulocytes by restraint stress is noteworthy. Extrathymic T cells were previously found to contain self-reactive forbidden clones as estimated by anti-Vβ mAbs in conjunction with the Mls system, and eventually killed not only syngeneic tumor cells but also rapidly proliferating self-cells (e.g., thymocytes, hepatocytes, and enterocytes) (1, 14, 27, 35). This result reminds us that cells infiltrating the joint of patients with rheumatoid arthritis are composed of granulocytes (80%) and CD57$^+$ T cells (15%), i.e., a human counterpart of extrathymic T cells (11, 26,

37). It is speculated that some tissues are destroyed by granulocytes then become a target for extrathymic T cells with self-reactivity.

Many investigators hypothesize that there is a marginal pool of granulocytes in some organ (6), because the response of granulocytes (i.e., granulocytosis seen in the periphery) is extremely quick. In this study, granulocytosis was seen in the blood as early as 8 h after the initiation of restraint stress. However, neither we nor other investigators have been able to determine such an organ, although we recently revealed that the bone marrow itself is a marginal pool. As shown in the Fig. 3A, it is obvious that the liver and spleen are not marginal pools. The life-span of granulocytes is very short (2 to 3 days). For example, under non-emergency states, 30 to 50% of granulocytes should be replaced by a new population. In this regard, the bone marrow itself has a great potential to produce a large number of granulocytes within a short time.

Histological examination did not reveal many granulocytes in the stomach of mice exposed to restraint stress (data not shown). However, a few granulocytes in the stomach were detected by flow cytometry. There is a possibility that granulocytes work within the vessels (2, 33) and, therefore, vessel dilatation and bleeding are first induced by stress. On the other hand, chronic stimuli of stress seem to induce the infiltration of granulocytes into the mucosal tissue of the stomach, as shown in the preparation of the resected stomach from patients with gastric ulcers. The histology of the fatty liver in mice exposed to resistant stress was also very interesting. We recently proposed the possibility that the formation of fatty liver is a major sign for severe stress (manuscript submitted for publication).

Since a large amount of anti-granulocyte mAb is available in rats (15, 30), we conducted an elimination experiment of granulocytes using this animal. The suppressive effect on the formation of gastric ulcers was striking after the elimination. In conjunction with a result from the pretreatment with G-CSF, granulocytes were found to be directly associated with ulcer formation. It is known that bacterial infection increases the level of granulocytes locally and in the body in general, and that bacteria and its components efficiently activate the function of granulocytes (10, 34, 36, 40). Taken together, it can be understood that *H. pylori* might be an important candidate for such stimuli. However, the present results showed that the background or basal conditions in humans and animals such as sympathetic nerve strain might also be important in the formation of gastric ulcers and the occurrence of other tissue damage.

Received 18 September 1997; and accepted 1 October 1997

REFERENCES

1. ARASE H., ARASE N., OGASAWARA K., GOOD R. A. and ONOE K. (1992) An $NK1.1^+CD4^+8^-$ single-positive thymocyte subpopulation that expresses a highly skewed T-cell antigen receptor $V\beta$ family. *Proc. Natl. Acad. Sci. USA* **89**, 6506–6510
2. ASAKO H., KUBES P., WALLACE J., GAGINELLA T., WOLF R. E. and GRANGER D. N. (1992) Indomethacin-induced leukocyte adhesion in mesenteric venules: role of lipoxygenase products. *Amer. J. Physiol.* **262**, G903–908
3. AXON A. T. (1993) *Helicobacter pylori* infection. *J. Antimicrob. Chemother.* **32**, Suppl., 61–68
4. BLASER M. J. (1990) *Helicobacter pylori* and the pathogenesis of gastroduodenal inflammation. *J. Infect. Dis.* **161**, 626–633
5. EDWARDS A. J., BACON T. H., ELMS C. A., VERARDI R., FELDER M. and KNIGHT S. C. (1984) Changes in the populations of lymphoid cells in human peripheral blood following physical exercise. *Clin. Exp. Immunol.* **58**, 420–427
6. FUKUDA M., MORODA T., TOYABE S., IIAI T., KAWACHI Y., TAKAHASHI-IWANAGA H., IWANAGA T., OKADA M. and ABO T. (1996) Granulocytosis induced by increasing sympathetic nerve activity contributes to the incidence of acute appendicitis. *Biomedical Res.* **17**, 171–181
7. FUKUDA Y., YAMAMOTO I., OKUI M., TONOKATSU Y. and SHIMOYAMA T. (1995) Combination therapies with a proton pump inhibitor for *Helicobacter pylori*-infected gastric ulcer patients. *J. Clin. Gastroenterol.* **20**, Suppl. 2, S132–135
8. GOOSSENS P. L., JOUIN H., MARCHAL G. and MILON G. (1990) Isolation and flow cytometric analysis of the free lymphomyeloid cells present in murine liver. *J. Immunol. Methods* **132**, 137–144
9. GRASSI G. M., SOMERS V. K., RENK W. S., ABBOUD F. M. and MARK A. L. (1989) Effects of alcohol intake on blood pressure and sympathetic nerve activity in normotensive humans: a preliminary report. *J. Hypertension* **7**, Suppl. 6, S20–21
10. HAN B.-G., KIM H.-S., RHEE K.-H., HAN H.-S. and CHUNG M.-H. (1995) Effects of rebamipide on gastric cell damage by *Helicobacter pylori*-stimulated human neutrophils. *Pharmacol. Res.* **32**, 201–207
11. HASHIMOTO S., TAKII Y., IIAI T., TSUCHIDA M., WATANABE H., SHINADA S., SHIBATA A. and ABO T. (1995) Characterization of $CD56^+$ T cells in humans: Their abundance in the liver and similarity to extrathymic T cells in mice. *Biomedical Res.* **16**, 1–9
12. IIAI T., WATANABE H., SEKI S., SUGIURA K., HIROKAWA K., UTSUYAMA M., TAKAHASHI-IWANAGA H., IWANAGA T., OHTEKI T. and ABO T. (1992) Ontogeny and development of extrathymic T cells in mouse liver. *Immunology* **77**, 556–563
13. IRELAND M. A., VANDONGEN R., DAVIDSON L., BEILIN L. J. and ROUSE I. L. (1984) Acute effects of moderate alcohol consumption on blood pressure and plasma catecholamines. *Clin. Sci.* **66**, 643–648

14. KAWACHI Y., WATANABE H., MORODA T., HAGA M., IIAI T., HATAKEYAMA K. and ABO T. (1995) Self-reactive T cell clones in a restricted population of IL-2 receptor β^+ cells expressing intermediate levels of the T cell receptor in the liver and other immune organs. *Eur. J. Immunol.* **25**, 2272-2278
15. KUDO C., YAMASHITA T., ARAKI A., TERASHITA M., WATANABE T., ATSUMI M., TAMURA M. and SENDO F. (1993) Modulation of *in vivo* immune response by selective depletion of neutrophils using a monoclonal antibody, RP-3. I. Inhibition by RP-3 treatment of the priming and effector phases of delayed type hypersensitivity to sheep red blood cells in rats. *J. Immunol.* **150**, 3728-3738
16. LABENZ J. and BORSCH G. (1994) Evidence for the essential role of *Helicobacter pylori* in gastric ulcer desease. *Gut* **35**, 19-22
17. LANDMANN R. M. A., MÜLLER F. B., PERINI C. H., WESP M., ERNE P. and BÜHLER E. R. (1984) Changes of immunoregulatory cells induced by psychological and physical stress: relationship to plasma catecholamines. *Clin. Exp. Immunol.* **58**, 127-135
18. MAIN J. and THOMAS T. (1990) Ethanol predominantly alters sodium influx in human leukocytes. *Clin. Sci.* **78**, 235-238
19. MAISEL A. S., HARRIS T., REARDEN C. A. and MICHEL M. C. (1990) β-Adrenergic receptors in lymphocyte subsets after exercise. Alterations in normal individuals and patients with congestive heart failure. *Circulation* **82**, 2003-2010
20. MAISEL A. S., KNOWLTON K. U., FOWLER P., REARDEN A., ZIEGLER M. G., MOTULSKY H. J., INSEL P. A. and MICHEL M. C. (1990) Adrenergic control of circulating lymphocyte subpopulations. Effect of congestive heart failure, dynamic exercise, and terbutaline treatment. *J. Clin. Invest.* **85**, 462-467
21. MCGUIGAN J. E. (1987) Peptic Ulcer. In *Harrison's Principles of Internal Medicine* (ed. MCGUIGAN J. E., BRAUNWALD E., ISSELFACHER K. J., PETERSDORF R. G., WILSON J. D., MARTIN J. B. and FAUCI A. S.) McGraw-Hill Book Company, New York, pp. 1239-1241
22. MILNE R., LOGAN R. P., HARWOOD D., MISIEWICZ J. J. and FORMAN D. (1995) *Helicobacter pylori* and upper gastrointestinal disease: a survey of gastroenterologists in the United Kingdom. *Gut* **37**, 314-318
23. MURRAY D. R., IRWIN M., REARDEN C. A., ZIEGLER M., MOTULSKY H. and MAISEL A. S. (1992) Sympathetic and immune interactions during dynamic exercise. Mediation via a β_2-adrenergic-dependent mechanism. *Circulation* **86**, 203-213
24. O'CONNOR H. J. (1994) The role of *Helicobacter pylori* in peptic ulcer disease. *Scand. J. Gastroenterol.* **201**, 11-15
25. OGAWA M., IIAI T., HIRAHARA H., TOMIYAMA K., KAWACHI Y., WATANABE H., SHIMOZI T. and ABO T. (1993) Immunologic states induced by starvation: Suppression of intrathymic T-cell differentiation but relative resistance of extrathymic T-cell differentiation. *Acta Med. Biol.* **41**, 177-187
26. OKADA T., IIAI T., KAWACHI Y., MORODA T., TAKII Y., HATAKEYAMA K. and ABO T. (1995) Origin of CD57$^+$ T cells which increase at tumor sites in patients with colorectal cancer. *Clin. Exp. Immunol.* **102**, 159-166
27. OSMAN Y., WATANABE T., KAWACHI Y., SATO K., OHTSUKA K., WATANABE H., HASHIMOTO S., MORIYAMA Y., SHIBATA A. and ABO T. (1995) Intermediate TCR cells with self-reactive clones are effector cells which induce syngeneic graft-versus-host disease in mice. *Cell. Immunol.* **166**, 172-186
28. RATGE D., WIEDEMANN A., KOHSE K. P. and WISSER H. (1988) Alterations of β-adrenoceptors on human leukocyte subsets induced by dynamic exercise: effect of prednisone. *Clin. Exp. Pharmacol. Physiol.* **15**, 43-54
29. SCHEDLOWSKI M., HOSCH W., OBERBECK R., BENSCHOP R. J., JACOBS R., RAAB H.-R. and SCHMIDT R. E. (1996) Catecholamines modulate human NK cell circulation and function via spleen-independent β_2-adrenergic mechanisms. *J. Immunol.* **156**, 93-99
30. SEKIYA S., GOTOH S., YAMASHITA T., WATANABE T., SAITOH S. and SENDO F. (1989) Selective depletion of rat neutrophils by *in vivo* administration of a monoclonal antibody. *J. Leukocyte Biol.* **46**, 96-102
31. SUGIYAMA T., HISANO K., OCHIAI T., FUJITA N., KOBAYASHI T., YABANA T., KUROKAWA I. and YACHI A. (1995) Lansoprazole versus lansoprazole plus amoxicillin treatment for eradication of *Helicobacter pylori* in patients with gastric ulcer. *J. Clin. Gastroenterol.* **20**, Suppl. 2, S104-106
32. SUNG J. J. Y., CHUNG S. C. S., LING T. K. W., YUNG M. Y., LEUNG V. K. S., NG E. K. W., LI M. K. K., CHENG A. F. B., and LI A. K. C. (1995) Antibacterial treatment of gastric ulcers associated with *Helicobacter pylori*. *N. Engl. J. Med.* **332**, 139-142
33. SUZUKI M., ASAKO H., KUBES P., JENNINGS S., CRISHAM M. B. and GRANGER D. N. (1991) Neutrophil-derived oxidants promote leukocyte adherence in postcapillary venules. *Microvascular Res.* **42**, 125-138
34. SUZUKI M., MIURA S., MORI M., KAI A., SUZUKI H., FUKUMURA D., SUEMATSU M. and TSUCHIYA M. (1994) Rebamipide, a novel antiulcer agent, attenuates *Helicobacter pylori* induced gastric mucosal cell injury associated with neutrophil derived oxidants. *Gut* **35**, 1375-1378
35. TAKAHASHI-IWANAGA H., IWANAGA T., SAKAMOTO Y. and FUJITA T. (1995) Ultrastructural and time-lapse observations of intraepithelial lymphocytes in the small intestine of the guinea pig: their possible role in the removal of effete enterocytes. *Cell Tissue Res.* **280**, 491-497
36. TAKEDA Y., WATANABE H., YONEHARA S., YAMASHITA T., SAITO S. and SENDO F. (1993) Rapid acceleration of neutrophil apoptosis by tumor necrosis factor-α. *Int. Immunol.* **5**, 691-694
37. TAKII Y., HASHIMOTO S., IIAI T., WATANABE H., HATAKEYAMA K. and ABO T. (1994) Increase in the proportion of granulated CD56$^+$ T cells in patients with malignancy. *Clin. Exp. Immunol.* **97**, 522-527
38. TANAKA T., TSUDO M., KARASUYAMA H., KITAMURA F., KONO T., HATAKEYAMA M., TANIGUCHI T. and MIYASAKA M. (1991) A novel monoclonal antibody against murine IL-2 receptor β-chain. Characterization of receptor expression in normal lymphoid cells and EL-4 cells. *J. Immunol.* **147**, 2222-2228
39. VAN TITS L. J. H., MICHEL M. C., GROSSE-WILDE H., HAPPEL M., ETGLER F.-W., SOLIMAN A. and BRODDE O.-E. (1990) Catecholamines increase lymphocyte β_2-adrenergic receptors via a β_2-adrenergic, spleen-dependent process. *Amer. J. Physiol.* **258**, E191-202
40. YUO A., KITAGAWA S., SUZUKI I., URABE A., OKABE T., SAITO M. and TAKAKU F. (1989) Tumor necrosis factor as an activator of human granulocytes. Potentiation of the metabolisms triggered by the Ca^{2+}-mobilizing agonists. *J. Immunol.* **142**, 1678-1684

LOW LEVEL OF MIXING OF PARTNER CELLS SEEN IN EXTRATHYMIC T CELLS IN THE LIVER AND INTESTINE OF PARABIOTIC MICE: ITS BIIOLOGICAL IMPLICATION

並体結合マウスの肝臓と腸における
胸腺外分化Ｔ細胞の中にパートナー細胞の混合度は低い：
その生物学的意味

European Journal of Immunology, 28: 3719-3729, 1998

chapter 10

Low level of mixing of partner cells seen in extrathymic T cells in the liver and intestine of parabiotic mice:its biiological implication

並体結合マウスの肝臓と腸における胸腺外分化T細胞の中にパートナー細胞の混合度は低い：その生物学的意味

Susumu Suzuki[1], Satoshi Sugahara[1], Takao Shimizu[2], Takashi Tada[2], Masahiro Minagawa[2], Satoshi Maruyama[2], Hisami Watanabe[1], Hisashi Saito[3], Hiromichi Ishikawa[3], Katsuyoshi Hatakeyama[2] and Toru Abo[1]

[1] Department of Immunology, Niigata University School of Medicine, Niigata, Japan
[2] First Department of Surgery, Niigata University School of Medicine, Niigata, Japan
[3] Department of Microbiology, Keio University School of Medicine, Tiokyo, Japan

【キーワード】

c-kit$^+$幹細胞／胸腺外分化T細胞／NK細胞／並体結合（パラビオーシス）／消化管

【要約】

近年、c-kit$^+$幹細胞が、成体マウスの肝臓と腸内で発見された。この幹細胞が肝臓や腸内で胸腺外分化T細胞を供給するか検証した。そこで、血液循環を共有するB6.Ly5.1とB6.Ly5.2の並体結合マウスを用いた。リンパ球が産生される場所を、抗Ly5.1と抗Ly5.2モノクローナル抗体を用いたフローサイトメトリー解析で確認した。末梢血、脾臓、リンパ節と肝臓におけるリンパ球は、結合14日後までは、B6.Ly5.1マウスでもB6.Ly5.2マウスでも、Ly5.1$^+$細胞とLy5.2$^+$細胞は同じ比率で混和していた。しかし、結合14日以降、肝臓と腸における胸腺外分化T細胞（NKT細胞）の混和の程度は減少した。胸腺T細胞でも同様の現象が見られた。浮遊細胞を用いたフローサイトメトリーの結果を、免疫組織化学染色のデータで確認することができた。本研究の結果より、肝臓と腸における胸腺外分化T細胞は、自身の前駆細胞（おそらく自身の幹細胞）から産生されている可能性が高まった。今、一つ重要な発見は、さまざまな部位において、個体におけるリンパ球サブセットの構成パターンが、そのパートナーのものと酷似していたことである。この結果は、特定のパートナー細胞だけが、個体の特定部位に移動することを意味すると解釈できる。

1.はじめに

近年、c-kit$^+$幹細胞が、マウスとヒトの肝臓と腸（胸腺外分化T細胞産生部位）に存在することが明らかになった［1-4］。マウスの肝臓と腸の胸腺外分化T細胞には、同じ特性を共有するだけでなく、顕著に異なる特性もある。すなわち、肝臓の胸腺外分化T細胞は、主にダブルネガティブ（DN）（CD4$^-$CD8$^-$）またはシングルポジティブ（CD4$^+$またはCD8$^+$）のいずれかを持つαβT細胞から構成される［5-8］。それに対して、腸の胸腺外分化T細胞は、ダブルポジティブ（DP）CD4$^+$8$^+$フェノタイプを持つγδT細胞とかなりの比率のαβT細胞から構成される［9-12］。この2種類のT細胞サブセットは、ある時点から分岐して系統発生的に進化

略語：DN：ダブル・ネガティブ　DP：ダブル・ポジティブ　IEL：上皮内リンパ球　LPL：粘膜固有層リンパ球　int：中等度

した可能性がある。この概念は、肝臓が胆汁を分泌するため腸が突起したものから進化したという事実に基づくものである［13, 14］。最近の研究において、c-kit$^+$ Lin$^-$ 細胞が、肝臓と腸から分離されたが、この細胞は、最終的には、それぞれ腸と肝臓において胸腺外分化T細胞を産生する能力を獲得した［2, 15, 16］。その他に明らかになったのは、肝臓の中のc-kit$^+$ Lin$^-$ 細胞は多能性であり（つまり、リンパ球だけでなく赤血球や骨髄細胞にも分化できる）、その一方、小腸と虫垂のそれらはより分化している前駆細胞（つまり、赤血球や骨髄細胞でなく必ずリンパ球様細胞になる）である。しかし、この幹細胞は骨髄由来であるのか、また、この胸腺外分化T細胞は、血液循環を通じて他の部位に移動するのであろうか、という疑問が残る。この問題を検証するべく、B6.Ly5.1マウスとB6.Ly5.2マウスとの並体結合を行なった［17-19］。リンパ球を混合させた後に、抗Ly5.1と抗Ly5.2モノクロナール抗体を用いて、リンパ球の由来をフローサイトメトリーで解析した。

2. 結果

2.1 幹細胞が腸において胸腺細胞と上皮内リンパ球を産生する

8週齢のマウス（B6.L1y5.1およびB6.Ly5.2）を用いて並体結合を行なった。細胞の起源を検証するためビオチン化した抗Ly5.1と抗L1y5.2モノクロナール抗体を用いた。並体結合3日後より、Ly5.2マウスの各臓器においてLy5.1$^+$ 細胞が出現した（Fig. 1A）。パートナーの細胞は3日後より出現し、14日後に末梢血、リンパ節、脾臓と肝臓において安定期（プラトー）に達した。この理由は、これら臓器に見られるリンパ球の起源は、骨髄（B細胞）と胸腺（T細胞）だからである。全く対照的に、胸腺においてパートナーの細胞（＜3.0％）は42日後まで

Figure.1

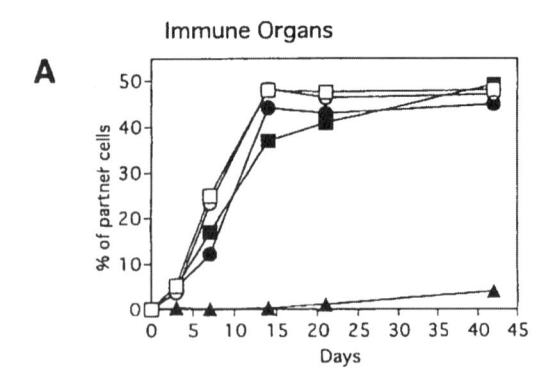

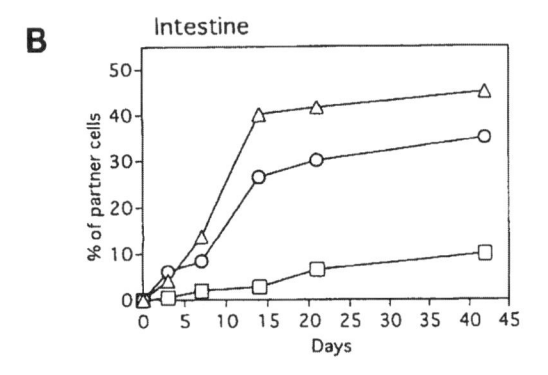

A Immune Organs

B Intestine

並体結合後の各個体マウスへのパートナー細胞の混入。(A)（■, 肝臓；●, 脾臓；▲, 胸腺；○, リンパ節；□, 末梢血）、(B) 腸の各部位（(□, IEL；○, LPL；△, パイエル板）。8週齢マウス（B6.Ly5.1およびB6.Ly5.2）を並体結合した。各時点において各免疫臓器と腸の各部位から細胞を採取した（各時点n=5）。Ly5.1マウスの場合、ビオチン化抗Ly5.2モノクロナール抗体でパートナー細胞との混入を確認した（Ly5.2マウスは抗Ly5.1モノクロナール抗体で確認）。

出現しなかった。推察されるのは、胸腺細胞の起源は、胸腺にもとから存在した胸腺の幹細胞であることである。成獣期（少なくとも本実験期間中）には、骨髄胸腺へ幹細胞が供給されない可能性がある。Ly5.1マウスの並体結合を行なっても、結果は同じであった（未発表データ）。性質が異なる腸内リンパ球を3箇所（上皮内部、粘膜固有層およびパイエル板）から採取することができた、そしてそれら細胞を分離して、特徴を検証した（Fig. 1B）。パイエル板のリンパ球は、パートナーの細胞とかなり混和し

Figure.2

A

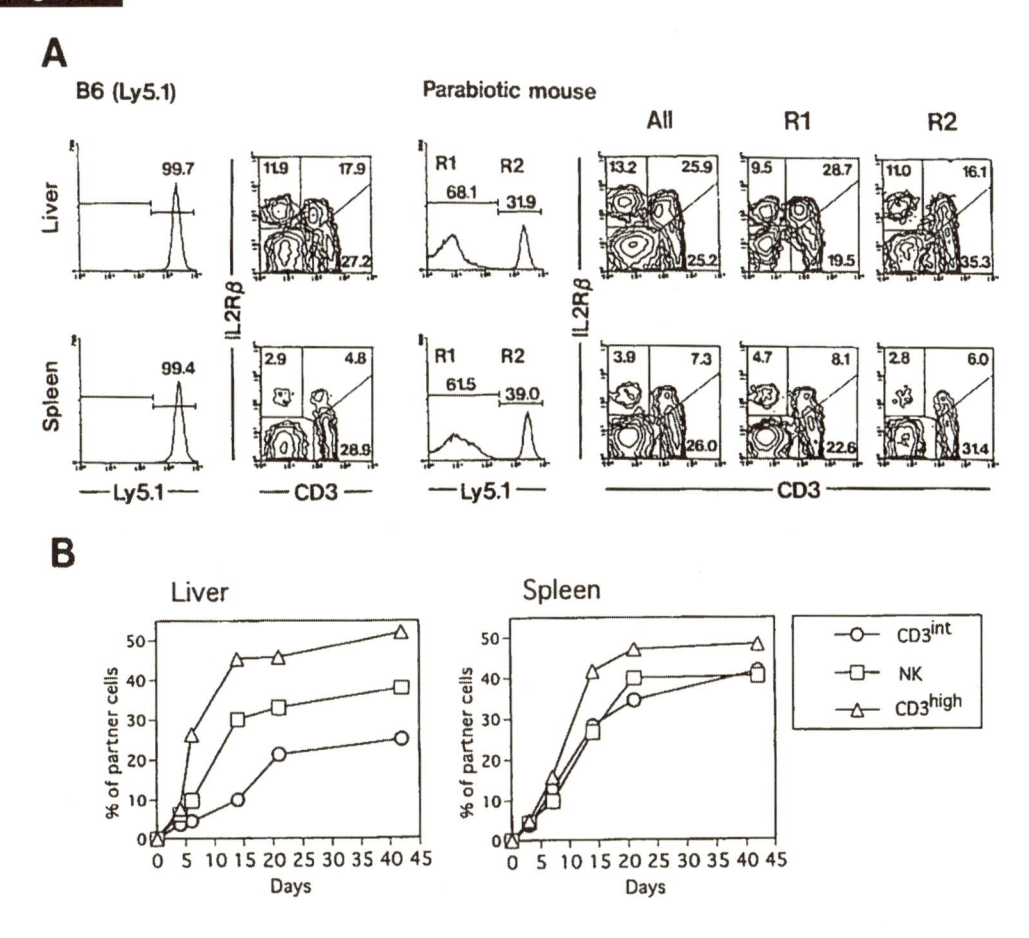

B6 (Ly5.1) / Parabiotic mouse

Liver / Spleen panels with axes Ly5.1, CD3, IL2Rβ. Values shown: Liver — 99.7; 11.9, 17.9, 27.2; R1 68.1, R2 31.9; All 13.2, 25.9, 25.8; R1 9.5, 28.7, 19.5; R2 11.0, 16.1, 35.3. Spleen — 99.4; 2.9, 4.8, 28.9; R1 61.5, R2 39.0; All 3.9, 7.3, 26.0; R1 4.7, 8.1, 22.6; R2 2.8, 6.0, 31.4.

B

Liver and Spleen graphs: % of partner cells vs Days (0–45). Series: ○ CD3^{int}, □ NK, △ CD3^{high}.

並体結合後、肝臓と脾臓の特定のリンパ球サブセットにパートナー細胞が混入する。(A) Ly5.2並体結合マウス (14日後) の三重染色 (CD3, IL-2Rβおよび Ly5.1)。(B) 肝臓と脾臓に存在する各リンパ球サブセット中のパートナー細胞の比率の経時的変化。各時点における細胞を採取し、三重染色を行なった。ゲーティングを行い、Ly5.2並体結合マウスにおける各リンパ球サブセット中の Ly5.1$^+$細胞の比率を測定した。経時的変化は、5匹の並体結合マウスの平均値を示す。

た (14日後40%) が、上皮内のリンパ球 (IEL) は、あまり混和しなかった (42日後7%)。粘膜固有層 (LPL) のリンパ球は、その中間であった (14日後26%) を示した。

2.2 自身の幹細胞から肝臓の NKT細胞が産生される

肝臓と脾臓におけるリンパ球サブセットの特徴を検証する実験を行なった (Fig. 2A)。正常マウス (B6.Ly5.1) の肝臓と脾臓におけるCD3$^-$IL-2Rβ$^+$NK細胞、CD3^{int}IL-2Rβ$^+$細胞 (胸腺外分3720化CD3^{int}細胞) およびCD3^{high}IL$^-$2Rβ$^-$細胞 (胸腺由来のCD3^{high}細胞) を同定した。肝臓において、NK細胞とCD3^{int}細胞が豊富であった。並体結合したLy5.2マウス (14日後) の脾臓と肝臓において見られたパートナーの細胞は、肝臓は31.9%、脾臓は39.0%であった。CD3、IL-2RβおよびLy5.1の三重染色を行い [2]、全体 (R1 +R2)、R1 (Ly5.1$^-$) とR2 (Ly.5.1$^+$) の染色パターンを比較した。染色パターンには違いがあり、特に肝臓におけるR1とR2とが異なっていた。つまり、R2におけるCD3^{int}細胞の比率はR1のものより少なかった。

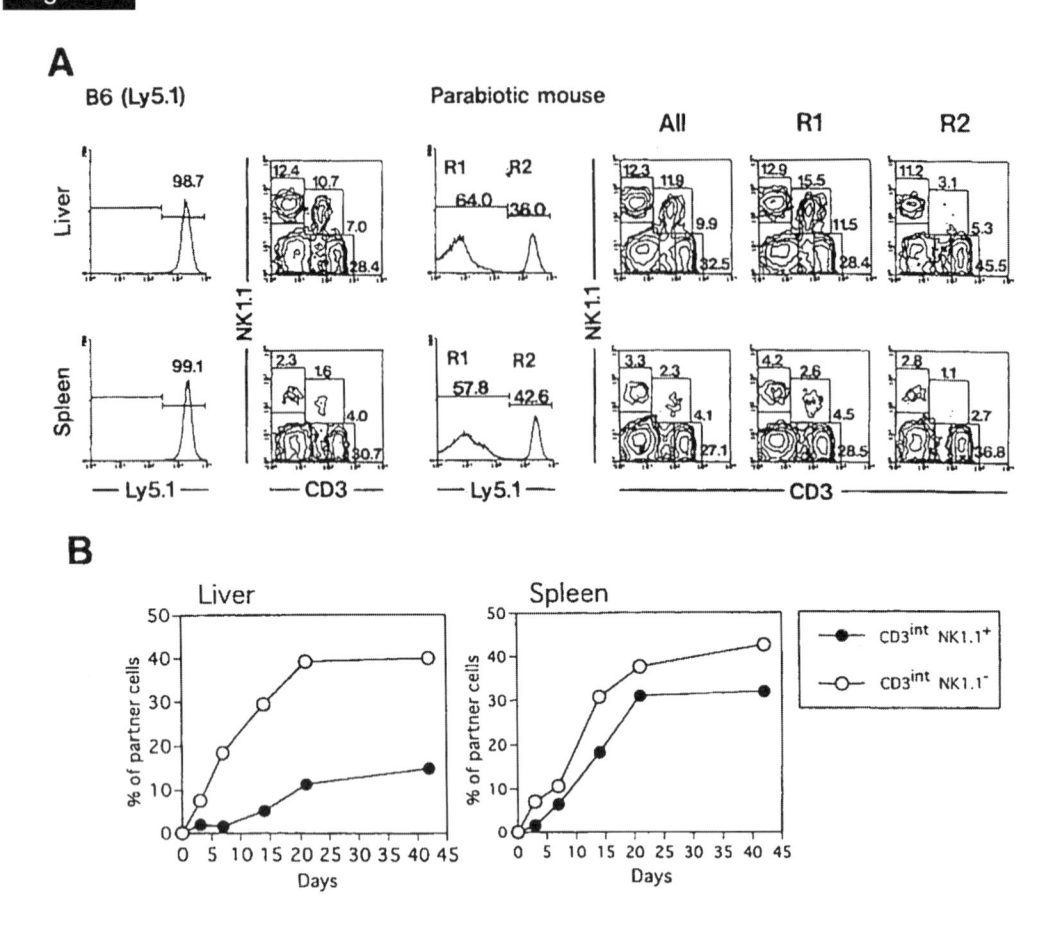

Figure.3

並体結合マウス肝臓の中にあるNK1.1⁺CD3^int細胞へパートナー細胞は混入困難である。(A) 並体結合マウス (14日後) の三重染色 (CD3, NK1.1およびLy5.1)。(B) 肝臓と脾臓に存在するNK1.1⁺CD3^int細胞の比率の経時的変化。各時点における細胞を採取し、三重染色を行なった。ゲーティングを行い、Ly5.2並体結合マウスにおける各リンパ球サブセット中のLy5.1⁺細胞の比率を測定した。経時的変化は、5匹の並体結合マウスの平均値を示す。

この点について、さまざまなリンパ球サブセットの構成の動態を検証した (Fig. 2B)。肝臓では、異なる混和パターンが見られた (CD3^high細胞>NK細胞>CD^int細胞)。この結果が示唆するのは、CD3^int細胞には肝臓で産生されるものもあるが、他の臓器で産生されるCD3^int細胞もあることである。同様の傾向が肝臓のNK細胞、脾臓のNK細胞とCD3^int細胞に見られた (脾臓は混和の程度がより低かった)。

以前、肝臓におけるCD3^intの約60%は、NK1.1⁺ (NKT細胞) であると報告した [81]。

それ故、NKT細胞に着目した (Fig. 3A)。正常マウス (B6.L1y5.1) のNK1.1⁺CD3^int細胞は、肝臓では多いが、脾臓ではそれほど多くはなかった。並体結合を行なったマウスにおいてもそうであった (全体R1+R2参照)。一方、肝臓でも脾臓でも、R1とR2の染色パターンに大きな相違が見られた。NK1.1⁺CD3^int細胞は、R1では多かったが、R2ではごく僅かだった。経時的変化を示す (Fig 3B)。肝臓におけるNK1.1⁺CD3^int細胞の混和の程度は低かった。同様の傾向が、脾臓におけるNK1.1⁺CD3^int細胞

Figure.4

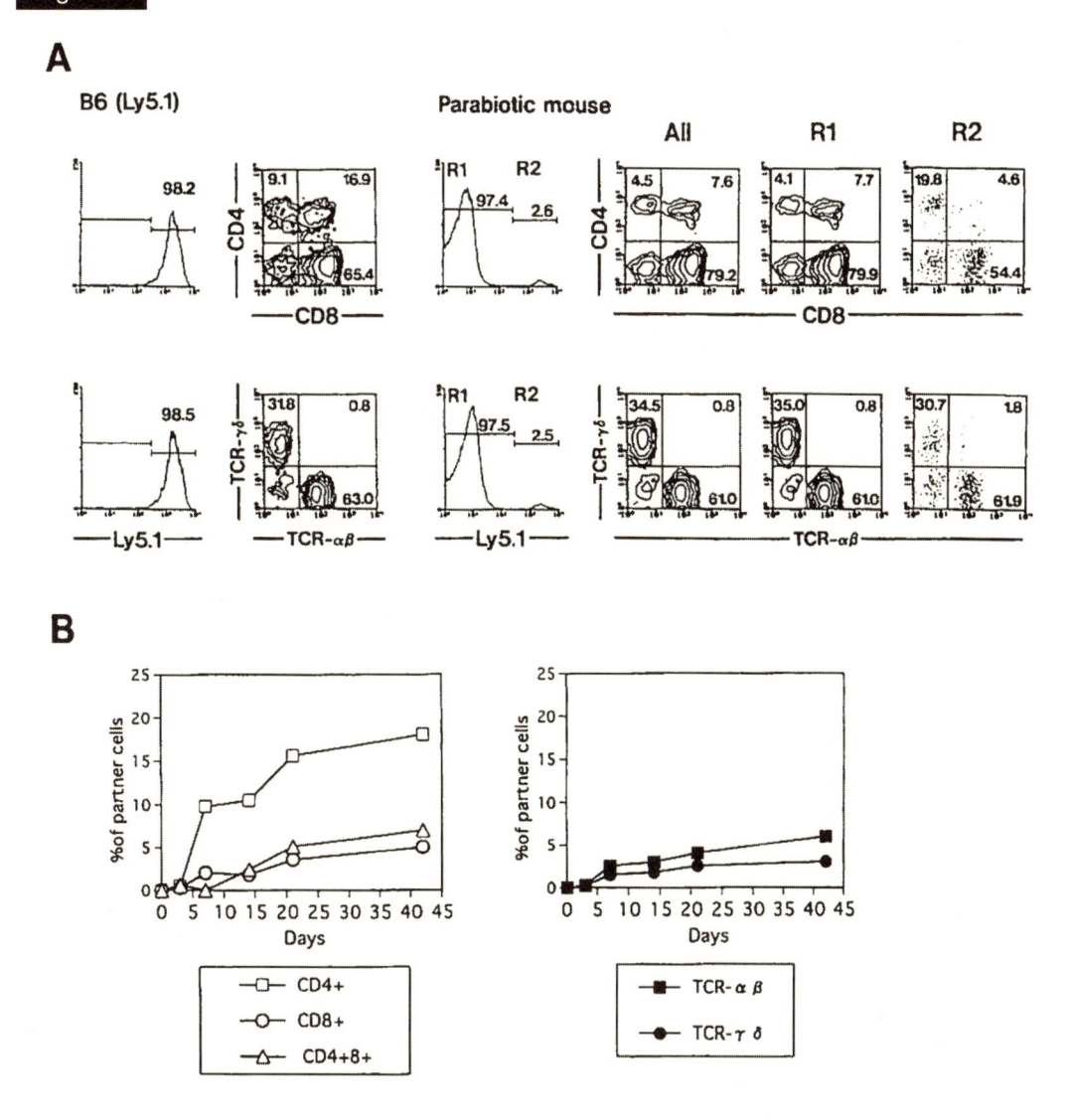

A

B6 (Ly5.1) / Parabiotic mouse / All / R1 / R2

B

並体結合マウスの腸に存在するIELの各リンパ球サブセットのうち、CD4⁺ IELサブセットのみにパートナー細胞が混入した。(A) 並体結合マウス（Ly5.2）（14日後）の三重染色（CD4, CD8およびLy5.1そしてTCR$\alpha\beta$, TCR$\gamma\delta$およびLy5.1）(B) 腸に存在するIELの各リンパ球サブセットにおけるパートナー細胞の比率の経時的変化。各時点における細胞を採取し、三重染色を行なった。ゲーティングを行い、Ly5.2並体結合マウスにおける各リンパ球サブセット中のLy5.1⁺細胞の比率を測定した。経時的変化は、5匹の並体結合マウスの平均値を示す。

で見られたが、混和の程度はより高かった。

2.3 腸におけるT細胞の更なる特徴

本研究において、腸におけるIELの更なる特徴の検証を行なった（Fig. 4A）。正常マウスB6.Ly5.1および並体結合したマウスB6.Ly5.2を用いて、IELの三重染色（CD4, CD8とLy5.1およびTCR$\alpha\beta$, TCR$\gamma\delta$とLy5.1）を行なった。正常マウスでは、IELにおいて、CD8⁺細胞はCD4⁺細胞より顕著に多かった。IEL独特の現象として、DP CD4⁺8⁺細胞が存在した。TCR$\alpha\beta$⁺細胞とTCR$\gamma\delta$⁺細胞の比率は、2：1であった。並体結合14日後のマウスにおいて

214

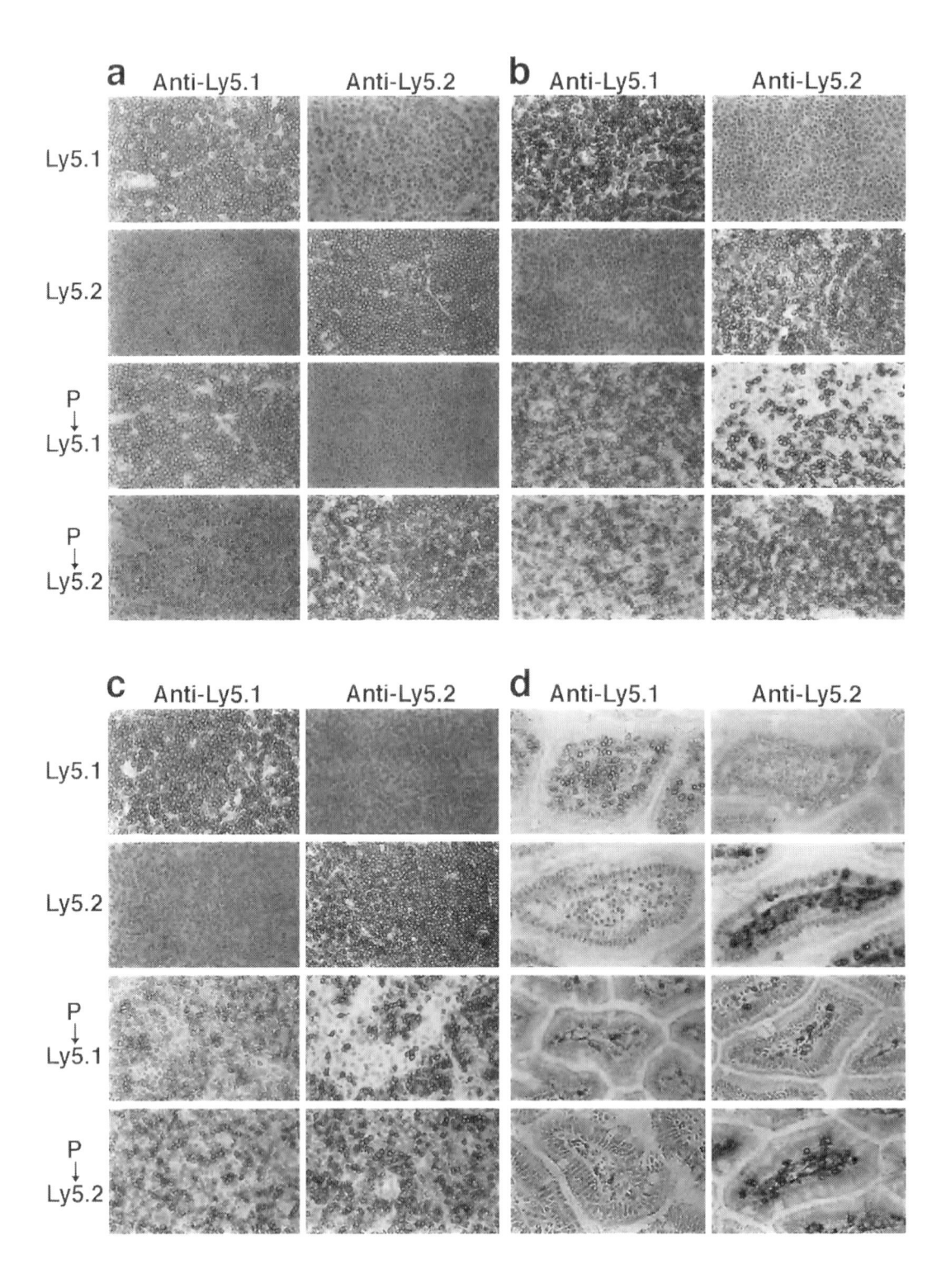

Figure.5

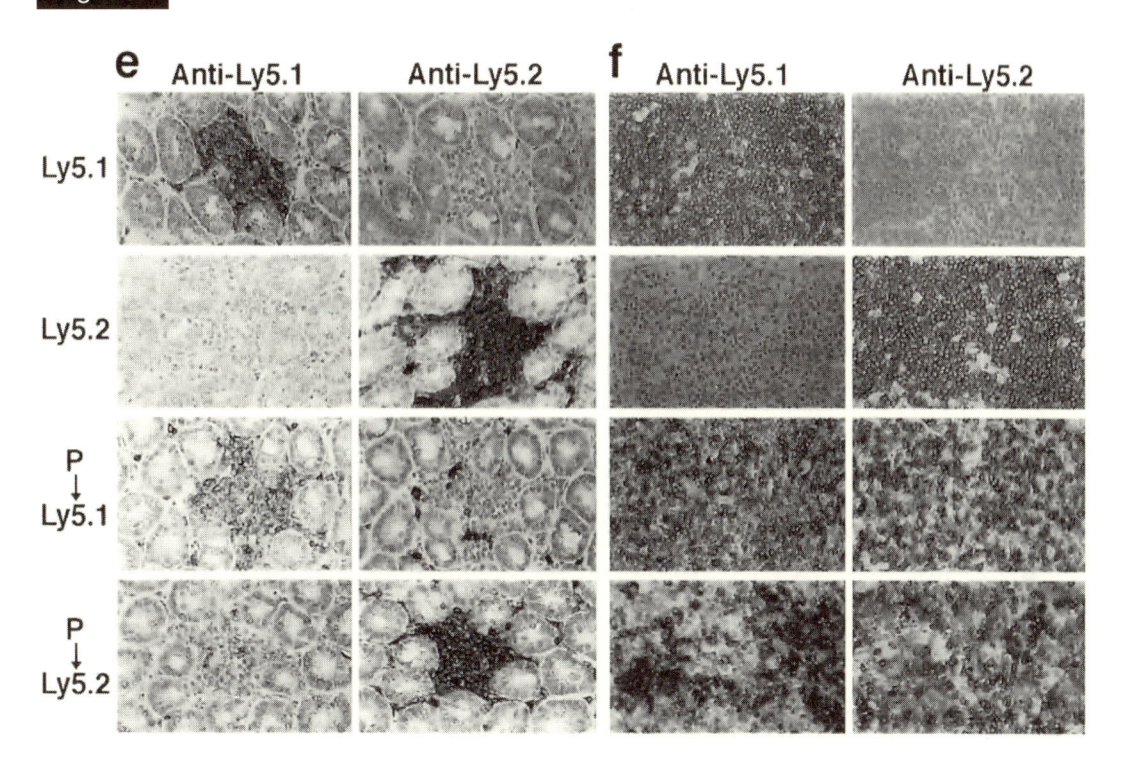

並体結合マウスにおけるLy5.1⁺とLy5.2⁺細胞の免疫組織化学的染色：胸腺（a）、脾臓（b）、リンパ節（c）、腸絨毛（d）、腸クリプトパッチ（e）および腸のパイエル板（f）（x400）。並体結合（P）Ly5.1とLy5.2マウスから標本採取を行い検証した（並体結合35日後）。それぞれの個体の中にパートナー細胞がどの程度諸器官に混入したか測定した。上段は、すべてLy5.1およびLy5.2マウス（並体結合ではないマウス）のコントロール染色である。

パートナーの細胞は極めて少なかった（< 3.0%）。そして全分画（R1＋R2）、R1分画とR2分画を比較した。R1とR2では、CD4⁺細胞における染色パターンに相違が見られた。IELの経時的変化を示す（Fig. 4B）。検証した全リンパ球サブセットの中で、パートナーの細胞はCD4⁺サブセットのみに見られた。しかし、比率はまだそれほど高くなかった（21日後15%）。この結果が示唆するのは、CD4⁺細胞の中には、胸腺外で産生されたものでないものが腸のIELの中にすら存在することである。

2.4 並体結合のマウスの組織の免疫組織化学染色

浮遊細胞を用いたフローサイトメトリー解析の結果を、並体結合のマウスの組織の免疫組織化学的染色を行い確認した（Fig. 5）。Ly5.1またはLy5.2マウスを用いて、Ly5.1またはLy5.2のコントロール染色を行なった（Fig. 5, 上）。並体結合実施35日後の並体結合マウス（Ly5.1とLy5.2）を用いた。胸腺では、抗Ly5.1モノクロナール抗体は、Ly5.1マウスの胸腺細胞だけを染色した；一方、抗Ly5.2モノクロナール抗体は、Ly5.2マウスの胸腺細胞だけを染色した。並体結合マウスでもこの通りであった。換言すると、並体結合したマウスの胸腺にはパートナー細胞は混和していなかった。

全く対照的に、並体結合したマウスの脾臓とリンパ節においてパートナー細胞はかなり混和していた。腸絨毛における結果は、大変興味深い：パートナーのリンパ球は、粘膜固有層でよく

混和したが、上皮内ではそうではなかった。そして、c-kit⁺幹細胞が特異的に存在すると知られているクリプトパッチに着目した [4]。クリプトパッチに混和したパートナー細胞は僅かであったが、リンパ球の大半は、この既存の前駆細胞に由来する。これが、並体結合で繋いだ両個体における結果である。最終実験では、パイエル板の検証を行なった。脾臓やリンパ節同様、どちらの個体のパイエル板にもパートナー細胞が多く混和していた。これらの結果の全ては、浮遊細胞を用いたフローサイトメトリー解析の結果と矛盾しない。肝臓のデータは提示しない。理由は、肝臓のほとんど肝細胞であり、染色をしてもあまり情報を得られなかったからである。

3. 考察

本研究では、並体結合マウス（B6.Ly5.1とB6.Ly5.2マウス）を用いて、各免疫臓器においてリンパ球サブセットがどのように産生されたか検証を行なった。局在するリンパ球またはリンパ球サブセットの中には、局所でその既存の前駆細胞から産生されるものがある可能性を示した。そのようなリンパ球の主なものには、肝臓のNKT細胞、腸のIELそして胸腺のT細胞がある。これらリンパ球の前駆細胞が、常に骨髄から供給されるのであるならば、本研究のような結果には至らなかっただろう。全く対照的に、並体結合14日後までに、末梢血、脾臓およびリンパ節における全リンパ球、そして肝臓と腸におけるいくつかのリンパ球サブセットでは、自分の細胞とパートナーの細胞の半々に混和していた。この部位にあるT細胞とB細胞はすべて、胸腺や骨髄で産生され、血液循環により常にそれぞれの部位に移動すると考えられる。パートナーの細胞が非常にゆるやかに混入した第3のリンパ球グループがあった。このリンパ球サブセットは、腸のLPLとCD4⁺ IEL細胞および肝臓のCD3^{int}細胞である。この部位のリンパ球には、胸腺由来のT細胞と局所で産生されるT細胞の二種類があると推測される。この結果を総合して考えると、特異的なリンパ球の中には、ある部位においてその場に局在する前駆細胞から産生されたものもあることが示唆される。胸腺外T細胞の寿命が非常に長いのであると（非常に成熟細胞を自己再生する能力が高い）、本結果は、必ずしもこの細胞が局在する前駆細胞から産生されたことを示すとは限らない。この問題は、非常に重要であるが、未だ解明されていない。しかし、肝臓と腸から採取したc-kit⁺幹細胞の実験結果から（腸と肝臓から分離したc-kit⁺Lin⁻細胞には、結局、幹細胞能があった [2, 15, 16]）、胸腺外分化T細胞の寿命が従来型T細胞より長いとは思えない。成熟細胞を自己再生する能力が遥かに高いとも思えない。しかし、この問題は、更に実験を深めて確認する必要がある。

本実験におけるもう一つの発見は、R2の比率（Ly5.1⁺細胞）の構成パターンが、いろいろな部位におけるR1の比率と酷似していたことであった。この結果は、特定の部位を目指す特定の細胞だけが、パートナー・マウスの特定の部位に移動することを意味すると解釈できる。

本研究は、c-kit⁺幹細胞が肝実質間隙（ディッセ腔）[2, 15] や腸のクリプトパッチ [4, 16] に存在するという近年の報告と矛盾しない。以前の研究において、正常マウス（B6.Ly5.1）の肝臓と骨髄から採取したc-kit⁺細胞を放射線照射（4Gy）したB6-SCIDマウス（Ly5.2）に移入した [2]。肝臓と骨髄から採取したc-kit⁺細胞を移入後、胸腺における全T細胞、肝臓における胸腺外T細胞そして骨髄における赤芽血糸と脊髄糸細胞が再構築された。本実験のプロトコルでは、通常は、骨髄のc-kit⁺細胞が、肝臓、腸または胸腺にさえ供給されることはない

可能性を明らかにした。同時に、正常マウス（Ly5.1）と放射線照射したマウス（Ly5.2）（1、3そして6Gy）を並体結合する実験を行なった。Ly5.2マウスに1Gyより強い放射線照射を行うと、Ly5.1$^+$ T細胞が、パートナー・マウスの胸腺（Ly5.2）に容易に見られた（未発表データ）。胸腺の幹細胞が損傷した場合、骨髄の幹細胞が胸腺の幹細胞と置き換わるという仮説は、実験結果から裏打ちされる。

以前、K.Hirokawaらの研究では[19]、同様の並体結合を用いた実験系で、パートナーの細胞がどこで産生されたかをThy1.1 and Thy1.2マーカーを組み合わせて検証した。しかし、Thy1抗原発現は、リンパ球集団の一部でしか確認できない。対照的に、多少のc-kit$^+$幹細胞以外は、Ly5抗原発現は、ほぼ全てのリンパ球集団で確認できる。この点については、本実験のプロトコルは、各免疫臓器における全てのリンパ球サブセット同定に役立つものである。さらに重要なことに、当時、胸腺外分化T細胞とそのc-kit$^+$幹細胞の概念は、まだなかった。その初期の研究は、胸腺細胞集団へパートナー細胞が非常にゆっくり混入することを示した[20-23]。先行研究では、c-kit$^+$前駆細胞の特定は胸腺で行われていた[20-23]。そこで、本研究では、危機的状況でない（前駆細胞の障害がない）場合、胸腺の前駆細胞が、未成熟および成熟した胸腺細胞を継続して産生している可能性を提案する。

その後、E. Donskyらの報告では[18]、並体結合（Thy1.1とThy1.2）をした各々の個体における胸腺には、ほとんどパートナー細胞が混入しなかったという結果だった。この報告と本研究における胸腺の結果はほぼ同じだが、その解釈は若干異なる。彼らの解釈では、出産後、一生、胸腺にある前駆細胞は、（おそらく骨髄由来の）血液由来前駆細胞である。我々の解釈では、肝臓と腸における胸腺外T細胞は肝臓と腸で局所産生されたものだが、その前駆細胞は、血液由来の前駆細胞でもある。既述したもう一つの可能性は、前駆細胞が肝臓と腸だけでなく胸腺の中にも存在していることである。胸腺の場合、前駆細胞がパートナー・マウスの胸腺に混入することは、非常に困難だった。つまり、IL-2Rα$^+$CD3$^-$細胞を静脈注射しても、パートナー・マウスの胸腺には定着しなかった。しかし、IL-2Rα$^+$CD3$^-$細胞を直接胸腔内へ移入すると、成熟したT細胞が胸腺で産生された（原稿準備中）。したがって、胸腺細胞の前駆細胞はすべて、T細胞系列統に分化限定されるのである。このように、この細胞が血液循環を通じて再び胸腺に入ることは困難である。一方、骨髄と肝臓から採取されたc-kit$^+$幹細胞は、まだ多分化能を失わず、血球の種類は分化限定されていない。この細胞は容易に胸腺に入ることができる。腸から分離されたc-kit$^+$幹細胞には、肝臓と胸腺のc-kit$^+$幹細胞の中間の特徴がある。このように、腸のc-kit$^+$幹細胞は胸腺に入ることができたが、通常のDP CD4$^+$8$^+$細胞は産生されることはなかった[15]。

近年、Poussierらの報告[24]では、腸のIELは、並体結合のLy5.1とLy5.2マウスで互いに混和しないので、腸のIELは独自な分化をし、胸腺非依存性であるという結論に達した。しかし、腸において自身の幹細胞からIELが産生される可能性には言及していない。なぜならば、当時、腸にc-kit$^+$幹細胞が存在するとは報告されていなかったからである。クリプトパッチの免疫組織化学的な染色データは、腸にc-kit$^+$幹細胞が存在することを示すので大変興味深い[4, 16]、パートナー細胞も多少腸に存在した。c-kit$^+$細胞の中には、胸腺の場合のように、時間をかけて骨髄から移動して来る可能性を排除できない。

胸腺外で分化したCD3^{int}細胞には、NK1.1$^+$とNK1.1$^-$フェノタイプを持つ2つのサブセッ

トが存在すると以前報告した[8]。どちらのCD3^{int}細胞のサブセットにも、Mls系における自己応答禁止クローンがある[25, 26]。最近の研究でマウスにおけるNK1.1$^+$CD3^{int}細胞はヒトにおいてCD56$^+$ T細胞に相当し、マウスにおけるNK1.1$^-$CD3^{int}細胞はヒトにおいてCD57$^+$ T細胞に相当するという可能性を提案した[27, 28]。このように、マウスとヒトにおいて、前者（NK1.1$^+$CD3int細胞，CD56$^+$ T細胞）は、肝臓と子宮に存在する、一方、後者（NK1.1$^-$CD3^{int}細胞，CD57$^+$ T細胞）は、骨髄に存在する。本研究より、以下の考えも検証できた。それは肝臓のNK1.1$^+$CD3^{int}細胞は、パートナー細胞とあまり混和しなかったが、肝臓のNK1.1$^-$CD3^{int}細胞はよく混和したことである（主に骨髄由来であるため）。腸のLPLとIELがどこで産生されるかの結論は出ていない[9-12]。本研究の結果から、大多数のIELとクリプトパッチの細胞は、腸で産生されるが、CD4$^+$ IELの中には他の部位（おそらく胸腺）で産生されるものもあると結論を出した。同様に、腸のLPLも、他の部位で産生されたリンパ球を含んでいる。リンパ球サブセットの中には、胸腺外分化したものがあるとしても、血液循環によりもとの場所に移動して定着する可能性もある。

最後に、一つ推測として、肝臓、腸や胸腺におけるc-kit$^+$幹細胞のほとんどは、胎生期の卵黄嚢、胎児肝臓または骨髄に由来する可能性である。常在しているマクロファージは、独特な部位（例、肝臓、肺と脳）に存在するので、幹細胞に関するこの概念には説得力がありそうだ。この場合、前駆細胞は、胎生期にそれぞれの部位に移動する可能性がある[29-33]。

4. 材料と方法

4.1 マウス

本研究では、C57BL/6（B6.Ly5.2, H-2^b）およびC57BL/6-Ly5.1（B6.Ly5.1, H-2^b）マウスを使用した。C57BL/6-Ly5.1（B6.Ly5.1, H-2^b）マウスは当初K. Kishihara博士（生体防御医学研究所，九州大学，福岡，日本）より寄与された後、新潟大学の動物施設にて飼育した。すべてのマウスは、SPF（特定病原体未感染）環境下で飼育した。

4.2 並体結合

定法により8週齢のマウス（B6.L1y5.1およびB6.Ly5.2）を用いて並体結合を行なった[18]。ストレスにより胸腺が萎縮した並体結合マウスは、実験から排除した。

4.3 細胞分離

定法により肝単核球を分離した[2]。略述すると、摘出した肝臓を200-ゲージ・ステンレス・スチール・メッシュで濾し、5mM Hepes培養液および2%非働化仔牛血清を添加したEagle MEM培養液（日水製薬（株），東京，日本）に浮遊させた。培養液で一度洗浄した後、細胞を15ml 35%パーコール溶液（Pharmacia Fine Chemicals, Piscataway, NJ）に再懸濁させ、比重遠心分離（2000rpm，15分間）を行い分別した[34]。分離した細胞塊を溶血用溶液（155mM NH4Cl,10mM KHCO3,1mM EDTA-Na,170mM Tris, PH7.3）に再懸濁させた。脾臓、胸腺と鼠径リンパ節をステンレス・スチール・メッシュで濾して脾臓細胞、胸腺細胞およびリンパ節のリンパ球を採取した。脾臓細胞は、溶血後に実験に使用した。

IEL、LPLおよびパイエル板を定法に従い、腸より採取した[35]。略述すると、摘出した小腸をPBSで洗浄し、腸管の内容物を排除した後、腸間膜とパイエル板を切除した。腸を縦方向に切開して得た切片（1-2cm）を、Dulbecco's PBSに入れ（20 ml, 5mM EDTA含，Ca^{2+}およびMg^{2+}不含）、恒温槽で振盪させた後（37℃，15分間）、上清を採取した。非連続

パーコール勾配（40%/80%）を用い、遠心分離（2800rpm，25分間）を行い、40%/80の中間層から細胞を採取した。

LPL採取のため、培養液にコラゲナーゼ（タイプII（90 U/ml））を添加して腸の酵素処理を行った。その後、浴槽で振盪させ（37℃，45-90分間）培養した。この腸を200-ゲージ・ステンレス・スチール・メッシュで漉し、培養液に懸濁した。細胞は、35%パーコール溶液を用いて分離した。

4.4 フローサイトメトリー解析

抗CD3（145-2C11）、抗-IL-2Rβ（TM-β1）、抗NK1.1（PK136）、抗CD4（RM4-5）、抗CD8（53-6.7）、抗TCRαβ（H57-597）と抗TCRγδ（GL3）モノクロナール抗体をPharMingen（San Diego、CA）より購入した[35]。マウス抗Ly5.1（A20.1.7）と抗Ly5.2（ALl-4A2）モノクロナール抗体は、T. Kina博士（京都大学，日本）の提供である。使用したモノクロナール抗体はすべて、FITC-（PE-またはビオチン-標識）である。ビオチン病識抗体は、TRl-COLOR標識ストレプトアビジン（Caltag Lab., San Francisco, CA）で発色させた。細胞をFACScan（Becton Dickinson Co., Mountain View, CA）を用いて分析した。モノクロナール抗体の非特異的結合を防ぐため、標識されたモノクロナール抗体で染色する前にCD32/16（24G2）抗体を加えた。死細胞をヨウ化プロピジウムで染色し、前方散乱光と側方散乱光でのゲーティングとを併用して除外した。

パートナー細胞の比率を、全集団または各サブセットのゲーティングを行い測定した（例、全CD3$^-$NK1.1$^+$細胞 中CD3$^-$NK1.1$^+$Ly5.2$^+$細胞の%）。平均±1SDを、5匹のマウスを用い算出した。各時点においてP<0.05であったので平均値の数字のみを図に記す。

4.5 免疫組織化学染色法

胸腺、腸間膜リンパ節および縦方向に切開した小腸と大腸（長さ10mm）をO.C.T.コンパウンド（Tissue-Tek, Miles Inc., Elkhart, IN）で包埋した）(-80℃)[4]。組織を6μmにクリオスタットで薄切し、ポリ-エル-リジンでコートしたスライドガラス（Matsunami Glass IND., LTD., Japan）に貼付した。組織切片を、冷風乾燥し、アセトンで固定した（室温 10分間）。一次抗体の非特異的結合を防ぐため、ブロック-エース（第日本住友製薬（株），大阪，日本）で前処理した（37℃，10分間）。そして、切片を、適度に希釈したラット、あるいはハムスター一次抗体でインキュベートした（37℃，30分間，または7℃，一晩）。PBSで3度洗浄した後、ビオチン標識ヤギ抗ラットIgG（Cedarlane LaboratoR1es Limited, Ontalio, Canada）または、ビオチン標識ヤギ抗ハムスター IgG（Vector LaboratoR1es, Inc., Burlingame, CA）でインキュベートした。その後、切片をPBSで3度洗浄し、アビジィン-ビオチン・ペルオキシダーゼ複合体（Vectastatin ABC kit; Vector LaboratoR1es, Inc.）でインキュベートした。

発色を、添付の説明書に従い、Vectastatin 3,3'-ジアミノベンジジン（DAB）サブストレート・キット（Vector LaboratoR1es, Inc.）を用いて行なった。切片を、顕微鏡検査のためヘマトキシリンで対比染色した。内在性ペルオキシダーゼを、0.3% H_2O_2と0.1% NaN_3溶液で不活性化した（室温10分間）。

謝辞

本研究は、文部科学省科学研究費補助金によるものである。原稿浄書について金子裕子氏に感謝する。

Low level of mixing of partner cells seen in extrathymic T cells in the liver and intestine of parabiotic mice: its biological implication

Susumu Suzuki[1], Satoshi Sugahara[1], Takao Shimizu[2], Takashi Tada[2], Masahiro Minagawa[2], Satoshi Maruyama[2], Hisami Watanabe[1], Hisashi Saito[3], Hiromichi Ishikawa[3], Katsuyoshi Hatakeyama[2] and Toru Abo[1]

[1] Department of Immunology, Niigata University School of Medicine, Niigata, Japan
[2] First Department of Surgery, Niigata University School of Medicine, Niigata, Japan
[3] Department of Microbiology, Keio University School of Medicine, Tokyo, Japan

c-kit$^+$ stem cells have recently been found in the liver and intestine of adult mice. We examined whether such stem cells give rise to extrathymic T cells in these organs *in situ*. To this end, we used parabiotic B6.Ly5.1 and B6.Ly5.2 mice, *i.e.* mice sharing the circulation. The origin of lymphocytes was identified by anti-Ly5.1 and anti-Ly5.2 monoclonal antibodies in conjunction with immunofluorescence assays. Lymphocytes in the blood, spleen, lymph nodes and liver had become a half-and-half mixture of Ly5.1$^+$ and Ly5.2$^+$ cells in both individuals by day 14. However, this level of mixing decreased in extrathymic T cells in the liver (*i.e.* NK T cells) and intestine by day 14 and thereafter. The same was observed in T cells of the thymus. The data from immunohistochemical staining supported the results of immunofluorescence assays for suspension cells. The present results raise the possibility that extrathymic T cells in the liver and intestine may arise from their own pre-existing precursor cells, possibly from their own stem cells. Another important finding was that the composition pattern of lymphocyte subsets in one individual was quite similar to that in its partner at various sites. This result was interpreted to mean that only selected partner cells migrate to specific sites in the other partner individual.

Received	24/4/98
Revised	28/7/98
Accepted	28/7/98

Key words: c-kit$^+$ stem cell / Extrathymic T cell / NK T cell / Parabiosis / Digestive tract

1 Introduction

It has recently been shown that c-kit$^+$ stem cell exist in the liver and intestine, *i.e.* sites of extrathymic T cell generation, of mice and humans [1–4]. Extrathymic T cells in the liver and intestine of mice not only share the same properties but also have some distinguishing properties. Namely, extrathymic T cells in the liver mainly comprise αβ T cells with double-negative (DN) CD4$^-$8$^-$ and single-positive CD4$^+$ or CD8$^+$ phenotypes [5–8], whereas those in the intestine contain γδ T cells and a significant proportion of αβ T cells with double-positive (DP) CD4$^+$8$^+$ phenotype [9–12]. The phylogenetic development of these two T cell subsets might have been separated at a certain point of time. This concept arises from the fact that the liver developed as a projection of the intestine for the secretion of bile [13, 14]. In recent studies, c-kit$^+$ Lin$^-$ cells were isolated from the liver and intestine and eventually gained the ability to give rise to extrathymic T cells in the corresponding organs [2, 15, 16]. Moreover, c-kit$^+$ Lin$^-$ cells in the liver were found to be pluripotent (*i.e.* able to generate erythroid and myeloid cells as well as lymphoid cells), whereas those in the small intestine and appendix were oligopotent (*i.e.* committed to become lymphoid cells but not erythroid and myeloid cells). However, there is still a question as to whether such stem cells originate in the bone marrow and whether such extrathymic T cells migrate to other sites through the circulation. To investigate this subject, we used parabiotic B6.Ly5.1 and B6.Ly5.2 mice [17–19]. After the mixing of lymphocytes, their origins were identified by anti-Ly5.1 and anti-Ly5.2 mAb in conjunction with immunofluorescence assays.

[I 18272]

Abbreviations: DN: Double-negative **DP:** Double-positive **IEL:** Intraepithelial lymphocytes **LPL:** Lamina propria lymphocytes **int:** Intermediate

© WILEY-VCH Verlag GmbH, D-69451 Weinheim, 1998

0014-2980/98/1111-3719$17.50+.50/0

2 Results

2.1 Generation of thymocytes and intraepithelial lymphocytes in the intestine by their own stem cells

B6.Ly5.1 and B6.Ly5.2 mice at the age of 8 weeks were used for parabiosis. Biotinylated anti-Ly5.1 and anti-Ly5.2 mAb were used to identify cell origins. From day 3 after parabiosis, the appearance of Ly5.1$^+$ cells in various organs of Ly5.2 mice was examined (Fig. 1A). The appearance of partner cells began on day 3 and reached a plateau on day 14 in the blood, lymph nodes, spleen and liver. This was due to the origin of such lymphocytes in these organs being the bone marrow (B cells) and the thymus (T cells). In sharp contrast, there was no appearance of partner cells (< 3.0 %) in the thymus up to day 42. It is speculated that thymocytes arose from their own stem cells which pre-existed in the thymus. There might be no supply of stem cells from the bone marrow to the thymus in adulthood (*i.e.* at least during this experimental period). The same result was produced in Ly5.1 parabiotic mice (data not shown).

Since intestinal lymphocytes with different properties could be isolated from three sites (*i.e.* the intraepithelium, lamina propria, and Peyer's patches), they were independently isolated and characterized (Fig. 1B). Lymphocytes in the Peyer's patches mixed well with partner cells (40 % on day 14), whereas intraepithelial lymphocytes (IEL) did not mix well (7 % at day 42). Lymphocytes in the lamina propria (LPL) showed an intermediate pattern (26 % on day 14).

2.2 Generation of NK T cells in the liver from their own stem cells

The experiments were extended to the characterization of lymphocyte subsets in the liver and spleen (Fig. 2A). In normal B6.Ly5.1 mice, CD3$^-$ IL-2Rβ^+ NK cells, CD3^{int} IL-2Rβ^+ cells (*i.e.* CD3^{int} cells of extrathymic origin), and CD3^{high} IL-2Rβ^- cells (*i.e.* CD3^{high} cells of thymic origin) were identified in both the liver and spleen. NK and CD3^{int} cells were abundant in the liver. In parabiotic Ly5.2 mice (day 14), 31.9 % and 39.0 % of partner cells appeared in the liver and spleen, respectively. By three-color staining of CD3, IL-2Rβ, and Ly5.1 [2], the staining patterns of the whole fraction (R1 + R2), the R1 fraction (Ly5.1$^-$), and the R2 fraction (Ly.5.1$^+$) were compared. There were some differences in the staining patterns, especially between R1 and R2 in the liver, namely, the proportion of CD3^{int} cells in R2 was smaller than that in R1. In this regard, the kinetics of the composition of various lymphocyte subsets was studied (Fig. 2B). In the liver, there were different mixture patterns, *i.e.* CD3^{high} cells > NK cells > CD3^{int} cells. These results suggest that some CD3^{int} cells were generated *in situ* in the liver but that the other CD3^{int} cells originated in other organs. A similar tendency was true of NK cells of the liver, and of NK cells and CD3^{int} cells of the spleen (the level of mixing was lower in this organ).

In a previous study, we reported that approximately 60 % of CD3^{int} cells in the liver are NK1.1$^+$ (*i.e.* NK T cells) [8]. Therefore, attention was then focused on NK T cells (Fig. 3A). There were many NK1.1$^+$ CD3^{int} cells in the liver and a few NK1.1$^+$ CD3^{int} cells in the spleen of normal B6.Ly5.1 mice. This was also the case in parabiotic mice

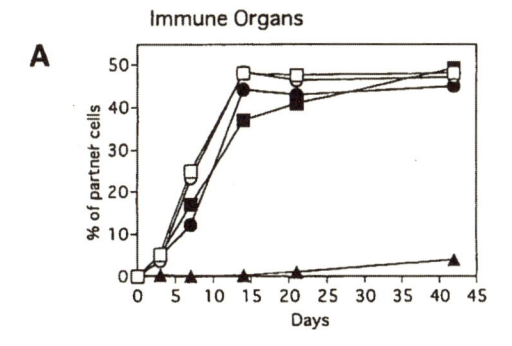

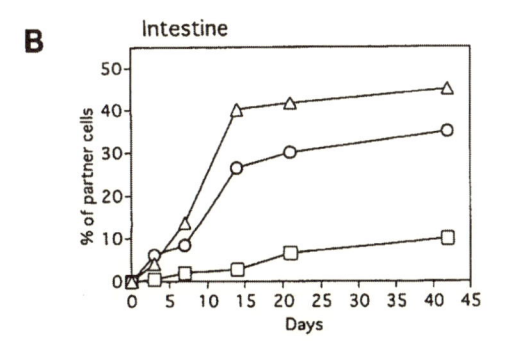

Figure 1. Entrance of partner cells into each individual mouse after parabiosis. (A) Various immune organs (■, liver; ●, spleen; ▲, thymus; ○, lymph node; □, peripheral blood), (B) various sites in the intestine (□, IEL; ○, LPL; △, Peyer's patch). Parabiosis of B6.Ly5.1 and B6.Ly5.2 mice at the age of 8 weeks was produced. At the indicated time points, cells were isolated from various immune organs and various sites of the intestine (*n* = 5 at each time point). In the case of Ly5.1 mice, the entrance of partner cells was identified by biotinylated anti-Ly5.2 mAb and vice versa.

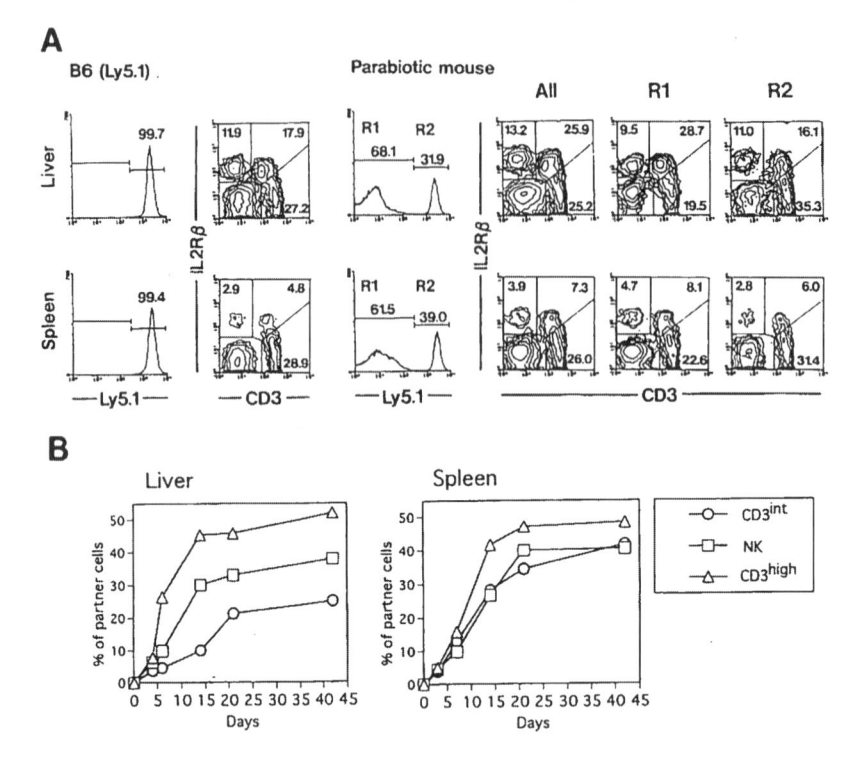

Figure 2. Entrance of partner cells into specific lymphocyte subsets in the liver and spleen after parabiosis. (A) Three-color staining for CD3, IL-2Rβ, and Ly5.1 in Ly5.2 parabiotic mice (day 14). (B) Kinetics of the proportion of partner cells in various lymphocyte subsets of the liver and spleen. Cells were isolated at the indicated time points and three-color staining was performed. By gated analysis, the proportions of Ly5.1⁺ cells in various lymphocyte subsets of Ly5.2 parabiotic mice were determined. Kinetics were produced from the mean of five parabiotic mice.

(see whole fraction of R1 + R2). On the other hand, there was a large difference in staining patterns between R1 and R2 in both the liver and spleen. NK1.1⁺CD3^{int} cells were abundant in R1 but were extremely few in R2. The kinetic data are represented in Fig. 3B. NK1.1⁺CD3^{int} cells in the liver showed a low level of mixing. A similar tendency was seen in NK1.1⁺CD3^{int} cells of the spleen, although the level of mixing was higher.

2.3 Further characterization of intestinal T cells

In this experiment, IEL in the intestine were further characterized (Fig. 4A). Three-color staining of IEL for CD4, CD8 and Ly5.1, and for TCRαβ, TCRγδ and Ly5.1 was conducted in normal B6.Ly5.1 mice and parabiotic Ly5.2 mice. As shown in normal mice, CD8⁺ cells were much more abundant than CD4⁺ cells in IEL. DP CD4⁺8⁺ cells were uniquely seen in IEL. TCRαβ⁺ and TCRγδ⁺ cells were present at a 2:1 ratio. When parabiotic mice (day 14) were observed, there were very few partner cells (< 3.0 %). Then the whole fraction (R1 + R2), the R1 fraction, and the R2 fraction were compared. A difference of staining patterns between R1 and R2 was seen in CD4⁺ cells. The kinetic data for IEL are represented in Fig. 4B. Among all tested lymphocyte subsets, the partner cells entered only the CD4⁺ subset. However, the proportion was still not so high (up to 15 % on day 21). This result suggests that some CD4⁺ cells were not of extrathymic origin, even in intestinal IEL.

2.4 Immunohistochemical staining of the tissues in parabiotic mice

To confirm the data from immunofluorescence assays of suspension cells, immunohistochemical staining of the tissues in parabiotics was conducted (Fig. 5). Control

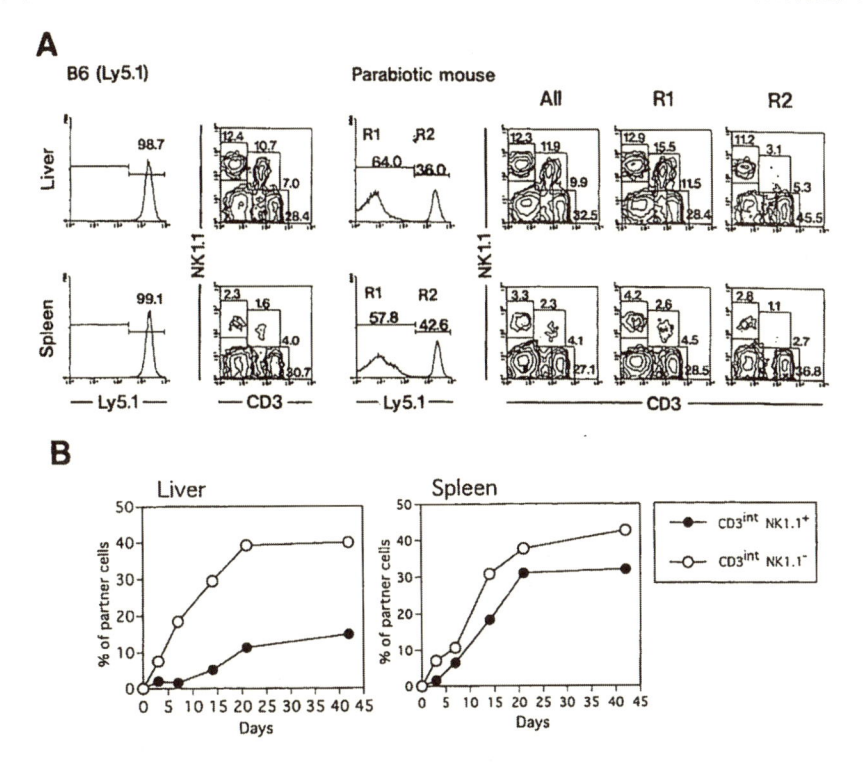

Figure 3. Difficulty of the entrance of partner cells into NK1.1$^+$CD3^{int} cells in the liver of parabiotic mice. (A) Three-color staining for CD3, NK1.1, and Ly5.1 in parabiotic mice (day 14). (B) Kinetics of the proportion of NK1.1$^+$CD3^{int} cells in the liver and spleen. Cells were isolated at the indicated time points and three-color staining was performed. By gated analysis, the proportions of Ly5.1$^+$ cells in various lymphocyte subsets of Ly5.2 parabiotic mice were determined. Kinetics were produced from the mean of five parabiotic mice.

staining for Ly5.1 or Ly5.2 was done by using Ly5.1 or Ly5.2 mice (Fig. 5, upper half of each figure). Parabiotic Ly5.1 and Ly5.2 mice were used on day 35 after the parabiotic operation. As shown in the thymus, anti-Ly5.1 mAb stained only thymocytes of Ly5.1 mice while anti-Ly5.2 mAb stained only thymocytes of Ly5.2 mice. This was also the case with parabiotic mice. In other words, there was no mixture of partner cells in the thymus of the parabiotic individuals.

In sharp contrast, the partner cells mixed well in the spleen and lymph nodes of the parabiotic individuals. In the case of intestinal villi, the result was very interesting: the partner lymphocytes mixed well in the lamina propria but not in the intraepithelia. Attention was then focused on the cryptopatches where c-kit$^+$ stem cells are known to exist preferentially [4]. Although a few partner cells mixed in the cryptopatches, the majority of lymphocytes originated from their own pre-existing precursors. This was true in both parabiotic individuals. In a final set of experiments, the Peyer's patches were examined. Similar to the case of the spleen and lymph nodes, partner cells mixed well in the Peyer's patches of each individual. All of these results are compatible with the data obtained from immunofluorescence assays for suspension cells. The data of the liver are not shown, because the figure contained mostly hepatocytes and the staining yielded little information.

3 Discussion

In this study we used parabiosis of B6.Ly5.1 and B6.Ly5.2 mice to identify how lymphocyte subsets are generated in various immune organs. We demonstrated that some lymphocytes or some lymphocyte subsets localized at specific sites might be generated *in situ* from their own pre-existing precursor cells. Such major lym-

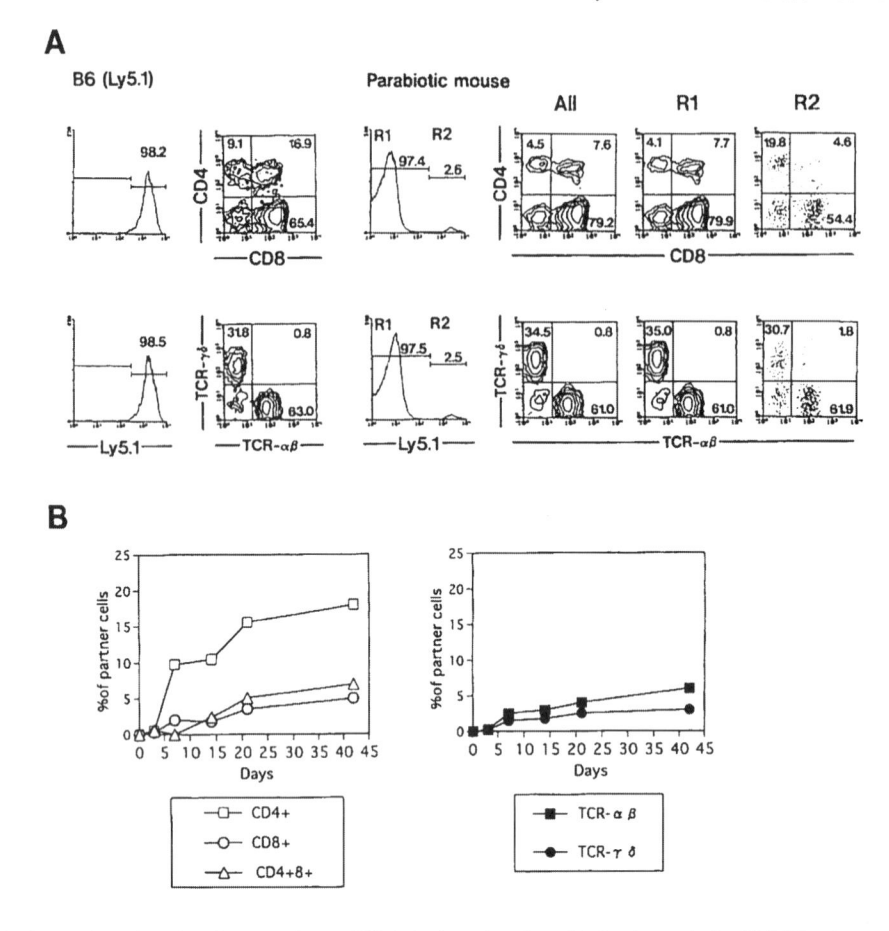

Figure 4. Among the various lymphocyte subsets of IEL in the intestine of parabiotic mice, only the CD4+ IEL subset was entered by partner cells. (A) Three-color staining for CD4, CD8, and Ly5.1 and that for TCRαβ, TCRγδ, and Ly5.1 in Ly5.2 parabiotic mice (day 14). (B) Kinetics of the proportion of partner cells in various lymphocyte subsets in IEL of the intestine. Cells were isolated at the indicated time points and three-color staining was performed. By gated analysis, the proportion of Ly5.1+ cells in various lymphocyte subsets of Ly5.2 parabiotic mice was determined. Kinetics were produced from the mean of five parabiotic mice.

phocytes included NK T cells in the liver, IEL in the intestine, and T cells in the thymus. If precursor cells for these lymphocytes are consistently supplied from the bone marrow, the present phenomenon would not have occurred. In sharp contrast, all lymphocytes in the blood, spleen, and lymph nodes, and some lymphocyte subsets in the liver and intestine had become a half-and-half mixture of their own cells and partner cells by day 14 after parabiosis. It is conceivable that all T and B cells at these sites come continuously from the thymus and bone marrow, respectively, through the circulation. There was a third group of lymphocytes in which the entrance of partner cells occurred very slowly. Such lymphocyte subsets included LPL and CD4+ IEL cells in the intestine, and CD3^{int} cells in the liver. It is speculated that lymphocytes at these sites comprise both T cells derived from the thymus and T cells generated *in situ*. Taken together, these findings indicate that some specific lymphocytes are generated *in situ* their own pre-existing precursor cells.

If extrathymic T cells have an extraordinarily long lifespan (including an extraordinarily high self-renewal capability of mature cells), the present data do not necessarily suggest that they are generated *in situ* from their own pre-existing precursors. We feel that this question is very important and as yet unsolved. However, concern-

	Anti-Ly5.1	Anti-Ly5.2
a		
Ly5.1		
Ly5.2		
P→Ly5.1		
P→Ly5.2		

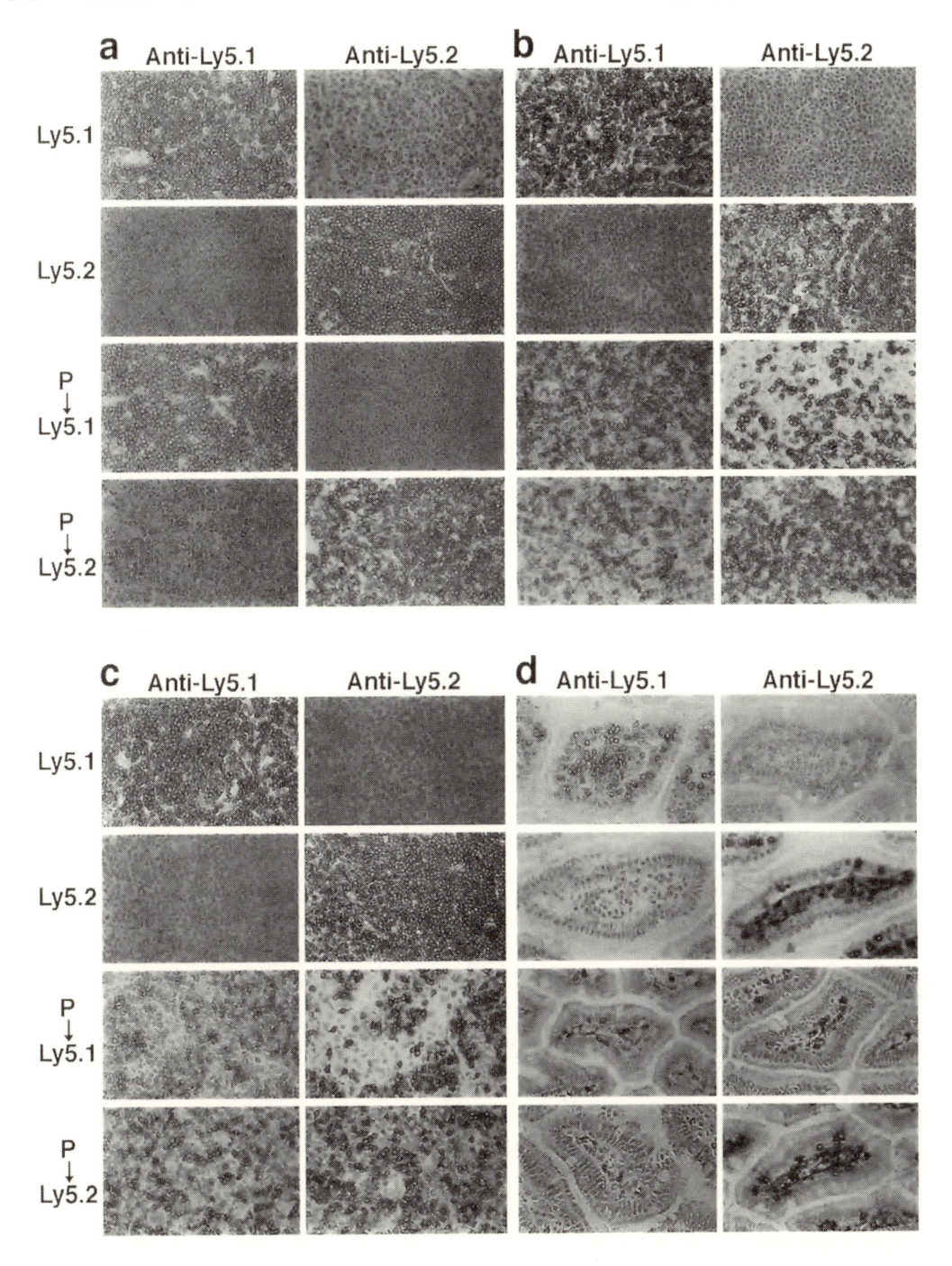

	Anti-Ly5.1	Anti-Ly5.2
b		
Ly5.1		
Ly5.2		
P→Ly5.1		
P→Ly5.2		

	Anti-Ly5.1	Anti-Ly5.2
c		
Ly5.1		
Ly5.2		
P→Ly5.1		
P→Ly5.2		

	Anti-Ly5.1	Anti-Ly5.2
d		
Ly5.1		
Ly5.2		
P→Ly5.1		
P→Ly5.2		

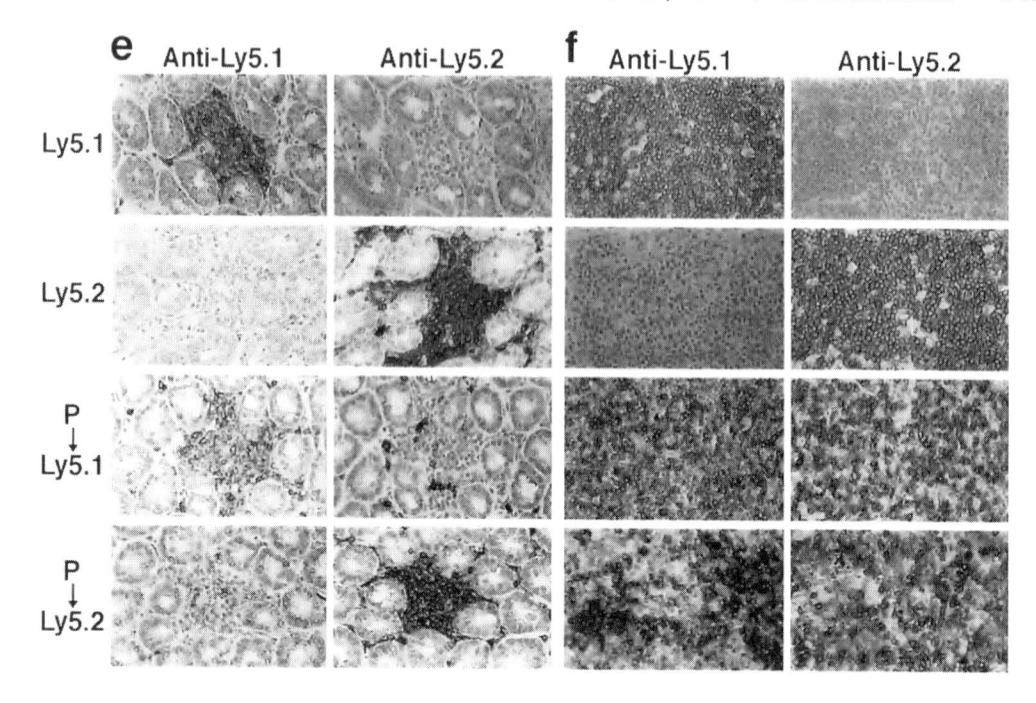

Figure 5. Immunohistochemical staining for Ly5.1⁺ and Ly5.2⁺ cells in the thymus (a), spleen (b), lymph nodes (c), intestinal villi (d), intestinal cryptopatches (e), and intestinal Peyer's patches (f) of parabiotic mice (×400). Samples from parabiotic (P) Ly5.1 and Ly5.2 mice were examined on day 35 after a parabiotic operation. Each individual was examined for the degree to which partner cells entered each organ. Control stainings of Ly5.1 and Ly5.2 mice (non-parabiotic mice) are always shown in parallel at the top of the figures.

ing the results from the experiments of c-kit⁺ Lin⁻ stem cells isolated from the liver and intestine (such c-kit⁺ Lin⁻ cells isolated from the liver and intestine eventually had stem cell capability) [2, 15, 16], we do not think that extrathymic T cells have a longer life-span nor a much higher capability of self-renewal of mature cells than conventional T cells. However, this subject should be confirmed further by ongoing experiments.

Another important finding of this experiment was that the composition pattern of the R2 fraction (Ly5.1⁺ cells) was quite similar to that of the R1 fraction at various sites. This result was interpreted to mean that only selected partner cells which should home in on the corresponding sites migrate to specific sites of another partner individual.

The present study was conducted in line with recent evidence that c-kit⁺ stem cells exist in the parenchymal space of the liver [2, 15] and in the cryptopatches of the intestine [4, 16]. In a previous study, we isolated c-kit⁺ cells from the liver and bone marrow of normal B6.Ly5.1 mice and injected them into 4 Gy-irradiated B6-SCID mice (Ly5.2) [2]. The injected c-kit⁺ cells isolated from the liver and bone marrow reconstituted all T cells in the thymus, extrathymic T cells in the liver, and erythroid and myeloid cells in the bone marrow. By using the present experimental protocol, we demonstrated that c-kit⁺ cells in the bone marrow might not always supply c-kit⁺ stem cells to the liver, intestine, or even the thymus under normal conditions. In a parallel study, we produced parabiosis of normal Ly5.1 mice and irradiated Ly5.2 mice (1, 3 and 6 Gy). When Ly5.2 mice were irradiated with more than 1 Gy, Ly5.1⁺ T cells easily appeared in the thymus of Ly5.2 partner mice (our unpublished observation). These results support the hypothesis that the stem cells in the thymus are replaced by the stem cells from the bone marrow when thymic stem cells are impaired.

In an earlier study by K. Hirokawa et al. [19], a similar experimental protocol of parabiosis was used and the origin of partner cells was identified by markers of a combination of Thy1.1 and Thy1.2. However, the expression of Thy1 antigens is limited to subpopulations of lymphocytes. In contrast, Ly5 antigens are expressed on almost all lymphocytes, except some c-kit$^+$ stem cells. In this regard, this experimental protocol was useful for the determination of all lymphocyte subsets in various immune organs. More importantly, the concept of extrathymic T cells and their own c-kit$^+$ stem cells had not yet been introduced at that time. In that earlier study, it was shown that the entrance of partner cells into thymocyte populations occurred very slowly. c-kit$^+$ precursor cells were identified in the thymus in earlier studies [20–23]. We therefore proposed the possibility that, in the absence of emergency conditions (i.e. the impairment of precursor cells), precursor cells in the thymus continuously give rise to immature and mature thymocytes.

Subsequently, E. Donsky et al. [18] reported the fact that only a few partner cells entered the thymus of each individual of parabiotic Thy1.1 and Thy1.2 mice. Although their results for the thymus were almost the same as ours, their interpretations are somewhat different. They speculated that intrathymic precursors are blood-borne precursors (possibly bone marrow-derived) throughout postnatal life. If we understand their speculation, extrathymic T cells in the liver and intestine are generated in situ but their precursor cells are also blood-borne precursors. Another possibility which we have already mentioned is that precursor cells pre-exist in the thymus as well as the liver and intestine. In the case of the thymus, it was very difficult to obtain such precursor cells which are able to enter the thymus of other mice. Namely, an i.v. injection of IL-2Rα$^+$ CD3$^-$ cells did not home to the thymus of other mice. However, injection of such IL-2Rα$^+$ CD3$^-$ cells by an intrathymic route gave in situ rise to mature T cells (manuscript in preparation). Therefore, all precursor cells for thymocytes are already committed to a T cell lineage. It is thus difficult for them to enter the thymus again through the circulation. On the other hand, c-kit$^+$ stem cells isolated from the bone marrow and liver are still pluripotent and are not committed to any types of blood cells. They can easily enter the thymus. c-kit$^+$ stem cells isolated from the intestine have an intermediate characteristics between those of the liver and thymus. Thus, intestinal c-kit$^+$ stem cells were able to enter the thymus but did not give rise to regular DP CD4$^+$8$^+$ cells [15].

In a recent study, Poussier et al. [24] reported that IEL in the intestine did not mix with each other in parabiotic Ly5.1 and Ly5.2 mice. They concluded that the development of IEL in the intestine is thymus independent. However, they did not mention the possibility of the generation of IEL from their own stem cells in the intestine. This was because there had been no report on the existence of c-kit$^+$ stem cells in the intestine at that time. The data from immunohistochemical staining for the cryptopatches showing that c-kit$^+$ stem cells in the intestine are present [4, 16] were very interesting, in that they showed that a few partner cells were present at that site. We cannot exclude the possibility that some c-kit$^+$ cells come from the bone marrow very slowly, similar to the case of the thymus.

We previously reported the existence of two subsets with NK1.1$^+$ and NK1.1$^-$ phenotype among CD3^{int} cells of extrathymic origin [8]. Both subsets of CD3^{int} cells comprise self-reactive forbidden clones in the Mls system [25, 26]. In a recent study, we proposed the possibility that NK1.1$^+$CD3^{int} cells in mice correspond to CD56$^+$ T cells in humans while NK1.1$^-$CD3^{int} cells in mice correspond to CD57$^+$ T cells in humans [27, 28]. Thus, the former cells exist in the liver and uterus, whereas the latter cells exist in the bone marrow in mice and humans. The present data also support this notion, because NK1.1$^+$CD3^{int} cells in the liver did not mix well with partner cells, but NK1.1$^-$CD3^{int} cells in the liver did mix well (due to being mainly of bone marrow origin).

The origin of LPL and IEL in the intestine has remained controversial [9–12]. Based on the findings of this study, we conclude that the majority of IEL and cryptopatch cells are of intestinal origin but that some CD4$^+$ IEL may originate at other sites, possibly the thymus. Similarly, LPL in the intestine also contain lymphocytes that come from other sites. There is also the possibility that even if some lymphocyte subsets are of extrathymic origin, they may circulate and home to their original place through the circulation.

Finally, one speculation is that the majority of c-kit$^+$ stem cells in the liver, intestine, and thymus might come from the yolk sack, fetal liver, or bone marrow during fetal stages. This concept for stem cells seems plausible, because many resident macrophages are primarily present at unique sites such as the liver, lung and brain. In these cases, their precursor cells may migrate to corresponding sites during fetal development [29–33]. There is a possibility that a similar migration of stem cells for lymphocytes occurs during fetal development.

4 Materials and methods

4.1 Mice

C57BL/6 (B6.Ly5.2, H-2^b) and C57BL/6-Ly5.1 (B6.Ly5.1, H-2^b) mice were used in this study. The latter mice were originally provided by Dr. K. Kishihara (Medical Institute of Bioregulation, Kyushu University, Fukuoka, Japan) and were

4.2 Parabiosis

Parabiosis of B6.Ly5.1 and B6.Ly5.2 mice at the age of 8 weeks was produced as described previously [18]. A few individual parabiotic mice that suffered from stress which resulted in thymic atrophy were eliminated from the experiments.

4.3 Cell preparation

Hepatic mononuclear cells were isolated by a method described previously [2]. Briefly, the liver was removed, pressed through 200-gauge stainless steel mesh, and suspended in Eagle's MEM medium (Nissui Pharmaceutical Co., Tokyo, Japan) supplemented with 5 mM Hepes and 2% heat-inactivated newborn calf serum. After being washed once with medium, the cells were fractionated by centrifugation in 15 ml of 35% Percoll solution (Pharmacia Fine Chemicals, Piscataway, NJ) for 15 min at 2000 rpm [34]. The pellet was resuspended in erythrocyte lysing solution (155 mM NH_4Cl, 10 mM $KHCO_3$, 1 mM EDTA-Na, 170 mM Tris, pH 7.3). The splenocytes, thymocytes and lymph node lymphocytes were obtained by forcing the spleen, thymus, and inguinal lymph nodes through stainless steel mesh. Splenocytes were used after erythrocyte lysing.

IEL, LPL and Peyer's patches were collected from the intestine according to the method described previously [35]. Briefly, the small intestine was removed and flushed with PBS to eliminate luminal contents. The mesentery and Peyer's patches were then resected. The intestine was opened longitudinally and cut into 1–2-cm fragments. These fragments were incubated for 15 min in 20 ml Ca^{2+}- and Mg^{2+}-free Dulbecco's PBS containing 5 mM EDTA, in a 37 °C shaking water bath. The supernatant was then collected. The cell suspensions were collected and centrifuged in a discontinuous 40%/80% Percoll gradient at 2800 rpm for 25 min. Cells from the 40%/80% interface were collected.

LPL were prepared after the digestion of intestine with collagenase type II at a concentration of 90 U/ml in the medium. Samples were incubated for 45–90 min in a 37 °C shaking water bath. Digested intestine was then pressed through 200-gauge stainless steel mesh and suspended in the medium. Cells were fractionated by the 35% Percoll solution.

4.4 Immunofluorescence assays

For flow cytometric analysis, anti-CD3 (145-2C11), anti-IL-2Rβ (TM-β1), anti-NK1.1 (PK136), anti-CD4 (RM4-5), anti-CD8 (53-6.7), anti-TCRαβ (H57-597), and anti-TCRγδ (GL3) mAb were purchased from PharMingen (San Diego, CA) [35]. Mouse anti-Ly5.1 (A20.1.7) and anti-Ly5.2 (ALI-4A2) mAb were provided by Dr. T. Kina (Kyoto University, Japan). All mAb were used in a FITC-, PE- or biotin-conjugated form. Biotinylated reagents were developed with TRI-COLOR-conjugated streptavidin (Caltag Lab., San Francisco, CA). Cells were analyzed by FACScan (Becton Dickinson Co., Mountain View, CA). To prevent nonspecific binding of mAb, CD32/16 (24G2) was added before staining with labeled mAb. Dead cells were excluded by forward scatter, side scatter and propidium iodide gating.

The percentages of partner cells were determined by the gated analysis of the whole population or each subset (e.g. % of $CD3^-NK1.1^+Ly5.2^+$ cells among total $CD3^-NK1.1^+$ cells). Mean and 1 SD were calculated from five mice. Since the variation of 1 SD was less than 5% at each point in time, only the mean is represented in the figures.

4.5 Immunohistochemical procedure

The thymus, the mesenteric lymph nodes, and ~ 10 mm in length of the longitudinally opened small and large intestines were embedded in O.C.T. compound (Tissue-Tek, Miles Inc., Elkhart, IN) at $-80\,°C$ [4]. The tissue segments were sectioned with a cryostat at 6 μm and applied to poly-L-lysine-coated glass slides (Matsunami Glass IND., LTD., Japan). The tissue sections that had been air-dried and fixed in acetone for 10 min at room temperature were pre-incubated with Block-ace (Dainippon Pharmaceutical Co., Osaka, Japan) for 10 min at 37 °C to block nonspecific binding of the primary mAb. The sections were then incubated with appropriately diluted primary rat or hamster mAb for 30 min at 37 °C or overnight at 7 °C, and rinsed three times with PBS, followed by incubation with biotin-conjugated goat anti-rat IgG (Cedarlane Laboratories Limited, Ontario, Canada) or with biotin-conjugated goat anti-hamster IgG (Vector Laboratories, Inc., Burlingame, CA). Subsequently, the sections were washed three times with PBS and then incubated with avidin-biotin peroxidase complexes (Vectastatin ABC kit; Vector Laboratories, Inc.). Histochemical color development was achieved by a Vectastatin 3,3'-diaminobenzidine (DAB) substrate kit (Vector Laboratories, Inc.) according to the manufacturer's instructions. The sections were counterstained with hematoxylin for microscopy. Endogenous peroxidase activity was blocked with 0.3% H_2O_2 and 0.1% NaN_3 in distilled water for 10 min at room temperature.

Acknowledgments: This work was supported by a Grant-in-Aid for Scientific Research and Cancer Research from the Ministry of Education, Science, and Culture, Japan. We wish to thank Mrs. Yuko Kaneko for preparation of the manuscript.

5 References

1 Taniguchi, H., Toyoshima, T., Fukao, K. and Nakauchi, H., Presence of hematopoietic stem cells in the adult liver. *Nature Med.* 1996. **2:** 198–203.

2 Watanabe, H., Miyaji, C., Seki, S. and Abo, T., c-kit+ stem cells and thymocyte precursors in the livers of adult mice. *J. Exp. Med.* 1996. **184:** 687–693.

3 Starzl, T. E., Murase, N., Thomson, A. and Demetris, A. J., Liver transplants contribute to their own success. *Nature Med.* 1996. **2:** 163–165.

4 Kanamori, Y., Ishimaru, K., Nanno, M., Maki, K., Ikuta, K., Nariuchi, H. and Ishikawa, H., Identification of novel lymphoid tissues in murine intestinal mucosa where clusters of c-kit+ IL-7R+ Thy1+ lympho-hemopoietic progenitors develop. *J. Exp. Med.* 1996. **184:** 1449–1459.

5 Abo, T., Ohteki, T., Seki, S., Koyamada, N., Yoshikai, Y., Masuda, T., Rikiishi, H. and Kumagai, K., The appearance of T cells bearing self-reactive T cell receptor in the livers of mice injected with bacteria. *J. Exp. Med.* 1991. **174:** 417–424.

6 Seki, S., Abo, T., Ohteki, T., Sugiura, K. and Kumagai, K., Unusual $\alpha\beta$-T cells expanded in autoimmune *lpr* mice are probably a counterpart of normal T cell in the liver. *J. Immunol.* 1991. **147:** 1214–1221.

7 Sato, K., Ohtsuka, K., Hasegawa, K., Yamagiwa, S., Watanabe, H., Asakura, H. and Abo, T., Evidence for extrathymic generation of intermediate TCR cells in the liver revealed in thymectomized, irradiated mice subjected to bone marrow transplantation. *J. Exp. Med.* 1995. **182:** 759–767.

8 Watanabe, H., Miyaji, C., Kawachi, Y., Iiai, T., Ohtsuka, K., Iwanaga, T., Takahashi-Iwanaga, H. and Abo, T., Relationships between intermediate TCR cells and NK1.1+ T cells in various immune organs. NK1.1+ T cells are present within a population of intermediate TCR cells. *J. Immunol.* 1995. **155:** 2972–2983.

9 Ferguson, A. and Parrott, D. M., The effect of antigen deprivation on thymus-dependent and thymus-independent lymphocytes in the small intestine of the mouse. *Clin. Exp. Immunol.* 1972. **12:** 477–488.

10 Mosley, R. L., Styre, D. and Klein, J. R., Differentiation and functional maturation of bone marrow-derived intestinal epithelial T cells expressing membrane T cell receptor in athymic radiation chimeras. *J. Immunol.* 1990. **145:** 1369–1375.

11 Bandeira, A., Itohara, S., Bonneville, M., Burlen-Defranoux, O., Mota-Santos, T., Coutinho, A. and Tonegawa, S., Extrathymic origin of intestinal intraepithelial lymphocytes bearing T-cell antigen receptor gamma delta. *Proc. Natl. Acad. Sci. USA* 1991. **88:** 43–47.

12 Rocha, B., Vassalli, P. and Guy-Grand, D., The Vβ repertoire of mouse gut homodimeric α CD8+ intraepithelial T cell receptor α/β+ lymphocytes reveals a major extrathymic pathway of T cell differentiation. *J. Exp. Med.* 1991. **173:** 483–486.

13 Abo, T., Watanabe, H., Iiai, T., Kimura, M., Ohtsuka, K., Sato, K., Ogawa, M., Hirahara, H., Hashimoto, S., Sekikawa, H. and Seki, S., Extrathymic pathways of T-cell differentiation in the liver and other organs. *Int. Rev. Immunol.* 1994. **11:** 61–102.

14 Abo, T., Watanabe, H., Sato, K., Iiai, T., Moroda, T., Takeda, K. and Seki, S., Extrathymic pathways of T-cell differentiation in the liver and other organs. *Nat. Immun.* 1995. **14:** 173–187.

15 Yamagiwa, S., Sugahara, S., Shimizu, T., Iwanaga, T., Yoshida, Y., Honda, S., Watanabe, H., Suzuki, K., Asakura, H. and Abo, T., The primary site of CD4− 8− B220+ $\alpha\beta$ T cells in *lpr* mice – the appendix in normal mice. *J. Immunol.* 1998. **160:** 2665–2674.

16 Saito, H., Kanamori, Y., Takemori, T., Nariuchi, H., Kubota, E., Takahashi-Iwanaga, H., Iwanaga, T. and Ishikawa, H., Generation of intestinal T cells from progenitors residing in gut cryptopatches. *Science* 1998. **280:** 275–278.

17 Scheid, M. P. and Triglia, D., Further description of the Ly-5 system. *Immunogenetics* 1979. **9:** 423–433.

18 Donskoy, E. and Goldschneider, I., Thymocytopoiesis is maintained by blood-borne precursors throughout postnatal life: a study in parabiotic mice. *J. Immunol.* 1992. **148:** 1604–1612.

19 Hirokawa, K., Utsuyama, M. and Sado, T., Immunohistological analysis of immigration of thymocyte-precursors into the thymus: evidence for immigration of peripheral T cells into the thymic medulla. *Cell Immunol.* 1989. **119:** 160–170.

20 Godfrey, D. I., Zlotnik, A. and Suda, T., Phenotypic and functional characterization of c-kit expression during intrathymic T cell development. *J. Immunol.* 1992. **149:** 2281–2285.

21 Schmitt, C., Ktorza, S., Sarun, S., Blanc, C., Jong, R. D. and Debre, P., CD34-expressing human thymocyte precursors proliferate in response to interleukin-7 but have lost myeloid differentiation potential. *Blood* 1993. **82:** 3675–3685.

22 Ktorza, S., Sarun, S., Rieux-Laucat, F., de Villartay, J. P., Debre, P. and Schmitt, C., CD34-positive early human thymocytes: T cell receptor and cytokine receptor gene expression. *Eur. J. Immunol.* 1995. **25:** 2471–2478.

23 Sanchez, M. J., Muench, M. O., Roncarolo, M. G., Lanier, L. L. and Phillips, J. H., Identification of a common T/Natural killer cell progenitor in human fetal thymus. *J. Exp. Med.* 1994. **180**: 569–576.

24 Poussier, P., Edouard, P., Lee, C., Binnie, M. and Julius, M., Thymus-independent development and negative selection of T cells expressing T cell receptor α/β in the intestinal epithelium: evidence for distinct circulation patterns of gut- and thymus-derived T lymphocytes. *J. Exp. Med.* 1992. **176**: 187–199.

25 Kawachi, Y., Watanabe, H., Moroda, T., Haga, M., Iiai, T., Hatakeyama, K. and Abo, T., Self-reactive T cell clones in a restricted population of IL-2 receptor β+ cells expressing intermediate levels of the T cell receptor in the liver and other immune organs. *Eur. J. Immunol.* 1995. **25**: 2272–2278.

26 Moroda, T., Iiai, T., Kawachi, Y., Kawamura, T., Hatakeyama, K. and Abo, T., Restricted appearance of self-reactive clones into T cell receptor intermediate cells in neonatally thymectomized mice with autoimmune disease. *Eur. J. Immunol.* 1996. **26**: 3084–3091.

27 Takii, Y., Hashimoto, S., Iiai, T., Watanabe, H., Hatakeyama, K. and Abo, T., Increase in the proportion of granulated CD56+ T cells in patients with malignancy. *Clin. Exp. Immunol.* 1994. **97**: 522–527.

28 Okada, T., Iiai, T., Kawachi, Y., Moroda, T., Takii, Y., Hatakeyama, K. and Abo, T., Origin of CD57+ T cells which increase at tumour sites in patients with colorectal cancer. *Clin. Exp. Immunol.* 1995. **102**: 159–166.

29 Shibata, Y., Bautista, A. P., Pennington, S. N., Humes, J. L. and Volkman, A., Eicosanoid production by peritoneal and splenic macrophages in mice depleted of bone marrow by ^{89}Sr. *Am. J. Pathol.* 1987. **127**: 75–82.

30 Shibata, Y., Dempsey, W. L., Morahan, P. S. and Volkman, A., Selectively eliminated blood monocytes and splenic suppressor macrophages in mice depleted of bone marrow by strontium 89. *J. Leukoc. Biol.* 1985. **38**: 659–669.

31 Shibata, Y. and Volkman, A., The effect of bone marrow depletion on prostaglandin E-producing suppressor macrophages in mouse spleen. *J. Immunol.* 1985. **135**: 3897–3904.

32 Naito, M. and Takahashi, K., The role of Kupffer cells in glucan-induced granuloma formation in the liver of mice depleted of blood monocytes by administration of strontium-89. *Lab. Invest.* 1991. **64**: 664–674.

33 Yamamoto, T., Naito, M., Moriyama, H., Umezu, H., Matsuo, H., Kiwada, H. and Arakawa, M., Repopulation of murine Kupffer cells after intravenous administration of liposome-encapsulated dichloromethylene diphosphonate. *Am. J. Pathol.* 1996. **149**: 1271–1286.

34 Goossens, P. L., Jouin, H., Marchal, G. and Milon, G., Isolation and flow cytometric analysis of the free lymphomyeloid cells present in murine liver. *J. Immunol. Methods* 1990. **132**: 137–144.

35 Ohtsuka, K., Iiai, T., Watanabe, H., Tanaka, T., Miyasaka, M., Sato, K., Asakura, H. and Abo, T., Similarities and differences between extrathymic T cells residing in mouse liver and intestine. *Cell Immunol.* 1994. **153**: 52–66.

Correspondence: Toru Abo, Department of Immunology, Niigata University School of Medicine, Niigata 951-8510, Japan
Fax: +81-2 27-07 66
e-mail: immunol2@med.niigata-u.ac.jp

Administration of Glucocorticoids Markedly Increases the Numbers of Granulocytes and Extrathymic T cells in the Bone Marrow

糖質コルチコイド投与による顕著な骨髄内顆粒球および胸腺外分化T細胞数の増加

Cellular Immunology, 194: 28-35, 1999

chapter 11

Administration of Glucocorticoids Markedly Increases the Numbers of Granulocytes and Extrathymic T cells in the Bone Marrow[1]

糖質コルチコイド投与による顕著な骨髄内顆粒球および
胸腺外分化T細胞数の増加

Satoshi Maruyama,*,† Masahiro Minagawa,*,† Takao Shimizu,*,† Hiroshi Oya,*,† Satoshi Yamamoto,*,†
Nobuyuki Musha,† Wataru Abo,‡ Anura Weerasinghe,* Katsuyoshi Hatakeyama,† and Toru Abo*[2]

*Department of Immunology and †First Department of Surgery, Niigata University School of Medicine, Niigata, Japan;
and ‡Aomori Central Hospital, Aomori, Japan

Received November 12, 1998; accepted March 9, 1999

【要約】

　糖質コルチコイド（ステロイドホルモン）は、抗炎症剤として広く使われている。しかし、臨床医はしばしば、副作用（例、潰瘍や組織損傷）に遭遇する。本研究では、糖質コルチコイドのこのような副作用がどのように起きるか、マウスを用いた実験を行い検証した。ヒドロコルチゾンを二週間毎日マウスに投与したところ（0.5または1.0mg/日/匹）重篤な白血球減少が免疫臓器に出現した。しかし、顆粒球数（Gr-1$^+$Mac-1$^+$）は骨髄と末梢血で増加した。これは、骨髄での骨髄造血能が上昇したのが一因であろう。Ca^{2+}インフラックスと超酸化物産生が示唆するように、顆粒球は数が増加するだけでなく、機能も活性化されていた。胸腺における古いT細胞（CD3^{int}IL-2Rβ$^+$）の比率と骨髄における古いT細胞の数も、増加した。ヒドロコルチゾン投与を行なったマウスは、ストレスに過敏になった。故に、このマウスに拘束ストレス（12時間）を与えると、胃潰瘍が見られた。この結果が示すのは、おそらく、顆粒球の超酸化物産生と古いT細胞の自己応答を通じて、活性化した顆粒球と古いT細胞には、ステロイド潰瘍と組織の損傷をもたらすメカニズムを有する可能性である。

はじめに

　糖質コルチコイドには強力な抗炎症作用があると広く知られている。故に、気管支喘息、アトピー性皮膚炎、ある種の自己免疫疾患などの治療薬に使用される（1-4）。リンパ球の免疫を抑制する影響に加え、顆粒球の機能抑制（例、貪食やアポトーシスの抑制）が、好中球、好塩基球などの細胞において幅広く報告されている（5-12）。しかし、糖質コルチコイドを長期間または高用量使用すると、潰瘍や組織損傷等の副作用が出現することもある（13-23）。ステロイドの副作用が見られた患者の末梢血では顆粒球高値が示されるという臨床研究を報告した（未発表データ）。

　糖質コルチコイド使用により顆粒球増多がど

---

[1] This work was supported by a Grant-in-Aid for Scientific Re-search and Cancer Research from the Ministry of Education, Science, and Culture, Japan.

[2] To whom correspondence should addressed.

[3] 略語：MNC, 単核球、CD3int cells; intermediate CD3 細胞；BM, 骨髄　PB, 末梢血

のように末梢に出現するか検証するべく、糖質コルチコイドをマウスに高用量投与し、骨髄と肝臓における造血能を測定した。この実験プロトコルは、骨髄にだけでなく肝臓にも多分化能幹細胞があり、胸腺外分化T細胞に加えて顆粒球が産生される事実に基づく（24, 25）。糖質コルチコイドの過剰や連続投与は、骨髄内での顆粒球と胸腺外分化T細胞（intermediate TCR細胞）の産生を加速させることが証明された。胸腺内代替経路でも産生されるので、intermediate TCR細胞（TCR^{int}細胞）[3]は、古いT細胞とも呼ばれる（26, 27）。さらに、そのような顆粒球は、活性化状態であることが明らかになった。糖質コルチコイドの過剰投与により、各免疫臓器において、顕著なリンパ球減少が起こったが、それとは反対に骨髄と末梢では、顆粒球の数と機能が増大した。従って、このように活性化した古いT細胞と活性化した顆粒球が原因で、生体の粘膜や組織損傷が出現することが推測される。

材料と方法

マウスとヒドロコルチゾン投与

本研究では、8週齢のC3H/HeNマウス（すべて日本チャールズ・リバー（株）, 日本, 厚木）より購入後、新潟大学動物施設内にて特定病原体未感染下で飼育）を使用した。このマウスに、二週間、毎日、0.5または1mg/匹量のヒドロコルチゾン（Sigma Chemical Co., St. Louis, MO）を皮下投与した。

拘束ストレス

マウスをステンレススチールメッシュで12時間拘束した。通常のマウスでは、胃潰瘍発症に24時間を要する（28）。

細胞調整

ヒドロコルチゾン投与2週間後、マウス各臓器より単核球（MNC）を採取した。肝臓単核球を、定法により分離した（29）。略述すると、エーテル麻酔し、マウスに心採血を行い脱血した。単核球採取にあたり、摘出した肝臓を200ゲージ・ステンレススチールメッシュで濾し、5mM Hepes（日水製薬（株）, 日本, 東京）と2%非働化仔牛血清を添加したEagle's MEM培養液中に懸濁させた。培養液で一度洗浄した後、細胞ペレットを、培養液の中に再懸濁させた。単核球を、肝実質細胞、肝細胞の核やクッパー細胞から、パーコール（100U/mlヘパリンを含む35%パーコール溶液）の勾配を利用し分離した（30）。

脾臓と胸腺を200-ゲージ・ステンレス・スチール・メッシュで濾し、脾臓細胞と胸腺細胞を採取した；脾臓の赤血球を0.83% NH$_4$Cl-Tris緩衝液を用い溶血した（pH 7.6）（29）。培養液で大腿骨内を洗浄して骨髄細胞を採取した。末梢血中単核球採取には、室温にて2%のデキストランに沈降させた（40-50分）後、上清の採取を行なった。赤血球は、NH$_4$Cl-Tris緩衝液を用い除去した。

フローサイトメトリー解析

細胞表面のフェノタイプをモノクロナール抗体を使用した二重免疫蛍光染色テストを行い分析した（31）。FITC、R-フィコエリトリン（R-PE）、またはビオチン標識抗CD3（145-2C11）、抗IL-2Rβ（TM-β1）および抗顆粒球（Gr-1, 6-8C5）モノクロナール抗体は、Pharmingen Co.（San Diego、CA）から購入した。FITC標識抗マクロファージ（Mac-1）モノクロナール抗体（Caltag Laboratories, San Francisco, CA）も使用した。ビオチン標識抗体は、PE標識アビディン（Caltag Laboratories）で発色させた。蛍光陽性の細胞を、FACScan（Becton-Dickinson, Mountain View, CA）を用いて解析した。

フローサイトメトリーを用いた骨髄細胞の細胞質内 Ca^{2+} の測定

骨髄細胞（2×10^6／本）をFluo-3/AM $1\mu M$（Molecular Probes, Eugene, OR）を用いて暗所で培養した（37℃，30分）。骨髄細胞の顆粒球のフローサイトメトリー解析（FACScan）を、前方／側方散乱または蛍光反応を用いて行なった。ゲーティングの際、顆粒球マーカー用いて必ず確認した。ゲーティングをした顆粒球の細胞質の遊離 Ca^{2+} 濃度を、Fluo-3蛍光を用い測定した。Fluo-3陽性細胞は、アルゴン・レーザー488nmで励起され、525nm蛍光の測定を行なった。刺激されていない細胞のFluo-3蛍光（基礎蛍光）は任意レベルにセットした。細胞を暗所でプレ培養し（24℃ 10分）、基礎蛍光測定後、細胞にfMLP（白血球遊走因子：Formyl Methionyl Leucyl Phenylalanine, Sigma Chemical Co.）を添加し刺激した。

ルミノール依存性蛍光反応

ルミノール依存性蛍光反応は、ルミノフォトメータ（TD-4000; Labo Science,Tokyo, Japan）を使用して超酸化物（厳密には H_2O_2 とミエロペロキシダーゼ放出）産生の指標として測定した。呼吸性バーストによるオキシダーゼ系の活性化から生ずる超酸化物産生を、ルミノール依存性蛍光反応で測定できる（33）。細胞を（2×10^6）、緩衝液II（$50\mu l$）（10mM Hepes, 5mM KCl,145mM NaClおよび5.5mM ブドウ糖（pH 7.4））に懸濁させた。この細胞に、ルミノール溶液（$100\mu l$）と緩衝液I（$100\mu l$）を加えた。緩衝液Iの成分は、緩衝液II に1mM $CaCl_2$ およびホルボール－ミリスチン酸塩アセテート（PMA; $20\mu g$）（$50\mu l$）（Sigma Chemical Co., St Louis, Missouri）を加えたものである。蛍光反応には、ルミノフォトメータで10分間、相対発光量を測定した。

血漿カテコラミン値

血漿をアドレナリンとノルアドレナリン値の計測に用いた。定法に従い、値を高速液体クロマトグラフィー（HPLC）法を用いて分析した（34）。検体におけるばらつきを1検体をいくつかに分けて前もって測定したが、各実験におけるばらつきは、アドレナリンで2 pg/ml、ノルアドレナリンで<10 pg/mlであった。

統計分析

有意性差検定には、スチューデントのt検定を用いた。

結果

糖質コルチコイド連続投与による白血球減少

マウスに、2週間毎日0.5または1mg/匹量のヒドロコルチゾンを投与した（Fig. 1）。肝臓、脾臓と胸腺から分離した白血球総数は、顕著に減少した（$P < 0.01$）、一方、骨髄や末梢血における白血球総数に変化は見られなかった。

糖質コルチコイドを投与したマウスの各免疫臓器における全般的な顆粒球の増加

Gr-1とMac-1の二重染色を行い（35）、顆粒球（Gr-1$^+$Mac-1$^+$）およびマクロファージ（Gr-1$^-$Mac-1$^+$）を同時に検証した（Fig. 2A）。対照群では、顆粒球とマクロファージの比率は、肝臓と脾臓におけるごく僅かであったが、骨髄と末梢血での比率は大きかった。胸腺では全く確認できなかった。ヒドロコルチゾンを二週間投与したところ、投与量に比例して、胸腺を除くすべての臓器で顆粒球の比率が増加した。

肝臓のNK細胞と胸腺のCD3^{int}細胞は糖質コルチコイド耐性である

CD3とIL-2Rβの二重染色を行い（36）、NK細胞（CD3$^-$IL-2Rβ$^+$）、胸腺外分化T細胞（CD3^{int}IL-2Rβ$^+$）および従来のT細胞（CD3^{high}IL-2Rβ$^-$）を解析した（Fig. 2B）。第1に、NK細胞（17.8%）と胸腺外分化T細胞

Figure.1

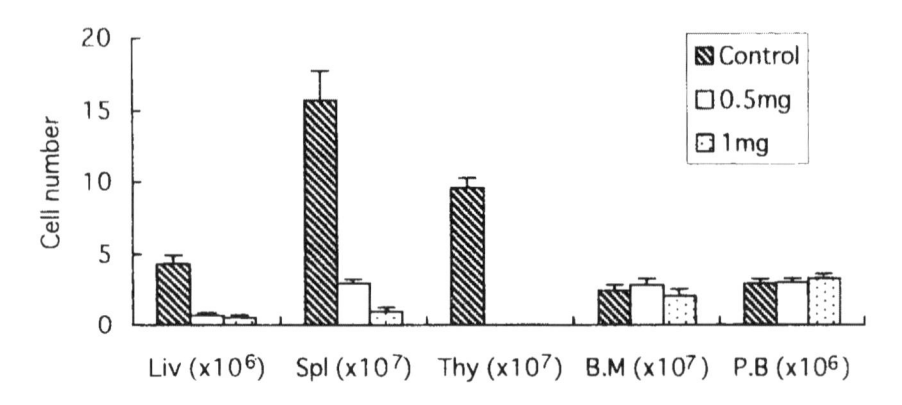

ヒドロコルチゾンの投与前後に、白血球総数をマウス諸免疫臓器において測定した。マウスに、2週間毎日0.5または1mg/匹のヒドロコルチゾンを投与した。平均値±1 SDを4匹のマウスを用いて算出した。

Figure.3

ヒドロコルチゾン投与したマウスにおいて、骨髄と末梢血の顆粒球数および骨髄における古いT細胞数が増加した。平均値±SDを4匹のマウスを用いて算出した。

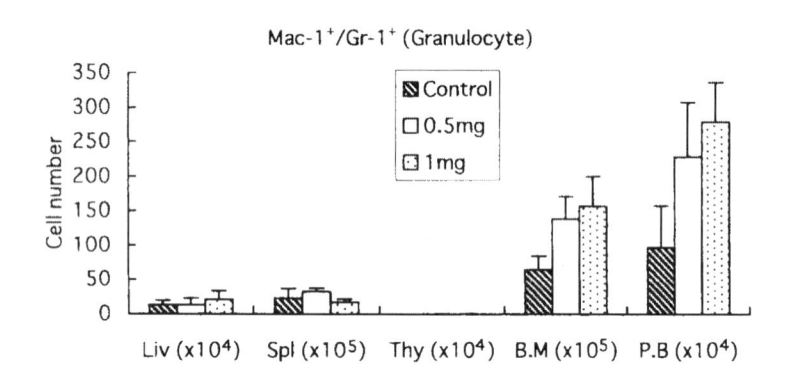

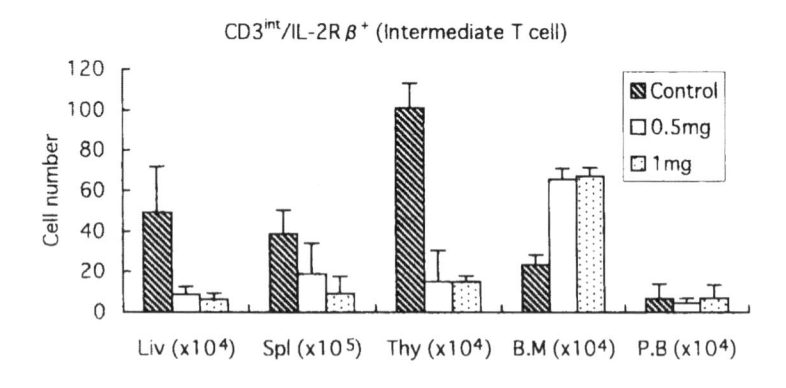

(17.9%)は、対照群マウスの肝臓に豊富であった。ヒドロコルチゾンを投与した後、NK細胞の比率が増加する傾向を示した。脾臓細胞数は顕著な減少を示したが、脾臓におけるリンパ球サブセットの分画には変化が見られなかった。

先行研究の通り(37)、胸腺細胞には、CD3⁻、CD3^{dull}とCD3^{high}細胞があり(Fig. 2対照群マウス)、すべての細胞においてIL-2Rβの発現は見られなかった。CD3^{int}IL-2Rβ^{+}細胞は、対照群マウスにおいて非常に少数(1.3%)であった

Figure.2

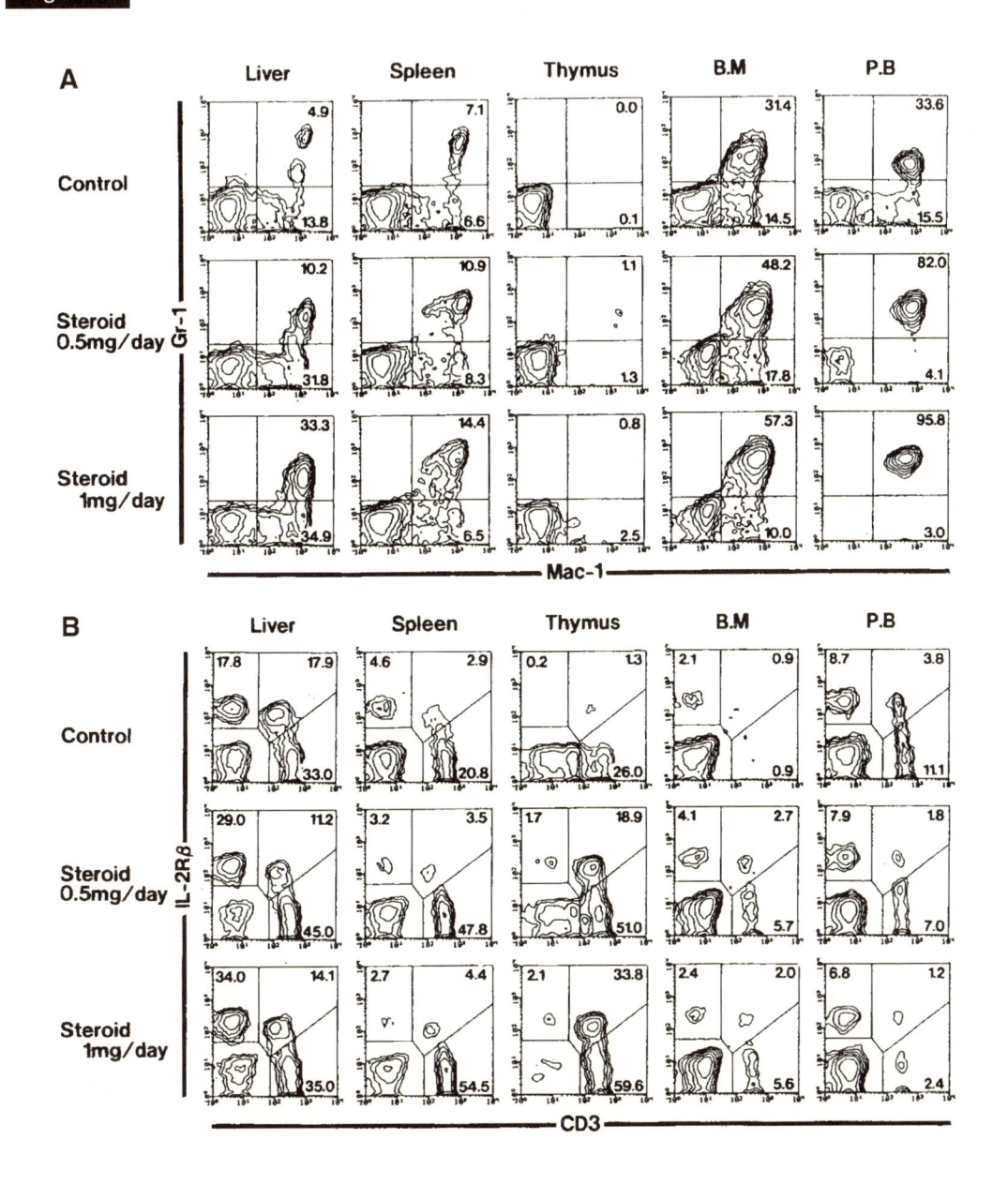

ヒドロコルチゾン投与の前後のマウスにおける細胞のフェノタイプ (A)Gr-1とMac-1の二重染色。(B)CD3とIL-2Rβの二重染色。マウスに、2週間毎日0.5または1mg/匹量のヒドロコルチゾンを投与した。3度実験を行なった典型例を示す。各分画内の数値は蛍光陽性細胞の比率を示す。

(Fig. 2)。一方、実験（ヒドロコルチゾン投与）群では、CD3^{int}IL-2Rβ$^+$細胞の比率は33.8%まで増加した。骨髄と末梢血において、リンパ球サブセットの染色パターンは変化しなかった。

糖質コルチコイドの顆粒球と胸腺外分化T細胞の絶対数に対する影響

白血球分画から顆粒球（Gr-1$^+$Mac-1$^+$）と胸腺外分化T細胞（CD3^{int}IL-2Rβ$^+$）の絶対数を算出した（図3）。平均値±1SDを4匹のマウス

Figure.4

対照群と実験（ヒドロコルチゾン投与）群マウスの骨髄細胞のCa^{2+}インフラックス値。平均蛍光ベースラインは、fMLP刺激なしの対照群マウスにおける骨髄細胞のCa^{2+}流入を示す。実験群（ヒドロコルチゾン投与）マウスにおける骨髄細胞からのCa^{2+}インフラックスのベースラインは、同じであった。3度実験を行なった典型例を示す。骨髄細胞にfMLP刺激を与えると、両群の間に平均蛍光の顕著な相違が出現した。実験群マウスの骨髄の顆粒球は、活性化状態であった。

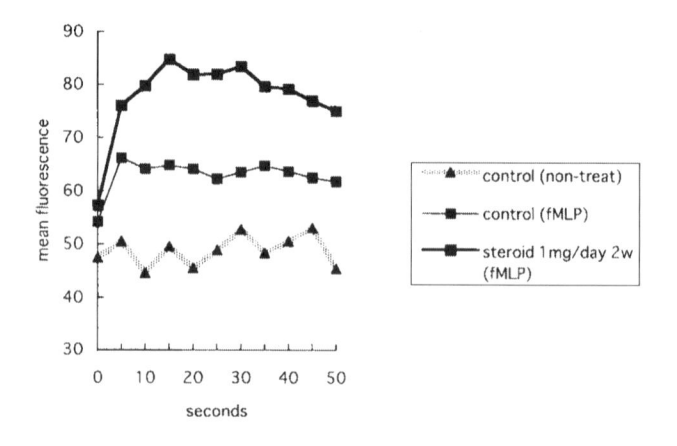

Figure.5

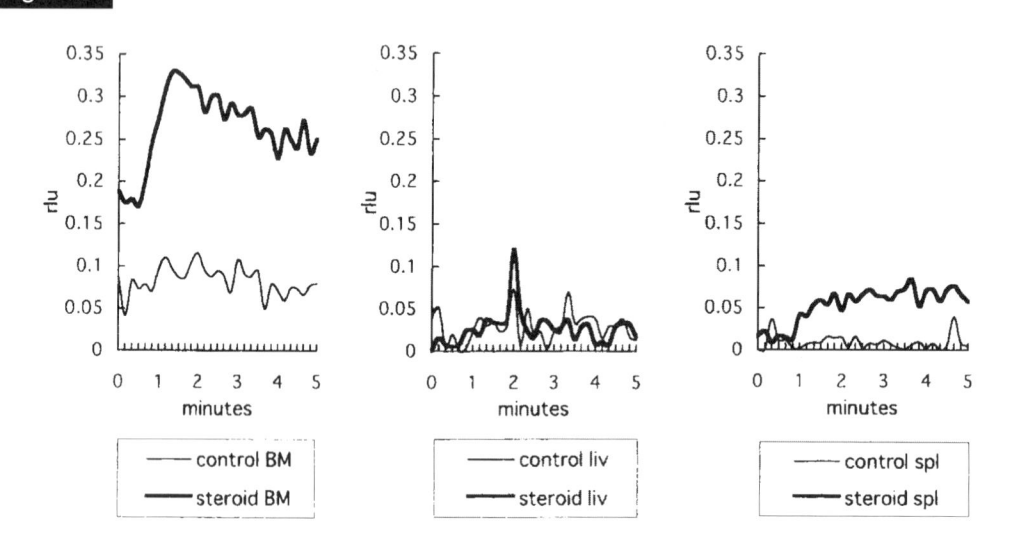

対照群および実験（ヒドロコルチゾン投与）群マウスの骨髄細胞、肝単核球と脾臓細胞における超酸化物産生。超酸化物産生をfMLP刺激後、ケミルミネセンスを用い測定した。3度実験を行なった典型例を示す。

を用いて算出した。骨髄と末梢血中における顆粒球数は、実験（ヒドロコルチゾン投与）群において投与量に比例して増加した（P<0.05）。一方、胸腺外分化T細胞は、骨髄以外のすべての臓器で減少したが（P<0.01）、骨髄では増加した（P < 0.05）。

糖質コルチコイドは、骨髄内における顆粒球の機能を活性化させる

骨髄内での顆粒球数の増加によりその機能が活性化されるか、fMLP刺激後のCa^{2+}インフラックス測定を行い検証した（Fig. 4）。対照群および実験（ヒドロコルチゾン投与）群マウスの骨髄顆粒球の蛍光ベースラインは同じであった（ボトムラインとする）。しかし、fMLPで刺激を与えると、実験（ヒドロコルチゾン投与）群マウスの骨髄顆粒球は対照群マウスものより高いCa^{2+}インフラックスを示した。同じ刺激を与えて、活性化した顆粒球が超酸化物を産生したかどうか検証した（Fig. 5）。実験（ヒドロコルチゾン投与）群マウスの骨髄から分離した細胞（脾臓細胞もある程度）の超酸化物産生の高いレベルを示した。

Table.I

糖質コルチコイド投与しても血清カテコラミン値は変化しなかった。

Mice[a]	Serum concentration of catecholamines (pg/ml)	
	Adrenaline	Noradrenaline
Control	15,386 ± 678[b]	16,794 ± 896
Steroid (0.5 mg/day/mouse)	16,383 ± 453	18,832 ± 746
Steroid (1 mg/day/mouse)	10,209 ± 1095	10,170 ± 1134

[a] マウスに、2週間毎日上記量のヒドロコルチゾンを投与した。
[b] いずれも統計的有意差を示さなかった（P＞0.05）。

血清カテコラミン値は、ヒドロコルチゾンを投与しても変化しなかった

最近の一連の研究（34, 38-40）において、交感神経緊張またはアドレナリン（ノルアドレナリン）投与により、顆粒球の数と機能が増加することが明らかになった。そこで、ヒドロコルチゾンの連続投与により交感神経系の刺激が起こるか検証した（Table I）。血清中アドレナリンとノルアドレナリン値を測定した。ヒドロコルチゾンのいずれの濃度においても有意差は観察されなかった。

ヒドロコルチゾン投与群マウスは、ストレスの影響を受けやすい

活性化した顆粒球がその後の組織損傷に関与したかどうか検証した。そこで、対照群および実験（ヒドロコルチゾン投与）群マウスに拘束ストレス（12時間）を与えた（Fig. 6）。正常マウスの胃潰瘍発症には24時間を要するとの報告がある（28）。対照群では、全く胃潰瘍は見られなかった（Fig. 6A）。全く対照的に、ヒドロコルチゾンを1mg/匹、2週間、毎日予め投与した実験群マウスでは、12時間で数多くの潰瘍が見られた（Fig. 6B）。これは、実験（ヒドロコルチゾン投与）群全マウス（n=6）において確認できた。

Figure.6

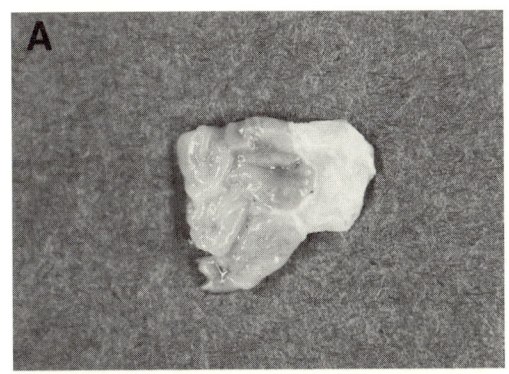

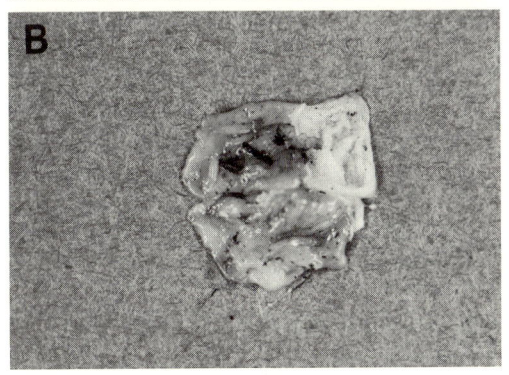

ヒドロコルチゾン投与を行ったマウスにおける胃潰瘍形成。（A）対照群。（B）実験（ヒドロコルチゾン投与）群マウス。対照群および実験（ヒドロコルチゾン投与）群マウス（どちらもn=6）に拘束ストレス（12時間）を与えた。実験（ヒドロコルチゾン投与）群マウスの全てに激しい胃潰瘍が見られた。

考察

本研究により糖質コルチコイドを連続投与すると顆粒球と胸腺外分化T細胞の数と機能が上昇することが明らかになった。顆粒球数の増加は末梢血だけでなく骨髄にもみられた。これは、骨髄造血そのものが更新しているようであった。先行研究と本研究に示すように（41）、糖質コルチコイド投与により全免疫臓器において顕著にリンパ球が減少するが、そこで、糖質コルチコイドは広く抗炎症剤として広く使用されている（1-4）。しかし、糖質コルチコイドには副作用もある（13-23）。本研究は、顆粒球と胸腺外分化T（または古いT）細胞に対する影響

は、薬剤の副作用と関係するメカニズムと考えられる可能性を示唆する。本研究の最後に、実験（ヒドロコルチゾン投与）群マウスは、拘束ストレスに曝された際、胃潰瘍が発症したことを示した。

最近の研究において、成年マウス肝臓にはc-kit$^+$幹細胞を有することを報告したが、この肝c-kit$^+$幹細胞は、顆粒球と胸腺外分化T細胞を産生する（24, 25）。従来型T細胞（胸腺で産生され肝臓に移動してきた）は主として肝類洞に存在する（42）。対照的に、顆粒球と胸腺外分化T細胞（肝臓で産生される）は、実質に存在する。ヒドロコルチゾンを投与すると、肝臓と骨髄において顆粒球（Gr-1$^+$Mac-1$^+$）の比率が上昇した。しかし、肝臓の顆粒球数の増加は、骨髄のものほど顕著ではなかった。換言すると、骨髄の造血能が主に糖質コルチコイド投与により増大したのであった。

本研究が示すのは、ヒドロコルチゾン投与により、胸腺において古いT細胞（CD3^{int}IL-2Rβ^+）の比率が上昇し、骨髄において細胞数が増加することである。以前にも報告したが（26, 27, 43）、胸腺内代替経路と同様に、肝臓や骨髄で古いT細胞（CD3^{int}IL-2Rβ^+）の産生が起こる。一方、従来型T細胞（CD3^{high}IL-2Rβ^+）は、胸腺内のT細胞分化の主経路で産生される（44-49）。従来型T細胞と古いT細胞の特徴の違いは、ダブルネガティブ（CD4$^-$8$^-$）細胞と自己応答性クローンの存在である（26, 27, 43）。これら古いT細胞は、増殖が速い自己細胞（例、胸腺細胞、肝細胞と腸上皮細胞）に対して自己応答性を示すことができる（50, 51）。超酸化物産生と組織破壊をすることができる活性化した顆粒球（52, 53）のみならず、自己応答性を持つ古いT細胞は、糖質コルチコイドで潰瘍が発症するような副作用に関与する可能性がある。

糖質コルチコイドを連続投与すると顆粒球が活性化することを次の二つの指標より確認できた；Ca^{2+}インフラックスと超酸化物産生である。先行研究のように（32）、Ca^{2+}インフラックスの値が高いと、fMLP刺激後の超酸化物産生が上昇する。このように考えると、活性化した顆粒球は、潰瘍発症や組織破壊の原因である可能性がある。ヒトを対象にした予備研究を行なったところ、ステロイド潰瘍患者の小腸などの炎症粘膜組織から顆粒球やCD56$^+$T細胞（ヒトにおける胸腺外分化T細胞）（54, 55）を大量に採取できた（未発表データ）。

現時点では、糖質コルチコイドにより顆粒球が増多する真の基礎メカニズムは不詳である。顆粒球表面にはアドレナリン受容体があり、カテコラミンを投与すると活性化するので（34, 38-40）、対照群および実験（ヒドロコルチゾン投与）群マウスの血清カテコラミン値を測定した。しかし、二群のマウスに違いは見られなかった。G-CSFやGM-CSFなどサイトカインの中には、この現象と関係しているものがある可能性がある。予備研究を行ったところ、過剰なヒドロコルチゾンは、組織停滞し、酸化コレステロールに変性することが明らかになった（未発表データ）。諸ステロイドホルモンは、コレステロール構造を有する。この点から、ステロイドホルモンの性質が有害な酸化物質になることを考慮する必要がある。

糖質コルチコイドは、リンパ球の免疫を抑制する機能があることや顆粒球を抑制する機能に作用するという報告が多数ある（4-12）。これまでの論旨をまとめると、本研究は、ステロイドホルモン投与により顆粒球の機能を強化する、そして、おそらく酸化したステロイドホルモンが、生体に停滞すると、近年、確認されたリンパ球集団（CD3^{int}細胞）が増加することを示した最初の研究である。

謝辞

渡辺正子氏の浄書と橋本哲夫氏の動物飼育に感謝する。

Administration of Glucocorticoids Markedly Increases the Numbers of Granulocytes and Extrathymic T Cells in the Bone Marrow[1]

Satoshi Maruyama,*,† Masahiro Minagawa,*,† Takao Shimizu,*,† Hiroshi Oya,*,† Satoshi Yamamoto,*,† Nobuyuki Musha,† Wataru Abo,‡ Anura Weerasinghe,* Katsuyoshi Hatakeyama,† and Toru Abo*,[2]

*Department of Immunology and †First Department of Surgery, Niigata University School of Medicine, Niigata, Japan; and ‡Aomori Central Hospital, Aomori, Japan

Received November 12, 1998; accepted March 9, 1999

Glucocorticoids, steroid hormones, are widely used as an anti-inflammatory drug. However, clinicians have sometimes encountered adverse drug reactions such as ulcers and tissue damage. In this study, we investigated how such adverse reactions of glucocorticoids are evoked, using an experimental mice model. When hydrocortisone (0.5 or 1.0 mg/day/mouse) was administered daily for 2 weeks, severe leukocytopenia was induced in all immune system organs. However, granulocytes (Gr-1$^+$Mac-1$^+$) were increased in number in the bone marrow and peripheral blood. This seemed to be due to an elevated level of myelopoiesis in the bone marrow. As well as increasing in number, granulocytes were functionally activated as estimated by the Ca^{2+} influx and superoxide production. The proportion of primordial T cells (CD3^{int}IL-2Rβ^+) in the thymus and the number of primordial T cells in the bone marrow also increased. Mice administered hydrocortisone became susceptible to stress. Thus, these mice showed gastric ulcers when they were exposed to restraint stress for 12 h. These results suggest that activated granulocytes and primordial T cells might provide a mechanism involved in steroid ulcers and tissue damage, possibly through the superoxide production of granulocytes and the autoreactivity of primordial T cells. © 1999 Academic Press

INTRODUCTION

It is widely known that glucocorticoids have a potent anti-inflammatory function. Therefore, they are used as therapeutic agents in cases of bronchial asthma, atopic dermatitis, certain autoimmune diseases, etc. (1–4). An immunosuppressive effect on lymphocytes and also an inhibitory function on granulocytes (e.g., suppression of phagocytosis and apoptosis) have been widely reported in neutrophils, basophils, and other cells (5–12). However, glucocorticoids sometimes induce adverse drug reactions, such as ulcers and tissue damage, when they are used for a long time or at high doses (13–23). In clinical studies, we have observed that affected patients show an elevated level of granulocytes in the peripheral blood (our unpublished observation).

To investigate how granulocytosis is induced in the periphery by the use of glucocorticoids, we treated mice with glucocorticoids at high doses and examined myelopoiesis in the bone marrow and liver. This protocol is based on the fact that not only the bone marrow but also the liver contains pluripotent stem cells that produce granulocytes as well as extrathymic T cells (24, 25). It was demonstrated that excessive and continuous administration of glucocorticoids accelerated the generation of granulocytes and extrathymic T cells (i.e., intermediate TCR cells) in the bone marrow. Since intermediate TCR cells (TCR^{int} cells)[3] are also generated by an alternative intrathymic pathway, we sometimes call them primordial T cells (26, 27). Moreover, such granulocytes were found to be in an activated state. Although excessive administration of glucocorticoids induced profound lymphocytopenia in various immune system organs, it inversely increased the number and function of granulocytes in the bone marrow and periphery. It is therefore speculated that such activated granulocytes together with activated primordial T cells then induce mucosal and/or tissue damage in hosts.

MATERIALS AND METHODS

Mice and hydrocortisone injection. Eight-week-old C3H/HeN mice, fed under specific pathogen-free conditions in our laboratory, were used for this study. All

---
[1] This work was supported by a Grant-in-Aid for Scientific Research and Cancer Research from the Ministry of Education, Science, and Culture, Japan.
[2] To whom correspondence should addressed.

[3] Abbreviations used: MNC, mononuclear cells, CD3^{int} cells; intermediate CD3 cells; BM, bone marrow; PB, peripheral blood.

mice were originally obtained from Charles River Japan, Inc. (Atsugi, Japan). Mice were injected with hydrocortisone subcutaneously (Sigma Chemical Co., St. Louis, MO) daily for 2 weeks at a concentration of 0.5 or 1 mg/day/mouse.

Restraint stress. Mice were exposed to stainless steel mesh for 12 h. In the case of normal mice, 24 h is required to induce gastric ulcers (28).

Cell preparation. Mononuclear cells (MNC) were harvested from various organs of mice 2 weeks after hydrocortisone administration. Hepatic MNC were isolated by a method described elsewhere (29). Briefly, mice anesthetized with ether were sacrificed by total exsanguination via a cardiac puncture. To obtain MNC, the liver was removed, pressed through 200-gauge stainless steel mesh, and then suspended in Eagle's MEM supplemented with 5 mM Hepes (Nissui Pharmaceutical Co., Tokyo, Japan) and 2% heat-inactivated newborn calf serum. After being washed with the medium once, the cell pellet was resuspended in the medium. MNC were isolated from parenchymal hepatocytes, the nuclei of hepatocytes, and Kupffer cells by the Percoll (35% Percoll containing 100 U/ml heparin) gradient method (30).

Splenocytes and thymocytes were obtained by pressing the spleen and thymus through 200-gauge steel mesh; erythrocytes in the spleen were lysed by 0.83% NH_4Cl–Tris buffer (pH 7.6) (29). Bone marrow cells were obtained by flushing femurs with the medium. Blood MNC were collected by 2% dextran sedimentation for 40–50 min at room temperature and then the supernatant was harvested. Erythrocytes were also eliminated by the NH_4Cl–Tris buffer.

Immunofluorescence test. The surface phenotypes of cells were analyzed using mAbs in conjunction with a two-color immunofluorescence test (31). FITC, R-phycoerythrin (R-PE), or biotin-conjugated anti-CD3 (145-2C11), anti-IL-2Rβ (TM-β1), and anti-granulocyte (Gr-1, RB6-8C5) mAbs were obtained from Pharmingen Co. (San Diego, CA). An FITC-conjugated anti-macrophage (Mac-1) mAb (Caltag Laboratories, San Francisco, CA) was also used. Biotin-conjugated reagents were developed with PE-conjugated avidin (Caltag Laboratories). The fluorescence-positive cells were analyzed with a FACScan (Becton-Dickinson, Mountain View, CA).

Measurement of cytosolic Ca^{2+} in bone marrow cells by flow cytometry. Bone marrow cells (2×10^6 cells/tube) were incubated for 30 min at 37°C in the dark with Fluo-3/AM (Molecular Probes, Eugene, OR) at a concentration of 1 μM (32). Flow cytometric analysis (FACScan) of bone marrow cells allows granulocytes to be identified by their forward/side scatter or fluorescence characteristics. Gate settings were always verified with the help of the granulocyte marker. The concentration of cytosolic free Ca^{2+} in the gated granulocytes was measured using Fluo-3 fluorescence. Fluo-3-loaded cells were excited with an argon laser at 488 nm and fluorescence was measured at 525 nm. The Fluo-3 fluorescence of unstimulated cells (basal fluorescence) was set at an arbitrary level. Cells were preincubated at 24°C in the dark for 10 min. After measurement of basal fluorescence, cells were stimulated by the addition of fMLP (Sigma Chemical Co.).

Luminol-dependent chemiluminescence. Luminol-dependent chemiluminescence was determined as an indicator of superoxide production (more accurately H_2O_2 and myeloperoxidase release) by a lumiphotometer (TD-4000; Labo Science, Tokyo, Japan). Superoxide production resulting from the activation of the respiratory burst oxidase system can be measured by the luminol-dependent chemiluminescence response (33). Cells (2×10^6) were suspended in 50 μl of buffer II, consisting of 10 mM Hepes, 5 mM KCl, 145 mM NaCl, and 5.5 mM glucose (pH 7.4). To the cells were added 100 μl of luminol solution and 100 μl of buffer I, consisting of buffer II supplemented with 1 mM $CaCl_2$, and 50 μl of phorbol myristate acetate (PMA; 20 μg/ml)

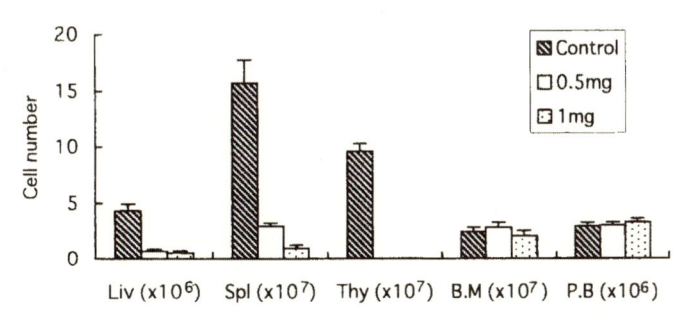

FIG. 1. The number of leukocytes yielded by various immune system organs of mice before and after administration of hydrocortisone. Mice were injected with hydrocortisone daily for 2 weeks at a concentration of 0.5 or 1 mg/day/mouse. The mean and SD are for four mice.

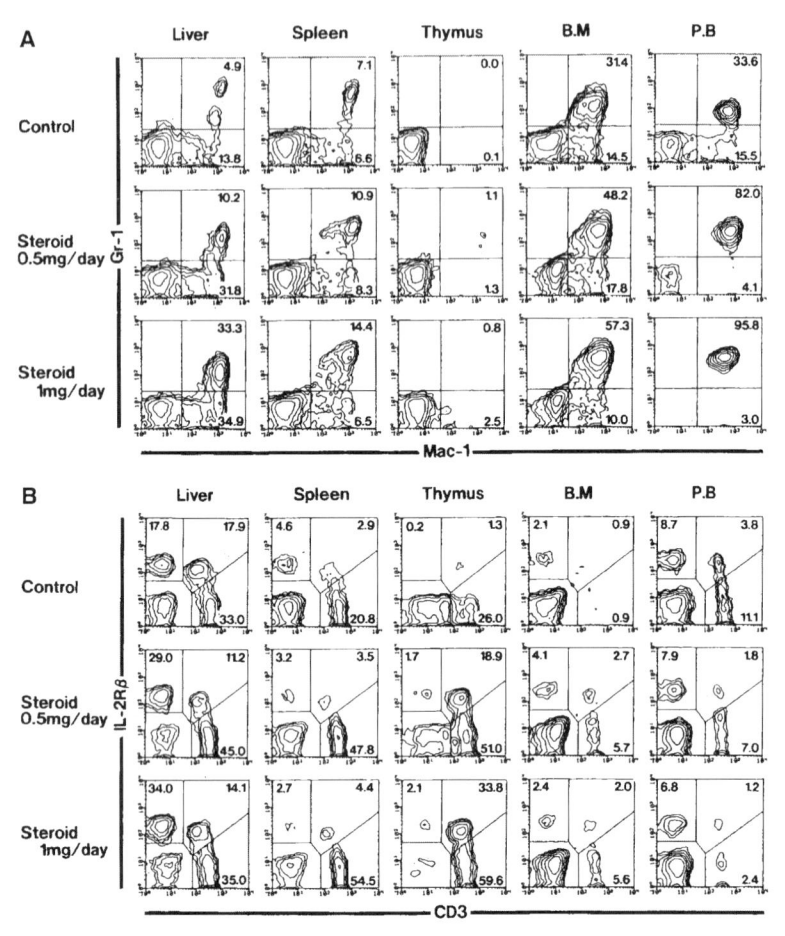

FIG. 2. Phenotypic characterization of cells in mice before and after administration of hydrocortisone. (A) Two-color staining for Gr-1 and Mac-1. (B) Two-color staining for CD3 and IL-2Rβ. Mice were injected with hydrocortisone daily for 2 weeks at a concentration of 0.5 or 1 mg/day/mouse. Representative results of three experiments are depicted. The numbers in the figure represent the percentages of fluorescence-positive cells in the corresponding areas.

(Sigma Chemical Co.). Chemiluminescence was monitored by the lumiphotometer for 10 min and is expressed in relative light units.

Serum level of catecholamines. Plasma was used to measure the concentration of adrenaline and noradrenaline. The concentrations were analyzed by the high-performance liquid chromatography (HPLC) system, as described elsewhere (34). Preliminary experiments of separate aliquots in one sample showed us that experiment-to-experiment variation was <2 pg/ml for adrenaline and <10 pg/ml for noradrenaline.

Statistical analysis. Statistical significance was analyzed by using Student's t test.

RESULTS

Leukocytopenia induced by continuous administration of glucocorticoids. Mice were was subcutaneously administered hydrocortisone daily for 2 weeks at a concentration of 0.5 or 1 mg/day/mouse (Fig. 1). The numbers of leukocytes isolated from the liver, spleen, and thymus were profoundly reduced ($P < 0.01$), whereas those from the bone marrow and peripheral blood remained unchanged.

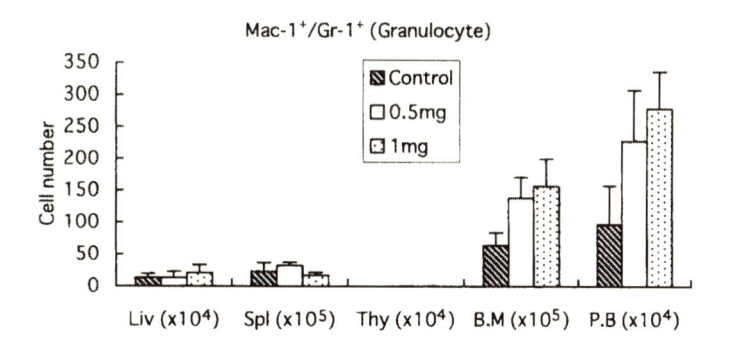

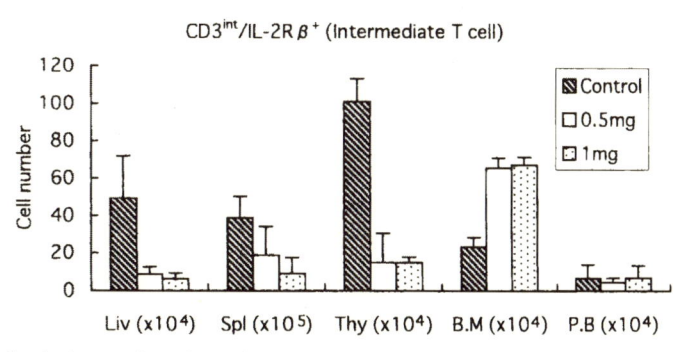

FIG. 3. Increase in the absolute numbers of granulocytes in the bone marrow and peripheral blood and in the absolute number of primordial T cells in the bone marrow of mice administered hydrocortisone. The mean and SD are for four mice.

Generalized expansion of granulocytes in various immune system organs of mice administered glucocorticoids. By two-color staining for Gr-1 and Mac-1 (35), granulocytes (Gr-1$^+$Mac-1$^+$) and macrophages (Gr-1$^-$Mac-1$^+$) were simultaneously identified (Fig. 2A). In control mice, a small proportion of granulocytes and macrophages was identified in the liver and spleen, and a large proportion was identified in the bone marrow and peripheral blood; none were found in the thymus. When hydrocortisone was administered for 2 weeks, the proportion of granulocytes increased in all organs tested, except the thymus, in a dose-dependent manner.

NK cells in the liver and CD3^{int} cells in the thymus are glucocorticoid-resistant. By two-color staining for CD3 and IL-2Rβ (36), NK cells (CD3$^-$IL-2Rβ$^+$), extrathymic T cells (CD3^{int}IL-2Rβ$^+$), and conventional T cells (CD3^{high}IL-2Rβ$^-$) were identified (Fig. 2B). Primarily, NK cells (17.8%) and extrathymic T cells (17.9%) were abundant in the liver of control mice. After the administration of hydrocortisone, the proportion of NK cells tended to increase. Although the number of splenocytes decreased prominently, the distribution pattern of lymphocyte subsets remained unchanged in the spleen. As already reported (37) and shown in Fig. 2 (see control mice), thymocytes comprised CD3$^-$, CD3^{dull}, and CD3^{high} cells, all lacking the expression of IL-2Rβ. CD3^{int}IL-2Rβ$^+$ cells were an extremely minor population in normal mice (1.3% in Fig. 2). On the other hand, after the administration of hydrocortisone, the proportion of CD3^{int}IL-2Rβ$^+$ cells increased to 33.8%.

In the bone marrow and peripheral blood, the staining pattern of lymphocyte subsets remained unchanged.

Effect of glucocorticoids on the absolute numbers of granulocytes and extrathymic T cells. In addition to the proportion of leukocytes, the absolute numbers of granulocytes (Gr-1$^+$Mac-1$^+$) and extrathymic T cells (CD3^{int}IL-2Rβ$^+$) were calculated (Fig. 3). The data are for four mice and are represented as the mean and one SD. The absolute numbers of granulocytes in the bone marrow and peripheral blood increased in a dose-dependent manner with hydrocortisone administration ($P < 0.05$). In contrast, the absolute number of extra-

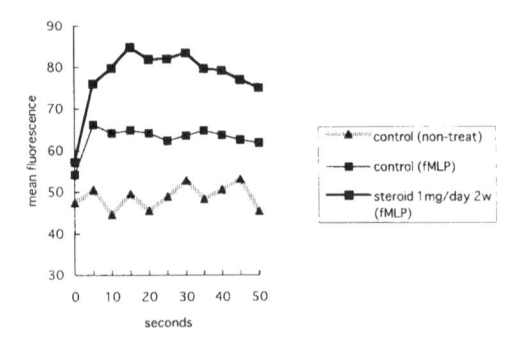

FIG. 4. Ca^{2+} influx in bone marrow cells in control and hydrocortisone-treated mice. The baseline of mean fluorescence shows the Ca^{2+} influx from bone marrow cells in control mice without fMLP stimulation. The baseline of Ca^{2+} influx from bone marrow cells in hydrocortisone-treated mice was the same. Representative results of three experiments are depicted. When bone marrow cells were stimulated with fMLP, a clear difference of the mean fluorescence emerged between control and treated mice. Granulocytes in the bone marrow of treated mice were in an activated state.

TABLE 1
Administration of Glucocorticoids Did Not Change the Serum Concentration of Catecholamines

Mice[a]	Serum concentration of catecholamines (pg/ml)	
	Adrenaline	Noradrenaline
Control	15,386 ± 678[b]	16,794 ± 896
Steroid (0.5 mg/day/mouse)	16,383 ± 453	18,832 ± 746
Steroid (1 mg/day/mouse)	10,209 ± 1095	10,170 ± 1134

[a] Mice were administered hydrocortisone at the indicated concentrations daily for 2 weeks.
[b] None of the changes were statistically significant ($P > 0.05$).

thymic T cells decreased in all organs ($P < 0.01$), except the bone marrow, where they increased ($P < 0.05$).

Glucocorticoids activate the function of granulocytes in the bone marrow. We tested whether the increase in the number of granulocytes in the bone marrow was accompanied by functional activation, using Ca^{2+} influx after fMLP stimulation (Fig. 4). Baseline fluorescence of bone marrow granulocytes from control and hydrocortisone-treated mice was the same (bottom line). However, bone marrow granulocytes in hydrocortisone-treated mice showed a higher level of Ca^{2+} influx than that in control mice, when stimulated with fMLP.

Using the same stimulus, it was examined whether superoxides were produced by activated granulocytes (Fig. 5). Cells isolated from the bone marrow (and to some extent, those from the spleen) of hydrocortisone-treated mice showed an elevated level of superoxide production.

Serum catecholamine levels are not changed by the administration of hydrocortisone. In a series of recent studies (34, 38–40), we demonstrated that sympathetic nerve activation or the administration of adrenaline (and noradrenalin) itself increased granulocyte number and function. Hence, we examined whether continuous administration of hydrocortisone stimulated the sympathetic nervous system (Table 1). Serum levels of adrenaline and noradrenaline were measured. A statistical difference was not observed at any concentration of hydrocortisone.

Mice administered hydrocortisone are susceptible to stress. It was then examined whether activated granulocytes were eventually associated with tissue damage. For this purpose, control and hydrocortisone-treated mice were exposed to restraint stress for 12 h (Fig. 6). It was reported that 24 h is required to induce

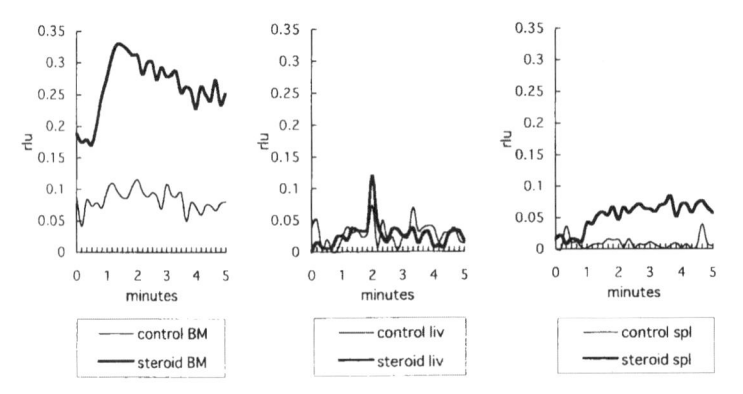

FIG. 5. Superoxide production in bone marrow cells, liver cells, and splenocytes from control and hydrocortisone-treated mice. Superoxide production was estimated by chemiluminescence after fMLP stimulation. Representative results of three experiments are depicted.

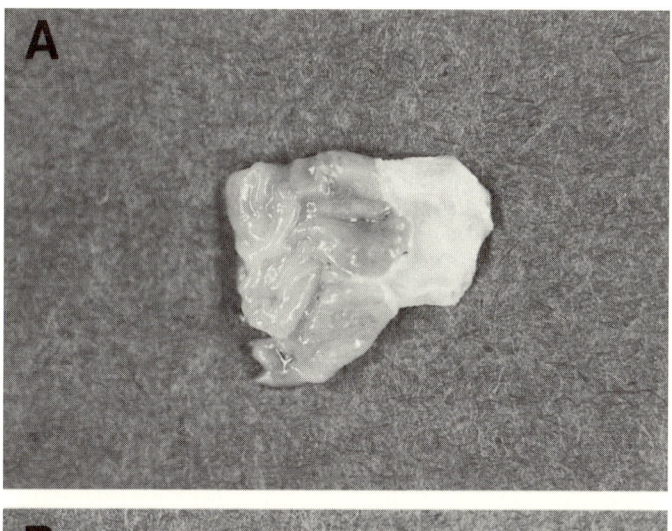

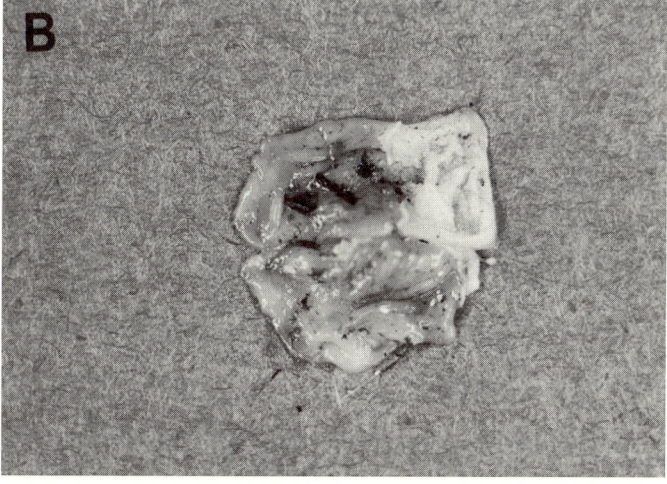

FIG. 6. Gastric ulcer formation in mice administered hydrocortisone. (A) Control mice. (B) Hydrocortisone-treated mice. Control and hydrocortisone-treated mice (six mice each) were exposed to restraint stress for 12 h. All hydrocortisone-treated mice showed severe gastric ulcers.

gastric ulcers in normal mice (28). In the case of control mice, we could not see any ulcers in the stomach (Fig. 6A). In sharp contrast, mice that were pretreated with hydrocortisone (1 mg/day/mouse) for 2 weeks showed many ulcers in the stomach for 12 h (Fig. 6B). This was true in all six hydrocortisone-treated mice.

DISCUSSION

In the present study, we demonstrated that the continuous administration of glucocorticoids increased granulocyte and extrathymic T cell number and function. Since the increase in the number of granulocytes was seen not only in the peripheral blood but also in the bone marrow, myelopoiesis itself seemed to be augmented. The adminstration of glucocorticoids induces severe lymphocytopenia in all immune organs as shown previously (41) and in this study, and therefore glucocorticoids are widely used as anti-inflammatory drugs (1–4). However, they cause some adverse drug reactions (13–23). The present study suggests that the effect on granulocytes and extrathymic T (or primordial T) cells might be considered a mechanism involved in such adverse reactions. In a final portion of the present experiments, we showed that hydrocortisone-treated mice fell victim to gastric ulcers when they were exposed to restraint stress.

In a recent study, we reported that the adult liver in mice contains c-kit$^+$ stem cells, which then give rise to granuloycytes and extrathymic T cells (24, 25). Conventional T cells, which are seen in the liver but migrate from the thymus, are present mainly in the sinusoidal lumen (42). In contrast, granulocytes and extrathymic T cells, which are generated in the liver, are present in the parenchymal space. The proportion of granulocytes (Gr-1$^+$Mac-1$^+$) was increased in the liver and in the bone marrow by the administration of hydrocortisone. However, the increase in the absolute number of granulocytes in the liver was not as marked as in the bone marrow. In other words, myelopoiesis in the bone marrow was augmented mainly by the administration of glucocorticoids.

This study indicates that the administration of hydrocortisone increases the proportion of primordial T cells (CD3^{int}IL-2Rβ^+) in the thymus and increases the absolute number in the bone marrow. As reported previously (26, 27, 43), primordial T cells (CD3^{int}IL-2Rβ^+) are generated extrathymically in the liver and bone marrow, as well as by an alternative intrathymic pathway. On the other hand, conventional T cells (CD3^{high}IL-2Rβ^-) are generated through the mainstream of T-cell differentiation in the thymus (44–49). Some characteristics of primordial T cells that differ from those of conventional T cells include double-negative CD4$^-$8$^-$ cells and self-reactive clones (26, 27, 43). These primordial T cells are able to mediate autoreactivity against rapidly proliferating self-cells (e.g., thymocytes, hepatocytes, and intestinal epithelial cells) (50, 51). Together with activated granulocytes showing superoxide production and the ability to damage tissue (52, 53), the autoreactivity of these primordial T cells might contribute to adverse reactions such as ulcers obtained with glucocorticoids.

Activation of granulocytes induced by the continuous administration of glucocorticoids was confirmed by two indicators, Ca^{2+} influx and superoxide production. As shown previously (32), the elevated level of Ca^{2+} influx results in an augmented level of superoxide production after fMLP stimulation. As we speculate above, such activated granulocytes might be responsible for the formation of ulcers and tissue damage. In a preliminary study in humans, we have been able to isolate many granulocytes and CD56$^+$ T cells (a human counterpart of extrathymic T cells) (54, 55) from inflammatory mucosal tissue (e.g., the small intestine) in patients with steroid ulcers (our unpublished observation).

As present, we do not know the actual mechanisms underlying granulocytosis induced by glucocorticoids. Since granulocytes bear surface adrenergic receptors and are activated by the administration of catecholamines (34, 38–40), we measured the serum level of catecholamines in control and hydrocortisone-treated mice. However, there were no differences between these mice. There is a possibility that some cytokines such as G-CSF and GM-CSF might be associated with the present phenomenon. In a preliminary study, we found that hydrocortisone, which was dosed excessively, stagnated in the tissue and turned to oxidized cholesterols (our unpublished observation). Steroid homones originate from a cholesterol structure. In this regard, we must consider their nature to be that of harmful oxidized substances.

There have been many reports that glucocorticoids mediate immunosuppressive function against lymphocytes and inhibitory function against granulocytes (4–12). A review of the literature indicates that this is the first study demonstrating a potentiation of granulocyte function by a steroid hormone and an increase in a recently identified lymphocyte population, CD3^{int} cells, possibly when their oxidized form remains for a long time in the body.

ACKNOWLEDGMENTS

We thank Mrs. Masako Watanabe for preparation of the manuscript and Mr. Tetuso Hashimoto for animal maintenance.

REFERENCES

1. Menkes, C. J., *Br. J. Rheumatol.* **32**(Suppl. 3), 14, 1993.
2. Sebaldt, R. J., *J. Rheumatol.* **15**, 200, 1988.
3. Schleimer, R. P., *Annu. Rev. Pharmacol. Toxicol.* **25**, 381, 1985.
4. Cohn, L. A., *Semin. Vet. Med. Surg.* **12**, 150, 1997.
5. Sayama, S., Yoshida, R., Oku, T., Imanishi, J., Kishida, T., and Hayaishi, O., *Proc. Natl. Acad. Sci. USA* **78**, 7327, 1981.
6. Schleimer, R. P., Lichtenstein, L. M., and Gillespie. E., *Nature* **292**, 454, 1981.
7. Zak-Nejmark, T., Jankowska, R., Malolepszy, J., Jutel, M., Kraus-Filarska, M., and Nadobna, G., *Arch. Immunol. Ther. Exp.* **44**, 77, 1996.
8. Sendo, F., Tsuchida, H., Takeda, Y., Gon, S., Takei, H., Kato, T., Hachiya, O., and Watanabe, H., *Hum. Cell* **9**, 215, 1996.
9. Tjandra, K., Kubes, P., Rioux, K., Swain, M. G., *Am. J. Physiol.* **270**, G821, 1996.
10. Burton, J. L., and Kehrli, M. E., Jr., *Am. J. Vet. Res.* **56**, 997, 1995.
11. Liles, W. C., Dale, D. C., and Klebanoff, S. J., *Blood* **86**, 3181, 1995.
12. Cox, G., *J. Immunol.* **154**, 4719, 1995.
13. Elks, J., *Br. J. Dermatol.* **94** (Suppl. 12), 3, 1976.
14. Bach, G. L., *Int. J. Clin. Pharm. Ther. Toxicol.* **7**, 198, 1973.
15. Kountz, D. S., and Clark, C. L., *Am. Family Physician* **55**, 521, 1997.
16. Frauman, A. G., *Adv. Drug React. Toxicol. Rev.* **15**, 203, 1996.
17. Allen, D. B., *Endocrinol. Metab. Clin. North. Am.* **25**, 699, 1996.
18. Spahn, J. D., and Kamada, A. K., *Pediatr. Rev.* **16**, 266, 1995.
19. Imam, A. P., and Halpern, G. M., *Allerg. Immunopathol.* **22**, 250, 1994.

20. Melo-Gomes, J. A., *J. Rheumatol. Suppl.* **37**, 35, 1993.
21. Kusunoki, M., Moeslein, G., Shoji, Y., Fujita, S., Yanagi, H., Sakanoue, Y., Saito, N., and Utsunomiya, J., *Dis. Colon Rect.* **35**, 1003, 1992.
22. Bianchi-Porro, G., and Pace, F., *Baill. Clin. Gastroenterol.* **2**, 309, 1988.
23. Black, H. E., *Toxicol. Pathol.* **16**, 213, 1988.
24. Watanabe, H., Miyaji, C., Seki, S., and Abo, T., *J. Exp. Med.* **184**, 687, 1996.
25. Yamagiwa, S., Sugahara, S., Shimizu, T., Iwanaga, T., Yoshida, Y., Honda, S., Watanabe, H., Suzuki, S., Asakura, H., and Abo, T., *J. Immunol.* **160**, 2665, 1998.
26. Kawachi, Y., Watanabe, H., Moroda, T., Haga, M., Iiai, T., Hatakeyama, K., and Abo, T., *Eur. J. Immunol.* **25**, 2272, 1995.
27. Kawachi, Y., Arai, K., Moroda, T., Kawamura, T., Umezu, H., Naito, M., Ohtsuka, K., Hasegawa, K., Takahashi-Iwanaga, H., Iwanaga, T., Shults, L. D., Watanabe, H., and Abo, T., *Eur. J. Immunol.* **25**, 3452, 1995.
28. Fukuda, M., Moroda, T., Toyabe, S., Iiai, T., Kawachi, Y., Takahashi-Iwanaga, H., Iwanaga, T., Okada, M., and Abo, T., *Biomed. Res.* **17**, 171, 1996.
29. Watanabe, H., Miyaji, C., Kawachi, Y., Iiai, T., Ohtsuka, K., Iwanaga, T., Takahashi-Iwanaga, H., and Abo, T., *J. Immunol.* **155**, 2972, 1995.
30. Goossens, P. L., Jouin, H., Marchal, G., and Milon, G., *J. Immunol. Methods* **132**, 137, 1990.
31. Osman, Y., Watanabe, T., Kawachi, Y., Sato, K., Ohtsuka, K., Watanabe, H., Hashimoto, S., Moriyama, Y., Shibata, A., and Abo, T., *Cell. Immunol.* **166**, 172, 1995.
32. Yamamura, S., Arai, K., Toyabe, S., Takahashi, E. H., and Abo, T., *Cell. Immunol.* **173**, 303, 1996.
33. Yoshikawa, H., Kawamura, K., Fujita, M., Tsukada, H., Arakawa, M., and Mitsuyama, M., *Infect. Immun.* **61**, 1334, 1993.
34. Suzuki, S., Toyabe, S., Moroda, T., Tada, T., Tsukahara, A., Iiai, T., Minagawa, M., Maruyama, S., Hatakeyama, K., Endoh, K., and Abo, T., *Clin. Exp. Immunol.* **110**, 500, 1997.
35. Honda, S., Takeda, K., Narita, J., Koya, T., Kawamura, T., Kuwano, Y., Watanabe, H., Arakawa, M., and Abo, T., *Cell. Immunol.* **177**, 144, 1997.
36. Moroda, T., Kawachi, Y., Iiai, T., Tsukahara, A., Suzuki, S., Tada, T., Watanabe, H., Hatakeyama, K., and Abo, T., *Immunology* **91**, 88, 1997.
37. Tsukahara, A., Moroda, T., Iiai, T., Suzuki, S., Tada, T., Hatakeyama, K., and Abo, T., *Eur. J. Immunol.* **27**, 361, 1997.
38. Tsukahara, A., Tada, T., Suzuki, S., Iiai, T., Moroda, T., Maruyama, S., Minagawa, M., Musha, N., Shimizu, T., Hatakeyama, K., and Abo, T., *Biomed. Res.* **18**, 237, 1997.
39. Kawamura, T., Toyabe, S., Moroda, T., Iiai, T., Takahashi-Iwanaga, H., Fukuda, M., Watanabe, H., Sekikawa, H., Seki, S., and Abo, T., *Hepatology* **26**, 1567, 1997.
40. Moroda, T., Iiai, T., Tsukahara, A., Fukuda, M., Suzuki, S., Tada, T., Hatakeyama, K., and Abo, T., *Biomed. Res.* **18**, 423, 1997.
41. Hirahara, H., Ogawa, M., Kimura, M., Iiai, T., Tsuchida, M., Hanawa, H, Watanabe, H., and Abo, T., *Cell. Immunol.* **153**, 401, 1994.
42. Iiai, T., Kawachi, Y., Hirahara, H., Haga, M., Takahashi-Iwanaga, H., Iwanaga, T., Arai, K., Hatakeyama, K., and Abo, T., *Biomed. Res.* **15**, 101, 1994.
43. Sato, K., Ohtsuka, K., Hasegawa, K., Yamagiwa, S., Watanabe, H., Iwanaga, T., Takahashi-Iwanaga, H., Asakura, H., and Abo, T., *J. Exp. Med.* **182**, 759, 1995.
44. Crispe, I. N., Moore, M. W., Husmann, L. A., Smith, L., Bevan, M. J., and Shimonkevitz, R. P., *Nature* **329**, 336, 1987.
45. Egerton, M., and Scollay, R., *Int. Immunol.* **2**, 157, 1990.
46. Bendelac, A., *Curr. Opin. Immunol.* **7**, 367, 1995.
47. MacDonald, H. R., *J. Exp. Med.* **182**, 633, 1995.
48. Bix, M., and Locksley, R. M., *J. Immunol.* **155**, 1020, 1995.
49. Vicari, A. P., and Zlotnik, A., *Immunol. Today* **17**, 71, 1996.
50. Kawamura, T., Kawachi, Y., Moroda, T., Weerashinghe, A., Iiai, T., Seki, S., Takada, G., and Abo, T., *Immunology* **89**, 68, 1996.
51. Moroda, T., Iiai, T., Kawachi, Y., Kawamura, T., Hatakeyama, K., and Abo, T., *Eur. J. Immunol.* **26**, 3084, 1997.
52. Suzuki, M., Asako, H., Kubes, P., Jennings, S., Crishan, M. B., and Granger, D. N., *Microvasc. Res.* **42**, 125, 1991.
53. Takeda, Y., Watanabe, H., Yonehara, S., Yamashita, T., Saito, S., and Sendo, F., *Int. Immunol.* **5**, 691, 1993.
54. Takii, Y., Hashimoto, S., Iiai, T., Watanabe, H., Hatakeyama, K., and Abo, T., *Clin. Exp. Immunol.* **97**, 522, 1994.
55. Okada, T., Iiai, T., Kawachi, Y., Moroda, T., Takii, Y., Hatakeyama, K., and Abo, T., *Clin. Exp. Immunol.* **102**, 159, 1995.

Suppressive Effect of Antiulcer Agents on Granulocytes — A Role for Granulocytes in Gastric Ulcer Formation

抗潰瘍剤の顆粒球抑制作用
──胃潰瘍発症における顆粒球の役割

Digestive Diseases and Sciences 45: 1786-1791, 2000

chapter 12

Suppressive Effect of Antiulcer Agents on Granulocytes
— A Role for Granulocytes in Gastric Ulcer Formation

抗潰瘍剤の顆粒球抑制作用——胃潰瘍発症における顆粒球の役割

TOSHIHIKO KAWAMURA, MD, CHIKAKO MIYAJI, SHINICHI TOYABE, MD, MINORU FUKUDA, MD, HISAMI WATANABE, PhD, and TORU ABO, MD

From the Department of Immunology, Niigata University School of Medicine, Niigata, Japan.

【キーワード】

胃潰瘍、H_2ブロッカー、プロトンポンプ阻害剤、顆粒球、ストレス

【要約】

臨床医の多くが、H_2ブロッカーとプロトンポンプ阻害剤の制酸剤効果により胃潰瘍を改善できると信じてきた。今回、これらの制酸剤の顆粒球に対する作用を検証した。1週間H_2ブロッカーまたはプロトンポンプ阻害剤を投与された胃潰瘍患者の、顆粒球数と超酸化物産生を検証した。顆粒球の動態を測定するため、マウスに24時間、拘束ストレスを与えた。ヒトとマウスにおいてH_2ブロッカーにより顆粒球数は減少したのに対して、プロトンポンプ阻害剤により超酸化物産生が抑制された。胃潰瘍治癒におけるH_2ブロッカーとプロトンポンプ阻害剤の主な機能は、顆粒球を抑制する効果であるようだ。この場合、ストレスにより骨髄から胃粘膜まで顆粒球の遊走が促進される。胃潰瘍発症における顆粒球の役割を説明することができれば、「胃酸-ペプシン説」と「ヘリコバクター・ピロリ菌説」の間を埋めることができる。

胃潰瘍発症に関係するメカニズムについては、議論の余地がある。しかし、臨床医の多くは、胃潰瘍患者に、制酸剤（例えばアルミニウム・ケイ酸塩、水酸化マグネシウム、H_2ブロッカー（1-4）やプロトンポンプ阻害剤（PPI）（5-8）を処方する。H_2ブロッカーとプロトンポンプ阻害剤（PPI）という二種類の薬剤により、最終的には、劇的に胃潰瘍が改善される患者が見られる。臨床医の多くの間では、H_2ブロッカーとPPIの持つ制酸効果が胃潰瘍を改善すると長い間信じられてきた。しかし、これら薬剤は、胃全摘術後の患者の吻合部潰瘍にも効果的であるが、これらの患者には、塩酸（HCl）を分泌する壁細胞はない。ヘリコバクター・ピロリ感染の有無にかかわらず、胃潰瘍周辺の粘膜に常に顆粒球の存在が見られたので、顆粒球に対するH_2ブロッカーとプロトンポンプ阻害剤の効果を検証した。

ヒトとマウスにおいて、H_2ブロッカーで顆粒球の数が減少した一方、PPIで顆粒球の機能（超酸化物産生）が抑制させたことを今回、報告する。全く対照的に、H_2ブロッカーでは顆粒球の機能は抑制されない一方、PPIでは顆粒球の数は減少しなかった。顆粒球の表面にはアド

Manuscript received May 6, 1999; accepted December 31, 1999.
Address for reprint requests: Dr. T. Abo, Department of Immunology, Niigata University School of Medicine, Asahimachi-757, Niigata 851-8510, Japan.

レナリン受容体（9-11）が存在し、交感神経緊張下では活性化するという最近の報告（12-14）も考慮すると、本研究の結果は、胃粘膜への顆粒球の蓄積が胃潰瘍の病因として重要である可能性を示唆する。胃潰瘍患者の場合、心身のストレスまたは細菌感染（例えば、ヘリコバクター・ピロリ）が原因で交感神経緊張が出現する可能性がある。

材料と方法

患者と治療

胃潰瘍患者（n=16，年齢20-58歳）、胃潰瘍治療前の患者を対象とした。8人の患者にH_2ブロッカー（塩酸ロキサチジン・アセテート75mg／日；帝国臓器製薬（株），東京，日本）を経口投与し、残り8人の患者には1週間プロトンポンプ阻害剤（ランソプラゾール30mg／日；武田薬品工業（株），東京，日本）を経口投与した。同年齢の健康な被験者(n=16)に、H_2ブロッカーまたはPPIを経口投与した。血液中の顆粒球の比率を投薬前後に測定した。

ルミノール依存性化学発光反応

ルミノール依存性化学発光反応は、ルミノフォトメータ（TD-4000; Labo Science, Tokyo, Japan）を使用して超酸化物産生の指標とした（15, 16）。細胞は、濃度10^8/mlで緩衝液II（50μl）（10mM HEPES, 5m KCl, 145mM NaClおよび5.5mM ブドウ糖（pH 7.4））に懸濁させた。この細胞に、ルミノール溶液（100μl）と緩衝液I（100μl）に1mM $CaCl_2$ およびホルボール・ミリスチン酸塩アセテート（PMA）（20μg/ml）（50μl）（Sigma Chemical Co., St Louis, Missouri）を加えた。超酸化物によるルミノール依存性化学反応には、ルミノフォトメータで10分間、相対発光量を測定した。

H_2受容体mRNAの検出

逆転写ポリメラーゼ連鎖反応（RT-PCR）法にて、H_2受容体のmRNAを検出した。トータルRNAは、リンパ球、顆粒球、心筋および胃粘膜より抽出した（17）。H_2受容体検出に使用したプライマーを以下記す；sense 5'-GTGCTGCCCTTCTCTGCCATCTAC-3'およびantisense 5'-TTGTGCTCCCCTGATGGTGGCTGC-3'。mRNAの完全性を確認するため、β-アクチンのmRNAも測定した。

マウス実験

マウスに、3日間H_2ブロッカー（塩酸ロキサチジン・アセテート0.4mg／日／匹）またはPPI（ランソプラゾール0.1mg／日／匹）を経口投与した。実験終了3日前、実験群のうち一群には、G-CSF（10μg／匹）を投与した。ヒト組み換え型G-CSF（キリンビール（株），東京，日本）を本実験では使用した。顆粒球比率を抗顆粒球抗体（Gr-1; PharMingen、San Diego、California）を用いフローサイトメトリー解析により測定した（15）。マウスに、拘束ストレスを与えた（8時間および24時間）（18）。本実験において顆粒球数は、$Gr-1^+$細胞の比率と骨髄、血液、肝臓および胃粘膜の白血球総数を用いて算出した。定法に従い、胃粘膜の白血球はコラゲナーゼ処理法を用いて採取した（18）。

結果

統計分析

有意差検定には、対応あるt検定またはスチューデントt検定を用いた。

H_2ブロッカーによる顆粒球数減少

胃潰瘍患者（A）と同年齢の健康な被験者（B）に1週間H_2ブロッカーまたはPPIを投与した（Figure 1）。以前の報告同様（18）、胃潰瘍患者の末梢血では顆粒球比率（60-70%）は、同年齢の健康被験者のもの（50-60%）と比較して、増加傾向を示した。胃潰瘍患者に1週間H_2ブロッカーを投与すると、顆粒球比率は正常レ

Figure.1

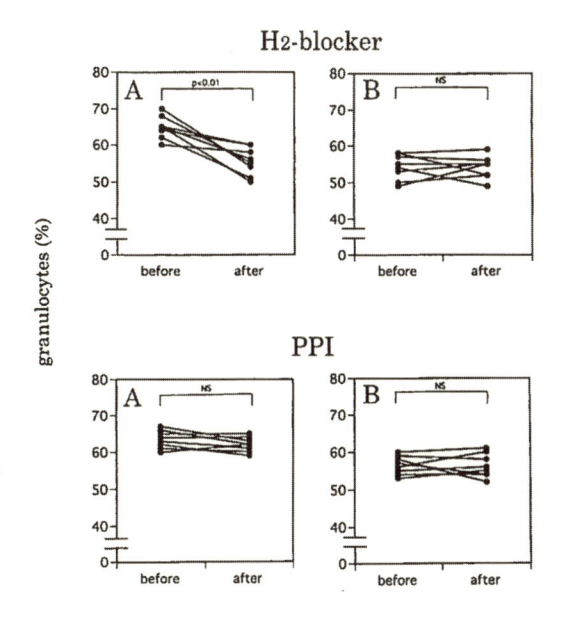

PPI抑制剤でなく、H₂ブロッカーの投与による胃潰瘍患者の顆粒球数の正常化。胃潰瘍患者（A）と健常対照者（B）に1週間H₂ブロッカーまたはPPIを投与して、その前後に末梢血中の顆粒球比率を測定した。H₂ブロッカー群の被験者とPPI群の被験者は異なる。胃潰瘍患者では、主として顆粒球高値が見られた。

Figure.2

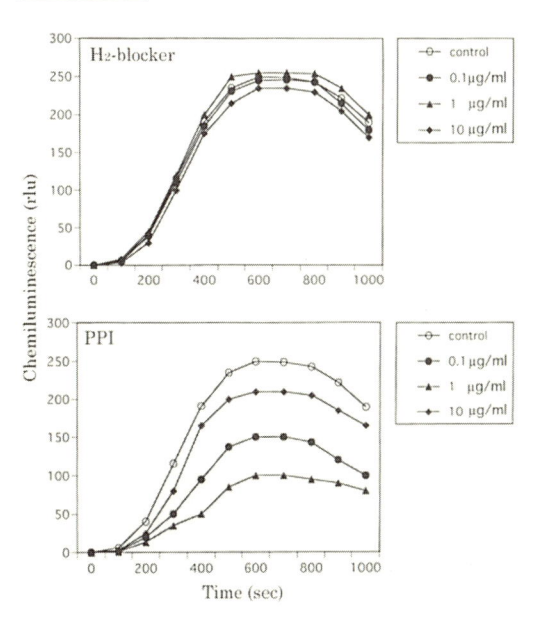

H₂ブロッカーでなく、PPIによる顆粒球の超酸化物産生の抑制。胃潰瘍患者3名から分離した顆粒球を使用した。顆粒球の超酸化物産生を、PMAによる刺激後に化学発光反応法で測定した。顆粒球の培養を予め行った（37℃、60分間）。H₂ブロッカーまたはPPIの濃度は表示の通りである。3回行なった実験の代表的なデータを示す。

ベル（$P < 0.01$）に低下した。一方、同年齢の健康被験者において、顆粒球比率はそのような減少を示さなかった（$P>0.05$）。胃潰瘍患者がPPIを服用しても、血中顆粒球比率は減少しなかった（$P> 0.05$）。同年齢の健康被験者でも同様であった。

PPIによる顆粒球の超酸化物産生の抑制

上記の実験より、H₂ブロッカーとPPIとで顆粒球数に対する影響が違うことが明らかになった。しかし、両剤により最終的には胃潰瘍を改善した（19-22）。薬剤が顆粒球の機能にもたらす影響を検証するために、ホルボール・ミリステート・アセテート（PMA）で刺激を与え顆粒球の超酸化物産生を測定した（Figure 2）。ルミノール依存性化学発光反応を測定し、ルミノフォトメータによる超酸化物産生（より正確には、H_2O_2とミエロペルオキシダーゼ放出）の指標とした（15）。胃潰瘍患者より顆粒球のみを採取し、各濃度のH₂ブロッカーまたはPPIを加え37℃、1時間培養した。H₂ブロッカーは、超酸化物産生に対し全く影響を示さなかった。対照的に、PPIは特に、濃度1μg/mlにおいて超酸化物産生抑制を示した。

顆粒球表面のH₂受容体発現

H₂ブロッカーは、どのように顆粒球数を減少させたのだろうか。H₂ブロッカーは、胃粘膜の壁細胞からの塩酸（HCl）分泌に対してH₂受容体を介して作用する（1-4）。そこで、顆粒球のH₂受容体の有無を検証した（Figure 3）。逆転写酵素（RT）-PCR方法を用いて、H₂受容体のmRNAを検出した。トータルRNAをヒトの4部位（リンパ球、顆粒球、心筋および胃粘膜）

Figure.3

H₂-receptor / β-actin
lymphocytes, granulocytes, cardiac muscle, gastric mucosa

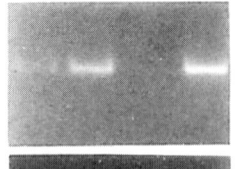

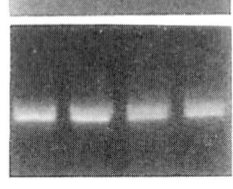

顆粒球のH₂受容体mRNAの検出。顆粒球のH₂レセプター発現を確認するためRT-PCR法を利用した。トータルRNAを、リンパ球、顆粒球、心筋と胃粘膜より抽出した（陽性対照）。

より採取して検証した。胃粘膜同様、顆粒球においてH₂受容体mRNAが発現していた。

動物（マウス）実験の結果を検証する

マウスを用いてH₂ブロッカーが顆粒球数を抑制する作用を実験した（Figure 4）。対照群およびG-CSF（18）で前処理した実験群のマウスの血中顆粒球比率を測定した。対照群マウスにおける血中顆粒球比率は、低値であった（20%）。3日間H₂ブロッカー（0.4mg/日/匹）またはPPI（0.1mg/日/匹）を投与した実験群マウスの数値も同様であった（Figure 4AおよびB）。しかし、G-CSF（10μg/マウス、実験終了3日前に1度投与）で前処理したマウスの血中顆粒球は高値であり（50%）、H₂ブロッカー投与により比率の減少が示された。ヒトの場合も同様に、血中顆粒球値が上昇した場合のみH₂ブロッカーの効果が見られた。PPIは、顆粒球比率に対し全く効果を示さなかった。

ストレスによる顆粒球遊走の加速

本研究の最終段階では、マウスにおける顆粒球の遊走を検証した。マウスに拘束ストレスを与え（18）、骨髄（BM）、末梢血、肝臓および胃など各器官における顆粒球数を測定した（Figure 4C）。マウスに与えたストレスは8時間と24時間である。興味深いことに、顆粒球数は、顆粒球を産生する骨髄においてストレス初期（8時間）で減少した。対照的に、顆粒球数は、末梢血、肝臓では、ストレス初期（8時間）で増加し、その後（24時間）胃で増加した。

考察

本研究において、抗潰瘍剤（H₂ブロッカーとPPI）がヒトとマウスで顆粒球に独特の影響を及ぼすことを証明した。このように、H₂ブロッカーは血中顆粒球数を減少させたが、プロトンポンプ阻害剤は顆粒球の機能（超酸化物産生）を抑制した。興味深いことに、H₂ブロッカーでは超酸化物産生を抑制せず、PPIでは顆粒球数は減少しなかった。胃粘膜付近で活性化した顆粒球の数と機能が、胃潰瘍形成の原因と密接な関連があるようである（18）。本研究の結果により、H₂ブロッカーとPPIの治療効果における実際のメカニズムが初めて明らかになった。

臨床医の多くは、健常人と比較して一般に胃潰瘍患者の胃酸分泌率は正常であるか減少していることに気付いている（23）。しかし、胃潰瘍治療おいて、制酸剤（特にH₂ブロッカー（1-4）とPPI（5-8））が、100%ではないものの、たいがい、効果を発揮する。H₂ブロッカーとPPIは、制酸剤としての作用よりもむしろ顆粒球に対する作用を通じて胃潰瘍を改善しているのではないかと仮定できる。H₂ブロッカーは、顆粒球上のH₂受容体を通じて顆粒球数を減少

Figure.4

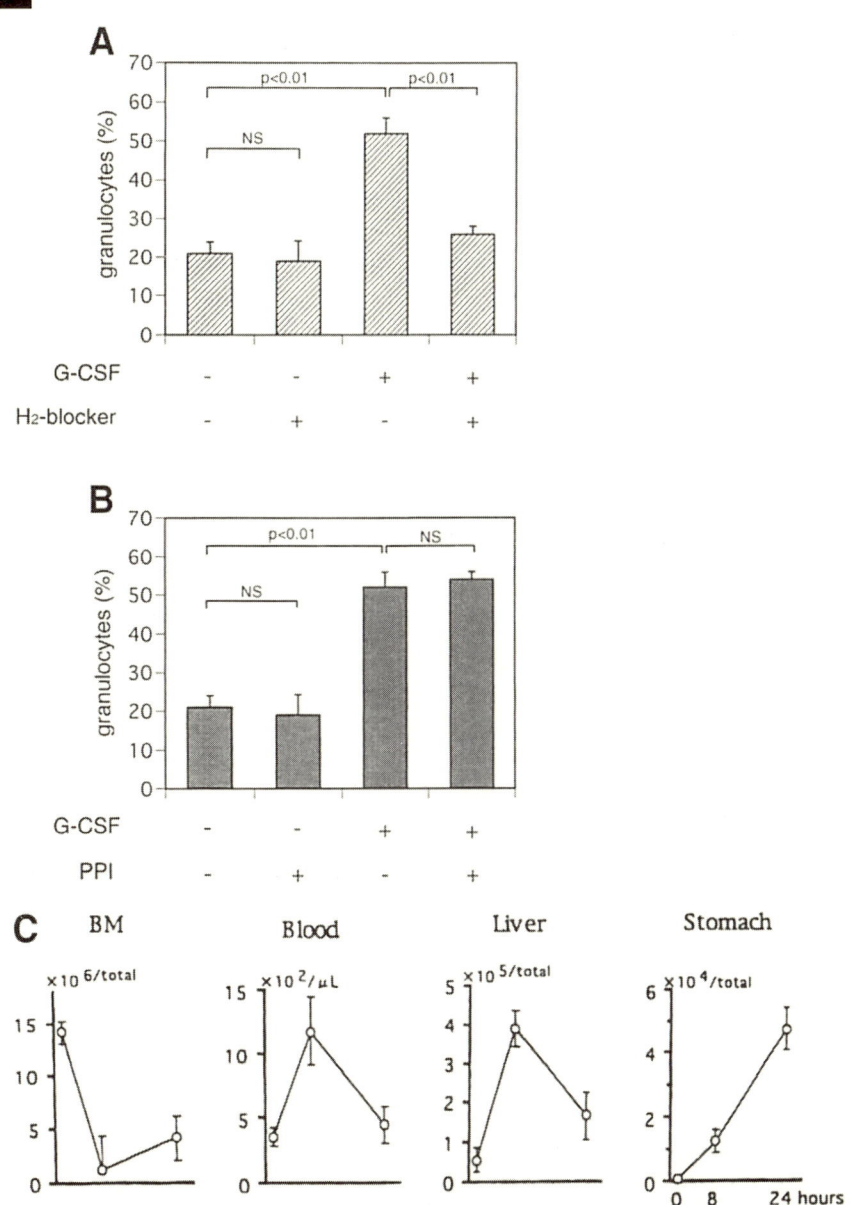

マウス実験における顆粒球動態の検証。(A) H_2ブロッカーの影響；(B) プロトンポンプ阻害剤の影響；(C) 拘束ストレスの影響。正常マウスとG-CSF処理したマウスを使用した。実験終了3日前に、マウスにヒト組み換え型G-CSF（10μg/匹）を投与し、血中顆粒球数を増加させた。骨髄で産生された顆粒球がどのようにして器官や粘膜へ移動して行くかを調べるためにマウスに拘束ストレス（8時間と24時間）を与えた。各器官の顆粒球数は、白血球総数とフローサイトメトリー解析による顆粒球比率（Gr-1$^+$）を用いて算出した。

させている可能性があり、一方、PPIは、顆粒球の機能を抑制しているのである。

　研究者の多くは、胃潰瘍発症の「胃酸―ペプシン説」に対して疑問を抱いた。というのは、迷走神経切除（1940年代に行われた）では患者（24-26）で胃潰瘍が改善されなかったからである（24-26）。しかし、J.W. Blackが発見した制酸剤H_2ブロッカーが胃潰瘍の治療に非常に効

果的だったので、そのような疑問は封印された（27, 28）。しかし、その後、研究者の中には（Blackを含む）は、H_2ブロッカーの投与が患者の末梢の顆粒球数が減少することに気づいた者ものもいた。顆粒球上に対するH_2ブロッカーのそのような副作用は、広く知られている。そこで、顆粒球に対するこのH_2ブロッカーのこの作用が実は治療メカニズムであると提唱する。

「胃酸－ペプシン説」が、長い間、胃潰瘍の病因を説明するものとして残った理由がもうひとつある。胃潰瘍患者には、常に胃酸の過剰分泌が見られるわけではないが、空腹時、胃酸分泌と疼痛が出現する。これらの現象は飢餓からの防御として起こると考えられてきた。実際、食物を摂取すると症状が緩解する。胃酸分泌は疼痛（空の胃が運動するため）を伴うので、胃潰瘍発症の原因を見誤ったのである。

これらのことから、胃潰瘍発症の「顆粒球説」を提唱する。表面にアドレナリン受容体を持つ顆粒球が（交感神経緊張により活性化されるが（9-11）、故に胃潰瘍が出現するのである（18）。最近の研究において、ヘリコバクター・ピロリ菌感染が、胃潰瘍発症の一因に挙げられた（29-32）。しかし、この「ヘリコバクター・ピロリ菌説」は不完全である。これまで述べたように、胃潰瘍患者の中にはこの菌に感染していない人もおり、また、健康人の多くはヘリコバクター・ピロリ菌に感染している。「胃潰瘍の顆粒球説」を用いると、胃潰瘍の全症例をこの概念を用いて説明できる可能性がある。ヘリコバクター・ピロリ感染は、顆粒球を刺激する第二の要因として重要である。交感神経緊張は、精神的ストレス、働き過ぎ、細菌感染、NSAID投与（17）やこれら要因の組合せなど多くの原因で出現する。

本研究の動物実験（マウス）で示したように、顆粒球動態（骨髄 → 血液循環 → 粘膜）は、「胃潰瘍の顆粒球説」を理解するのに重要である。ストレスが継続して慢性化するならば、骨髄内における顆粒球産生自体が増加して（15）、末梢血同様、組織内において顆粒球値が上昇する（Figure 1）。本研究により、抗潰瘍剤であるH_2ブロッカーとPPIの治療の基本をしっかり理解できる。「胃潰瘍の顆粒球説」を用いると、H_2ブロッカーとPPIがなぜ胃酸を分泌する壁細胞を全て失った胃全摘患者でも、吻合部潰瘍が改善するかについて説明できる。

胃潰瘍形成に顆粒球が関与することを示唆する論文は複数ある（33-35）。しかし、これら論文の著者は胃潰瘍形成の第二の要因として顆粒球の影響を考慮している、あるいは、顆粒球の影響と「胃酸―ペプシン説」との若干の混同が見られた。この点、本論文は、潰瘍形成の基本的メカニズムについて顆粒球の正確な役割を証明するものである。

謝辞

本研究は、文部科学省科学研究費補助金によるものである。原稿浄書について渡辺正子氏に感謝する。

Suppressive Effect of Antiulcer Agents on Granulocytes—A Role for Granulocytes in Gastric Ulcer Formation

TOSHIHIKO KAWAMURA, MD, CHIKAKO MIYAJI, SHINICHI TOYABE, MD, MINORU FUKUDA, MD, HISAMI WATANABE, PhD, and TORU ABO, MD

Many clinicians have believed that H_2-blockers and proton pump inhibitors ameliorate gastric ulcers via their antacid function. We examined the effects of these antacids on granulocytes. Gastric ulcer patients were administered an H_2-blocker or proton pump inhibitor for a week and the number of granulocytes and the superoxide production were examined. To determine the trafficking of granulocytes, mice were exposed to restraint stress for 24 hr. The H_2-blocker decreased the number of granulocytes, while the proton pump inhibitor suppressed their superoxide production in humans and mice. The major function of H_2-blockers and proton pump inhibitors in curing gastric ulcers seems to be their suppressive effects on granulocytes. In this case, stress accelerates the trafficking of granulocytes from the bone marrow to the gastric mucosa. If we demonstrate a role for granulocytes in gastric ulcer formation, an gap in the acid–pepsin theory and the *Helicobacter pylori* theory is filled in.

KEY WORDS: gastric ulcer; H_2-blocker; proton pump inhibitor; granulocyte; stress.

The mechanisms involved in gastric ulcer formation remain controversial. However, for gastric ulcer patients, many clinicians prescribe antacids such as aluminum silicate, magnesium hydroxide, H_2-blockers (1–4), and proton pump inhibitors (PPI) (5–8). The latter two drugs, in particular, eventually ameliorate gastric ulcers in some patients. Many clinicians have long believed that H_2-blockers and PPI ameliorate gastric ulcers via their antacid function. However, these drugs are also effective on the junctional ulcers in patients who have undergone total gastrectomy. These patients lack parietal cells that secrete HCl. Since we always encountered granulocytes in the mucosa around gastric ulcers with or without *Helicobacter pylori* infection, the effects of H_2-blockers and proton pump inhibitors on granulocytes were examined.

We report here, that an H_2-blocker decreased the number of granulocytes while a PPI suppressed the function (i.e., superoxide production) of granulocytes in humans and mice. In sharp contrast, the H_2-blocker did not suppress the function of granulocytes and the PPI did not decrease the number of granulocytes. In conjunction with recent results that granulocytes carry surface adrenergic receptors (9–11) and are activated by sympathetic nerve stimulation (12–14), the present results suggest that the accumulation of granulocytes in the gastric mucosa might be important in the pathogenesis of gastric ulcers. Sympathetic nerve activation in such patients might be induced by mental and physical stress or bacterial infection (eg, *H. pylori*).

MATERIALS AND METHODS

Patients and Therapy. Gastric ulcer patients ($n = 16$, ages 20–58) who had not previously been treated, were

Manuscript received May 6, 1999; accepted December 31, 1999.
From the Department of Immunology, Niigata University School of Medicine, Niigata, Japan.
Address for reprint requests: Dr. T. Abo, Department of Immunology, Niigata University School of Medicine, Asahimachi-757, Niigata 851-8510, Japan.

selected. Eight patients were orally administered an H_2-blocker (75 mg/day of roxatidine acetate hydrochloride; Teikoku Zoki, Tokyo, Japan) and the other eight patients were orally administered a proton pump inhibitor (30 mg/day of lansoprazole; Takeda Chemical, Tokyo, Japan) for a week. Age-matched healthy volunteers ($n = 16$) were administered an H_2-blocker or a PPI. The proportions of granulocytes in the blood were measured before and after treatment.

Luminol-Dependent Chemiluminescence. Luminol-dependent chemiluminescence was applied as an indicator of superoxide production using a lumiphotometer (TD-4000; Labo Science, Tokyo, Japan) (15, 16). Cells were suspended to yield 10^8/ml in 50 µl of buffer II, consisting of 10 mM HEPES, 5 mM KCl, 145 mM NaCl, and 5.5 mM glucose (pH 7.4). To the cells were added 100 µl of luminol solution and 100 µl of buffer I consisting of buffer II supplemented with 1 mM $CaCl_2$ and 50 µl of phorbol myristate acetate (PMA) (20 µg/ml) (Sigma Chemical Co., St Louis, Missouri). Chemiluminescence was monitored by the lumiphotometer for 10 min and expressed in relative light units.

Detection of mRNA of H_2-Receptors. The reverse transcriptase-polymerase chain reaction (RT-PCR) method was applied to detect mRNA of H_2-receptors. Total RNA was extracted from lymphocytes, granulocytes, cardiac muscle, and gastric mucosa (17). The primers used for H_2-receptors were as follows: sense 5'-GTGCTGCCCTTCTCTGC-CATCTAC-3' and antisense 5'-TTTGTGCTCCCCTGAT-GGTGGCTGC-3'. To confirm the intactness of mRNA, mRNA of β-actin was also examined.

Mouse Studies. Mice were orally administered with an H_2-blocker (0.4 mg/day/mouse of roxatidine acetate hydrochloride) or a PPI (0.1 mg/day/mouse of lansoprazole) for three days. One group of mice was pretreated with G-CSF (10 µg/mouse, one injection three days before being killed). Human recombinant G-CSF (Kirin Beer Co., Tokyo, Japan) was used for this experiment. The proportion of granulocytes was determined by anti-granulocyte antibody (Gr-1; PharMingen, San Diego, California) in conjunction with an immunofluorescence test (15). Mice were exposed to restraint stress for 8 and 24 hr (18). In this experiment, the number of granulocytes was calculated from the proportion of Gr-1$^+$ cells and the number of total cells in the bone marrow, blood, liver, and gastric mucosa. Cells from the gastric mucosa were obtained by the collagenase digestion method, as previously reported (18).

Statistical Analysis. Differences were determined by the paired t test or Student's t test.

RESULTS

Decrease in Number of Granulocytes by H_2-Blocker. Gastric ulcer patients (A) and age-matched healthy subjects (B) were administered either an H_2-blocker or PPI for a week (Figure 1). As shown previously (18) as well as in this figure, the proportion of granulocytes (60–70%) in the peripheral blood of gastric ulcer patients tended to increase in comparison with those (50–60%) of age-matched healthy

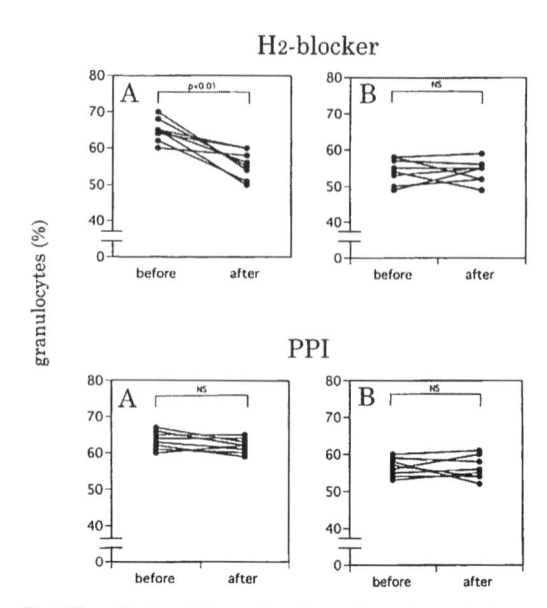

Fig 1. Normalization of the number of granulocytes in gastric ulcer patients by the administration of an H_2-blocker, but not a PPI inhibitor. Gastric ulcer patients (A) and healthy controls (B) were administered either an H_2-blocker or a PPI for a week. The proportion of granulocytes in the blood was determined before and after treatment. Subjects in the H_2-blocker group and those in the PPI group were different individuals. Gastric ulcer patients primarily showed a high level of granulocytes.

subjects. When gastric ulcer patients were administered an H_2-blocker for a week, the proportion of granulocytes decreased to a normal level ($P < 0.01$). On the other hand, age-matched control subjects did not show such a decrease in the proportion of granulocytes ($P > 0.05$). When gastric ulcer patients were administered a PPI, the proportion of granulocytes in the blood did not decrease ($P > 0.05$). This was also true in the case of age-matched control subjects.

Suppression of Superoxide Production of Granulocytes by PPI. The aforementioned experiments revealed a difference in effects on the number of granulocytes between an H_2-blocker and a PPI. However, both drugs eventually ameriolated gastric ulcers (19–22). To determine their functional effects on granulocytes, superoxide production of granulocytes upon stimulation with phorbol myristate acetate (PMA) was examined (Figure 2). Luminol-dependent chemiluminescence was determined as an indicator of superoxide production (more accurately H_2O_2 and myeloperoxidase release) by lumiphotometer (15). Purified granulocytes were prepared from gastric ul-

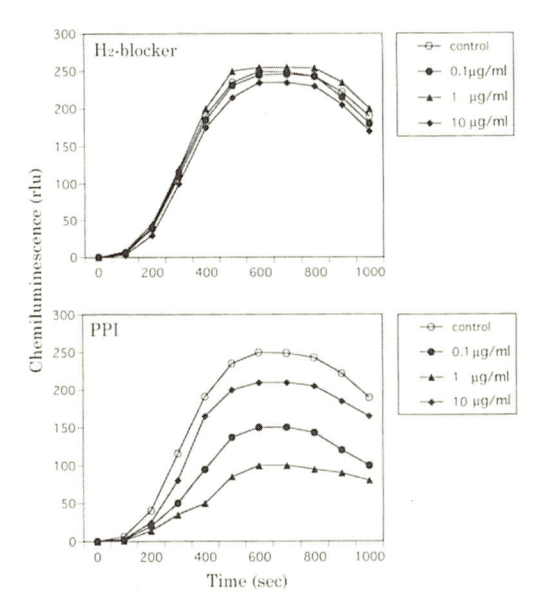

Fig 2. Suppression of the superoxide production from granulocytes by a PPI, but not an H$_2$-blocker. Granulocytes isolated from three gastric ulcer patients were used. Superoxide production from granulocytes was measured *in vitro* by the chemiluminescence method after stimulation with PMA. The preincubation of granulocytes at 37°C for 60 min was conducted at the indicated concentrations of an H$_2$-blocker or PPI. The data shown here are representative of three experiments.

cer patients and preincubated with the indicated concentrations of an H$_2$-blocker or a PPI at 37°C for 1 hr. The H$_2$-blocker did not show any effects on superoxide production. In contrast, the PPI suppressed superoxide production, especially at a concentration of 1 μg/ml.

Expression of H$_2$-Receptors on Granulocytes. The question was raised as to how the H$_2$-blocker decreased the number of granulocytes. HCl secretion from parietal cells in the gastric mucosa is mediated through H$_2$-receptors (1–4). It was therefore determined whether granulocytes carried H$_2$-receptors (Figure 3). The reverse transcriptase (RT)-PCR method was applied to detect mRNA of H$_2$-receptors. Total RNAs were isolated from four sources of human materials, including lymphocytes, granulocytes, cardiac muscle, and gastric mucosa. Granulocytes as well as gastric mucosa showed prominent signs of mRNA of H$_2$-receptors.

Confirmation of Results in a Mouse Study. By using mouse materials, the suppressive effects of an H$_2$-blocker on the number of granulocytes were examined (Figure 4). In the blood of normal mice and

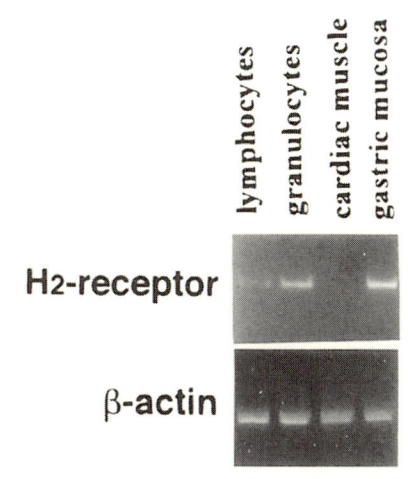

Fig 3. Detection of the signs of H$_2$-receptor mRNA in granulocytes. To identify the expression of H$_2$-receptors in granulocytes, the RT-PCR method was applied. Total RNAs were extracted from lymphocytes, granulocytes, cardiac muscle, and gastric mucosa (a positive control).

mice pretreated with G-CSF (18), the proportion of granulocytes was enumerated. The proportion of granulocytes in the blood of normal mice was low (20%). This was also the case in mice treated with an H$_2$-blocker (0.4 mg/day/mouse) or PPI (0.1 mg/day/mouse) for three days (Figure 4A and B). However, mice pretreated with G-CSF (10 μg/mouse, one injection three days before being killed) and that had an elevated level of granulocytes (50%) in the blood showed a decreased proportion in the case of the H$_2$-blocker. Similar to the case in humans, the H$_2$-blocker was only effective when there were elevated levels of granulocytes in the blood. The PPI did not show any effects on the proportion of granulocytes.

Accelerated Trafficking of Granulocytes by Stress. In a final portion of these experiments, we investigated the trafficking of granulocytes in mice. Mice were exposed to restraint stress (18) and the number of granulocytes determined in various organs, including the bone marrow (BM), blood, liver, and stomach (Figure 4C). Mice were killed 8 and 24 hr after exposure. Interestingly, the number of granulocytes decreased in the bone marrow, where granulocytes are generated, 8 hr after exposure, while in contrast, the number of granulocytes in the blood and liver increased in this early phase of stress (8 hr) and that in the stomach increased in the late phase (24 hr).

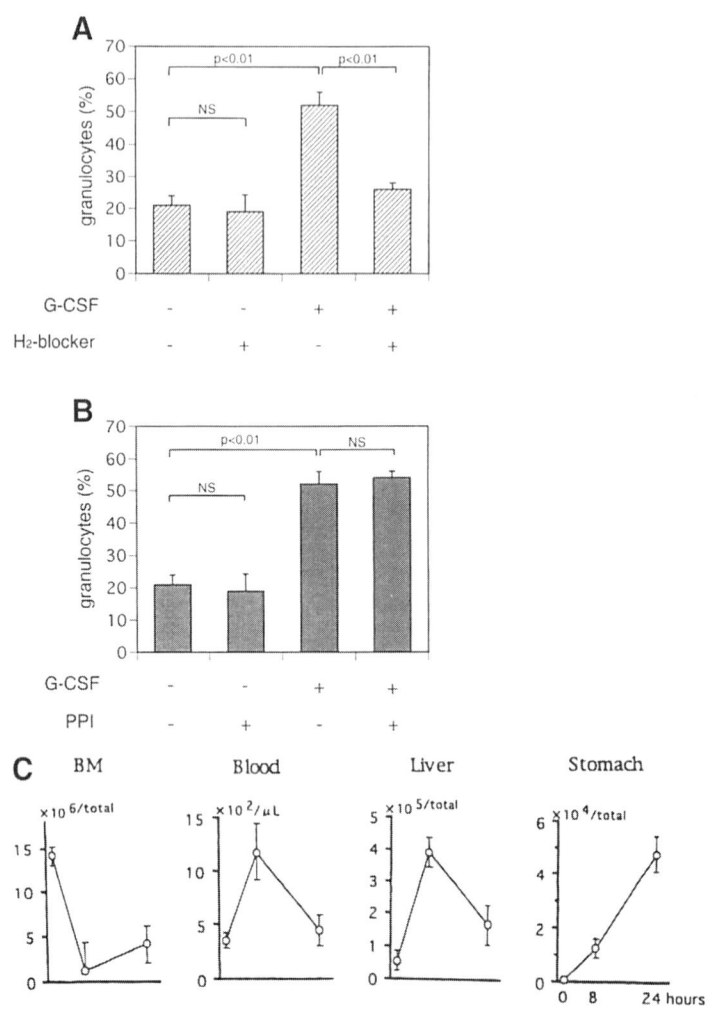

Fig 4. Confirmation of the kinetics of granulocyte behavior in a mouse study. (A) Effect of an H_2-blocker; (B) effect of a proton pump inhibitor; (C) effect of restraint stress. We used normal mice and mice treated with G-CSF. To increase the numbers of granulocytes in the blood, mice were administered with human recombinant G-CSF (10 μg/mouse) three days before killing. To determine how granulocytes (which were produced in the bone marrow) behave in the circulation, organs, and mucosa, mice were exposed to restrain stress for 8 and 24 hr. The number of granulocytes in each organ was determined by the cell yield of leukocytes and the proportion of granulocytes (Gr-1+) as shown by an immunofluorescence test.

DISCUSSION

In the present study, we demonstrated that antiulcer agents, an H_2-blocker and a PPI, had unique effects on granulocytes in humans and mice. Thus, an H_2-blocker decreased the number of granulocytes in the blood, whereas a proton pump inhibitor suppressed the function (ie, superoxide production) of granulocytes. Interestingly, the H_2-blocker did not suppress the superoxide production and the PPI did not decrease the number. Granulocytes activated in number and function around the gastric mucosa appear to be intimately related to the pathogenesis of gastric ulcer formation (18). The present results revealed for the first time the actual mechanisms involved in the therapeutic effects of H_2-blockers and PPIs.

Many clinicians know that gastric ulcer patients generally have acid secretory rates that are normal or reduced, when compared with such rates in healthy individuals (23). However, antacids, especially H_2-blockers (1–4) and PPI (5–8), are often, but not always, effective in gastric ulcer treatment. We postulate that H_2-blockers and PPIs ameliorate gastric ulcers via their action against granulocytes rather than via their action as antacids. In the case of H_2-blockers, they may decrease the number of granulocytes through H_2-receptors on granulocytes. In the case of PPIs, they suppress the function of granulocytes.

Many investigators have questioned the acid–pepsin theory of gastric ulcer formation, because vagotomy, used as treatment in the 1940s, did not ameliorate gastric ulcers in patients (24–26). However, the discovery of H_2-blockers by J.W. Black overcame such suspicion, because this antacid was highly effective in the treatment of gastric ulcers (27, 28). Thereafter, however, some investigators, including Black, noticed that the administration of H_2-blockers decreases the number of granulocytes in the periphery of patients. Such adverse effects of H_2-blockers on granulocytes are widely known. We now propose that this effect of H_2-blockers on granulocytes is actually a therapeutic mechanism.

There is another reason why the acid–pepsin theory has remained as an explanation of the pathogenesis of gastric ulcers for a long time. Although gastric ulcer patients do not show consistent acid hypersecretion, they sometimes manifest both acid secretion and pain when they become hungry. We have considered that these phenomena occur as protection from starvation. Indeed, food intake rescues them. Since the acid secretion is accompanied by pain (due to the movement of empty stomach), we have been misled as to the cause of gastric ulcer formation.

Given the above, we propose a granulocyte theory of gastric ulcer formation. Granulocytes, which carry surface adrenergic receptors, are therefore activated by sympathetic nerve stimulation (9–11) and subsequently induce gastric ulcers (18). In recent studies, *H. pylori* infection has been raised as one of the causes for gastric ulcer formation (29–32). However, this concept is incomplete. Thus, some gastric ulcer patients are free from this infection and many healthy individuals are infected with *H. pylori*. If we introduce the granulocyte theory of gastric ulcer formation, all cases of gastric ulcers might be explained by this concept. In this case, *H. pylori* infection is important as a secondary factor that stimulates granulocytes. Sympathetic nerve stimulation is induced by many causes, including mental stress, overwork, bacterial infection, NSAID administration (17), and a combination of such factors.

As shown in our mouse study, granulocyte trafficking (the bone marrow→the circulation→the mucosa) is important for understanding the granulocyte theory. If stress continues chronically, granulopoiesis itself increases in the bone marrow (15) and the levels of granulocytes in the periphery are elevated in various tissues, as well as in the blood (see Figure 1). This study enabled us to properly understand the therapeutic base of antiulcer agents, H_2-blockers, and PPIs. The proposed theory also explains why H_2-blockers and PPIs ameriolate the junction ulcers in patients with total gastrectomy who have lost all parietal cells for acid secretion.

Several papers have indicated the association of granulocytes in gastric ulcer formation (33–35). However, the authors of these papers seemed concerned with the effect of granulocytes as the secondary factor for gastric ulcer formation, or there has been some confusion between the effect of granulocytes and the acid–pepsin theory. In this regard, our paper determines a precise role of granulocytes in the mechanisms underlying ulcer formation.

ACKNOWLEDGMENTS

We thank Mrs. Masako Watanabe in preparation of the manuscript. This work was supported by a Grant-in-Aid for Scientific Research and Cancer Research from the Ministry of Education, Science and Culture, Japan.

REFERENCES

1. Lin JH: Pharmacokinetic and pharmacodynamic properties of histamine H_2-receptor antagonists. Relationship between intrinsic potency and effective plasma concentrations. Clin Pharmacokinet 20:218–236, 1991
2. Deakin M, Williams JG: Histamine H_2-receptor antagonists in peptic ulcer disease. Efficacy in healing peptic ulcers. Drugs 44:709–719, 1992
3. Feldman M, Richardson CT: Histamine H_2-receptor antagonists. Adv Intern Med 23:1–24, 1978
4. Rademaker JW, Hunt RH: Acid and barriers. Current research

and future developments for peptic ulcer therapy. Scand J Gastroenterol (Suppl)175:19–26, 1990
5. Garnett WR: Lansoprazole: A proton pump inhibitor. Ann Pharmacother 30:1425–1436, 1996
6. Brunner G: Proton-pump inhibitors are the treatment of choice in acid-related disease. Eur J Gastroenterol Hepatol 8(suppl 1):S9–S13, 1996
7. Langtry HD, Wilde MI: Lansoprazole. An update of its pharmacological properties and clinical efficacy in the management of acid-related disorders. Drugs 54:473–500, 1997
8. Franko TG, Richter JE: Proton-pump inhibitors of gastric acid-related disease. Clev Clin J Med 65:27–34, 1998
9. Tsukahara A, Tada T, Suzuki S, Iiai T, Moroda T, Maruyama S, Minagawa M, Musha N, Shimizu T, Hatakeyama K, Abo T: Adrenergic stimulation simultaneously induces the expansion of granulocytes and extrathymic T cells in mice. Biomed Res 18:237–246, 1997
10. Suzuki S, Toyabe S, Moroda T, Tada T, Tsukahara A, Iiai T, Minagawa M, Maruyama S, Hatakeyama K, Endo K, Abo T: Circadian rhythm of leukocytes and lymphocyte subsets and its possible correlation with the function of autonomic nervous system. Clin Exp Immunol 110:500–508, 1997
11. Kawamura T, Toyabe S, Moroda T, Iiai T, Takahashi-Iwanaga H, Fukuda M, Watanabe H, Sekikawa H, Seki S, Abo T: Neonatal granulocytosis is a postpartum event which is seen in the liver as well as in the blood. Hepatology 26:1567–1572, 1997
12. Ratge D, Wiedemann A, Kohse KP, Wisser H: Alterations of β-adrenoceptors on human leukocyte subsets induced by dynamic exercise: Effect of prednisone. Clin Exp Pharm Phys 15:43–53, 1988
13. Maisel AS, Knowlton KU, Fowler P, Rearden A, Ziegler MD, Motulsky HJ, Insel PA, Michel MC: Adrenergic control of circulating lymphocyte subpopulations. Effects of congestive heart failure, dynamic exercise, and terbutaline treatment. J Clin Invest 85:462–467, 1990
14. Murray DR, Irwin M, Rearden CA, Ziegler M, Motulsky H, Maisel AS: Sympathetic and immune interactions during dynamic exercise. Mediation via a β_2-adrenergic-dependent mechanism. Circulation 86:203–213, 1992
15. Yamamura S, Arai K, Toyabe S, Takahashi EH, Abo T: Simultaneous activation of granulocytes and extrathymic T cells in number and function by excessive administration of nonsteroidal anti-inflammatory drugs. Cell Immunol 173:303–311, 1996
16. Yoshikawa H, Kawamura I, Fujita M, Tsukada H, Arakawa M, Mitsuyama M: Membrane damage and interleukin-1 production in murine macrophages exposed to listeriolysin O. Infect Immun 61:1334–1339, 1993
17. Honda S, Takeda K, Narita J, Koya T, Kawamura T, Kuwano Y, Watanabe H, Arakawa M, Abo T: Expansion of an unusual population of Gr-1$^+$CD3^{int} cells in the lymph nodes and other peripheral organs of mice carrying the lpr gene. Cell Immunol 177:144–153, 1997
18. Moroda T, Iiai T, Tsukahara A, Fukuda M, Suzuki S, Tada T, Hatakeyama K, Abo T: Association of granulocytes with ulcer formation in the stomach of rodents exposed to restraint stress. Biomed Res 18:423–437, 1997
19. Lazzaroni M, Bianchi PG: Treatment of peptic ulcer in the elderly. Proton pump inhibitors and histamine H_2 receptor antagonists. Drugs Aging 9:251–261, 1996
20. Tryba M, Cook D: Current guidelines on stress ulcer prophylaxis. Drugs 54:581–596, 1997
21. Freston JW: Long-term acid control and proton pump inhibitors: Interactions and safety issues in perspective. Am J Gastroenterol 92(suppl 4):51S–55S, 1997
22. Spencer CM, Faulds D: Lansoprazole. A reappraisal of its pharmacodynamic and pharmacokinetic properties, and its therapeutic efficacy in acid-related disorders. Drugs 48:404–430, 1994
23. McGuigan JE: Peptic ulcer. *In* Principles of Internal Medicine. E Braunwald, KJ Isselbacher, JD Wilson, JB Martn, AS Fauci (eds.) New York, McGraw-Hill, 1987, pp 1246–1247
24. Witte CL: Is vagotomy and gastrectomy still justified for gastroduodenal ulcer? J Clin Gastroenterol 20:2–3, 1995
25. Lindsetmo RO, Johnsen R, Revhaug A: Abdominal and dyspeptic symptoms in patients with peptic ulcer treated medically or surgically. Br J Surg 85:845–849, 1998
26. Salimk AS: The mechanism of vagotomy-induced acute gastric mucosal injury in the rat. Am J Med Sci 297:343–347, 1989
27. Black JW, Duncan WAM, Durant CJ, Ganellin CR, Parsons EM: Definition and antagonism of histamine H_2-receptors. Nature 236:385–390, 1972
28. Wyllie JH, Hesselbo T, Black JW: Effects in man of histamine H_2-receptor blockade by burimamide. Lancet 2:1117–1120, 1972
29. Axon AT: *Helicobacter pylori* and the pathogenesis of gastroduodenal inflammation. Clin Exp Immunol 58:420–427, 1993
30. Blaser MJ: *Helicobacter pylori* and the pathogenesis of gastroduodenal inflammation. J Infect Dis 161:626–633, 1990
31. Labenz J, Borsch G. Evidence for the essential role of *Helicobacter pylori* in gastric ulcer disease. Gut 35:19–22, 1994
32. Milne R, Logan RP, Harwood D, Misiewicz JJ, Forman D: *Helicobacter pylori* and upper gastrointestinal disease: A survey of gastroenterologists in the United Kingdom. Gut 37:314–318, 1995
33. Okajima K, Koga S, Inoue M, Okabe H, Takatsuki K: Plasma levels of polymorphonuclear leukocyte elastase-α_1-proteinase inhibitor complex in patients with gastric ulcer. Clin Chim Acta 189:237–242, 1990
34. Liu W, Okajima K, Murakami K, Harada N, Isobe H, Irie T: Role of neutrophil elastase in stress-induced gastric mucosal injury in rats. J Lab Clin Med 132:432–439, 1998
35. Murakami K, Okajima K, Uchiba M, Harada N, Johno M, Okabe H, Takatsuki K: Rebamipide attenuates indomethacin-induced gastric mucosal lesion formation by inhibiting activation of leukocytes in rats. Dig Dis Sci 42:319–325, 1997

EXTRATHYMIC PATHWAYS OF T CELL DIFFERENTIATION

T細胞分化の胸腺外経路

Archivum Immunologiae et Therapiae Experimentalis, 49: 81-90, 2001

chapter 13

Extrathymic pathways of T cell differentiation

T細胞分化の胸腺外経路

TORU ABO*

Department of immunology, Niigata University School of Medicine, Niigata, Japan

【キーワード】

胸腺外分化T細胞、Intermediate T細胞、NKT細胞、肝臓、自己免疫疾患

【要約】

　胎児期の主要な造血器官は肝臓であることが知られているが、この器官における造血は誕生時に終了する。しかし、出生後でも肝臓にはc-kit$^+$幹細胞が存在し、胸腺外分化T細胞、NK細胞と顆粒球を分化させる。マウス肝臓で産生される胸腺外分化T細胞は、intermediateTCR（TCR^{int}）細胞と同定される。この細胞には、二つのサブセットがある；NK1.1$^+$TCR^{int}（NKT細胞）サブセットとNK1.1$^-$TCR^{int}サブセットである。胸腺外分化T細胞の数は、若年期にはわずかであるが、加齢に伴い増加する。胸腺外分化T細胞の数と機能も、ストレス、感染症、悪性腫瘍、妊娠、自己免疫疾患、慢性移植片対宿主（GVH）病等の場合に上昇する。そして、この条件下では、胸腺（通常型T細胞を産生する）におけるT細胞分化の主経路は反対に抑制を受ける。胸腺外分化T細胞は、自己応答禁止クローンで構成され、異常自己細胞に対する細胞傷害活性を介在する。従って、胸腺外分化T細胞は、異常自己細胞を排除するのに役立つ可能性がある。しかし、胸腺外分化T細胞の過剰な活性化は、特定の自己免疫疾患発症の原因である可能性もある。

はじめに

　これまで、ヒトとマウスの肝臓で、胸腺外分化T細胞の性質の特徴を研究してきた[34, 58, 60, 67, 78, 82]。従来のものとは異なるT細胞集団（例、ダブルネガティブ（DN）CD4$^-$8$^-$αβT細胞またはCD8$^+$γδT細胞）がマウスの肝臓に豊富であることを明らかにした後、これらの研究を開始した[2, 55, 56, 69]。これらのT細胞集団は、先天的に胸腺が欠損したヌードマウスの肝臓の中にも存在する[31, 68]。これらのT細胞は胸腺外経路で分化している可能性がある、また、肝臓がT細胞分化の胸腺外経路が活躍する主要な箇所の1つである可能性があると考えた。肝臓におけるDN αβT細胞とCD8$^+$γδT細胞には、共通の性質があることが判明した。共通の性質とは、IL-2Rβ$^+$、中等度のTCR発現（TCR^{int}）、NK1.1$^+$（約50%）、CD44$^+$、L-selectin$^-$等のフェ

略語：TCR^{int}細胞-intermediate TCR細胞，TCR^{high}細胞－TCR high細胞，NKT細胞－ナチュラルキラーT細胞，DN-ダブルネガティブ，DP-ダブルポジティブ．

*Correspondence to : Dr. Toru Abo, Department of immunology, Niigata University School of Medicine, Asahimachi-dori 1, Niigata 951-8510, Japan, Fax +81 25 227 0766 , e-mail: immunol2@med.niigata-u.ac.jp

ノタイプである[4,57,70]。これら細胞をTCR^{int}細胞と命名した。この基準を用いて、休止状態にある従来型T細胞（胸腺由来T細胞）をTCR^{high}細胞（IL-2Rβ^-, TCR^{high}, NK1.1$^-$, CD44$^-$, L-selectin$^+$等のフェノタイプ）と命名した。

これらの研究と同時に、2系統の齧歯類を用いて独特なT細胞の研究も行なった。当初、多くの研究者は、NK1.1抗原の発現の有無にかかわらず、DN CD4$^-$8$^-$ $\alpha\beta$T細胞を観察し特徴づけた。これらの細胞のうち少量が、胸腺[11,15,18,20,21,41,63,64,77,87,90]や、末梢（例、脾臓；[36,45,65,66,72]、リンパ節；[24,30]および骨髄；[62]）に存在することが明らかになった。その後、BENDELACらが以下の報告を行なった[7,9]：これらT細胞の中にはNK1.1抗原を発現するものも存在する。そして、これらNK1.1$^+$ $\alpha\beta$T細胞（DNとCD4$^+$ $\alpha\beta$T細胞を含む）は、CD1d（非MHC遺伝子をコード化したMHCクラスI様分子）を認識する。このようなT細胞を、ナチュラル・キラーT（NKT）細胞と命名した。その他、TANIGUCHI等による一連の研究では、サプレッサーT細胞ハイブリドーマの中に優先的に同一な変TCRα鎖（Vα14$^+$Jα281）を使用するようなVα14$^+$T細胞が肝臓、胸腺や他の器官に見られることが明らかになった[39,75]。谷口らは、全てではないにしても大部分のVα14$^+$ T細胞は、NKT細胞と一致し、胸腺外である肝臓において分化することをも示した[43]。

NKT細胞はTCR^{int}細胞サブセットに属している。TCR^{int}細胞には、NK1.1$^+$サブセットとNK1.1$^-$サブセットの二つがあり、特に肝臓と胸腺において両者の比率は1：1である[80,82]。さらに、TCR^{int}細胞（NKT細胞を含む）が胸腺外である肝臓内や胸腺内代替経路を通じて分化することが判明している[18,73]。対照的に、従来型T細胞は、胸腺内主経路を通じて分化する。これらの結果を考慮して、本総論では、フェノタイプ、形態学、機能および進化の面より、TCR^{int}細胞とNKT細胞の特徴を更に深く考察する。

TCR^{int}細胞とNKT細胞の組織局在

マウスにおいてTCR^{int}（CD3^{int}）細胞またはNKT細胞を同定するため、CD3とIL-2RβまたはCD3とNK1.1の二重染色を行った。NK細胞（IL-2Rβ^+CD3$^-$）、TCR^{int}細胞（IL-2Rβ^-CD3^{high}）そして従来型T細胞（IL-2Rβ^-CD3^{high}）を同定した。NK細胞もTCR^{int}細胞も、常にIL-2Rβを発現していたが、従来型T細胞は、IL-2Rβの発現が欠如していた。従来型T細胞は、系統進化の途上でリンパ球の休止形（IL-2R$\alpha^-\beta^-$）を獲得したと考えられる。抗原刺激をすると、従来型T細胞に高親和性IL-2R（IL-2R$\alpha^+\beta^+$）が発現する。この状況を反映して、原始リンパ球は他のリンパ球より反応が速い（NK細胞→TCR^{int}細胞→TCR^{high}細胞）[59]。しかし、これら細胞の中で、一番激しい反応を示すのは、TCR^{high}細胞である。

諸器官においてCD3^{int}細胞とNKT細胞の分布は、ほぼ同様であった、すなわち、両細胞とも肝臓に多かったが、他器官では数少なかった。しかし、測定を行った全器官において、NKT細胞の比率は、常にTCR^{int}細胞の比率より少なかった。NKT細胞におけるTCR$^-$CD3複合体（TCR^{int}細胞）が低密度である事実から考えると、NKT細胞は、TCR^{int}細胞集団の中に存在する。肝臓と胸腺においてTCR^{int}細胞の中のNKT細胞の比率は、>50%であった、ところが脾臓、リンパ節および骨髄においてTCR^{int}細胞の中のNKT細胞の比率は約20%であった[82]。

NK細胞、TCR^{int}細胞とTCR^{high}細胞のフェノタイプの特徴

NK/T細胞系のリンパ球の系統進化であろうと考えられる系統を示す：NK細胞→TCR^{int}細胞→TCR^{high}細胞である（Fig. 1）。進化して、

Figure.1

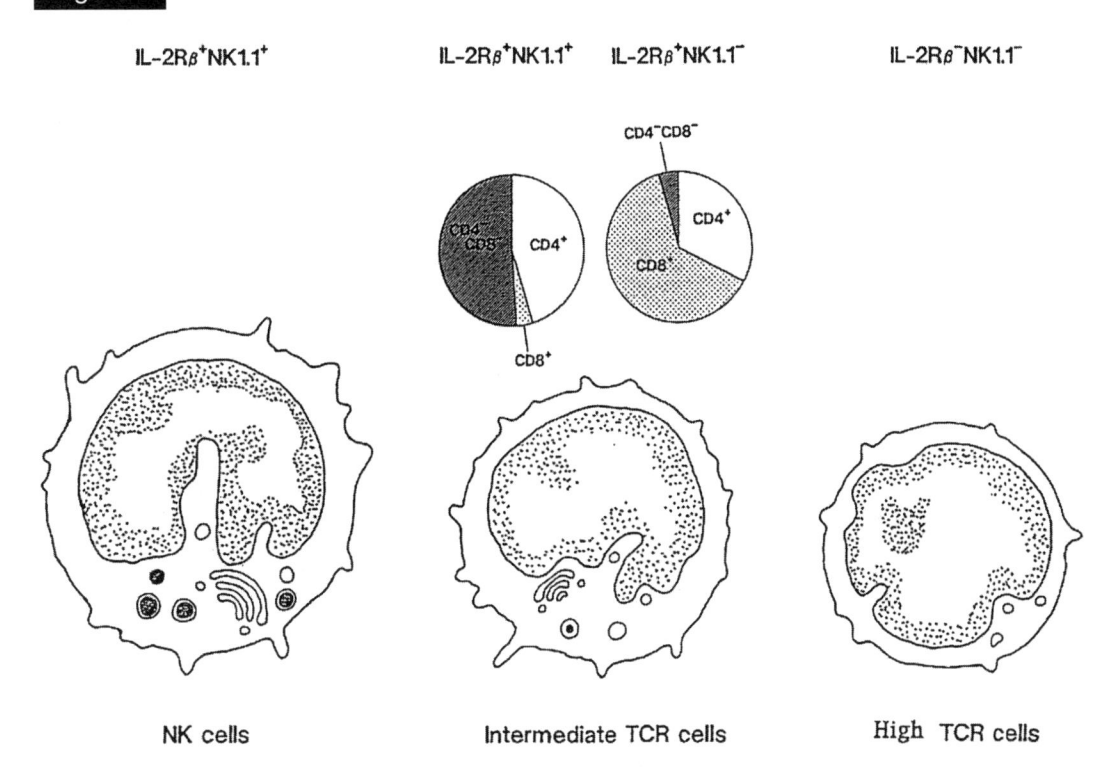

IL-2Rβ⁺NK1.1⁺　　　IL-2Rβ⁺NK1.1⁺　　IL-2Rβ⁺NK1.1⁻　　　IL-2Rβ⁻NK1.1⁻

NK cells　　　　　　Intermediate TCR cells　　　　High TCR cells

NK/T細胞系のリンパ球の系統進化的進化。TCR^{int}細胞は、IL-2Rβ⁺NK1.1⁺IL-2Rβ⁺NK1.1⁻サブセットで構成される。

リンパ球は休止型という形態とフェノタイプを獲得した。この変化により、充分に進化したT細胞は小型の休止型リンパ球の形態を有し、長い寿命を獲得した。対応する抗原に遭遇すると、ただちに休止型リンパ球は、細胞分裂をしてクローンを拡大する。この種のクローン増殖には、NK細胞を伴わず、TCR^{int}細胞がごく少量伴うのみと推定される。

　TCR^{int}細胞のサブセット、独特のフェノタイプの細胞集団で構成される（Fig. 1上）。IL-2Rβ⁺NK1.1⁺（NKT細胞）サブセットは、主としてDN CD4⁻8⁻細胞とCD4⁺細胞で構成されるのに対し、IL-2Rβ⁺NK1.1⁻サブセットは主としてCD8⁺細胞で構成される[34]。IL-2Rβ⁺NK1.1⁺サブセットは、IL-2Rβ⁺NK1.1⁻サブセットよりも原始的な形状であると推測される。興味深いことに前述のサブセット（NKT細胞）がCD1分子（非古典的あるいは、多様性のないMHCクラスⅠ様抗原）を認識すると報告された[7,9]。一方、TCR^{int}細胞の中のCD8⁺IL-2Rβ⁺NK1.1⁻細胞は、多様性MHCクラスⅠ抗原と共に数種のペプチドを認識するようである。胸腺が欠損しているヌードマウスの場合、TCR^{int}細胞とNKT細胞の数はわずかであるが、そのすべてはTCR^{int}細胞と分類される[31,68]。さらに、NKT細胞とNK1.1⁻TCR^{int}細胞はどちらもほとんど、DNまたはCD4⁺フェノタイプではなくCD8⁺フェノタイプを示す。

肝臓と胸腺におけるTCR^{int}細胞またはNKT細胞の分化

TCR^{int}細胞かNKT細胞がどのようにマウス体内で分化するかを知ることは興味深い。先天的に胸腺が欠損しているヌードマウスにおいて、T細胞はTCR^{int}細胞しかない。このことから、TCR^{int}細胞は、胸腺外で分化したことは明らかである[31, 68]。その主要な分化の場所は胸腺欠損マウスでも胸腺が正常であるマウスでも、肝臓であるようである（Fig. 2）。c-kit$^+$幹細胞は、肝臓の実質間隙に存在するが、この幹細胞が胸腺外分化T細胞を生成し、数多くリンパ系細胞群を形成したことをこれまでに証明した[54, 83]。このc-kit$^+$細胞には、リンパ系細胞のみでなく、顆粒球や赤血球などの他の血液細胞を産生する能力がある[83, 88]。胸腺外分化T細胞と顆粒球は、肝臓の実質間隙で分化し（赤血球は分化しない）、成熟後、類洞に移動する[78, 89]。IL-7は胸腺外T細胞の初期成熟のサイトカインとして機能するが[48]、IL-12、IL-15およびIL-18は機能を成熟させるサイトカインとして機能する可能性がある[6, 23, 26]。

TCR^{int}細胞やNKT細胞は、胸腺内代替経路でも分化される（Fig. 2上）。少量のTCR^{int}細胞とNKT細胞は、皮質の至る所に散在しているが、これらT細胞のほとんどは髄質内に存在する[38]。一方、従来型T細胞を分化させるT細胞分化の主経路は、皮質に存在する。肝臓における胸腺外分化T細胞と同様に、胸腺におけるTCR^{int}細胞とNKT細胞は、ダブルポジティ

Figure.2

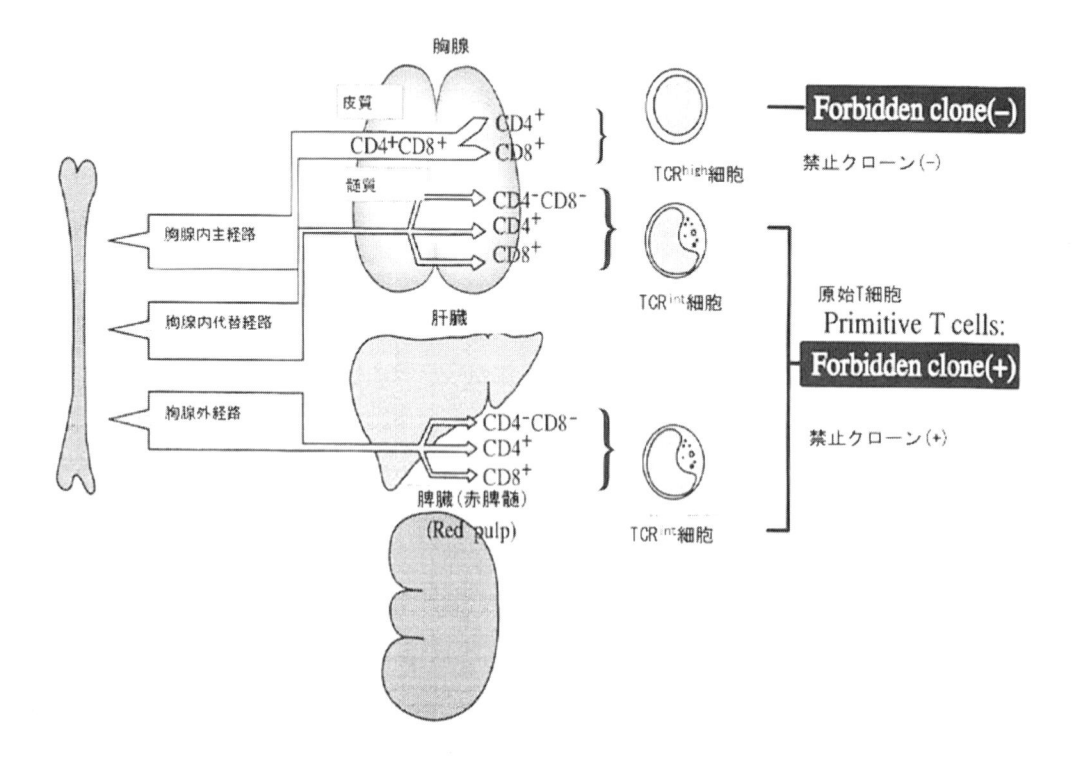

胸腺と肝臓におけるT細胞分化経路。胸腺内主経路は、DP CD4$^+$CD8$^+$細胞のステージを経て、従来型T細胞に分化する。この経路では、負の選択により禁止クローンを排除する。一方、胸腺内代替経路と肝臓（と脾臓）における胸腺外経路では、不完全な負の選択のため禁止クローンを含む原始的細胞が分化する。

Figure.3

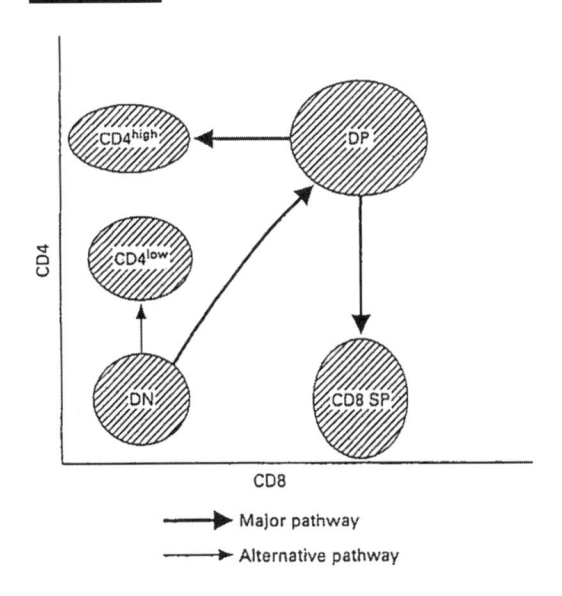

[図: 胸腺のT細胞分化の主要経路と代替経路の略図。縦軸CD4、横軸CD8。DN→CD4low→CD4high、DN→DP→CD4high（Major pathway）、DP→CD8 SP（Major pathway）、DN→DP（Alternative pathway）]

胸腺のT細胞分化の主要経路と代替経路の略図。胸腺には、主要経路とT細胞分化の代替経路がある。マウスが急性胸腺萎縮から回復する時、代替経路はむしろ顕著となる。

ブ（DP）CD4$^+$8$^+$期を経ずに分化し、3つのサブセット（DN CD4$^-$8$^-$、CD4$^+$およびCD8$^+$）が出現する[44]。TCR^{int}細胞やNKT細胞は、DP CD4$^+$8$^+$期を経過せず分化するので、Mls（マイナーリンパ球刺激抗原）システムで決定されるように、禁止クローンを排除する負の選択は、常に不完全である[49, 51, 60]。Mlsシステムの禁止クローンを同定するには、C57BL/6（B6）マウスや（B6マウスと他系のマウスをかけあわせた）F$_1$マウス以外のマウスを使用する必要がある。

T細胞分化の胸腺内代替経路は、若年期には限定的である。しかし、宿主の急性胸腺萎縮が回復する際、この経路は顕著になる（Fig. 3）。DN CD4$^-$8$^-$TCR$^-$細胞は、CD4^{low}TCR^{int}細胞またはDN TCR^{int}細胞に分化する[44]。より重要なことは、代替経路で産生されたこのTCR^{int}細胞は自己応答性を有することである。本研究において、放射線照射（6.5Gy）、または、ヒドロコルチゾン投与（10mg/匹）を行い急性胸腺萎縮マウスモデルとした。この他にも、何らかの微生物感染や身体的（または精神的）ストレスにより急性胸腺萎縮が出現すると考えられる。自己応答性TCR^{int}細胞の分化は、自己免疫疾患発症と密接な関係がある可能性を提唱する。胸腺萎縮からの回復期間にTCR^{int}細胞が顕著であるのは、通常型TCR^{high}細胞よりも回復が早いTCR^{int}細胞の回復が行われることが原因である。この回復期には、従来型T細胞の中に禁止クローンは見られなかったことを強調しなければならない[44, 49, 51]。NK1.1$^+$TCR^{int}細胞でも、NK1.1$^-$TCR^{int}細胞でも、この原始的T細胞の関連を自己免疫疾患の基本となるメカニズムとともに考慮する必要がある。

各部位において胸腺外分化T細胞が独立して分化する

TCR^{int}細胞やNKT細胞は、胸腺外である脾臓（おそらく赤脾髄）で分化する（Fig. 2）。TCR^{int}細胞とNKT細胞を産生する胸腺外経路は、体の複数部位に見られる。産生部位には、子宮[27, 28, 40, 42]、小腸[16, 17, 19, 25, 52]、や外分泌腺（例、唾液腺[74]や涙腺）がある。小腸には、CD8$\alpha\beta$ $\gamma\delta$T細胞とDP CD4$^+$8$^+$ $\alpha\beta$T細胞が独特に存在する。このすべての胸腺外分化T細胞では、NK1.1抗原の発現が見られない。系統進化において、ある時期には、肝臓と小腸の胸腺外分化T細胞は、同じように分化するが、その後、別々に分化する。虫垂の場合、自己免疫疾患モデルマウスMRL-*lpr/lpr*マウスにおいて独特のT細胞（B220$^+$T細胞）が見られる[88]。このT細胞は、胸腺外分化T細胞の可能性もある。

この節での最後の検討課題は、どのようにしてc-kit$^+$幹細胞が肝臓に供給されるかである。この質問に答えるべく、B6.Ly5.1系とB6.Ly5.2

系のマウスの並体結合を行なった[71, 74, 76]。フローサイトメトリーのゲーティング解析を行なったところ、並体結合を行なった後でも、肝臓におけるTCR^{int}細胞とNKT細胞は、パートナーのTCR^{int}細胞とNKT細胞との混在の程度が低いことが明らかになった。一方、すべての末梢免疫臓器（例、脾臓やリンパ節）における従来型T細胞は、並体結合14日後までに、マウス自身の細胞とそのパートナー細胞の1：1の混在となった。これは、脾臓とリンパ節における従来型T細胞が、脾臓やリンパ節以外の部位（胸腺）から来るという事実によるものである。肝臓においてc-kit$^+$幹細胞が一貫して骨髄由来であるならば、TCR^{int}細胞とNKT細胞はパートナーの細胞と十分に混在が起きていたはずである。しかし、そうではなかった。肝臓の中のc-kit$^+$幹細胞は、出生後、通常の状況では、骨髄由来ではないと結論づけられる。もちろん、肝臓においてc-kit$^+$幹細胞（例えば放射線照射によって）の機能を弱められた場合、機能が減弱した幹細胞は、骨髄の幹細胞と効率的に置き替えられる[71]。

胸腺でさえ、肝臓と同様にパートナー細胞との混和の程度は低かった[76]。換言すると、胸腺のc-kit$^+$幹細胞は、生後、骨髄から一貫して供給されるのではない。胸腺に存在するそのような幹細胞は、同様に胎児期にも胸腺に存在する可能性があるのである。

免疫機構の系統進化

胸腺外分化T細胞の概念により、免疫機構がどのように進化したかを明確に説明できるようになった（Fig. 4）。原始的な生物において基本的な生体防御機構は、マクロファージのみであった可能性がある。しかし、マクロファージの仲間の中には、貪食能を失い、接着分子（例えば、免疫グロブリン遺伝子スーパーファミリー）を利用して免疫機構を獲得してリンパ球

Figure.4

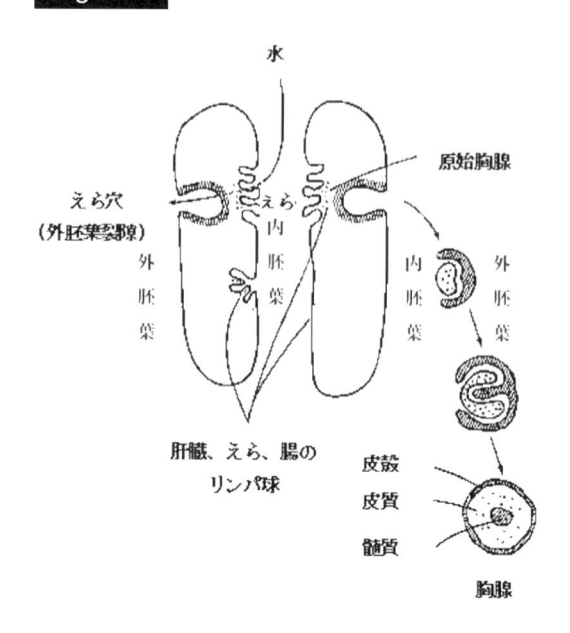

免疫臓器の系統進化的進化の図。原始免疫機構は、消化管と外胚葉で進化した可能性がある。その後、免疫機構は、腸から生まれた肝臓にも広まった。胸腺は、外胚葉の亀裂とえらとの組み合わせから生まれた。

様細胞へと進化したものもあった。免疫機構が進化した部位は、消化管（または腸）と外胚葉であろう。実際、消化管上部には原始胸腺（えらとえらの下にあるリンパ球様細胞）が生まれ、消化管下部には腸管免疫機構が生まれた。肝臓は腸から進化したので、肝臓にも腸にも原始的なリンパ球（例、NK細胞や胸腺外分化T細胞）が存在する。小腸における胸腺外分化T細胞の場合、ほぼすべての小腸におけるT細胞は、NKマーカー（NK1.1）を失った：NKT細胞は、マウスの小腸には存在しない。さらに、小腸における胸腺外分化T細胞は、すべてではないが、TCRを高発現（TCR^{high}）しており、αβT細胞の場合、CD4$^+$8$^+$フェノタイプを獲得した[16, 17, 19, 25, 52]。この腸に見られる独特なT細胞の進化は、腸という部位が抗原刺激を受ける頻度が高いからかもしれない。一方、肝臓、そし

て大腸は、NKマーカーを持つT細胞（NKT細胞）を含む[57]。すなわち、肝臓と大腸には、進化途上の胸腺外分化T細胞が存在するのである。

原始胸腺の場合、えら穴（外胚葉の亀裂）は生物が上陸した時、えらと結合した。従って、正常な胸腺は、必ず外胚葉組織でできている[3]。胸腺において、被膜と髄質が外胚葉由来の部位である。この外胚葉組織は、自己応答性クローンを排除する負の選択にとても重要である。髄質にT細胞が分化する胸腺内代替経路が存在する理由を、図を用いて説明する（Fig. 4）：髄質（外胚葉由来）には、外胚葉（皮膚）由来の古い胸腺外経路が存在する。マウスとヒトにおいてさえ、皮下には胸腺外分化T細胞が多く存在する。皮膚の遺伝子の異常があれば、先天的に胸腺が欠損しているヌードマウス同様、胸腺自体の形成も損なわれる。

NK細胞とNKT細胞による抗原認識

NK細胞は、主にMHC抗原がない自己細胞（例、悪性腫瘍細胞）を認識するのに対し、NKT細胞は、多様性のないMHCクラスI様抗原の中のいくつかの自己抗原を認識することが知られている。この多様性のないMHCクラスI様抗原には、CD1d（非MHCにコード化されたMHCクラスI様分子）とTリンパ球（MHCにコード化されたMHCクラスI抗原）がある[8,33,84]。一方、ヒトで多様性のないMHCクラスI抗原には、CD1抗原（CD1a、CD1b、CD1cおよびCD1dがある）と個人間で多様性のないHLAクラスI抗原（HLA-E、-Fおよび-Gを含む）がある。TCR^{int}細胞の中には、他にもサブセット（NK1.1$^-$ TCR^{int}）がある[82]。このサブセットは、多様性のないMHCクラスI抗原と多能性のあるMHCクラスI抗原とともに、いくつかの自己抗原を認識するようである。このNK1.1$^-$ TCR^{int}細胞の機能の詳細は、不明である。

ヒトの場合、CD56$^+$T細胞はNK1.1$^+$$TCR^{int}$細胞と一致する可能性がある一方、CD57$^+$T細胞は、NK1.1$^-$$TCR^{int}$細胞と一致する可能性がある[53,60,78]。この概念の根拠は、これら細胞の細胞傷害活性機能と局在である。例えば、CD56$^+$T細胞は、強力な細胞傷害活性を有する。また、実際、CD56$^+$T細胞は主に肝臓で分化するが、CD57$^+$T細胞は主に骨髄で分化する。白血病患者は化学療法を受けた後、骨髄移植を受けるが、この時、新たに生まれるT細胞はCD57$^+$T細胞である[22,29,32]。マウスとヒトにおいて、これらのNKマーカーがあるT細胞の形態は全て顆粒を持つリンパ球である[47,82]。

NK1.1$^+$$TCR^{int}$細胞（NKT細胞）が自己抗原を認識する際、抗原提示細胞のほぼ全てはCD1d分子を使用するようだ[7,9]。この場合、そのような抗原は糖脂質、α-ガラクトシルセラミド（α-GalCer）[10,12]である。CD1d分子は、α-GalCer等の抗原だけでなく、ペプチド抗原もNKT細胞に提示することがある[79]。CD1d分子はNK細胞抑制受容体（NKIRまたはLy-49A）と相互作用して、NK細胞に対して細胞傷害活性機能を抑圧するシグナルを提示することが報告されている[13]。NKT細胞とCD1d分子と間の相互関係に加えて、これらのNKT細胞のほぼ全ては、TCRαβにはVα14Jα281の不変鎖を使用する[39,43,75]。しかし、Vα14Jα281鎖を使用しないNKT細胞の中には、CD1d分子と一緒に自己抗原を認識することがあるものの存在が明らかになった[14]。

TCR^{int}細胞とTCR^{high}細胞分化の相互変化

出生時、肝臓やその他器官のTCR^{int}細胞やNKT細胞の数は、非常に少ない[31]。これらのリンパ球は、マウスの場合、4週齢前後に肝臓と胸腺に現れる。その後、TCR^{int}細胞とNKT細胞の数と比率は、加齢に伴い（特に胸腺退縮に伴い）増加する[80]。換言すると、肝臓における

T細胞分化の胸腺外経路とT細胞分化の胸腺内代替経路は、胸腺内T細胞分化の主経路と、反比例の関係にあるようである。さらに重要なことは、このことは、加齢のみならず、感染[2,59]、ストレス[50,81]、妊娠[37,46]、悪性腫瘍[35]、慢性GVH病[61,85,86]等にも見られる。若年期でさえ、これらの状況下では、急性胸腺萎縮が出現し、肝臓や胸腺で同時にTCR^{int}細胞の分化が増加する。考えられるのは、この免疫機構の変化は、宿主が上述の緊急事態を乗り越える際に、重要である可能性である。TCR^{int}細胞とNKT細胞が作用する自己応答性細胞傷害活性は、異常な自己細胞を排除するため不可欠である可能性がある。異常な自己細胞は緊急事態に出現するのである。しかし、このような反応が長期化もしくは、激し過ぎる場合には、TCR^{int}細胞やNKT細胞の産生が過剰活性化されてしまう可能性がある。これらの原始的T細胞は、全て自己応答禁止クローンで構成されていて、自己反応性細胞傷害活性に作用するが[34,51,82]、この時、生体は、自己免疫疾患発症の危険に直面している[5,85]。

これらの免疫抑制状況下でさえ胸腺や末梢の従来型T細胞（TCR^{high}細胞）には、禁止クローン見られないことを強調する必要がある[44,49,51]。換言すると、自己応答性反応に関与しているのは、TCR^{int}細胞（NK1.1$^+$TCR^{int}細胞とNK1.1$^-$TCR^{int}細胞のサブセットを含む）のみである可能性がある。

謝辞

金子裕子氏の浄書に感謝する。

Referances

（原文参照）

Review

Extrathymic Pathways of T Cell Differentiation

Toru Abo*

Department of Immunology, Niigata University School of Medicine, Niigata, Japan

Abstract. It is known that the liver is a major hematopoietic organ at fetal stages, but the hematopoiesis of this organ ceases at birth. However, the liver is still found to comprise c-kit+ stem cells and gives rise to extrathymic T cells, NK cells, and even granulocytes after birth. Extrathymic T cells generated in the liver of mice are identified as intermediate TCR (TCR^{int}) cells, which include the NK1.1+TCR^{int} (i.e. NKT cells) and NK1.1−TCR^{int} subsets. Although extrathymic T cells are few in number during youth, they increase in number with advancing age. The number and function of extrathymic T cells are also elevated under conditions of stress, infections, malignancy, pregnancy, autoimmune diseases, chronic GVH diseases, etc. Under these conditions, the mainstream of T cell differentiation in the thymus, which produces conventional T cells, is inversely suppressed. Extrathymic T cells comprise self-reactive forbidden clones and mediate cytotoxicity against abnormal self-cells. Therefore, they might be beneficial for the elimination of such cells. However, over-activation of extrathymic T cells might be responsible for the onset of certain autoimmune diseases.

Key words: extrathymic T cells; intermediate TCR cells; NKT cells; liver; autoimmune diseases.

Introduction

We have been characterizing the nature of extrathymic T cells in the liver of humans and mice[34, 58, 60, 67, 78, 82]. We initiated these studies since we found that unusual T cell populations, such as double-negative (DN) CD4−8− αβT cells or CD8+ γδT cells, are abundant in the liver of mice[2, 55, 56, 69]. These T cell populations also exist in the liver of congenitally athymic nude mice[31, 68]. We speculated that these T cells might be generated through extrathymic pathways and that the liver might be one of the major sites for the extrathymic pathways of T cell differentiation. We have determined that both DN αβT cells and CD8+ γδT cells in the liver share common properties, including the phenotypes of IL-2Rβ+, intermediate TCR (TCR^{int}), NK1.1+ (approximately 50%), CD44+, L-selectin−, etc.[4, 57, 70]. We term them TCR^{int} cells. Based on these criteria, conventional T cells (i.e. thymus-derived T cells) are termed TCR^{high} cells, carrying the phenotypes of IL-2Rβ−, TCR^{high}, NK1.1−, CD44−, L-selectin+, etc., under resting conditions.

In parallel with these studies, two series of murine studies on unusual T cells were ongoing. First, many investigators observed and characterized DN CD4−8− αβT cells with or without the expression of NK1.1 antigen. A small number of these cells were found to be present in the thymus[11, 15, 18, 20, 21, 41, 63, 64, 77, 87, 90] and periphery, e.g. the spleen[36, 45, 65, 66, 72], lymph nodes[24, 30] and bone marrow[62]. Subsequently, Bendelac

---
Abbreviations used: TCR^{int} cells – intermediate TCR cells, TCR^{high} cells – high TCR cells, NKT cells – natural killer T cells, DN – double-negative, DP – double-positive.
* Correspondence to: Dr. Toru Abo, Department of Immunology, Niigata University School of Medicine, Asahimachi-dori 1, Niigata 951-8510, Japan, fax: +81 25 227 0766, e-mail: immunol2@med.niigata-u.ac.jp

et al.[7, 9] reported that some of these T cells express the NK1.1 antigen and that these NK1.1+ αβT cells, including DN and CD4+ αβT cells, recognize non-MHC gene-encoded MHC class I-like molecules, CD1d. These T cells are termed natural killer T (NKT) cells. In another series of studies by Taniguchi and his colleagues, it was found that some suppressor T cell hybridomas preferentially use an invariant TCRα chain, Vα14-Jα281, and that such Vα14+ T cells are detected in the liver, thymus and other organs[39, 75]. They also demonstrated that most Vα14+ T cells, if not all, coincide with NKT cells and are extrathymically generated in the liver[43].

NKT cells belong to a subset of TCR^{int} cells, i.e. TCR^{int} cells consist of both NK1.1+ and NK1.1- subsets at a ratio of 1:1, especially in the liver and thymus[80, 82]. Moreover, it has been found that TCR^{int} cells (including NKT cells) are generated extrathymically in the liver and through an alternative intrathymic pathway[18, 73]. In contrast, conventional T cells are generated through the mainstream of T cell differentiation in the thymus. In light of these findings, we further characterize TCR^{int} cells and NKT cells in the liver and other organs in terms of their phenotype, morphology, function and development in this review.

Tissue Distribution of TCR^{int} Cells and NKT Cells

Two-color staining for CD3 and IL-2Rβ or for CD3 and NK1.1 was conducted to identify TCR^{int} (CD3^{int}) cells or NKT cells in mice. NK cells were identified as IL-2Rβ+CD3-, TCR^{int} cells as IL-2Rβ+CD3^{int}, and conventional T cells as IL-2Rβ-CD3^{high}. Both NK cells and TCR^{int} cells consistently express IL-2Rβ, while conventional T cells lack the expression of IL-2Rβ[82]. It is conceivable that conventional T cells acquired a resting form of lymphocytes in phylogeny (i.e. IL-2Rα-β-). After antigenic stimulation they begin to express a high affinity IL-2R (i.e. IL-2Rα+β+). Reflecting this situation, primitive lymphocytes respond more quickly than others (NK cells→TCR^{int} cells→TCR^{high} cells)[59]. Among these, however, the magnitude of response is the greatest in TCR^{high} cells.

The distribution of CD3^{int} cells and NKT cells in various organs was almost the same, namely, both were abundant in the liver but few in number in other organs. However, the proportion of NKT cells was always smaller than that of TCR^{int} cells in all tested organs. Concerning the fact that NKT cells had a lower density of TCR-CD3 complex (i.e. TCR^{int} cells), NKT cells are present within the population of TCR^{int} cells. The pro-

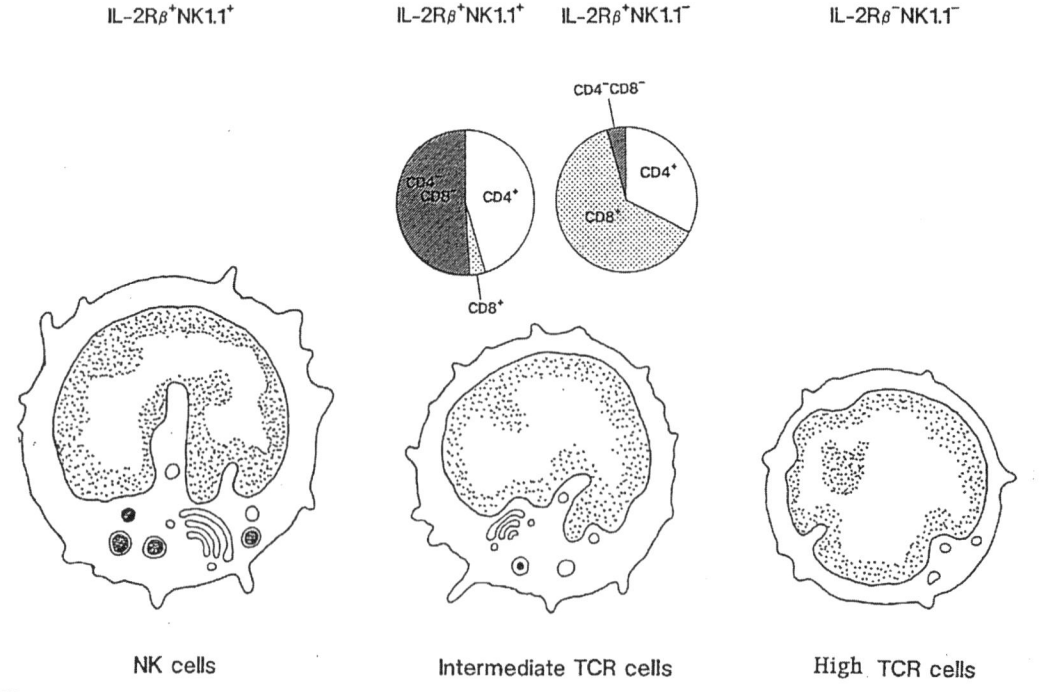

Fig. 1. Phylogenetic development of lymphocytes of a NK/T cell lineage. TCR^{int} cells comprise IL-2Rβ+NK1.1+ and IL-2Rβ+NK1.1- subsets

portion of NKT cells among TCR^{int} cells was >50% in the liver and thymus, whereas that of NKT cells among TCR^{int} cells was approximately 20% in the spleen, lymph nodes and bone marrow[82].

Characterization of the Phenotype of NK Cells, TCR^{int} Cells and TCR^{high} Cells

A possible line of the phylogenic development of lymphocytes of a NK/T cell lineage is represented: NK cells→TCR^{int} cells→TCR^{high} cells (Fig. 1). Depending on the development, lymphocytes acquired a resting form of morphology and phenotype. According to this change, well-developed T cells have the morphology of small resting lymphocytes and acquire a long life-span. Once they encounter corresponding antigens, they undergo cell-division to expand the clones. It is presumed that this kind of clonal expansion is not accompanied by NK cells and is only slightly accompanied by TCR^{int} cells.

The subsets of TCR^{int} cells comprise cells with a distinct phenotype (see the top of Fig. 1). The IL-2Rβ$^+$NK1.1$^+$ subset (i.e. NKT cells) mainly consists of DN CD4$^-$8$^-$ cells and CD4$^+$ cells, whereas the IL-2Rβ$^+$NK1.1$^-$ subset mainly consists of CD8$^+$ cells[34]. It is speculated that the IL-2Rβ$^+$NK1.1$^+$ subset is a more primitive form than the IL-2Rβ$^+$NK1.1$^-$ subset. Interestingly, it has been reported that the former subset, namely NKT cells, recognize CD1 molecules (i.e. a non-classical or monomorphic MHC class I-like antigen)[7,9]. On the other hand, the CD8$^+$IL-2Rβ$^+$NK1.1$^-$ cells among TCR^{int} cells seem to recognize some peptides together with a polymorphic MHC class I antigen. In the case of athymic nude mice, TCR^{int} cells and NKT cells are few in number, although all of them are classified as TCR^{int} cells[31,68]. Moreover, the majority of both NKT cells and NK1.1$^-$TCR^{int} cells express the CD8$^+$ phenotype instead of the DN or CD4$^+$ phenotype.

Differentiation of TCR^{int} Cells or NKT Cells in the Liver and Thymus

It is interesting to know how TCR^{int} cells or NKT cells are generated in the bodies of mice. Since all T cells in congenitally athymic nude mice are TCR^{int} cells, it is obvious that TCR^{int} cells are generated extrathymically[31,68]. In both athymic mice and normal eu-

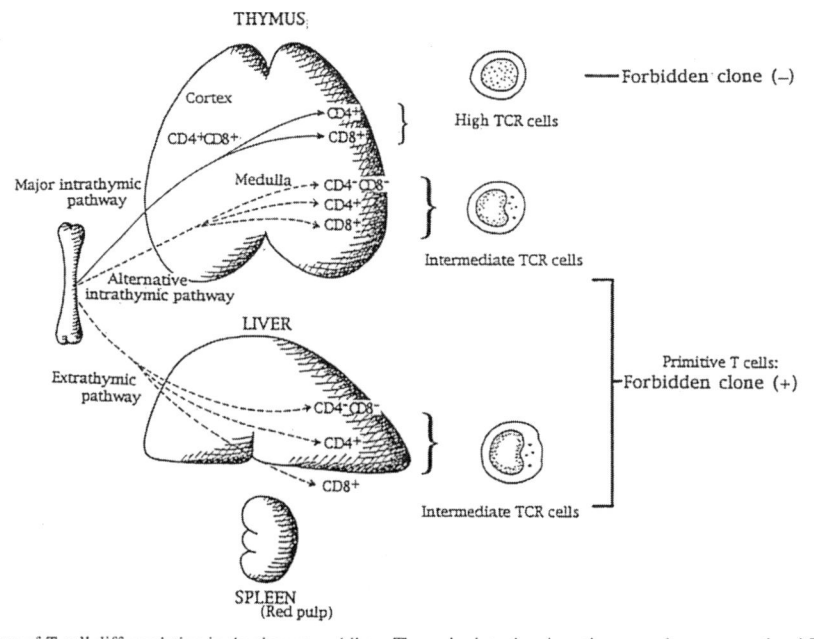

Fig. 2. Pathways of T cell differentiation in the thymus and liver. The major intrathymic pathway produces conventional T cells through a stage of DP CD4$^+$8$^+$ cells. This pathway eliminates forbidden clones by negative selection. On the other hand, an alternative intrathymic pathway and the extrathymic pathways in the liver (and spleen) produce primitive T cells which contain forbidden clones due to incomplete negative selection

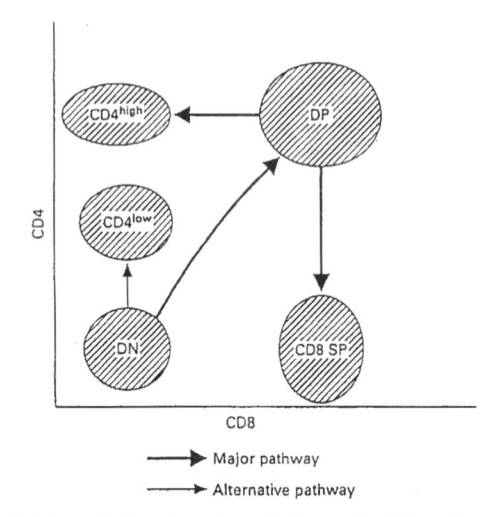

Fig. 3. Schema for the major pathway (mainstream) and alternative pathway of T cell differentiation in the thymus. The thymus comprises both the major pathway (the mainstream) and an alternative pathway of T cell differentiation: the alternative pathway becomes rather prominent when mice are recovering from acute thymic atrophy

thymic mice, the major site appears to be the liver (Fig. 2). We have demonstrated that c-kit⁺ stem cells exist in the parenchymal space of the liver and that such stem cells give rise to extrathymic T cells, forming clusters of many lymphoid cells[54, 83]. These c-kit⁺ cells have the potential to give rise not only to lymphoid cells, but also to other hematopoietic cells such as granulocytes and erythrocytes[83, 88]. Extrathymic T cells and granulocytes, but not erythrocytes, are generated in the parenchymal space of the liver and then migrate to the sinusoidal lumen after maturation[78, 89]. IL-7 functions as a cytokine for the initial maturation of extrathymic T cells[48], but IL-12, IL-15 and IL-18 may function as cytokines for the functional maturation[6, 23, 26].

TCR^{int} cells or NKT cells are also generated through an alternative intrathymic pathway (Fig. 2 top). Although a few TCR^{int} cells and NKT cells are scattered throughout the cortex region, the majority of these T cells exists in the medullary region[38]. On the other hand, the mainstream of T cell differentiation for the generation of conventional T cells occurs in the cortex region. Similar to the case of extrathymic T cells in the liver, TCR^{int} cells and NKT cells in the thymus are generated into three subsets, i.e. DN CD4⁻8⁻, CD4⁺ and CD8⁺, without passing through a double-positive (DP) CD4⁺8⁺ stage[44]. Since TCR^{high} cells and NKT cells are generated without passing through a DP CD4⁺8⁺ stage,

their negative selection for the elimination of forbidden clones is always incomplete, as determined in the Mls system[49, 51, 60]. To detect the forbidden clones in the Mls system, we have to use mice other than C57BL/6 (B6) mice or (B6×other strains) F₁ mice.

The alternative pathway of T cell differentiation in the thymus is minor in youth. However, this pathway becomes prominent when the hosts recover from acute thymic atrophy (Fig. 3). DN CD4⁻8⁻ TCR⁻ cells become CD4^{low}TCR^{int} cells or DN TCR^{int} cells[44]. More importantly, these TCR^{int} cells generated through the alternative pathway contain self-reactivity. In these experiments, we induced acute thymic atrophy by irradiation (6.5 Gy) or by the administration of hydrocortisone (10 mg/mouse). In addition of these conditions, it is speculated that some microbial infections or physical (or mental) stress could induce acute thymic atrophy. We propose the possibility that the generation of self-reactive TCR^{int} cells might be intimately associated with the onset of autoimmune diseases. The prominence of TCR^{int} cells during recovery from thymic atrophy is due to the recovery of the TCR^{int} cells, which is quicker than that of conventional TCR^{high} cells. It should be emphasized that there was no leakage of forbidden clones into conventional T cells at this time[44, 49, 51]. Irrespective of NK1.1⁺TCR^{int} cells or NK1.1⁻TCR^{int} cells, the association of these primordial T cells should be concerned with the mechanism underlying autoimmune diseases.

Independent Generation of Extrathymic T Cells in Various Sites

TCR^{int} cells or NKT cells are also generated extrathymically in the spleen (possibly the red pulp region) (Fig. 2). The extrathymic pathways for the generation of TCR^{int} cells and NKT cells occur at multiple sites in the body[34]. Such sites include the uterus[27, 28, 40, 42], small intestine[16, 17, 19, 25, 52], and exocrine glands such as the salivary glands[74] and lacrimal glands. In the small intestine, CD8αβ γδT cells and DP CD4⁺8⁺ αβT cells are uniquely present. All of these extrathymic T cells lack the expression of NK1.1 antigen. In certain phylogenic periods, extrathymic T cells in the liver and small intestine develop in a similar way, but then develop independently. In the case of the appendix, an unusual population of T cells (i.e. B220⁺T cells) seen in autoimmune MRL-lpr/lpr mice are present[88]. This T cell population might also be extrathymic T cells.

A final question in this section is how c-kit⁺ stem cells are supplied to the liver. To answer this question, we prepared B6.Ly5.1 and B6.Ly5.2 strains of parabiotic mice[71, 74, 76]. By gated analysis in immunofluorescence tests, we found that TCR^{int} cells and NKT cells in the liver showed a low mixture of partner cells after parabiosis. On the other hand, conventional T cells in all peripheral immune organs (e.g. the spleen and lymph nodes) became a half-and-half mixture of a mouse's own cells and his partner's cells by 14 days after parabiosis. This is due to the fact that conventional T cells in the spleen and lymph nodes come from another site, the thymus. If c-kit$^+$ stem cells in the liver are consistently supplied from the bone marrow, TCR^{int} cells and NKT cells should have mixed well with partner cells. However, this was not the case. It is concluded that c-kit$^+$ stem cells in the liver are not supplied from the bone marrow under normal conditions after birth. Of course, if c-kit$^+$ stem cells are impaired in the liver (e.g. by irradiation), such stem cells are efficiently replaced by those of the bone marrow[71].

A similar low mixture of partner cells was seen even in the thymus[76]. In other words, c-kit$^+$ stem cells in the thymus are not consistently supplied from the bone marrow after birth. It is speculated that such stem cells existing in the thymus might home to the thymus at fetal stages as well.

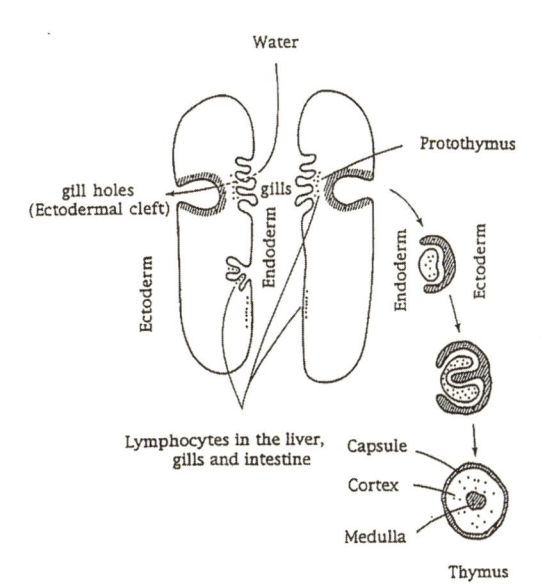

Fig. 4. Diagram of how the immune organs developed in phylogeny. The primary immune system might have developed in the digestive tract and the ectoderm. Subsequently, the immune system was distributed to the liver, which originated from the intestine. The thymus originated from a combination of the gills with the ectodermal cleft

Phylogeny of the Immune System

The concept of extrathymic T cells has given us a clearer picture of how the immune system was developed (Fig. 4). The fundamental host defense system in underdeveloped living creatures might have consisted only of macrophages. However, some groups of macrophages developed into lymphoid cells which lost their phagocytic function but acquired an immune system by use of some adhesion molecules (e.g. the immunoglobulin gene superfamily). Such sites for the development of the immune system might be the digestive tract (or intestine) and the ectoderm. Indeed, the upper portion in the digestive tract gave rise to the protothymus (i.e. the gills and lymphoid cells under the gills), whereas the lower portion in the digestive tract gave rise to the intestinal immune system. Since the liver developed from the intestine, both the liver and intestine became the sites for the presence of primitive lymphocytes such as NK cells and extrathymic T cells. In the case of extrathymic T cells in the small intestine, almost all T cells at this site lost a NK marker, NK1.1: NKT cells are absent in the small intestine of mice. Morover, they acquired a high density of TCR (TCR^{high}) and, if not completely, acquired the DP CD4$^+$8$^+$ phenotype in the case of αβT cells[16, 17, 19, 25, 52]. This unique development of T cells which occurred in the intestine might be due to the high frequency of antigenic stimulation at this site. On the other hand, extrathymic T cells in the liver and even in the large intestine still comprise T cells with the NK marker (i.e. NKT cells)[57]: these organs still carry a less-developed subset of extrathymic T cells.

In the case of the protothymus, the gill holes (i.e. the ectodermal cleft) combined with the gills when living creatures went onto land. Therefore, the intact thymus always consists of ectodermal tissues[3]. Such sites are the capsule and medulla of the thymus. These ectodermal tissues are extremely important for negative selection to eliminate self-reactive clones. This schema (Fig. 4) also explains the reason why the medullary region comprises an alternative intrathymic pathway for T cell differentiation: the medulla, which is derived from the ectoderm, still contains the ancient extrathymic pathway of ectodermal (skin) origin. Even in mice and humans, many extrathymic T cells are present under the skin. If there is a genetic abnormality of the skin, the formation of the thymus itself is also impaired, as shown in congenitally athymic nude mice.

Antigen Recognition by NK Cells and NKT Cells

It is known that NK cells mainly recognize MHC antigen-losing self-cells (e.g. malignant tumor cells) while NKT cells recognize some self-antigens in the context with monomorphic MHC class I (-like) antigens. These monomorphic MHC class I (-like) antigens include a non-MHC-encoded MHC class I-like molecule, CD1d, and a MHC-encoded MHC class I antigen, T lymphocytes[8, 33, 84]. On the other hand, human monomorphic MHC class I (-like) antigens include CD1 antigens (including CD1a, CD1b, CD1c, and CD1d) and non-classical HLA class I antigens (including HLA-E, -F, and –G). There is another subset, NK1.1⁻TCR^{int}, among TCR^{int} cells[82]. This subset seems to recognize some self-antigens in the context of both monomorphic and polymorphic MHC class I antigens. Details of the function of these NK1.1⁻TCR^{int} cells remain to be further investigated.

In the case of humans, CD56⁺T cells may correspond to NK1.1⁺TCR^{int} cells, while CD57⁺T cells may correspond to NK1.1⁻TCR^{int} cells[53, 60, 78]. This notion is based on their cytotoxic function and cell distribution, e.g. CD56⁺T cells have potent cytotoxicity, and in the fact that CD56⁺T cells are mainly generated in the liver, but CD57⁺T cells are mainly generated in the bone marrow. When patients with leukemia receive bone marrow transplantation after chemotherapy, newly recovered T cells are known to be CD57⁺T cells[22, 29, 32]. All of these T cells with NK markers in mice and humans have the morphology of granular lymphocytes[47, 82].

When NK1.1⁺TCR^{int} cells (NKT cells) recognize some self-antigens, almost all of the antigen presenting cells seem to use the CD1d molecule[7, 9]. In this case, one such antigen is a glycolipid, α-galactosylceramide (α-GalCer)[10, 12]. The CD1d molecule presents not only antigens such as α-GalCer, but also some peptide antigens to NKT cells[79]. It is reported that the CD1d molecule interacts with NK cell inhibitory receptors (NKIR or Ly-49A) and presents suppressive signals of the cytotoxic function to NK cells[13]. In addition to a cross relationship between NKT cells and the CD1d molecule, almost all of these NKT cells use an invariant chain of Vα14Jα281 for TCRαβ[39, 43, 75]. However, some NK⁻ T cells using non-Vα14Jα281 chains have been found to recognize some self-antigens in the context of the CD1d molecule[14].

Reciprocal Change of the Differentiation in TCR^{int} Cells and TCR^{high} Cells

The number of TCR^{int} cells and NKT cells is extremely low in the liver and other organs at birth[31]. These lymphocytes become detectable in the liver and thymus approximately 4 weeks after birth in mice. Thereafter, the number and proportion of TCR^{int} cells and NKT cells increase with advancing age, especially in parallel with thymic involution[80]. In other words, the extrathymic pathway of T cell differentiation in the liver and an alternative intrathymic pathway of T cell differentiation appear to be inversely regulated in comparison with the mainstream of T cell differentiation in the thymus. More importantly, this is not only the case in aging, but also in the cases of infections[1, 2, 59], stress[50, 81], pregnancy[37, 46], malignancy[35], chronic GVH diseases[61, 85, 86], etc. Even in youth, these conditions induce acute thymic atrophy and simultaneously augment the differentiation of TCR^{int} cells in the liver and thymus. It is conceivable that this switching of the immune system might be important in overcoming the above-mentioned emergencies in hosts, in that the autoreactive cytotoxicity mediated by TCR^{int} cells and NKT cells might be essential for the elimination of abnormal self-cells which are generated under the conditions of emergency. However, if these responses are continued for too long or are too strong, the generation of TCR^{int} cells or NKT cells might be over-activated. Since these primordial T cells always comprise self-reactive forbidden clones and mediate self-reactive cytotoxicity[34, 51, 82], such hosts are in danger of falling victim to autoimmune diseases[5, 85]. We have to emphasize that, even under these immunosuppressive conditions, there is no leakage of forbidden clones into conventional T cells (i.e. TCR^{high} cells) in the thymus and periphery[44, 49, 51]. In other words, the autoreactive responses might be events mediated only by TCR^{int} cells, including their subsets of NK1.1⁺TCR^{int} cells and NK1.1⁻TCR^{int} cells.

Acknowledgment. We would like to thank Mrs. Yuko Kaneko for preparation of the manuscript.

References

1. ABO T., KUSUMI A., SEKI S., OHTEKI T., SUGIURA K., MASUDA T., RIKIISHI H., IIAI T. and KUMAGAI K. (1992): Activation of extrathymic T cells in the liver and reciprocal inactivation of intrathymic T cells by bacterial stimulation. Cell. Immunol., 142, 125–136.
2. ABO T., OHTEKI T., SEKI S., KOYAMADA N., YOSHIKAI Y.,

MASUDA T., RIKIISHI H. and KUMAGAI K. (1991): The appearance of T cells bearing self-reactive T cell receptor in the livers of mice injected with bacteria. J. Exp. Med., 174, 417–424.
3. ABO T., WATANABE H., SATO K., IIAI T., MORODA T., TAKEDA K. and SEKI S. (1995): Extrathymic T cells stand at an intermediate phylogenetic position between natural killer cells and thymus-derived T cells. Nat. Immun., 14, 173–187.
4. ARAI K., IIAI T., NAKAYAMA M., HASEGAWA K., SATO K., OHTSUKA K., WATANABE H., HANYU T., TAKAHASHI H. E. and ABO T. (1995): Adhesion molecules on intermediate TCR cells. I. Unique expression of adhesion molecules, $CD44^+$L-selectin$^-$, on intermediate TCR cells in the liver and the modulation of their adhesion by hyaluronic acid. Immunology, 84, 64–71.
5. ARAI K., YAMAMURA S., HANYU T., TAKAHASHI H. E., UMEZU H., WATANABE H. and ABO T. (1996): Extrathymic differentiation of resident T cells in the joints of mice with collagen-induced arthritis. J. Immunol., 157, 5170–5177.
6. BARBULESCU K., BECKER C., SCHLAAK J. F., SCHMITT E., MEYER ZUM BUSCHENFELD K.-H. and NEURATH M. F. (1998): IL-12 and IL-18 differentially regulate the transcriptional activity of the human IFN-γ promoter in primary $CD4^+$ T lymphocytes. J. Immunol., 160, 3642–3648.
7. BENDELAC A. (1995): Positive selection of mouse NK^+ T cells by CD1-expressing cortical thymocytes. J. Exp. Med., 182, 2091–2096.
8. BENDELAC A. (1995): CD1: presenting unusual antigens to unusual T lymphocytes. Science, 269, 185–186.
9. BENDELAC A., LANTZ O., QUIMBY M. E., YEWDELL J. W., BENNINK J. R. and BRUTKIEWICZ R. R. (1995): CD1 recognition by mouse NK^+ T lymphocytes. Science, 268, 863–865.
0. BROSSAY L., NAIDENKO O., BURDIN N., MATSUDA J., SAKAI T. and KRONENBERG M. (1998): Structural requirements for galactosylceramide recognition by CD1-restricted NK T cells. J. Immunol., 161, 5124–5128.
1. BUDD R. C., MIESCHER G. C., HOW R. C., LEES R. K., BRON C. and MACDONALD H. R. (1987): Developmentally regulated expression of T cell receptor β chain variable domains in immature thymocytes. J. Exp. Med., 166, 577–582.
2. BURDIN N., BROSSAY L., KOEZUKA Y., SMILEY S. T., GRUSBY M. J., GUI M., TANIGUCHI M., HAYAKAWA K. and KRONENBERG M. (1998): Selective ability of mouse CD1 to present glycolipids: α-galactosylceramide specifically stimulates Vα 14$^+$NK T lymphocytes. J. Immunol., 161, 3271–3281.
3. CHANG C. S., BROSSAY L., KRONENBERG M. and KANE K. P. (1999): The murine nonclassical class I major histocompatibility complex-like CD1.1 molecule protects target cells from lymphokine-activated killer cell cytolysis. J. Exp. Med., 189, 483–491.
4. CHIU Y.-H., JAYAWARDENA J., WEISS A., LEE D., PARK S.-H., VARSAT A. D. and BENDELAC A. (1999): Distinct subsets of CD1d-restricted T cells recognize self-antigens loaded in different cellular compartments. J. Exp. Med., 189, 103–110.
5. CRISPE I. N., MOORE M. W., HUSMANN L. A., SMITH L., BEVAN M. J. and SHIMONKEVITZ R. P. (1987): Differentiation potential of subsets of $CD4^-8^-$ thymocytes. Nature, 329, 336–339.
6. DE GEUS B., VAN DEN ENDEN M., COOLEN C., NAGELKERKEN L., VAN DEN HIJDEN P. and ROZING J. (1990): Phenotype of intraepithelial lymphocytes in euthymic and athymic mice: implications for differentiation of cells bearing a CD3-associated γδ T cell receptor. Eur. J. Immunol., 20, 291–298.
7. EBERT E. C. (1990): Intraepithelial lymphocytes: interferon-gamma production and suppressor/cytotoxic activities. Clin. Exp. Immunol., 82, 81–85.
18. EGERTON M. and SCOLLAY R. (1990): Intrathymic selection of murine TCR αβ$^+$ $CD4^-CD8^-$ thymocytes. Int. Immunol., 2, 157–163.
19. FERGUSON A. and PARROTT D. M. V. (1972): The effect of antigen deprivation on thymus-dependent and thymus-independent lymphocytes in the small intestine of the mouse. Clin. Exp. Immunol., 12, 477–488.
20. FOWLKES B. J., KRUISBEEK A. M., TON-THAT H., WESTON M. A., COLIGAN J. E., SCHWARTZ R. H. and PARDOLL D. M. (1987): A novel population of T-cell receptor αβ-bearing thymocytes which predominantly expresses a single Vβ gene family. Nature, 329, 251–254.
21. GOFF L. K. and HUBY R. D. J. (1992): Characterization of constitutive and strain-dependent subsets of $CD45RA^+$ cells in the thymus. Int. Immunol., 4, 1303–1311.
22. GOROCHOV G., DEBRE P., LEBLOND V., SADAT-SOWTI B., SIGAUX F. and AUTRAN B. (1994): Oligoclonal expansion of $CD8^+CD57^+$ T cells with restricted T-cell receptor β chain variability after bone marrow transplantation. Blood, 83, 587–595.
23. GRABSTEIN K. H., EISENMAN J., SHANEBECK K., RAUCH C., SRINIVASAN S., FUNG V., BEERS C., RICHARDSON J., SCHOENBORN M. A., AHDIEH M., JOHNSON L., ALDERSON M. R., WATSON J. D., ANDERSON D. M. and GIRI J. G. (1994): Cloning of a T cell growth factor that interacts with the β chain of the interleukin-2 receptor. Science, 264, 965–968.
24. GUIDOS C. J., WEISSMAN I. L. and ADKINS B. (1989): Developmental potential of $CD4^-8^-$ thymocytes: peripheral progeny include mature $CD4^-8^-$ T cells bearing αβ T cell receptor. J. Immunol., 142, 3773–3780.
25. GUY-GRAND D., CERF-BENSUSSAN N., MALISSEN B., MALASSIS-SERIS M., BRIOTTET C. and VASSALLI P. (1991): Two gut intraepithelial $CD8^+$ lymphocyte populations with different T cell receptors. A role for the gut epithelium in T cell differentiation. J. Exp. Med., 173, 471–481.
26. HASHIMOTO W., TAKADA K., ANZAI R., OGASAWARA K., SAKIHARA H., SUGIURA K., SEKI S. and KUMAGAI K. (1995): Cytotoxic NK1.1 Ag^+ αβ T cells with intermediate TCR induced in the liver of mice by IL-12. J. Immunol., 154, 4333–4340.
27. HAYAKAWA S., SAITO S., NEMOTO N., CHISHIMA F., AKIYAMA K., SHIRAISHI H., HAYAKAWA J., SUZUKI M. K., FUJII K. T., ICHIJO M., SAKURAI I. and SATOH K. (1994): Expression of recombinase-activation genes (RAG-1 and -2) in human decidual mononuclear cells. J. Immunol., 153, 4934–4939.
28. HEYBORN K. D., FU Y. X., KALATARADI H., REARDON C., ROARK C., EYSTER C., VOLLMER M., BORN W. and O'BRIEN R. L. (1993): Evidence that murine Vγ5 and γp-TCR$^+$ lymphocytes are derived from a common distinct lineage. J. Immunol., 151, 4523–4527.
29. HILBE W., EISTERER W., SCHMID C., STARZ I., SILLY H., DUBA C., LUDESCHER C. and THALER J. (1994): Bone marrow lymphocyte subsets in myelodysplastic syndromes. J. Clin. Pathol., 47, 505–507.
30. HUANG L. and CRISPE I. N. (1992): Distinctive selection mechanisms govern the T cell receptor repertoire of peripheral $CD4^-CD8^-$ αβ T cells. J. Exp. Med., 176, 699–706.
31. IIAI T., WATANABE H., SEKI S., SUGIURA K., HIROKAWA K., UTSUYAMA M., TAKAHASHI-IWANAGA H., IWANAGA T., OHTEKI T. and ABO T. (1992): Ontogeny and development of extrathymic T cells in mouse liver. Immunology, 77, 556–563.

32. IZQUIERDO M., BALBOA M. A., FERNANDEZ-RANADA J. M., FIGUERA A., TORRES A., IRIONDO A. and LOPEZ-BOTET M. (1990): Relation between the increase of circulating $CD3^+CD57^-$ lymphocytes and T cell dysfunction in recipients of bone marrow transplantation. Clin. Exp. Immmunol., 82, 145–150.
33. JOYCE S., NEGISHI I., BOESTEANU A., DESILVA A. D., SHARMA P., CHORNEY M. J., LOH D. Y. and KAER L. V. (1996): Expansion of natural (NK1$^+$) T cells that express $\alpha\beta$ T cell receptors in transporters associated with antigen presentation-1 null and thymus leukemia antigen positive mice. J. Exp. Med., 184, 1579–1584.
34. KAWACHI Y., WATANABE H., MORODA T., HAGA M., IIAI T., HATAKEYAMA K. and ABO T. (1995): Self-reactive T cell clones in a restricted population of IL-2 receptor β^+ cells expressing intermediate levels of the T cell receptor in the liver and other immune organs. Eur. J. Immunol., 25, 2272–2278.
35. KAWAMURA T., SEKI S., TAKEDA K., NARITA J., EBE Y., NAITO M., HIRAIDE H. and ABO T. (1999): Protective effect of NK1.1$^+$ T cells as well as NK cells against intraperitoneal tumors in mice. Cell. Immunol., 193, 219–225.
36. KIKLY K. and DENNERT G. (1992): Evidence for extrathymic development of TNK cells. NK1$^+$CD3$^+$ cells responsible for acute marrow graft rejection are present in thymus-deficient mice. J. Immunol., 149, 403–412.
37. KIMURA M., HANAWA H., WATANABE H., OGAWA M. and ABO T. (1995): Synchronous expansion of intermediate TCR cells in the liver and uterus during pregnancy. Cell. Immunol., 162, 16–25.
38. KIMURA M., WATANABE H., OHTSUKA K., IIAI T., TSUCHIDA M., SATO S. and ABO T. (1993): Radioresistance of intermediate TCR cells and their localization in the body of mice revealed by irradiation. Microbiol. Immunol., 37, 641–652.
39. KOSEKI H., ASANO H., INABA T., MIYASHITA K., MORIWAKI K., LINDAHL K. F., MIZUTANI Y., IMAI K. and TANIGUCHI M. (1991): Dominant expression of a distinctive V14$^+$ T-cell antigen receptor α chain in mice. Proc. Natl. Acad. Sci. USA, 88, 7518–7522.
40. LACHAPELLE M. H., MIRON P., HEMMINGS R. and ROY D. C. (1996): Endometrial T, B, and NK cells in patients with recurrent spontaneous abortion. Altered profile and pregnancy outcome. J. Immunol. 156, 4027–4034.
41. LEVITSKY H. I., GOLUMBEK P. T. and PARDOLL D. M. (1991): The fate of CD4$^-$8$^-$ T cell receptor-$\alpha\beta^+$ thymocytes. J. Immunol., 146, 1113–1117.
42. LIN H., MOSMANN T. R., GUIBERT L., TUNTIPOPIPAT S. and WEGNANN T. G. (1993): Synthesis of T helper 2-type cytokines at the maternal-fetal interface. J. Immunol., 151, 4562–4573.
43. MAKINO Y., YAMAGATA N., SASHO T., ADACHI Y., KANNO R., KOSEKI H., KANNO M. and TANIGUCHI M. (1993): Extrathymic development of Vα14 – positive T cells. J. Exp. Med., 177, 1399–1408.
44. MARUYAMA S., TSUKAHARA A., SUZUKI S., TADA T., MINAGAWA M., WATANABE H., HATAKEYAMA K. and ABO T. (1999): Quick recovery in the generation of self-reactive CD4^{low} NKT cells by an alternative intrathymic pathway when restored from acute thymic atrophy. Clin. Exp. Immunol., 117, 587–595.
45. MIENO M., SUTO R., OBATA Y., UDONO H., TAKAHASHI T., SHIKU H. and NAKAYAMA E. (1991): CD4$^-$8$^-$ T cells receptor $\alpha\beta$ T cell: generation of an *in vitro* major histocompatibility complex I specific cytotoxic T lymphocyte response and allogeneic tumor rejection. J. Exp. Med., 174, 193–201.
46. MINAGAWA M., NARITA J., TADA T., MARUYAMA S., SHIMIZU T., BANNAI M., OYA H., HATAKEYAMA K. and ABO T. (1999): Mechanisms underlying immunologic states during pregnancy: possible association of the sympathetic nervous system. Cell. Immunol., 196, 1–13.
47. MIYAJI C., WATANABE H., MINAGAWA M., TOMA H., NOHARA Y., NOZAKI H., SATO Y. and ABO T. (1997): Numerical and functional characteristics of lymphocyte subsets in centenarians. J. Clin. Immunol., 17, 420–429.
48. MIYAJI C., WATANABE H., OSMAN Y., KUWANO Y. and ABO T. (1996): A comparison of proliferative response to IL-7 and expression of IL-7 receptors in intermediate TCR cells of the liver, spleen, and thymus. Cell. Immunol., 169, 159–165.
49. MORODA T., IIAI T., KAWACHI Y., KAWAMURA T., HATAKEYAMA K. and ABO T. (1996): Restricted appearance of self-reactive clones into intermediate T cell receptor cells in neonatally thymectomized mice with autoimmune disease. Eur. J. Immunol., 26, 3084–3091.
50. MORODA T., IIAI T., TSUKAHARA A., FUKUDA M., SUZUKI S., TADA T., HATAKEYAMA K. and ABO T. (1997): Association of granulocytes with ulcer formation in the stomach of rodents exposed to restraint stress. Biomed. Res., 18, 423–437.
51. MORODA T., KAWACHI Y., IIAI T., TSUKAHARA A., SUZUKI S., TADA T., WATANABE H., HATAKEYAMA K. and ABO T. (1997): Self-reactive forbidden clones are confined to pathways of intermediate T cell receptor cell differentiation even under immunosuppressive conditions. Immunology, 91, 88–94.
52. MOSLEY R. L., STYRE D. and KLEIN J. R. (1990): Differentiation and functional maturation of bone marrow-derived intestinal epithelial T cells expression membrane T cell receptor in athymic radiation chimeras. J. Immunol., 145, 1369–1375.
53. MUSHA N., YOSHIDA Y., SUGAHARA S., YAMAGIWA S., KOYA T., WATANABE H., HATEKEYAMA K. and ABO T. (1998): Expansion of CD56$^+$NK T and $\gamma\delta$T cells from cord blood of human neonates. Clin. Exp. Immmunol., 113, 220–228.
54. NARITA J., MIYAJI C., WATANABE H., HONDA S., KOYA T., UMEZU H., USHIKI T., SUGAHARA S., KAWAMURA T., ARAKAWA M. and ABO T. (1998): Differentiation of forbidden T cell clones and granulocytes in the parenchymal space of the liver in mice treated with estrogen. Cell. Immunol., 185, 1–13.
55. OHTEKI T., ABO T., SEKI T., KOBATA T., YAGITA H., OKUMURA K. and KUMAGAI K. (1991): Predominant appearance of $\gamma\delta$T lymphocytes in the liver of mice after birth. Eur. J. Immunol., 21, 1733–1740.
56. OHTEKI T., SEKI S., ABO T. and KUMAGAI K. (1990): Liver is a possible site for the proliferation of abnormal CD3$^+$4$^-$8$^-$ double-negative lymphocytes in autoimmune MRL-*lpr/lpr* mice. J. Exp. Med., 172, 7–12.
57. OHTSUKA K., HASEGAWA K., YAMAGIWA S., SATO K., NAKAYAMA M., WATANABE H., SAKURA H. and ABO T. (1996): Intraepithelial lymphocytes in colon have similar properties to intraepithelial lymphocytes in small intestine and hepatic intermediate TCR cells. Digest. Dis. Sci., 41, 902–911.
58. OHTSUKA K., IIAI T., WATANABE H., TANAKA T., MIYASAKA M., SATO K., ASAKURA H. and ABO T. (1994): Similarities and differences between extrathymic T cells residing in mouse liver and intestine. Cell. Immunol., 153, 52–66.
59. OHTSUKA K., SATO K., WATANABE H., KIMURA M., ASAKURA H. and ABO T. (1995): Unique order of the lymphocyte subset induction in the liver and intestine of mice during *Listeria monocytogenes* infection. Cell. Immunol., 161, 112–124.

60. OKADA T., IIAI T., KAWACHI Y., MORODA T., TAKII Y., HATAKEYAMA K. and ABO T. (1995): Origin of CD57$^+$ T cells which increase at tumour sites in patients with colorectal cancer. Clin. Exp. Immunol., 102, 159–166.
61. OSMAN Y., WATANABE T., KAWACHI Y., SATO K., OHTSUKA K., WATANABE H., HASHIMOTO S., MORIYAMA Y., SHIBATA A. and ABO T. (1995): Intermediate TCR cells with self-reactive clones are effector cells which induce syngeneic graft-versus-host disease in mice. Cell. Immunol., 166, 172–186.
62. PALATHUMPAT V., JONES D. S., HOLM B., WANG H., LIANG O. and STROBER S. (1992): Studies of CD4$^-$CD8$^-$ $\alpha\beta$ bone marrow T cells with suppressor activity. J. Immunol., 148, 373–380.
63. PAPIERNIK M. and PONTOUX C. (1990): In vivo and in vitro repertoire of CD3$^+$CD4$^-$CD8$^-$ thymocytes. Int. Immunol., 2, 407–412.
64. PEARSE M., GALLAGHER P., WILSON A., WU L., FISICARO N., MILLER J. F. A. P., SCOLLAY R. and SHORTMAN K. (1988): Molecular characterization of T-cell antigen receptor expression by subsets of CD4$^-$CD8$^-$ murine thymocytes. Proc. Natl. Acad. Sci. USA, 85, 6082–6086.
65. PRUD'HOMME G. J., BOCARRO D. C. and LUKE E. C. H. (1991): Clonal deletion and autoreactivity in extrathymic CD4$^-$CD8$^-$ (double negative) T cell receptor-α/β T cells. J. Immunol., 147, 3314–3318.
66. REIMANN J., BELLAN A. and CONRADT P. (1988): Development autoreactive L3T4$^+$ T cells from double-negative (L3T4$^-$/Ly-2$^-$) Thy-1$^+$ spleen cells of normal mice. Eur. J. Immunol., 18, 989–999.
67. SATO K., OHTSUKA K., HASEGAWA K., YAMAGIWA S., WATANABE H., ASAKURA H. and ABO T. (1995): Evidence for extrathymic generation of intermediate TCR cells in the liver revealed in thymectomized, irradiated mice subjected to bone marrow transplantation. J. Exp. Med., 182, 759–767.
68. SATO K., OHTSUKA K., WATANABE H., ASAKURA H. and ABO T. (1993): Detailed characterizaiton of $\gamma\delta$T cells within the organs in mice: Classification into three groups. Immunology, 80, 380–387.
69. SEKI S., ABO T., MASUDA T., OHTEKI T., KANNO A., TAKEDA A., RIKIISHI H., NAGURA H. and KUMAGAI K. (1990): Identification of activated T cell receptor $\gamma\delta$ lymphocytes in the liver of tumor-bearing hosts. J. Clin. Invest., 86, 409–415.
70. SEKI S., ABO T., OHTEKI T., SUGIURA K. and KUMAGAI K. (1991): Unusual $\alpha\beta$ T cells expanded in autoimmune lpr mice are probably a counterpart of normal T cells in the liver. J. Immunol., 147, 1214–1221.
71. SHIMIZU T., SUGAHARA S., OYA H., MARUYAMA S., MINAGAWA M., BANNAI M., HATAKEYAMA K. and ABO T. (1999): The majority of lymphocytes in the bone marrow, thymus and extrathymic T cells in the liver are generated in situ from their own preexisting precursors. Microbiol. Immunol., 43, 595–608.
72. SKINNER M. A., SAMBHARA S. R., BENVENISTE P. and MILLER R. G. (1992): Characterization of $\alpha\beta^+$ CD4$^-$CD8$^-$ CTL lines isolated from mixed lymphocyte cultures of adult mouse spleen cells. Cell. Immunol., 139, 375–385.
73. SUDA T. and ZLOTNIK A. (1993): Origin, differentiation, and repertoire selection of CD3$^+$CD4$^-$CD8$^-$ thymocytes bearing either $\alpha\beta$ or $\gamma\delta$ T cell receptors. J. Immunol., 150, 447–455.
74. SUGAHARA S., SHIMIZU T., YOSHIDA Y., AIBA T., YAMAGIWA S., ASAKURA H. and ABO T. (1999): Extrathymic derivation of gut lymphocytes in parabiotic mice. Immunology, 96, 57–65.
75. SUMIDA T., TAKEI I. and TANIGUCHI M. (1984): Activation of acceptor-suppressor hybridoma with antigen specific suppressor T cell factor of two-chain type: requirement of the antigen- and the I- J-restricting specificity. J. Immunol., 133, 1131–1136.
76. SUZUKI S., SUGAHARA S., SHIMIZU T., TADA T., MINAGAWA M., MARUYAMA S., WATANABE H., SAITO H., ISHIKAWA H., HATAKEYAMA K. and ABO T. (1998): Low level of mixing of partner cells seen in extrathymic T cells in the liver and intestine of parabiotic mice: Its biological implication. Eur. J. Immunol., 28, 3719–3729.
77. TAKAHAMA Y., KOSUGI A. and SINGER A. (1991): Phenotype, ontogeny, and repertoire of CD4$^-$CD8$^-$ T cell receptor $\alpha\beta^+$ thymocytes. Variable influence of self-antigens of T cell receptor Vβ usage. J. Immunol., 146, 1134–1141.
78. TAKII Y., HASHIMOTO S., IIAI T., WATANABE H., HATAKEYAMA K. and ABO T. (1994): Increase in the proportion of granulated CD56$^+$ T cells in patients with malignancy. Clin. Exp. Immunol., 97, 522–527.
79. TANGRI S., BROSSAY L., BURDIN N., LEE D. J., CORR M. and KRONENBERG M. (1998): Presentation of peptide antigens by mouse CD1 requires endosomal localization and protein antigen processing. Proc. Natl. Acad. Sci. USA, 95, 14314–14319.
80. TSUKAHARA A., SEKI S., IIAI T., MORODA T., WATANABE H., SUZUKI S., TADA T., HIRAIDE H., HATAKEYAMA K. and ABO T. (1997): Mouse liver T cells: their change with aging and in comparison with peripheral T cells. Hepatology, 26, 301–309.
81. TSUKAHARA A., TADA T., SUZUKI S., IIAI T., MORODA T., MARUYAMA S., MINAGAWA M., MUSHA N., SHIMIZU T., HATAKEYAMA K. and ABO T. (1997): Adrenergic stimulation simultaneously induces the expansion of granulocytes and extrathymic T cells in mice. Biomed. Res., 18, 237–246.
82. WATANABE H., MIYAJI C., KAWACHI Y., IIAI T., OHTSUKA K., IWANAGA T., TAKAHASHI-IWANAGA H. and ABO T. (1995): Relationships between intermediate TCR cells and NK1.1$^+$ T cells in various immune organs. NK1.1$^+$T cells are present within a population of intermediate TCR cells. J. Immunol., 155, 2972–2983.
83. WATANABE H., MIYAJI C., SEKI S. and ABO T. (1996): c-kit$^+$ stem cells and thymocyte precursors in the livers of adult mice. J. Exp. Med., 184, 687–693.
84. WATANABE H., OHTSUKA K., OBATA Y., IIAI T., KIMURA M., TAKAHASHI T., HIROKAWA K., UTSUYAMA M. and ABO T. (1993): Generalized expansion of extrathymic T cells in various immune organs of TL-transgenic mice. Biomed. Res., 14, 273–288.
85. WATANABE T., KAWAMURA T., KAWAMURA H., HAGA M., SHIRAI K., WATANABE H., EGUCHI S. and ABO T. (1997): Intermediate T-cell receptor cells in mouse lung. Their effector function to induce pneumonitis in mice with autoimmune-like graft--versus-host disease. J. Immunol., 158, 5805–5814.
86. WEERASINGHE A., KAWAMURA T., MORODA T., SEKI S., WATANABE H. and ABO T. (1998): Intermediate TCR cells can induce graft-versus-host disease after allogeneic bone marrow transplantation. Cell. Immunol., 185, 14–29.
87. WILSON A., EWING T., OWENS J., SCOLLAY R. and SHORTMAN K. (1988): T cell antigen receptor expression by subsets of Ly-2$^-$L3T4$^-$ (CD4$^-$CD8$^-$) thymocytes. J. Immunol., 140, 1470–1476.
88. YAMAGIWA S., SUGAHARA S., SHIMIZU T., IWANAGA T., YOSHIDA Y., HONDA S., WATANABE H., SUZUKI K., ASAKURA H. and

ABO T. (1998): The primary site of CD4⁻8⁻B220⁺ αβT cells in *lpr* mice – the appendix in normal mice. J. Immunol., **160**, 2665–2674.

89. YAMAMOTO S., SATO Y., SHIMIZU T., HALDER R. C., OYA H., BANNAI M., HATAKEYAMA K. and ABO T. (1999): Consistent infiltration of thymus-derived T cells into the parenchymal space of the liver in normal mice. Hepatology, **30**, 705–713.

90. ZLOTNIK A., GODFREY D. I., FISCHER M. and SUDA T. (1992): Cytokine production by mature and immature CD4⁻CD8⁻ T cells. αβT cell receptor⁺ CD4⁻CD8⁻ T cells produce IL-4. J. Immunol., **149**, 1211–1215.

Received in November 1999
Accepted in December 1999

Immunomodulation by the Autonomic Nervous System: Therapeutic Approach for Cancer, Collagen Diseases, and Inflammatory Bowel Diseases

自律神経系による免疫調節：がん、膠原病と炎症性腸疾患治療へのアプローチ

Therapeutic Apheresis, 6: 348-357, 2002

chapter **14**

Immunomodulation by the Autonomic Nervous System: Therapeutic Approach for Cancer, Collagen Diseases, and Inflammatory Bowel Diseases

自律神経系による免疫調節：がん、膠原病と炎症性腸疾患治療へのアプローチ

Toru Abo

Department of Immunology, Niigata University School of Medicine, Niigata, Japan

【キーワード】

白血球の自律神経支配—白血球—アドレナリン作動性—アセチルコリン作動性

【要約】

　ヒトでも動物でも、自律神経が白血球を支配する。交感神経が、顆粒球の数と機能を支配する一方、副交感神経がリンパ球の数と機能を支配する。これは顆粒球表面にはアドレナリン受容体が存在し、一方、リンパ球表面にはアセチルコリン受容体が存在するからである。この「白血球の自律神経支配」は生体防御に有益である可能性がある。しかし、自律神経がバランスを崩し、どちらか一方に傾いてしまうと、病気になってしまう。例えば、激しい身体的または精神的ストレス→交感神経緊張→顆粒球増多→組織破壊(膠原病、炎症性腸疾患やがん等)。「白血球の自律神経支配」を理解するならば、膠原病、炎症性腸疾患やがんにさえ新たなるアプローチがもたらされる。「白血球の自律神経支配」によるアプローチで、このような疾病ももはや不治ではないと信ずる。

はじめに

　多細胞生物は、自律神経系支配のおかげで、ある細胞が他の細胞とある行動をするため協調して働くことができるようになった。それ故、多くの細胞の表面には、アドレナリンもしくはアセチルコリン受容体が存在する。白血球もこの法則の例外ではない(1,2)。顆粒球とリンパ球(系統発生的にマクロファージから進化した主要な2つの白血球)には、それぞれアドレナリン受容体とアセチルコリン受容体が存在する(3,4)。従って、交感神経緊張では、顆粒球の数と機能が活性化するのに対し、副交感神経優位では、リンパ球の数と機能が活性化する。

　顆粒球の重要な役割は、貪食により細菌を処理することである。生体が活動する時、手足から体内に細菌が侵入する可能性が高まる。故に、交感神経緊張により顆粒球数が増加すると、体を細菌感染から防御するのに有益である。

　一方、リンパ球の重要な役割は、免疫機能によって微細な抗原処理を行うことである。微細な抗原とは、消化管において酵素により消化されたウイルス粒子や外来蛋白を含むものである。リンパ球は、消化管で系統学的に進化した(5)。消化管の機能は、副交感神経が支配する。故に、リンパ球は、消化管とともに副交感神経支配を受ける。体を微細な抗原の侵入から防御するため、リンパ球の数が増加することは、有益である。

　白血球に見られるこのような生物学的反応の

Figure.1

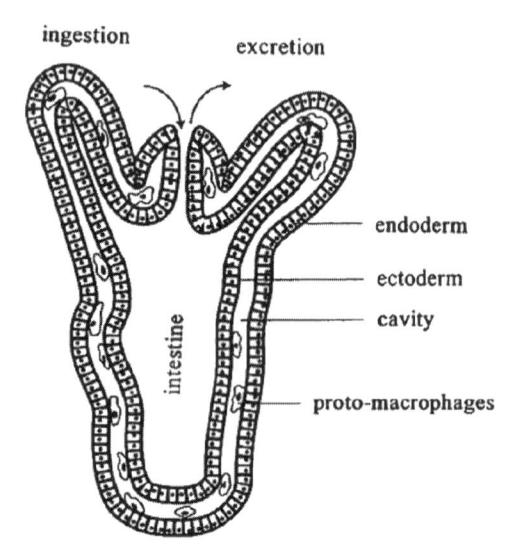

最初の多細胞生物で見られる外胚葉と内胚葉の隙間に存在する原始マクロファージを示す。白血球の起源はこの原始マクロファージであり、また、系統発生の進化において中胚葉性細胞が起源である。

Figure.2

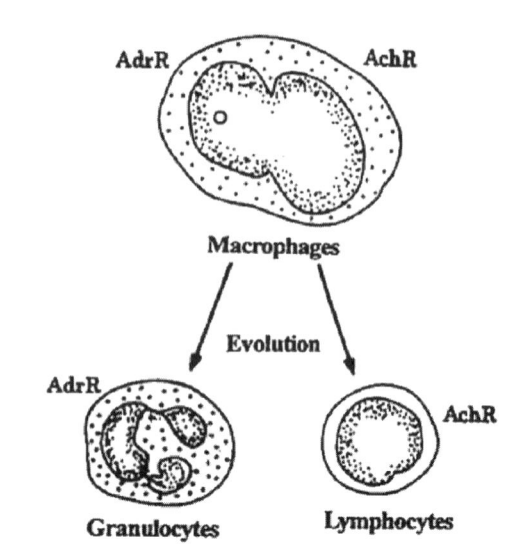

マクロファージから顆粒球とリンパ球が系統発生的に進化した可能性を示す。

ほぼ全ては、生体防御に重要な役割を演じている可能性がある。しかし、自律神経系がバランスを崩し一方向に傾くと、(つまり交感神経緊張または副交感神経優位になると)、顆粒球またはリンパ球の過剰な活性化が出現する。

白血球の系統発生の進化

最も原始的な多細胞生物は、外胚葉と内胚葉で構成されている。しかし、外胚葉と内胚葉の間隙に存在する原始マクロファージを忘れてはならない (Fig. 1)。原始マクロファージは、主に貪食脳を用いた生体防御に重要な役割を果たす (Fig. 1)。外胚葉や内胚葉に起源を持つ細胞の機能は、分化の過程で単細胞生物としての機能の多くを失った。対照的に、原始マクロファージは、単細胞生物としての機能を失わなかった。

原始マクロファージは、その後、血液細胞と中胚葉が起源である細胞に系統学的に分化した。原始マクロファージは、生体防御細胞(白血球)の起源としても重要である。原始マクロファージがマクロファージへ分化したのみならず、顆粒球およびリンパ球へとさらに進化した可能性がある (Fig. 2)。マクロファージが貪食能に特化し、多数の細胞質顆粒を得ることにより、顆粒球へ分化したと考えられる。一方、マクロファージは、他の方向へも分化した。マクロファージの中には、貪食能を失い、表面の接着分子を発達させたものもある。そのような接着分子の一つは、免疫グロブリン遺伝子スーパーファミリーの産物である。結果として、免疫機能を持つリンパ球に分化した。

ヒトの末梢血での白血球の構成は、マクロファージ、顆粒球およびリンパ球は、およそ各5%、60%および35%である。しかし、この白血球分画の比率は、自律神経系の影響を受け変化する(4)。

Figure.3

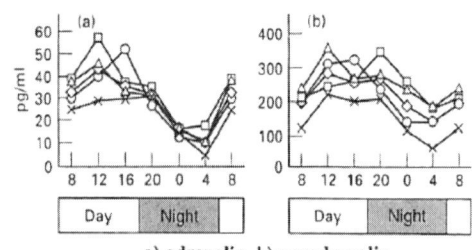

a) adrenalin, b) noradrenalin

健常人の血清中アドレナリン値とノルアドレナリン値の日内変動。(a)アドレナリンも(b)ノルアドレナリンも、昼間高く、夜間低い。

Figure.4

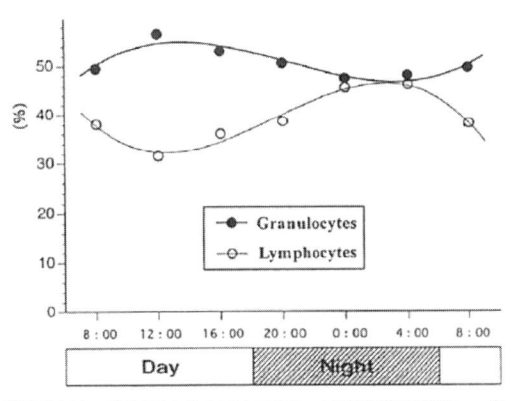

顆粒球とリンパ球の数と比率の日内変動。4時間毎(24時間)に、健常人の白血球分画を測定した。

白血球のアドレナリン受容体とアセチルアセチルコリン受容体

白血球と自律神経系の関係を解明するべく、白血球表面に存在するのは、アドレナリン受容体なのかアセチルアセチルコリン受容体なのか検証した (Fig. 2)。マクロファージ (血液中では単球) の細胞表面には、アドレナリン受容体もアセチルアセチルコリン受容体も存在するが、アドレナリン受容体とアセチルコリン受容体の密度が白血球の種類により異なることが明らかになった。すなわち、顆粒球の細胞表面には、高密度のアドレナリン受容体と低密度のアセチルアセチルコリン受容体が存在する一方、リンパ球の細胞表面には、高密度のアセチルアセチルコリン受容体と低密度のアドレナリン受容体が存在する (3,4)。これらの結果は、Saito の先行研究と一致する (1)。例えば、交感神経緊張下では、ヒトの血液や他の免疫器官では顆粒球の割合が高い可能性がある。この時、免疫抑制が起こり、リンパ球の減少が見られる。

顆粒球とリンパ球の生理的反応

ヒトは、昼間は活動的で、交感神経緊張の状態である。一方、ヒトは、夜間は活動的ではなく、副交感神経優位の状態である。自律神経の変動の状態を反映して、血清中アドレナリン値およびノルアドレナリン値は、昼間高く、夜間低い (Fig. 3)。このような自律神経系の日内変動が、ヒトの血液中の白血球分画に影響を及ぼすか検証した (4)。

白血球総数の変化は、1日を通して、ごくわずかであるが、顆粒球とリンパ球の数と比率は大きく変動した (Fig.4)。顆粒球の数と割合は、昼間に増加し、夜間に減少する。全く対照的に、リンパ球の数と割合は、昼間に減少し、夜間に増加する。この変化は、白血球表面にある受容体の発現が、アドレナリン受容体であるかアセチルアセチルコリン受容体であるかと一致している。

顆粒球は、骨髄で生まれ、血液循環で運ばれ、主に粘膜組織で最後を迎えることが知られている (6)。顆粒球の寿命は、BCL-2 遺伝子が欠損しているので非常に短命 (成熟後僅か2日) である。つまり、顆粒球の50%は、毎日、骨髄が供給する新しいものと交換されている。顆粒球の核の分葉は、アポトーシスへの進行状況を示している。研究を進めるうち、顆粒球の数の変化は、骨髄での顆粒球産生変化が原因であることが明らかとなった。

chapter 14

Figure.5

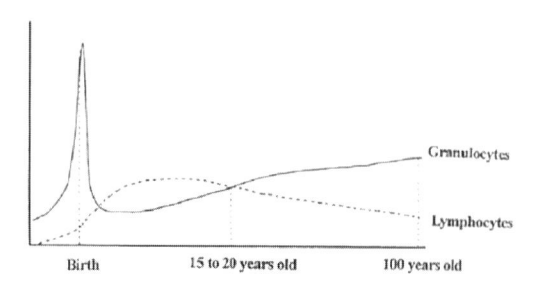

顆粒球数とリンパ球数の加齢変化。出生直後に、新生児顆粒球増多症が出現する。その後、15‐20歳までリンパ球増多が続く。リンパ球増多の時期は、先進国で長期化する傾向がある。この時期以降は、はっきりとした成人型の白血球分画（顆粒球：リンパ球）となる。

ヒト白血球分画における加齢変化

新生児の血液では、白血球総数高値、顆粒球増多症が見られることが知られている (Fig. 5)。これは、分娩後、新生児が肺呼吸を開始することが原因であることが明らかになった (7)。つまり、酸素ストレスにより交感神経緊張が誘導され、その結果、顆粒球増多症が出現するのである。

その後の小児の血液では、リンパ球優位が見られる。特に、1-4歳の子供では、リンパ球の数と比率の両方で顕著な増加が見られる、一方、5-15歳では、リンパ球と顆粒球の比率は、1:1である。15-20歳を過ぎると、リンパ球と顆粒球の比率は、大人のパターン（35％：60％）となる。加齢に伴い、顆粒球比率が徐々に増加するのである。

小児に見られるリンパ球増加は、副交感神経優位が原因である。小児における免疫状態は、発育というストレスを和らげるのに重要である可能性がある。何故なら、1-4歳の小児では体重増加が非常に顕著であるからだ。

年齢を重ねると、顆粒球増多が一般的になる(8)。これは、交感神経が優位になるためであるが、その原因は、酸化物質の蓄積である可能性がある。最近の研究において百寿者では、顆粒球の貪食能は増強したが、顆粒球の超酸化物産生は増加しなかったと報告した (9)。顆粒球機能の特異的変化には、高齢者の健康維持に有益であるものもある。いずれにせよ、リンパ球と顆粒球の比率が加齢に関連して変化するのは、自律神経系の影響がある可能性もある。この場合、ステロイドホルモン類が同時に関連している可能性も考えられる。

ストレスと胃潰瘍

ヒトとマウスにおいて、H_2ブロッカーにより顆粒球数が減少したのに対し、プロトンポンプ阻害剤 (PPI) による顆粒球機能（超酸化物産生）の抑制をしたと報告した (6)。

全く対照的に、H_2ブロッカーでは顆粒球の機能は抑制されなかった。そして、PPIでは顆粒球の数は減少しなかった。顆粒球表面にアドレナリン受容体が存在し、交感神経緊張時に活性化することを最近報告したが、これらの結果は、顆粒球が胃粘膜に集積することが胃潰瘍の発症機序として重要である可能性を示唆する。胃潰瘍患者の交感神経緊張の原因は、心身のストレスまたは細菌感染（ヘリコバクター・ピロリ）である可能性がある。

マウスを用いた実験を示すが、顆粒球移動（骨髄→血液循環→粘膜）が、「胃潰瘍の顆粒球説」を理解するのに重要である (Fig. 6)。ストレスが慢性的に継続すると、骨髄内で顆粒球産生自体が増加する。そして、末梢の顆粒球の数は血液中のみならず各組織中でも上昇する。本研究を一読すれば、抗潰瘍剤、H_2ブロッカーとPPIの治療の基礎を適切に理解できる。「胃潰瘍の顆粒球説」ならば、H_2ブロッカーとPPIにより、胃全摘術を受け、胃酸を分泌する壁細胞を全て失った患者であるのに吻合部潰瘍が改善する謎も説明できる。

上述のことより「胃潰瘍の顆粒球説」を提唱

Figure.6

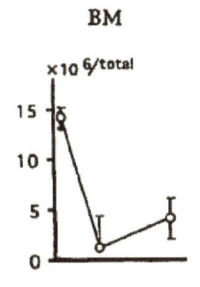

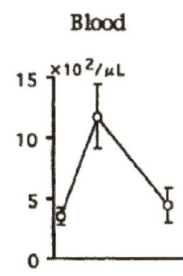

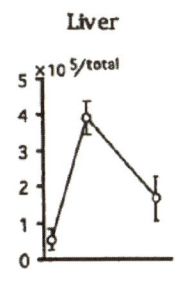

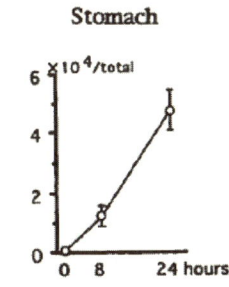

拘束ストレスを与えたマウスにおける独特の顆粒球動態。マウスに拘束ストレス(8時間と24時間)を与えた。顆粒球を、Gr-1モノクロナール抗体を用いたフローサイトメトリー解析によって分析した。

する(6)。細胞表面にアドレナリン受容体を持つ顆粒球が、交感神経緊張により活性化され、その後胃潰瘍発症が起こる。最近の研究において、「胃潰瘍のヘリコバクター・ピロリ感染説」が寄せられた(10-13)。しかし、この学説は不完全である。実際、胃潰瘍患者には、ヘリコバクター・ピロリに感染していない人もおり、健常人の多くは、ヘリコバクター・ピロリに感染しているのである。「胃潰瘍の顆粒球説」ならば、おそらく胃潰瘍の全症例を説明できるであろう。この場合、ヘリコバクター・ピロリ感染症が、顆粒球を刺激する第2の要因として重要である。交感神経緊張の原因は、数多くあり、精神的ストレス、働き過ぎ、細菌感染、非ステロイド性消炎鎮痛剤(NSAID)投与やこれら要因の組合せがある。

非ステロイド消炎鎮痛剤(NSAID)

非ステロイド消炎鎮痛剤(NSAID)は、疼痛、発熱、炎症を緩和することができるので、世界中の医師が最も多く処方する薬剤である。しかし、NSAIDには、時々、副作用(例、胃粘膜傷害や腎機能低下)が見られる。患者(例えば、関節リウマチ)にNSAIDを継続的に投与すると、交感神経緊張の徴候(例、高血圧、食欲不振、便秘、不眠、易疲労)が出現する。興味深い疑問は、副作用とNSAIDによる交感神経緊張との関連性である。

一連の最近の研究において、NSAID(例えば、インドメタシン、アスピリンやケトプロフェン)の投与によりマウスの骨髄内で顆粒球産生が増加することを証明した(14,15)。NSAIDを投与したマウスの末梢では、顆粒球と原始(古い免疫系の)リンパ球(NK細胞と胸腺外分化T細胞)の両方に、数と機能の活性化が認められた。これは、NSAIDによる交感神経緊張と、それに続いて起こる表面にアドレナリン受容体を持つ白血球の活性化が原因である可能性がある。NSAIDがシクロオキシゲナーゼ産生を阻害する結果、プロスタグランジン合成を阻害することは知られている。プロスタグランジンにはカテコラミンの産生を阻害する作用があるので、NSAIDにより常に交感神経緊張が出現する(Fig. 7)。

Figure.7

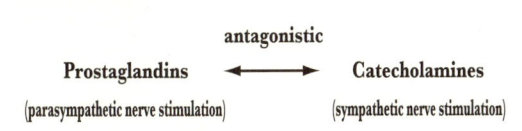

antagonistic
Prostaglandins ←→ Catecholamines
(parasympathetic nerve stimulation)　　(sympathetic nerve stimulation)

NSAIDがプロスタグランジン合成を抑制する結果、交感神経緊張が出現する。

NSAIDにより交感神経緊張が出現するメカニズム。

Figure.8

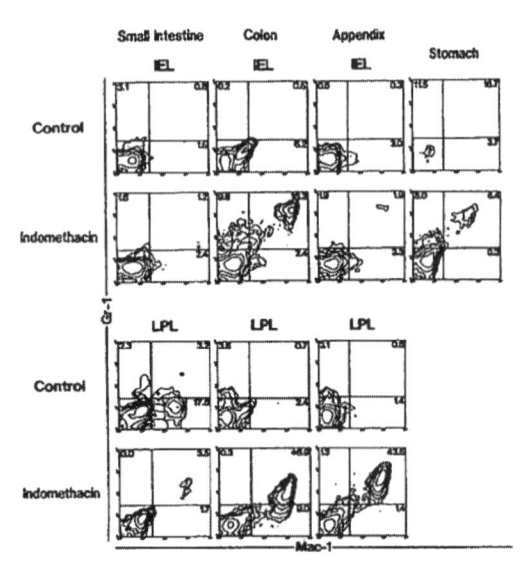

インドメタシンを投与したマウスでは全身で顆粒球の驚くべき増加が見られた。肝臓、脾臓および末梢血における白血球染色(下); 消化管における白血球染色(上)。Gr-1およびMac-1の二重染色を行い、顆粒球（Gr-1$^+$Mac-1$^+$）とマクロファージ（Gr-1$^-$Mac-1$^+$）を同定した。

本研究において、インドメタシンをマウスに投与したところ、胃のみならず大腸においても、重篤な腸疾患を認めた (Fig. 8)。顆粒球の厳しい浸潤がこの場合の腸疾患の特徴である。活性化した顆粒球は、組織破壊に関与することが知られている。そこで、NSAID(交感神経緊張の一因)は、顆粒球が関与する炎症の場合、消炎鎮痛剤と考えるべきではないとの結論に達した。NSAIDはむしろ炎症の原因である。

長期間、NSAIDは、多量もしくは長期投与すると、体内で顆粒球が広範囲にわたり増大するという基礎データ不在のまま処方されてきた。関節リウマチ患者の場合さえ、(経口投与でも経皮投与でも)NSAIDを長期投与すると、関節でも他の器官でも顆粒球が増多して、鎮痛の一方、関節破壊が促進されることが判明した(未発表データ)。換言すると、NSAID投与は、結果として顆粒球が関与する炎症を招く。もちろん、NSAIDを投与すれば、適切に、プロスタグランジンが大量産生されるリンパ球が関与する炎症を抑制する

(例、ウイルス感染時のカタル性炎症)。NSAIDを投与すると交感神経緊張が出現するため、長期間投与を続けると関連する様々な症状(例、末梢血液循環不全、消化管蠕動運動低下や潰瘍形成)が出現する。このように、NSAID使用に際しては、顆粒球増多およびその結果として生じる組織破壊に対して慎重に且つ注意を払う必要がある。

ステロイドホルモン

糖質コルチコイドには強力な抗炎症作用があることを広く知られている。従って、気管支喘息、アトピー性皮膚炎、ある種の自己免疫疾患等の治療薬として使用される。リンパ球の免疫抑制性効果のみならず顆粒球(好中球、好塩基球など)の抑制(例、貪食やアポトーシス抑制)など様々な報告があった。しかし、糖質コルチコイドを長期間もしくは多量に使用すると、副作用が出現することがある(例、潰瘍、組織破壊)(16)。臨床研究では、患者の末梢血中における顆粒球が上昇していた(未発表データ)。

糖質コルチコイド使用によりどのように顆粒球増多が起こるのか検証するため、マウスに多量の糖質コルチコイドを投与し、骨髄と肝臓における造血能を測定した(未発表データ)。この実験のプロトコルは、骨髄だけでなく肝臓にも、胸腺外分化T細胞および顆粒球の産生を行う多分化能幹細胞が存在するという事実に基づくものである。糖質コルチコイドを多量に長期投与すると、骨髄における顆粒球と胸腺外分化T細胞(intermediate TCR細胞、TCR^{int}細胞)の産生を促進することが明らかになった。TCR^{int}細胞は、代替胸腺内経路で産生されるので、原始的T細胞と呼ぶこともある。さらに、その場合、顆粒球は活性化状態であった。糖質

コルチコイドの過剰投与により諸免疫系器官において顕著なリンパ球減少症が出現したが、反対に骨髄と末梢血における顆粒球の数と機能は増大した。そこで、活性化した原始T細胞とこの活性化した顆粒球が、その後、体内の粘膜および/または組織破壊を引き起こすと推察できる。

現時点では、糖質コルチコイドによる顆粒球増多の基礎となる真の機序は不明である。顆粒球表面にはアドレナリン受容体が存在し、カテコラミンの投与により活性化する。そこで、対照群マウスとヒドロコルチゾン（コルチゾール）投与群マウスにおける血清カテコラミン値を測定した。しかし、二群のマウス間には差を認められなかった。サイトカイン（顆粒球コロニー刺激因子(G-CSF)や顆粒球・マクロファージコロニー刺激因子(GM-CSF)等）の中には、この現象と関連するものがある可能性がある。予備研究を行なったところ、過剰投与したヒドロコルチゾンは、組織に停留して酸化コレステロールに変性することを認めた（未発表データ）。ステロイドホルモンは、コレステロール骨格を持つ。この点について、ステロイドホルモンには、有害な酸化物質の性質を有すると考える必要がある。

膠原病または自己免疫疾患

研究者や臨床医の多くは、自己応答性禁止クローン（自己免疫疾患や膠原病の原因）は胸腺におけるT細胞分化に失敗して発生するのであろうと長期間信じてきた。しかし、胸腺内T細胞分化において、そのような分化の失敗は観察されない(17,18)。

自己免疫疾患を発症しやすいNZB/WF$_1$マウスにおいては、発症時に、より顕著な胸腺萎縮が出現する（未発表データ）。この結果が示すのは、T細胞分化の主経路は自己免疫状況下で抑制されることである。反対に、肝臓（胸腺外分化T細胞が存在）におけるリンパ球の数と腹腔内リンパ球（自己抗体産生B細胞またはB-1細胞が存在）の数は増加する。換言すると、T細胞分化の胸腺外経路（主に負の選択なしで自己応答性禁止クローンを産生する）は、自己免疫疾患または膠原病で活性化する。

この状況を反映して、関節リウマチ(RA)患者においてリンパ球（通常型TとB細胞）減少と顆粒球増多（交感神経緊張の結果）が決まって認められることが観察された(Table 1)。このような現象は、他の自己免疫疾患または膠原病（例、全身エリテマトーデス、橋本病、硬皮症、ベーチェット病）患者にも認められる。

自己免疫疾患または膠原病の主要な2つの原因は、感染症や精神または身体のストレスである(Fig. 9)。ウイルスでも細菌でも重篤な感染では、炎症のため組織破壊が起きる。この組織破壊により交感神経が緊張し、顆粒球増多や原始リンパ球（自然免疫）が出現する。組織破壊

Table.1

	n	No of WBC (/mm3)	% Cranulocytes	% Lymphocytes
Control	20	5620.0 ± 423.3	58.0 ± 3.4	33.2 ± 3.1
RA:CRP$^+$	25	7707.7 ± 621.4	71.7 ± 2.7	20.9 ± 2.2
RA:CRP$^-$	20	6228.6 ± 550.3	60.4 ± 3.8	31.2 ± 4.5

関節リウマチ患者の顆粒球増多とリンパ球減少

Figure.9

1) 感染 ⇒ 組織破壊 ⇔ 交感神経緊張
2) 精神的または身体的ストレス ⇒ 交感神経緊張 ⇔ 組織破壊

交感神経緊張は胸腺萎縮や自然免疫活性化を誘発する。

自己免疫疾患の原因とメカニズムの仮説を示す。組織破壊と交感神経緊張は互いに影響しあう。

Figure.10

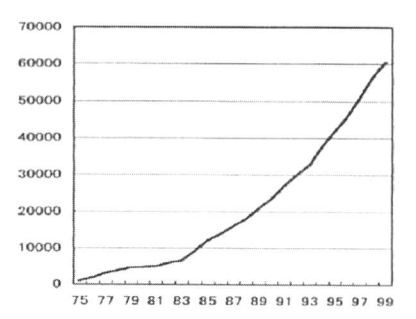

日本における潰瘍性大腸炎患者数の爆発的増加。1975年に、潰瘍性大腸炎が難病に指定され、この年から患者数が増加し始めた。

Figure.11

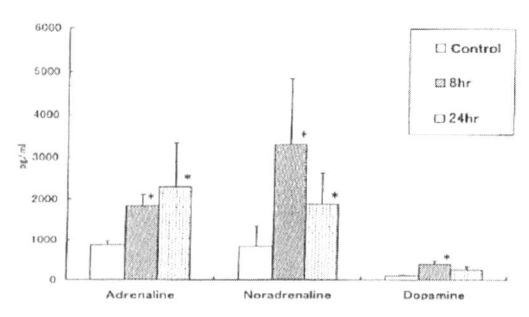

NSAID継続投与による交感神経緊張。インドメタシンを(0.5mg/匹)7日間、毎日投与した後、8日目に血清中カテコールアミン値を測定した。

が続けば、活性化した顆粒球は大量の炎症性サイトカイン(例、TNF α、IFN γや IL-6)だけでなく超酸化物を産生するので、組織破壊が加速する。この時、胸腺外分化T細胞(ヒトではCD56$^+$Tまたは CD57$^+$T 細胞)のみならず原始リンパ球も、変性した自己組織に対する自己応答性に反応し、また B-1 細胞は自己抗体を産生する(19)。

この反応は、変性した自己細胞を除去するのに役立つこともあるが、それ以外の場合には、組織破壊を加速させるので危険である。同様に、精神的もしくは身体的ストレスは自己免疫疾患の原因になる。というのは、このようなストレスが交感神経緊張を招くからだ。こうした交感神経緊張が起こった結果、顆粒球増多や組織破壊が起こる。実際、自己免疫疾患の患者の発症時には、このような心身のストレス(例、働き過ぎ)があることが多い。

交感神経が緊張すると、胸腺萎縮も出現するが、この時、胸腺における T 細胞分化の主経路の抑制が起こる(6)。反対に、NK 細胞、胸腺外分化 T 細胞や自己抗体産生 B-1 細胞(自然免疫の構成メンバー)といった原始リンパ球の活性化が起こる。また、原始リンパ球は、異常細胞や変性した自己細胞の除去を行うので、この反応は必ずしも生体に有害なわけではない。他の研究者も同様の提案を行なっている(20)。

自己免疫疾患または膠原病は重度の免疫抑制状態であることに気付けば、これらの病気のためには新しい治療的なアプローチが必要であることに気づく。免疫抑制剤やステロイドホルモンは、疾病を悪化させる。これらの薬剤使用が、これまで自己免疫疾患や膠原病の通常治療であった。低体温を招く NSAID は、これらの病気の治療にとっても危険である。このように、NSAID を使用すると、激しい交感神経緊張が起こる結果、顆粒球増多が見られる(14,15)。この現象は、NSAID の長期投与が原因である胃炎や胃潰瘍にも関連がある。

自己免疫疾患または膠原病では必ず炎症が見られ、疼痛、発熱、発赤、皮膚発疹、下痢等の症状を示す。これらの炎症の徴候は、組織破壊から回復を促す血液循環が促進した結果と考えなければならない。副交感神経優位は、これら徴候に関連している。実際にこの徴候を引き起こすのは、プロスタグランジン、ヒスタミン、セロトニン、アセチルコリン、ロイコトリエン等である。

免疫を抑制させる薬剤を使用するのではなく、血液循環、炎症、免疫機能を改善させる治療を選択する必要がある。その治療法とは、軽い運動、入浴、笑いや東洋医療（鍼灸や漢方薬）である。特に、鍼灸や漢方薬では、患者の副交感神経を刺激することができる (21)。

潰瘍性大腸炎(UC)とクローン病(CD)

1975 年、日本政府が潰瘍性大腸炎 (UC) を特定疾患に指定した後、患者数が増加した (Fig. 10)。その後、標準的治療としてアミノサリチル酸 (NSAID の一種) やステロイドホルモンを使用するような不適当な治療が定着したと考えられる。

本研究では、毎日マウスに NSAID(インドメタシン)(0.5mg/ 匹) を 7 日間投与し交感神経緊張の様子を検証した (Fig.11)。血清中カテコラミン値の顕著な増加がマウスに認められた。NSAID がプロスタグランジンを抑制することが、この結果に影響していると考えられる。このように、プロスタグランジンにはカテコラミンを抑制する作用がある。このようなインドメタシンによる交感神経緊張により、消化管のあちこちに顆粒球浸潤が見られた。大腸 → 胃 → 虫垂 → 小腸の順に顆粒球が浸潤していた。その結果から、NSAID は、胃だけでなく腸粘膜も重篤な組織破壊が起こる可能性もある。

NSAID が UC 患者の下痢と腹痛に効果を発揮するが、NSAID を長期間使用すると、患者の粘膜破壊が悪化すると容易に推測できる。UC 患者の大腸粘膜に顆粒球の炎症が見られるのに対し、クローン病 (CD) 患者の小腸粘膜にマクロファージ (やリンパ球) の炎症が見られることが、広く知られている。そこで、UC と CD の間にどのような病理学的相違が存在するか考察した (Fig. 12)。本研究では、血液中の白血球総数、顆粒球およびリンパ球の数と比率を比較した (UC, n =10; CD, n =17)。UC と同様に、

Figure.12

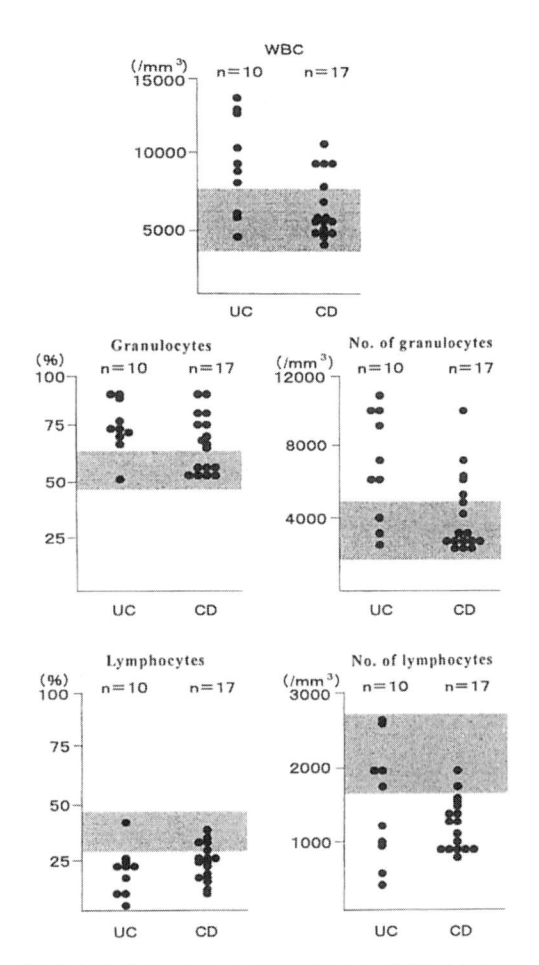

潰瘍性大腸炎(UC)とクローン病(CD)患者の白血球総数および顆粒球とリンパ球の数と比率を比較した。

CD でも、顆粒球の高値とリンパ球低値を示す患者が多かった。

換言すると、UC や CD の患者の血液においては同様の白血球分画のパターンを示し、交感神経緊張が示唆された。実際、この患者の中には瀕脈を示す患者が多かった。長期間 NSAID 投与すると、精神的ストレスと医原性のストレスが起こるが、このストレスがこのような交感神経緊張と顆粒球増多の原因となる可能性がある。しかし、末梢血の顆粒球は大腸に浸潤す

Figure.13

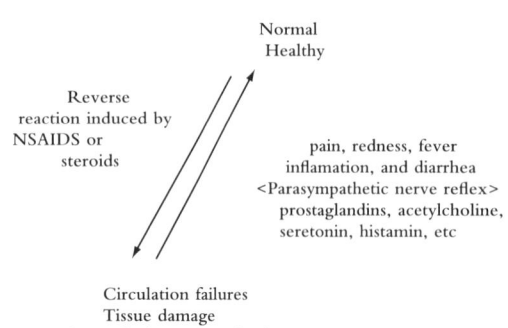

```
                    Normal
                    Healthy
        Reverse         ↗↙
    reaction induced by
      NSAIDS or           pain, redness, fever
       steroids           inflamation, and diarrhea
                          <Parasympathetic nerve reflex>
                          prostaglandins, acetylcholine,
                          seretonin, histamin, etc
                    ↓
                Circulation failures
                 Tissue damage
              <Sympathetic nerve activation>
```

血流障害と組織破壊からの治癒反応。過敏徴候は、むしろ副交感神経緊張による治癒反応である。NSAIDやステロイドホルモンの長期間投与は、体の中の大切な反応を抑制する。

るが、小腸には浸潤しない (Fig. 10)。その結果、小腸に固有のマクロファージとリンパ球のみが活性化して、小腸において肉芽腫を形成する。このことからも、UC患者よりもCD患者の発生率が低いことを説明できる。

これらの結果を考慮して、UCおよびCDのための新たな治療を以下、提案する。すなわち、顆粒球増多の原因となるサラゾスルファピリジン (Salazopyrin)、メサラジン (Pentasa) およびステロイド (Steroneam) の使用をやめる；精神的ストレスと食品に注意する：そして、副交感神経を刺激する (鍼灸、軽い運動、入浴、笑い等)。

病気からの治癒反応に伴う疼痛、発赤、発熱、炎症や下痢

激しい精神的・身体的なストレスを受けると、交感神経が緊張し、血流障害や組織破壊が起こる (Fig. 13)。血流障害と組織破壊から回復するために、速やかに副交感神経反射が起こり、疼痛、発赤、発熱、炎症や下痢が出現する。前述したように、プロスタグランジン、アセチルコリン、セロトニン、ヒスタミン等はこの反応と関連している。

NSAIDやステロイドホルモンを長期間使用すると、こういった治癒反応が全て停止してしまう。従って、薬剤を使い症状を抑えると症状がぶり返す。患者は、治癒反応を繰り返してしまうのである。

がん

これまでの研究の積み重ねから、がん遺伝子が正常細胞を悪性にすることが判明した。このがん遺伝子のほぼ全ては、正常な上皮細胞にもある増殖遺伝子と関連するというのは本当である。それならば、このがん遺伝子がどのように体内で活性化するのか考慮しなければならない。働き過ぎ、精神的ストレスまたは他の原因により、交感神経緊張が継続すると、激しい血流障害が起こる。実際、がん患者の血液では顆粒球が増加し、リンパ球が減少している (Fig. 14)。この時、顆粒球活性が原因で産生された超酸化物に曝露された細胞が死ぬ。そして、上皮細胞の再生が加速する。上皮細胞再生により、発がん率上昇やがん遺伝子のスイッチが入りやすくなることが考えられる。

持続的な顆粒球増多が発がんにつながる理由がもう一つある。交感神経緊張により顆粒球が増多する際、必ず免疫抑制 (細胞傷害性T細胞を含むリンパ球減少症) が現れる。NK細胞が、細胞質顆粒に有するパーフォリンを用いて悪性腫瘍細胞を殺傷することが知られている (22)。しかし、交感神経緊張の影響で、個体レベルでも細胞レベルでも分泌機構が抑制されるため、NK細胞のパーフォリンの分泌は抑制される。

これらの結果より、がん患者がいかに顆粒球増多とそれに伴う免疫抑制から逃れるかを考える必要がある。我々は、以下の方法を提案する：交感神経緊張の原因となる働き過ぎ、精神的ストレスあるいは交感神経緊張の原因となる長期間NSAID投与からの逃避；免疫を抑制するよ

りむしろ賦活化する治療をする(多くの抗がん剤では免疫が抑制される)。最近の研究で、血液中のリンパ球数が 1,800 -2,000/μL 以上あれば、肺がん、腎臓がん、子宮がん、乳腺ガンおよび転移性ガンなどの自然退縮の可能性があることが明らかになった。がん患者が、すでに抗がん剤または放射線治療を受けている場合、免疫を増強することは若干困難である可能性がある。免疫を増強するためには、鍼灸、漢方薬などの治療が役に立つ。抗がん剤や放射線治療のかわりに、上述した治療法を選択するならば、進行がん患者の 60% 以上に 1-2 年以内に自然退縮が現れるだろう。

終わりに

本総論は、膠原病、炎症性腸疾患およびがんの発症は、交感神経が過剰に緊張することが原因であることを強調するものである。これらの病気に共通している免疫状態は、免疫抑制である。

さらに、副交感神経の優位過剰が原因の病気もある。どのような病気かというと、アレルギー疾患(例、アトピー性皮膚炎、気管支喘息や花粉症)である。このような病気の患者は、リンパ球が多い段階では症状は目立たないが、顆粒球が増加すると症状が出る。換言すると、これらの患者はリンパ球が多いので、抗原や精神的ストレスにとても敏感であり治癒反応が起こる時、(交感神経緊張→副交感神経優位)不快な症状を示す。抗原や精神的ストレスを避けるだけでなく、副交感神経優位に体の状態を改善するような治療が必要である。抗ヒスタミン剤やステロイド剤のような抗アレルギー剤では、決してアレルギー疾患の完治は望めない。

Immunomodulation by the Autonomic Nervous System: Therapeutic Approach for Cancer, Collagen Diseases, and Inflammatory Bowel Diseases

Toru Abo and Toshihiko Kawamura

Department of Immunology, Niigata University School of Medicine, Niigata, Japan

Abstract: The distribution of leukocytes is regulated by the autonomic nervous system in humans and animals. The number and function of granulocytes are stimulated by sympathetic nerves whereas those of lymphocytes are stimulated by parasympathetic nerves. This is because granulocytes bear adrenergic receptors, but lymphocytes bear cholinergic receptors on the surface. These regulations may be beneficial to protect the body of living beings. However, when the autonomic nervous system deviates too much to one direction, we fall victim to certain diseases. For example, severe physical or mental stress → sympathetic nerve activation → granulocytosis → tissue damage, including collagen diseases, inflammatory bowel diseases, and cancer. If we introduce the concept of *immunomodulation by the autonomic nervous system*, a new approach for collagen diseases, inflammatory bowel diseases, and even cancer is raised. With this approach, we believe that these diseases are no longer incurable. **Key Words:** Immunomodulation—Autonomic nervous system—Regulation—Leukocytes—Adrenergic—Cholinergic

INTRODUCTION

The autonomic nervous system of multicellular organisms was developed to enable cooperation of one cell with others to achieve a single purpose of their behavior. Many cells, therefore, bear adrenergic or cholinergic receptors on the surface. Leukocytes are no exception to this rule (1,2). Granulocytes and lymphocytes, the two major types of leukocytes that developed from macrophages in phylogeny, bear adrenergic receptors and cholinergic receptors, respectively (3,4). In this regard, granulocytes are activated in number and function under sympathetic nerve stimulation whereas lymphocytes are so activated under parasympathetic nerve stimulation.

Granulocytes are important for processing bacteria by phagocytosis. When living beings behave actively, the frequency of the invasion of bacteria into the body from the hands and feet increases. Therefore, the increase in the number of granulocytes by the stimulation of sympathetic nerves is beneficial for protecting the body from bacterial infection.

On the other hand, lymphocytes are important for processing small antigens by immune functions. Such small antigens include viral particles and foreign proteins that are digested by enzymes in the digestive tract. Lymphocytes developed in phylogeny in the digestive tract (5). The functions of the digestive tract are regulated by parasympathetic nerves. Lymphocytes are therefore governed by parasympathetic nerves and act in parallel with the digestive tract. The increase in the number of lymphocytes is beneficial for protecting the body from the invasion of small antigens.

Almost all of these biological responses seen in leukocytes may play a pivotal role in protecting the bodies of living beings. However, if the autonomic nervous system deviates in one direction (i.e., overactivation of sympathetic nerves or overactivation of parasympathetic nerves), overactivation of granulocytes or lymphocytes results.

PHYLOGENETIC DEVELOPMENT OF LEUKOCYTES

The most primitive multicellular organisms consist of ectoderm and endoderm. However, the existence of protomacrophages in the space between the ecto-

Received July 2002.
Address correspondence and reprint requests to Dr. Toru Abo, Department of Immunology, Niigata University School of Medicine, Niigata 951-8510, Japan. E-mail: immunol2@med.niigata-u.ac.jp

derm and endoderm should not be forgotten (Fig. 1). These protomacrophages play an important role in self-defense, mainly by use of their phagocytic function. The cells of ectodermal and endodermal origins differentiated their functions and lost many of them as unicellular organisms. In contrast, such protomacrophages retain their functions as unicellular organisms.

Protomacrophages differentiated into blood cells and into cells of mesodermal origin in subsequent phylogenic development. These protomacrophages are also important as the origin of self-defense cells, namely, leukocytes. In addition to the differentiation of protomacrophages into macrophages, these protomacrophages might give rise to granulocytes and lymphocytes in phylogeny (Fig. 2). We consider that macrophages differentiated into granulocytes by refining their phagocytic function and acquiring numerous cytoplasmic granules. On the other hand, there was another direction of differentiation in macrophages. Some macrophages lost their phagocytic function and developed adhesion molecules on the surface. One family of such adhesion molecules is a product of the immunoglobulin gene superfamily. As a result, such macrophages differentiated into lymphocytes that have immune functions.

In the peripheral blood of humans, macrophages, granulocytes, and lymphocytes constitute approximately 5%, 60%, and 35% of the leukocytes, respectively. However, the ratio of these components among leukocytes varies because of the influence of the autonomic nervous system (4).

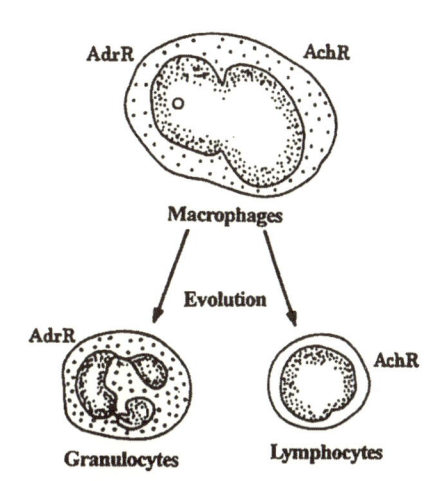

FIG. 2. Possible phylogenetic development of granulocytes and lymphoid cells from macrophages are shown.

ADRENERGIC AND CHOLINERGIC RECEPTORS ON LEUKOCYTES

To definitely reveal the relationship between leukocytes and the autonomic nervous system, we examined the possibility of the existence of adrenergic or cholinergic receptors on leukocytes (Fig. 2). Although macrophages (monocytes in the blood) bear both adrenergic and cholinergic receptors on the cell surface, the density of adrenergic receptors and cholinergic receptors was found to deviate depending on the subsets of leukocytes. Namely, granulocytes bear a high density of adrenergic receptors and a low density of cholinergic receptors on the cell surface whereas lymphocytes bear a high density of cholinergic receptors and a low density of adrenergic receptors on the cell surface (3,4). These results are in agreement with the previous findings produced by Saito (1). For example, if a person is under conditions of sympathetic nerve activation, he or she may carry a high level of granulocytes in the blood and other immune organs. At this time, his or her immunological state becomes suppressive, showing lymphocytopenia.

PHYSIOLOGICAL RESPONSES OF GRANULOCYTES AND LYMPHOCYTES

Humans are active and in a dominant state of sympathetic nerves in the daytime whereas they are inactive and in a dominant state of parasympathetic

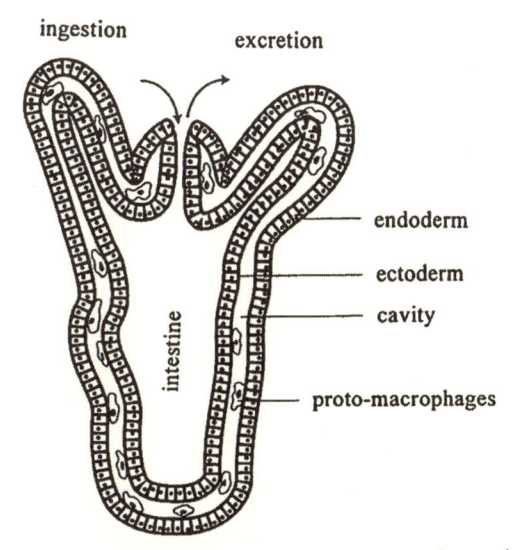

FIG. 1. Protomacrophages in the space between ectoderm and endoderm as seen in the most primitive multicellular organisms are shown. These protomacrophages were the origin of leukocytes, as well as the origin of mesodermal cells in phylogenetic development.

nerves at night. Reflecting these situations, serum levels of adrenaline and noradrenaline are high in the daytime but low at night (Fig. 3). We examined whether such circadian variation of the autonomic nervous system influences the distribution of leukocytes in the blood of humans (4).

Although the variation of whole leukocytes is minimal during the day, the number and proportion of granulocytes and lymphocytes vary significantly as seen in Fig. 4. The number and proportion of granulocytes increase in the daytime and decrease at night. In sharp contrast, the number and proportion of lymphocytes decrease in the daytime and increase at night. These variations coincide with the relationship between the expressions of adrenergic or cholinergic receptors on leukocytes.

It is known that granulocytes are produced in the bone marrow and die mainly in the mucosal tissues through the circulation (6). The lifespan of granulocytes is extremely short (only 2 days after maturation) because of the lack of use of the *bcl-2* gene. In other words, 50% of the granulocytes are replaced by newcomers from the bone marrow each day. The segmentation of their nucleus indicates ongoing apoptosis. Our subsequent study revealed that the variation in the number of granulocytes is produced by the variation in the magnitude of their generation in the bone marrow.

AGE-ASSOCIATED CHANGE IN THE DISTRIBUTION OF LEUKOCYTES IN HUMANS

It is known that a newborn baby shows an elevated level of total leukocytes in the blood, showing granulocytosis (Fig. 5). We found that this is the postpartum event induced by pulmonary respiration in newborns (7). Namely, oxygen stress induces the activation of sympathetic nerves and results in granulocytosis.

Subsequently, children show a dominant state of

FIG. 4. Circadian rhythm in the number and proportion of granulocytes and lymphocytes are shown. A healthy donor was examined as to various immunoparameters every 4 h (for 24 h).

lymphocytes in the blood. In particular, children from 1–4 years show prominent lymphocytosis in both number and proportion whereas those from 5–15 years have a 1:1 ratio of lymphocytes and granulocytes. After 15–20 years, the ratio of lymphocytes and granulocytes adopts an adult pattern (e.g., 35%:60%). As a function of age, the proportion of granulocytes increases gradually.

Lymphocytosis seen in children is induced by the dominant state of parasympathetic nerves. This immunological state in children may be important for the absorption of growing stress. Thus, the increase in body weight is extremely prominent in children between the ages of 1–4 years.

Granulocytosis becomes common in the elderly (8). This is due to the dominant state of the sympathetic nerves. Accumulation of oxidized substances may induce this dominant state of sympathetic nerves. In a recent study (9), we observed that the phagocytic function of granulocytes isolated from

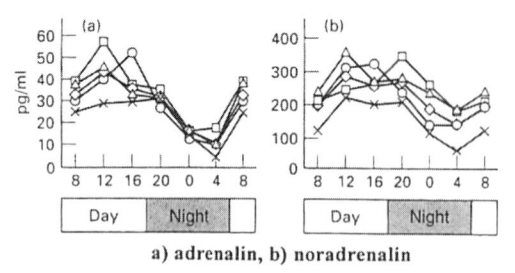

FIG. 3. Circadian rhythm in serum levels of adrenaline and noradrenaline in healthy persons are shown. Serum levels of adrenaline (a) and noradrenaline (b) are high in the daytime but low at night.

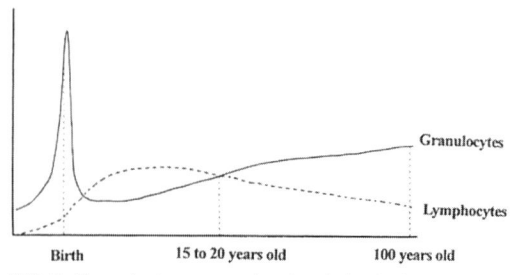

FIG. 5. Shown is the age-associated variation in the number of granulocytes and lymphocytes. Just after birth, neonatal granulocytosis is seen. Thereafter, lymphocytosis continues up to 15–20 years old. This age tends to increase in developed countries. After this age, the adult pattern of leukocytes (granulocytes:lymphocytes) becomes prominent.

centenarians increased whereas the superoxide production of granulocytes did not increase. Some specific variation of the function of granulocytes is beneficial for maintaining the health of the elderly. In any case, the age-associated variation in the ratio of lymphocytes and granulocytes may also be regulated by the autonomic nervous system. We do not deny the possibility of the concomitant association of steroid hormones with this phenomenon.

STRESS AND GASTRIC ULCER

We have reported that an H_2-blocker decreased the number of granulocytes whereas a proton pump inhibitor (PPI) suppressed the function (i.e., superoxide production) of granulocytes in humans and mice (6). In sharp contrast, the H_2-blocker did not suppress the function of granulocytes, and the PPI did not decrease the number of granulocytes. In conjunction with recent results that granulocytes carry surface adrenergic receptors and are activated by sympathetic nerve stimulation, these results suggest that the accumulation of granulocytes in the gastric mucosa might be important in the pathogenesis of gastric ulcers. Sympathetic nerve activation in such patients might be induced by mental and physical stress or bacterial infection (e.g., *Helicobacter pylori*).

As shown in a mouse study in Fig. 6, granulocyte trafficking (the bone marrow → the circulation → the mucosa) is important for understanding the granulocyte theory. If stress continues chronically, granulopoiesis itself increases in the bone marrow, and the levels of granulocytes in the periphery are elevated in various tissues as well as in the blood. This study enables us to properly understand the therapeutic base of antiulcer agents, H_2-blockers, and PPIs. The proposed theory also explains why H_2-blockers and PPIs ameliorate the junction ulcers in patients with total gastrectomy who have lost all parietal cells for acid secretion.

Given the preceding, we propose a granulocyte theory of gastric ulcer formation (6). Granulocytes, which carry surface adrenergic receptors, are therefore activated by sympathetic nerve stimulation and subsequently induce gastric ulcers. In recent studies, *H. pylori* infection has been raised as one of the causes of gastric ulcer formation (10–13). However, this concept is incomplete. Thus, some gastric ulcer patients are free from this infection, and many healthy individuals are infected with *H. pylori*. With the granulocyte theory of gastric ulcer formation, all cases of gastric ulcer can possibly be explained. In this case, *H. pylori* infection is important as a secondary factor that stimulates granulocytes. Sympathetic nerve stimulation is induced by many causes, including mental stress, overwork, bacterial infection, nonsteroidal anti-inflammatory drug (NSAID) administration, and a combination of such factors.

NSAIDS

NSAIDs are some of the most frequently prescribed drugs by doctors throughout the world because they can alleviate pain, fever, and inflammation. However, NSAIDs sometimes induce adverse drug reactions, such as stomach injury and deterioration of renal functions. If NSAIDs are continuously administered to patients (e.g., those with rheumatoid arthritis), they induce symptoms of sympathetic nerve activation (e.g., hypertension, anorexia, constipation, insomnia, easy fatigue). A question of interest is how adverse drug reactions and sympathetic nerve activation induced by NSAIDs are related.

In a series of recent studies (14,15), we demonstrated that the administration of NSAIDs (e.g., indomethacin, aspirin, and ketoprofen) augments granulopoiesis in the bone marrow of mice. In the periphery of these mice, both granulocytes and primordial lymphocytes (i.e., NK cells and extrathymic T cells) are activated in number and function. This might be due to the sympathetic nerve stimulation by NSAIDs and subsequent activation of these leukocytes that carry adrenergic receptors on the surface. It is known that NSAIDs inhibit the function of

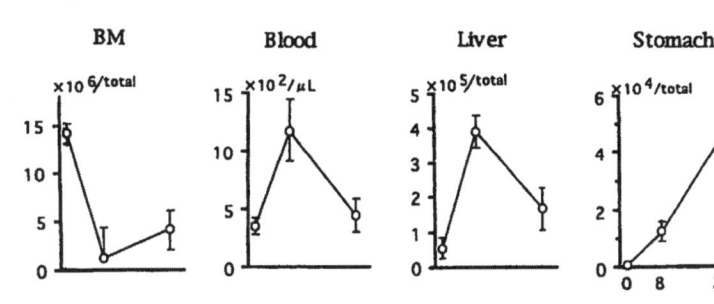

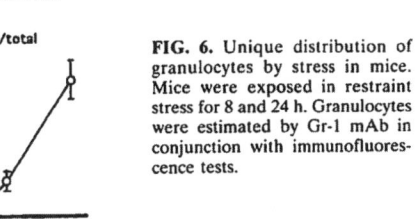

FIG. 6. Unique distribution of granulocytes by stress in mice. Mice were exposed in restraint stress for 8 and 24 h. Granulocytes were estimated by Gr-1 mAb in conjunction with immunofluorescence tests.

cyclooxygenase and result in the inhibition of prostaglandin synthesis. Because prostaglandins act as antagonists against the production of catecholamines, NSAIDs always induce an activated state of the sympathetic nervous system (Fig. 7).

In this study, we administered indomethacin to mice and induced severe enteropathy, not only in the stomach but also in the large intestine (Fig. 8). This enteropathy was characterized by severe infiltration of granulocytes. Activated granulocytes are known to be associated with tissue destruction. We therefore concluded that NSAIDs, which induce sympathetic nerve activation, should not be considered anti-inflammatory drugs (rather they are inflammation-inducing drugs) in the case of inflammation associated with granulocytes.

For a long time, NSAIDs have been prescribed in the absence of basic data showing that high or chronic doses of NSAID administration induce widespread expansion of granulocytes in the body. Even in the case of patients with rheumatoid arthritis, we have found that chronic doses of NSAIDs (not only by means of the oral route but also by means of the dermal route) induce granulocytosis in the joints as well as other organs and accelerate joint deformity in parallel with the loss of pain (our unpublished observation). In other words, the administration of NSAIDs results in granulocyte-related inflammation. Of course, the administration of NSAIDs appropriately suppresses the lymphocyte-associated inflammations in which prostaglandins are intensively produced (e.g., catarrhal inflammation with fever in viral infections). Because the administration of NSAIDs in parallel induces sympathetic nerve activation, chronic doses also induce many related signs such as the failure of peripheral circulation, paralysis of digestive tract movement, and ulcer formation. Thus, careful attention should be given to granulocytosis and resultant tissue damage when NSAIDs are used.

STEROID HORMONES

It is widely known that glucocorticoids have a potent anti-inflammatory function. Therefore, they are used as therapeutic agents in cases of bronchial

```
                    antagonistic
     Prostaglandins  ←——→  Catecholamines
(parasympathetic nerve stimulation)  (sympathetic nerve stimulation)

     NSAIDs suppress the synthesis of prostaglandins
         and result in sympathetic nerve stimulation.
```

FIG. 7. Mechanism by which NSAIDs induce sympathetic nerve activation are shown.

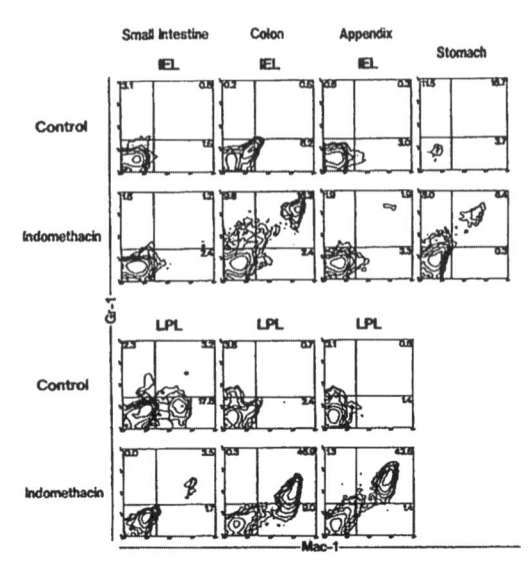

FIG. 8. Extraordinary expansion of granulocytes at generalized sites of mice administered indomethacin are shown: staining of leukocytes in the liver, spleen, and blood **(bottom)**; staining of leukocytes in the digestive tract **(top)**. Two-color staining for Gr-1 and Mac-1 was conducted to identify granulocytes (Gr-1$^+$Mac-1$^+$) and macrophages (Gr-1$^-$Mac-1$^+$).

asthma, atopic dermatitis, certain autoimmune diseases, etc. An immunosuppressive effect on lymphocytes and also inhibition of granulocytes (e.g., suppression of phagocytosis and apoptosis) has been widely reported in neutrophils, basophils, and other cells. However, glucocorticoids sometimes induce adverse drug reactions, such as ulcers and tissue damage, when they are used for a long time or at high doses (16). In clinical studies, we have observed that affected patients show an elevated level of granulocytes in the peripheral blood (our unpublished observation).

To investigate how granulocytosis is induced in the periphery by the use of glucocorticoids, we treated mice with glucocorticoids at high doses and examined myelopoiesis in the bone marrow and liver (data not shown). This protocol is based on the fact that not only the bone marrow but also the liver contains pluripotent stem cells that produce granulocytes as well as extrathymic T cells. It was demonstrated that excessive and continuous administration of glucocorticoids accelerated the generation of granulocytes and extrathymic T cells (i.e., intermediate TCR cells or TCR^{int} cells) in the bone marrow. Because TCR^{int} cells are also generated by an alternative intrathymic pathway, we sometimes call them primordial T cells. Moreover, such granulocytes were found to be in an activated state. Although excessive administration of glucocorticoids induced profound lymphocytopenia in various immune system organs, it inversely increased the number and function of granulocytes in the bone marrow and periphery. It is therefore speculated that such activated granulocytes together with activated primordial T cells then induce mucosal and/or tissue damage in hosts.

As present, we do not know the actual mechanisms underlying granulocytosis induced by glucocorticoids. Because granulocytes bear surface adrenergic receptors and are activated by the administration of catecholamines, we measured the serum level of catecholamines in control and hydrocortisone-treated mice. However, there were no differences between these groups of mice. There is a possibility that some cytokines such as granulocyte colony-stimulating factor (G-CSF) and granulocyte-macrophage colony-stimulating factor (GM-CSF) might be associated with this phenomenon. In a preliminary study, we found that hydrocortisone, which was given in excessive doses, stagnated in the tissue and turned to oxidized cholesterols (our unpublished observation). Steroid hormones originate from a cholesterol structure. In this regard, we must consider their nature to be that of harmful oxidized substances.

COLLAGEN DISEASES OR AUTOIMMUNE DISEASES

Many investigators and clinicians have long believed that self-reactive forbidden clones, which evoke autoimmune diseases or collagen diseases, may be generated through failure in T-cell differentiation in the thymus. However, we have never encountered such failure of intrathymic T-cell differentiation (17,18).

In autoimmune prone NZB/WF$_1$ mice, severe thymic atrophy is rather induced at the onset of disease (data not shown). This result suggests that the mainstream of T-cell differentiation is arrested under autoimmune conditions. Inversely, the number of lymphocytes in the liver (consisting of extrathymic T cells) and that of peritoneal exudate cells (consisting of autoantibody-producing B cells or B-1 cells) increase. In other words, the extrathymic pathway of T-cell differentiation, which primarily produces self-reaction forbidden clones without negative selection, is activated in autoimmune diseases or collagen diseases.

Reflecting these situations, we have always observed that lymphocytopenia (consisting of conventional T and B cells) and granulocytosis (resulting from sympathetic nerve stimulation) are accompanied in patients with rheumatoid arthritis (RA) (Table 1). Similar phenomena are also seen in patients with other autoimmune diseases or collagen diseases (e.g., systemic lupus erythematosus, Hashimoto's disease, scleroderma, Behçet's syndrome).

There are two major causes of autoimmune diseases or collagen diseases, namely, infections and mental or physical stress (Fig. 9). When viral or bacterial infection is severe, tissue damage is evoked by inflammation. Such tissue damage induces sympathetic nerve activation and results in granulocytosis and primitive lymphocytes (i.e., innate immunity). If tissue damage is continued, activated granulocytes produce superoxides as well as many inflammatory cytokines (e.g., TNFα, IFNγ, and IL-6), and accelerate tissue damage. At this time, primitive lymphocytes such as extrathymic T cells (i.e., CD56$^+$T or CD57$^+$T cells in humans) mediate autoreactivity against denatured self-tissue, and B-1 cells produce autoantibodies (19).

These responses are sometimes beneficial for the elimination of denatured self-cells, and at other times they are dangerous for the acceleration of tissue damage. Similarly, mental or physical stress becomes the cause of autoimmune diseases because such stress induces sympathetic nerve activation. Such sympathetic nerve activation then induces granulocytosis and results in tissue damage. Indeed, we are often able to see such mental and physical stress (e.g., overwork) at the onset of disease from patients with autoimmune diseases.

Sympathetic nerve activation also induces thymic atrophy which indicates the arrest of the mainstream T-cell differentiation in the thymus (6). Inversely, primitive lymphocytes such as NK cells, extrathymic T cells, and autoantibody-producing B-1 cells (i.e., constituents of innate immune system) are activated. Again, these responses are not always harmful to the body because these cells are responsible for the elimination of abnormal or denatured self-cells. A similar opinion is also proposed by other investigators (20).

If we notice that the immunological state of autoimmune diseases or collagen diseases is severe im-

TABLE 1. *Granulocytosis and lymphocytopenia in patients with rheumatoid arthritis*

	n	No. of WBC (/mm^3)	% Granulocytes	% Lymphocytes
Control	20	5620.0 ± 423.3	58.0 ± 3.4	33.2 ± 3.1
RA:CRP+	25	7707.7 ± 621.4	71.7 ± 2.7	20.9 ± 2.2
RA:CRP−	20	6228.6 ± 550.3	60.4 ± 3.8	31.2 ± 4.5

1) Infections → tissue damage ⇌ sympathetic nerve activation
2) Mental or physical stress → sympathetic nerve activation ⇌ tissue damage

Sympathetic nerve activation induces thymic atrophy and the activation of innate immune system.

FIG. 9. Possible causes and mechanisms underlying the onset of autoimmune diseases are shown. Tissue damage and sympathetic nerve activation influence each other.

munosuppression, a new therapeutic approach for these diseases is raised. Immunosuppressants and steroid hormones must worsen the diseases. This was a conventional therapy for autoimmune diseases or collagen diseases until the present. NSAIDs that reduce our body temperature are also dangerous for the treatment of these diseases. Thus, NSAIDs induce severe sympathetic nerve activation and result in granulocytosis (14,15). This phenomenon is also related to the gastritis and gastric ulcers induced by the long-lasting administration of NSAIDs.

We always encounter the inflammations of autoimmune diseases or collagen diseases showing pain, fever, redness, skin rash, diarrhea, etc. These inflammations should be considered a result of acceleration of circulation which induces the recovery from tissue damage. Parasympathetic nerve activation is related to these symptoms. Actual factors include prostaglandins, histamine, serotonin, acetylcholine, leukotrienes, etc.

Instead of the use of immunosuppressants, we have to select a therapy to increase circulation, inflammation, and immune functions. Such therapies include mild exercise, bathing, laughing, and the use of oriental medicine such as acupuncture and Chinese medicines. Especially, acupuncture and Chinese medicines induce the stimulation of parasympathetic nerves in patients (21).

ULCERATIVE COLITIS AND CROHN'S DISEASE

In 1975, ulcerative colitis (UC) was indicated as one of the specific diseases by the declaration of the Japanese government. The numbers of such patients increased thereafter (Fig. 10). We believe that an inappropriate therapy was fixed since then because the standard therapy is the use of aminosalicylic acid (one of NSAIDs) and steroid hormones.

In this experiment (Fig. 11), we examined how NSAIDs (indomethacin, 0.5 mg/day/mouse × 7 days in this experiment) stimulated sympathetic nerves. A prominent increase in the serum concentration of catecholamines was induced in mice. It is speculated that the suppression of prostaglandins by NSAIDs is related to this phenomenon. Thus, prostaglandin acts as the suppressive system against catecholamines.

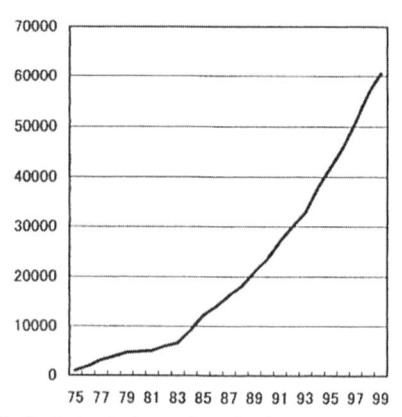

FIG. 10. Explosion in the number of patients with ulcerative colitis in Japan is shown. In 1975, ulcerative colitis was indicated as one of the incurable diseases. From that time, the number of patients began to increase.

Such sympathetic nerve stimulations induced by indomethacin then induced the infiltration of granulocytes into various sites of the digestive tract, showing the high magnitude in the colon → stomach → appendix → small intestine. This response reminds us of gastric mucosal damage and other damage induced by NSAIDs. These results further suggest that not only the stomach but also the colon mucosa may be a serious target of tissue damage by NSAIDs. Although NSAIDs suppress diarrhea and abdominal pain in patients with UC, the long-lasting use of NSAIDs is easily speculated to worsen the mucosal damage in these patients.

It is widely known that the inflammation of granulocytes is mainly observed in the mucosa of the large

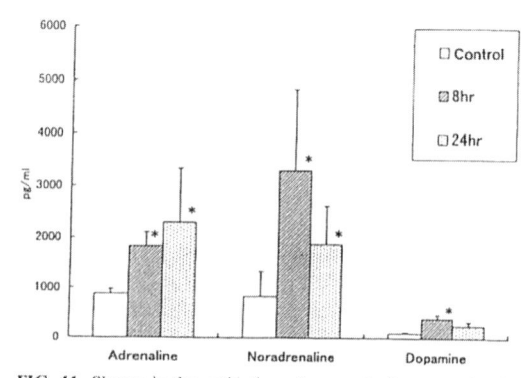

FIG. 11. Shown is the activation of sympathetic nerves by the continuous administration of NSAIDs. Indomethacin (0.5 mg/d/mouse) was administrated every day for 7 days. Serum levels of catecholamines were measured on day 8.

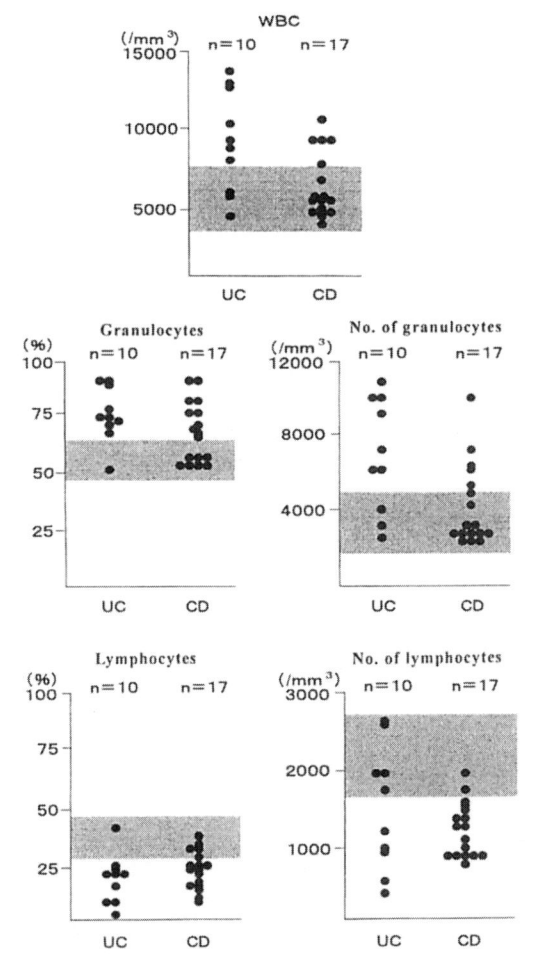

FIG. 12. Comparisons are shown of the number of whole leukocytes and the proportion and number of granulocytes and lymphocytes between patients with ulcerative colitis (UC) and Crohn's disease (CD).

intestine in patients with UC whereas the inflammation of macrophages (and lymphocytes) is observed in the mucosa of the small intestine in patients with Crohn's disease (CD). We then consider how this pathological difference is present between UC and CD (Fig. 12). In these experiments, we compared the number of whole leukocytes with the proportion and number of granulocytes and lymphocytes in the blood (UC, n = 10; CD, n = 17). Similar to the case of UC, many patients with CD showed an elevated level of granulocytes and a decreased level of lymphocytes.

In other words, patients with both UC and CD showed the same distribution pattern of leukocytes in the blood, suggesting sympathetic nerve activation. Indeed, many of these patients had tachycardia. Mental stress and iatrogenic stress from the long-lasting administration of NSAIDs might induce such sympathetic nerve activation and granulocytosis. However, peripheral granulocytes invade the large intestine whereas they do not invade the small intestine as shown in Fig. 10. As a result, only resident macrophages and lymphocytes are activated to make the granulomas in the small intestine. This situation also explains the lower incidence of patients with CD than those with UC.

In light of these findings, we propose a new therapeutic approach for UC and CD. It includes: cessation of salazosulfapyridine (Salazopyrin), mesalazine (Pentasa), and steroid (Steroneam), which induce granulocytosis; care for mental stress and foods; and stimulation of parasympathetic nerves (acupuncture, mild exercise, bathing, laughing, etc).

ACCOMPANYING PAIN, REDNESS, FEVER, INFLAMMATION, AND DIARRHEA IN THE RECOVERY RESPONSE FROM DISEASES

When we encounter severe mental or physical stress, circulation failure and tissue damage are induced by sympathetic nerve activation (Fig. 13). To recover circulation failure and tissue damage, parasympathetic nerve reflex is suddenly induced, accompanying pain, redness, fever, inflammation, and diarrhea. As already mentioned, prostaglandins, acetylcholine, serotonin, histamine, etc. are associated with these responses.

If we use NSAIDs or steroid hormones, especially for a long time, all recovery responses cease. Therefore, the suppression of symptoms and the reappear-

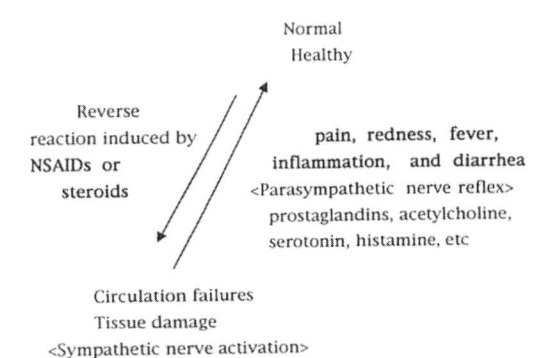

FIG. 13. Recovery responses from circulation failure and tissue damage are shown. Irritable symptoms are rather recovery responses with parasympathetic nerve activation. The long-lasting administration of NSAIDs and steroid hormones suppress such valuable responses in our body.

ance of recovery responses are repeated in the patients.

CANCER

Cumulative studies have revealed that there are many oncogenes that render normal cells malignant. It is also true that almost all of these oncogenes are related to the proliferation genes for normally growing epithelial cells. If this is the case, we have to consider how these oncogenes become active in the body. When a person is in a continuous state of sympathetic nerve activation because of overwork, mental stress, or other factors, severe granulocytosis and circulatory failure are induced. Indeed, cancer patients show an increased level of granulocytes and a decreased level of lymphocytes in the blood (Fig. 14). These conditions accelerate renewal of epithelial cells because of the death of cells exposed to superoxides produced by activated granulocytes. It is conceivable that the renewal of epithelial cells increases the incidence of oncogene onset.

There is another reason why continuous granulocytosis induces the onset of malignancy. Granulocytosis induced by sympathetic nerve activation is always accompanied by immunosuppression (i.e., lymphocytopenia including cytotoxic T cells). NK cells are known to kill malignant tumor cells by using perforin which exists in the cytoplasmic granules (22). However, the secretion of perforin by NK cells is suppressed under conditions of sympathetic nerve activation because sympathetic nerves are related to the suppressive effect of many secretion systems in the body and at the cellular level.

In light of these findings, we have to consider how cancer patients can escape from granulocytosis and accompanying immunosuppression. We propose the following: relief from overwork, mental stress, or the continuous administration of NSAIDs, all of which induce sympathetic nerve activation; treatment for immunopotentiation rather than for immunosuppression, namely, many anticancer drugs induce immunosuppression.

In recent studies, we found that >1,800 to 2,000 lymphocytes/μL of blood is a critical point to acquire a spontaneous regression of tumors, including lung cancer, kidney cancer, uterine cancer, mammary gland cancer, and metastatic cancers. If cancer patients were already exposed to anticancer drugs or irradiation, the immunopotentiation might be somewhat difficult. To support immunopotentiation, acupuncture, Chinese medicines, and other therapies are helpful. If we select the previously mentioned care for cancer patients instead of anticancer drugs or irradiation, more than 60% of such patients with advanced tumors show spontaneous regression within 1–2 years.

CLOSING REMARKS

In this review, we emphasize that the onset of collagen diseases, inflammatory bowel diseases, and cancer is induced by the overactivation of sympathetic nerves. The immunological state common to these diseases is immunosuppression.

In addition, there are certain diseases that are evoked by the overactivation of parasympathetic nerve activation. Such diseases include allergic diseases (e.g., atopic dermatitis, bronchial asthma, and pollen rhinitis). Patients with these diseases show lymphocytosis at the stage of no symptoms but granulocytosis at the diseased state. In other words, these patients are extremely sensitive to antigen exposure or mental stress because of the lymphocytosis and show unpleasant symptoms as recovery responses (sympathetic nerve activation → parasympathetic nerve activation). Not only the escape from antigen exposure (or mental stress) but also the improvement of parasympathetic nerve activated–conditions in the body should be required for therapy. Antiallergic drugs such as antihistamine drugs and steroid hormones never provide complete recovery from allergic diseases.

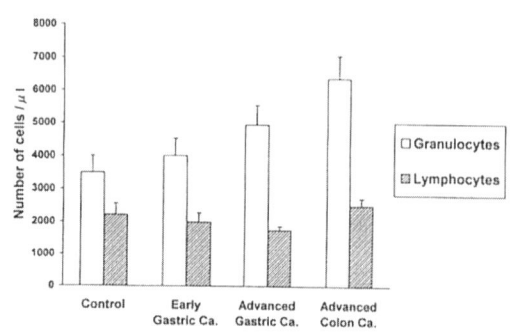

FIG. 14. Increased levels of granulocytes in cancer patients are shown. Early gastric cancer (n = 30), advanced gastric cancer (n = 30), and advanced colon cancer (n = 35).

REFERENCES

1. Saito A. Acute adaptational disturbances due to the imbalance of the autonomic nervous system. *Tohoku J Exp Med* 1971;103:71–92.
2. Saito A. Chronic adaptational disturbances due to the imbalance of the autonomic nervous system. *Tohoku J Exp Med* 1971;103:93–114.
3. Toyabe S, Iiai T, Fukuda M, Kawamura T, Suzuki S, Uchiyama M, Abo T. Identification of nicotinic acetylcholine re-

ceptors on lymphocytes in periphery as well as thymus in mice. *Immunology* 1997;92:201–5.
4. Suzuki S, Toyabe S, Moroda T, Tada T, Tsukahara A, Iiai T, Minagawa M, Maruyama S, Hatakeyama K, Endo K, Abo T. Circadian rhythm of leukocytes and lymphocyte subsets and its possible correlation with the function of autonomic nervous system. *Clin Exp Immunol* 1997;110:500–8.
5. Abo T, Kawamura T, Watanabe H. Physiological responses of extrathymic T cells in the liver. *Immunol Rev* 2000;174:135–49.
6. Kawamura T, Miyaji C, Toyabe S, Fukuda M, Watanabe H, Abo T. Suppressive effect of anti-ulcer agents on granulocytes–A role of granulocytes for gastric ulcer formation. *Digest Dis Sci* 2000;45:1786–91.
7. Kawamura T, Toyabe S, Moroda T, Iiai T, Takahashi-Iwanaga H, Fukuda M, Watanabe H, Sekikawa H, Seki S, Abo T. Neonatal granulocytosis is a postpartum event which is seen in the liver as well as in the blood. *Hepatology* 1997;26:1567–72.
8. Miyaji C, Watanabe H, Minagawa M, Toma H, Nohara Y, Nozaki H, Sato Y, Abo T. Numerical and functional characteristics of lymphocyte subsets in centenarians. *J Clin Immunol* 1997;17:420–9.
9. Miyaji C, Watanabe H, Toma H, Akisaka M, Tomiyama K, Sato Y, Abo T. Functional alteration of granulocytes, NK cells, and natural killer T cells in centenarians. *Human Immunol* 2000;61:908–16.
10. Axon AT. *Helicobacter pylori* and the pathogenesis of gastroduodenal inflammation. *Clin Exp Immunol* 1993;58:420–7.
11. Blaser MJ. *Helicobacter pylori* and the pathogenesis of gastroduodenal inflammation. *J Infect Dis* 1990;161:626–33.
12. Labenz J, Borsch G. Evidence for the essential role of *Helicobacter pylori* in gastric ulcer disease. *Gut* 1994;35:19–22.
13. Milne R, Logan RP, Harwood D, Misiewicz JJ, Forman D. *Helicobacter pylori* and upper gastrointestinal disease: a survey of gastroenterologists in the United Kingdom. *Gut* 1995;37:314–8.
14. Yamamura S, Arai K, Toyabe S, Takahashi EH, Abo T. Simultaneous activation of granulocytes and extrathymic T cells in number and function by excessive administration of nonsteroidal anti-inflammatory drugs. *Cell Immunol* 1996;173:303–11.
15. Yamagiwa S, Yoshida Y. Halder, Weerasinghe A, Sugahara S, Asakura H, Abo T. Mechanisms involved in the enteropathy induced by the administration of nonsteroidal anti-inflammatory drugs (NSAIDs). *Digest Dis Sci* 2001;46:192–9.
16. Maruyama S, Minagawa M, Shimizu T, Oya H, Yamamoto S, Musha N, Abo W, Weerasinghe A, Hatakeyama K, Abo T. Administration of glucocorticoids markedly increases the numbers of granulocytes and extrathymic T cells in the bone marrow. *Cell Immunol* 1999;194:28–35.
17. Kawachi Y, Watanabe H, Moroda T, Haga M, Iiai T, Hatakeyama K, Abo T. Self-reactive T cell clones in a restricted population of IL-2 receptor β+ cells expressing intermediate levels of the T cell receptor in the liver and other immune organs. *Eur J Immunol* 1995;25:2272–8.
18. Moroda T, Kawachi Y, Iiai T, Tsukahara A, Suzuki S, Tada T, Watanabe H, Hatakeyama K, Abo T. Self-reactive forbidden clones are confined to pathways of intermediate T cell receptor cell differentiation even under immunosuppressive conditions. *Immunology* 1997;91:88–94.
19. Arai K, Yamamura S, Seki S, Hanyu T, Takahashi H-E, Abo T. Increase of CD57+T cells in knee joints and adjacent bone marrow of rheumatoid arthritis (RA) patients: implication of an anti-inflammatory role. *Clin Exp Immunol* 1998;111:345–52.
20. Schwartz M, Cohen IR. Autoimmunity can benefit self-maintenance. *Immunol Today* 2000;21:265–8.
21. Mori H, Nishijo K, Kawamura H, Abo T. Unique immunomodulation by electro-acupuncture in humans possibly via stimulation of the autonomic nervous system. *Neurosci Lett* 2002;320:21–4.
22. Bannai M, Oya H, Kawamura T, Shimizu T, Kawamura H, Miyaji C, Watanabe H, Hatakeyama K, Abo T. Disparate effect of *beige* mutation on cytotoxic function between NK and NKT cells. *Immunology* 2000;100:165–9.

Stagnation of Steroid Hormones in Patients with Atopic Dermatitis and Unique Variation of Leukocyte Pattern during the Withdrawal Syndrome after Cessation of Steroid Ointment

アトピー性皮膚炎患者のステロイドホルモン停滞とステロイド軟膏中止後の禁断症状における独特の白血球分画

Biomedical Reseach, 24: 89-96, 2003

chapter 15

Stagnation of Steroid Hormones in Patients with Atopic Dermatitis and Unique Variation of Leukocyte Pattern during the Withdrawal Syndrome after Cessation of Steroid Ointment

アトピー性皮膚炎患者のステロイドホルモン停滞とステロイド軟膏中止後の禁断症状における独特の白血球分画

Minoru FUKUDA[1], Nobuaki KAWADA[2], Nobuyo KATOH[3], Hiroki KAMAMURA[4] and Toru ABO[4]

[1]Fukuda-iin, Niigata, [2]Department of Obstetrics and Gynecology, Uhrin Hospital, Fukushima, [3]Department of Public Health, Juntendo University School of Medicine, Tokyo and [4]Department of Immunology, Niigata University School of Medicine, Niigata Japan

【要約】

　アトピー性皮膚炎は、通常15-20歳くらいで寛解するが、20歳を超えても重症なままの患者も存在する。塗布した軟膏に含有されるステロイドホルモンが皮膚で停滞し、酸化コレステロールに変性し、これが循環不全や顆粒球が関与する炎症を誘発している可能性がある。今回、重症アトピー性皮膚炎患者が、ステロイドホルモン含有軟膏使用の中断後、数カ月以内に治癒成功したことを報告する。ステロイドホルモン含有軟膏を中断後、2-3週間、アトピー性皮膚炎患者は禁断症状に苦しむ。そこで、鍼治療を行なった。治療前、アトピー性皮膚炎患者の血液像は、顆粒球および好酸球の高値、リンパ球の低値が見られた。顆粒球数と比率は、交感神経緊張により増加することが知られている。ゆえに、アトピー性皮膚炎患者は、交感神経緊張状態であったことが示唆される。治療期間中、離脱症状のおかげで白血球分画はさらに悪化したが、炎症の寛解とともに白血球分画の正常化が見られた。このような結果より、現在不明である何らかの原因により、長期間ステロイド軟膏を使用したにアトピー性皮膚炎患者に異常な白血球分画(顆粒球増多)が出現し、そして、病気の寛解と同時にステロイドホルモン中断により白血球分画は正常化したことが明らかになった。

　アトピー性皮膚炎の発症は、幼児期が多く、思春期以前に自然治癒することもある(3,12)。もともと、幼児期の免疫レベルは高い(=リンパ球高値)(5)が、成長するにつれ、免疫レベルは低下する(9)。日本の15-20才において顆粒球値はリンパ球値より高い(未発表データ)。このように年齢により免疫系が変化することが、アトピー性皮膚炎の自然治癒の理由である可能性が推測できる。換言すると、アトピー性皮膚炎の多くは、成長とともにT細胞数が減少するので自然におさまるのである。

　通常は、このような経過をたどるが、アトピー性皮膚炎患者の中には自然治癒せず、逆に顔面の皮膚のひどい炎症や発赤の症状に苦しむ患者も存在する(3,12)。このような患者は、ステロイドホルモンを含む軟膏を局所に長期間使用している。このようなアトピー性皮膚炎の重症化は避けられないのだろうか、そして適切な治療法はあるのだろうか。

　軟膏に含有されるステロイドホルモンが、長期間、皮膚組織の中に残存すると、酸化されたコレステロールになると推測される。ステロイドホルモンは、コレステロール構造を有し、ステロイドホルモンを含有する軟膏を使用したアトピー性皮膚炎患者の皮膚は悪臭がする。このことは、酸化物質による組織への刺激や顆粒球

の浸潤を示唆する。このことを、動物実験で確認した(7)。酸化コレステロールは、局所に直接顆粒球の蓄積を引き起こす(未発表データ)。そのような顆粒球は、常在菌に対し反応した後、交感神経緊張の他にもサイトカイン(TNFα、IFNγ、G-CSF等)刺激によりますます活性化する。

過去4年間、我々は重症アトピー性皮膚炎患者の皮膚からこのような酸化物質の除去を試み、ほぼ全症例の治癒に成功した(＞95%)。この除去治療中、患者はステロイドホルモンの離脱症状に苦しむ。そこで、鍼治療を行なった。ステロイドホルモンが実際に副作用を有する事実を認識すれば、治療に成功している他の臨床医と同様に、(ステロイドホルモン依存である場合でさえ)多数の重症アトピー性皮膚炎患者の治療は可能であろう。現時点で、真の理由は断定できないが、重症アトピー性皮膚炎患者の治療中に起きる離脱症状に顆粒球増多が見られるのは興味深い。少なくとも重症アトピー性皮膚炎の症例においては、IgE、T細胞および好酸球の機能(1,20)のみならず顆粒球の機能をも考慮する必要がある。

材料と方法

患者

重症アトピー性皮膚炎患者(89名中、男性45歳、女性44歳、年齢12-28歳、平均19.9±6.0歳)を治療した。アトピー性皮膚炎の重症度は、既報に従い分類した(13)。文献(13)や(2)の報告のようにアトピー性皮膚炎の重症度の診断は容易ではない。アトピー性皮膚炎、最も簡便な分類法は、「軽度」、「中等度」、「重度」の分類である(13)。本研究において、ほぼ全患者(ほぼ100%)が数年間ステロイドホルモン含有軟膏を使用していて、少なくとも80%のアトピー性皮膚炎患者は「重症」と分類しなければならない。対応する年齢の対照群(n=100)を患者と白血球分画患者と比較するため設定した。

白血球分画

健常人(対照)と重症アトピー性皮膚炎患者において白血球の数(総白血球数)を測定した。顆粒球(好中球と好塩基球を含む)、好酸球とリンパ球比率の測定には、メイグリュンワルドギムザ染色を行なった。対照者と治療中の患者の血液よりデータを採取した。

尿中遊離カテコールアミン、バニリルマンデル酸(VMA)、17-ketosterolds(17-KS)及び17-OHコルチコステロイド(17-0HCS)測定

アトピー性皮膚炎患者(治療法前)13名と年齢が対応した健常人(対照)20名の採尿を行ない、24時間HPLC方法を用いてこれら物質の濃度(/リットル)を測定した(8)

脂質およびコレステロール測定

(血清中)脂質およびコレステロール測定値をSRL(Tokyo, Japan、http://www.SRL-inc.co.jp/)にて測定した。

鍼治療

患者への精神的サポートとして鍼治療を行なった。概略すると、手足末梢部を26-ゲージ針で刺鍼した；詳細すると、爪甲の角に刺鍼した際、若干の出血も見られた。この刺激は、副交感神経優位を引き起こし、末梢血流循環の回復、血圧低下、かゆみの軽減がみられた。治療中重篤な離脱症状や肝不全を示唆する血清トランスアミナーゼの上昇も出現することもあったが、このような重篤な場合には(治療した患者の10%未満)、生理食塩水(500ml利尿剤を含む)の輸液を一日1度、静注で行った(最多でも数回)。

統計解析

健常者とアトピー性皮膚炎患者間の有意差を、スチューデントのt検定を用い解析した。

| Table.1 | 健常者とアトピー性皮膚炎患者の白血球分布比較 |

Parameter	Healthy subjects (n=100)	Patients with severe atopic dermatitis (n=89)		
		Before therapy	2 wks after therapy	At discharge
Number of leukocytes[a]	6,500 ± 1,180	7,700 ± 1,800*	8,500 ± 2400*	7,500 ± 1800*
% Granulocytes	57.0 ± 9.2	59.5 ± 10.7	63.3 ± 10.9*	52.0 ± 10.3
% Eosinocytes	1.8 ± 1.0	11.8 ± 8.4*	13.1 ± 8.1*	13.7 ± 8.5*
% Lymphocytes	38.9 ± 5.2	27.8 ± 8.6*	22.6 ± 8.8*	34.2 ± 9.4

[a] Neurophils and basophils(not including eosinophils)
* $p<0.05$

結果

患者の免疫学的指標

重症アトピー性皮膚炎患者(n= 89)の免疫状態測定のため、末梢血を用い白血球総数と白血球比率を測定した(Table 1)。重症患者は、顔や体の他の部位のアトピー性皮膚炎に苦しみ、全患者に、数カ月 - 数年間、ステロイドホルモン含有軟膏の使用歴があった。本治療前、この患者たちは、何箇所か他の病院を受診していた。対照とするため、対応した年齢の健常人(n=100)の白血球分画も同時に測定した。治療前の重症アトピー患者には、白血球総数と好酸球比率上昇、リンパ球比率低下が見られた($P<0.05$)。白血球総数については、顆粒球数と好酸球数(リンパ球は該当しない)の上昇が示唆された($P<0.05$)。

尿中カテコラミン値

我々は、ヒトにおいても(5,8,15)マウスにおいても(4,10,22)交感神経系緊張により末梢血中や他の組織において顆粒球上昇が誘発されるとこれまでに報告した。従って、顆粒球高値を示す重症アトピー性皮膚炎患者は、交感神経緊張である可能性がある。このことは、大部分の患者に頻脈と不眠症が見られた事実からも明らかであった。生理的に分泌されるステロイドホルモンの代謝産物と同様に尿中のカテコールアミン値を測定したところ (Fig. 1)、患者の遊離カテコールアミンと VMA(カテコールアミンの代謝産物)は高値を示した(一日あたり)($P<0.05$)。17-KS 値は低値だが ($P<0.05$)、17-0HCS 値は、正常であった ($P<0.05$)。

血清中脂質とコレステロール値

停滞したステロイド由来の酸化コレステロールが交感神経緊張を誘発した可能性を検討すべく、脂質とコレステロールの血清レベルを測定した (Fig. 2)。測定したパラメータのうち、総脂質、総コレステロール、βリポタンパク、エステル型コレステロールおよび遊離コレステロールの値を対照群と患者群の間で比較した。しかし、患者群では、過酸化脂質(酸化コレステロールを含むことが知られている)値は、増加を示したものの、総胆汁酸値は減少を示した($P<0.01$)。

アトピー性皮膚炎の治癒

皮膚の中に残留した酸化コレステロールが蓄積しているという仮説に基づき、患者の治療を開始した。治療内容は、1) 軟膏使用中止、2) 鍼治療、そして、3) 精神的サポートである。治療開始二週間後、重症アトピー性皮膚炎患者に見られる白血球分画(顆粒球と好酸球の数増加)は、さらに顕著になった(Table 1)。すなわち、

Figure.1

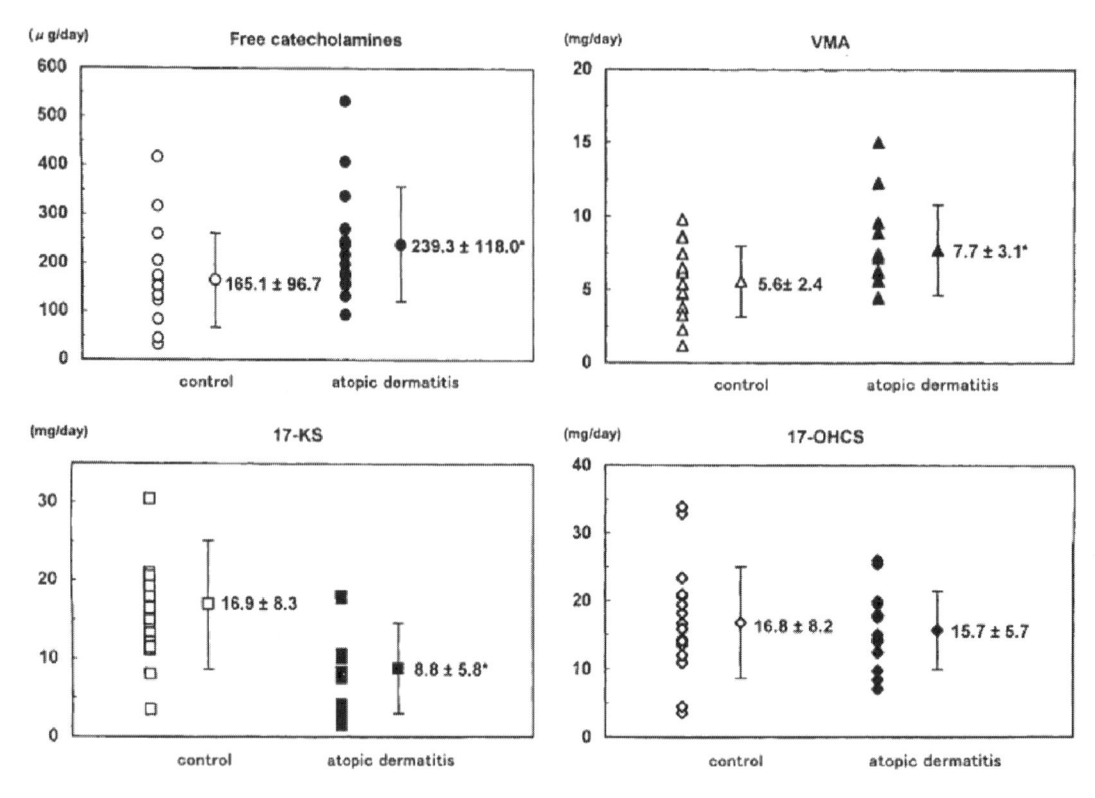

Free catecholamines (μg/day)
control: 165.1 ± 96.7
atopic dermatitis: 239.3 ± 118.0*

VMA (mg/day)
control: 5.6 ± 2.4
atopic dermatitis: 7.7 ± 3.1*

17-KS (mg/day)
control: 16.9 ± 8.3
atopic dermatitis: 8.8 ± 5.8*

17-OHCS (mg/day)
control: 16.8 ± 8.2
atopic dermatitis: 15.7 ± 5.7

健常者と患者の尿中に排泄された(/日)遊離カテコールアミン、VMA、17-KSおよび17-OHCS。重症アトピー性皮膚炎症患者(n=13)と年齢が対応した健常者(n=20)より尿を採取した。 P<0.05

離脱症状の大きな症状として、白血球分画の悪化が、炎症の重症化とともに出現したのである。しかし、このような症状は徐々に鎮静した(Table 1 と Fig. 3)。退院時、好酸球値以外の白血球分画は、ほぼ正常になった(Table 1 右)。Fig. 3のように、本治療では重症アトピー性皮膚炎の患者において著しい改善が見られた。治療に要した時間は、1ヵ月 - 5ヵ月である。しかしながら、患者のなかには、治療開始時の激しい離脱症状が原因で、ドロップ・アウトし治療を断念するものもいた(約5%)。患者の中には、治療終了後にさえ、アトピー性皮膚炎が散発的に増悪した(約20%)。しかし、このような症状は時間の経過とともに徐々に消滅した。適度な運動が増悪防止に非常に有効であると考え、我々は患者には運動を勧めた。

考察

最近の一連の研究において、我々は白血球の自律神経支配を報告してきた(4,5,8,10,15,17,22)。白血球の自律神経支配は、顆粒球表面にはアドレナリン受容体(11)が、リンパ球表面にはコリン受容体(17)が存在するためである。交感神経緊張になると、顆粒球数が増加し、顆粒球の機能が強化される。反対に、副交感神経優位になると、T細胞やB細胞のようなリンパ球数が増加し、リンパ球の機能が強化される。白血球分布が急速に変化するのは、白血球が非常に短命であるためである。則ち、顆粒球の寿命は成熟後二日のみである(10)。その上、交感神経緊張

Figure.2

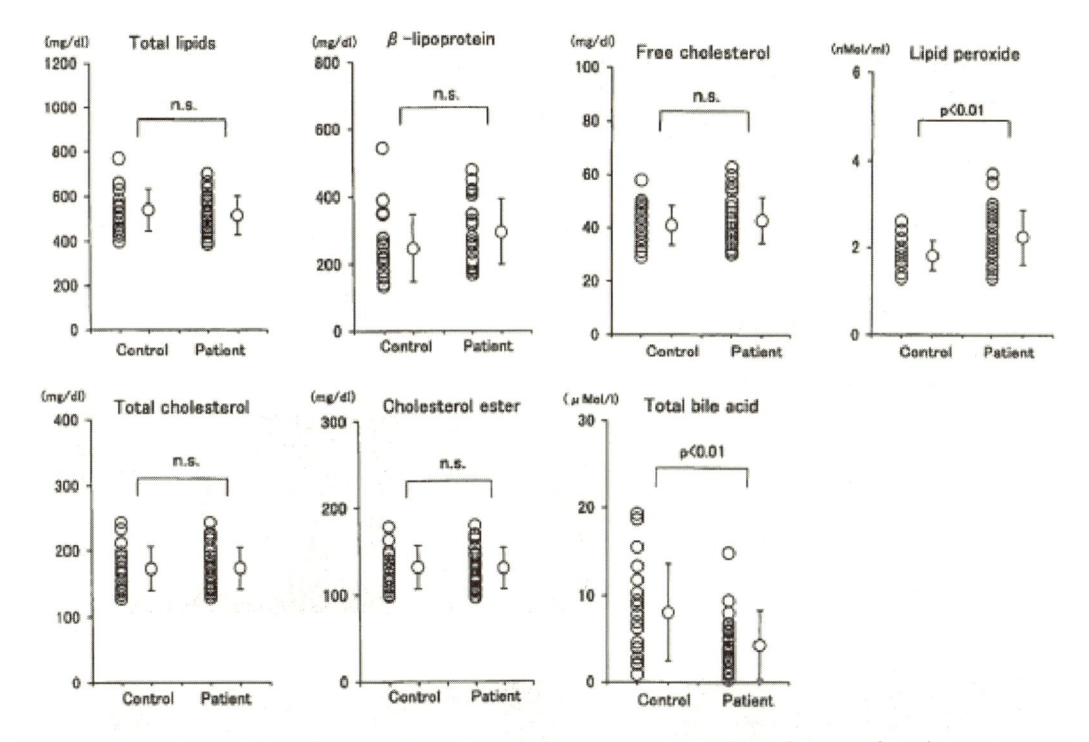

[Scatter plots comparing Control vs Patient for: Total lipids (n.s.), β-lipoprotein (n.s.), Free cholesterol (n.s.), Lipid peroxide (p<0.01), Total cholesterol (n.s.), Cholesterol ester (n.s.), Total bile acid (p<0.01)]

血清中脂質およびコレステロール値を健常者と重症アトピー性皮膚炎患者の間で比較した。重症アトピー性皮膚炎(n=29)と対応した年齢の健常者(n=19)より血液サンプルを採取し、脂質とコレステロールの血清値を測定した。患者において、過酸化脂質値は上昇したが、総胆汁酸値は減少した(P＜0.01)。

は、顆粒球遊走を加速する。つまり、骨髄に顆粒球はプールしてあるのだが、これが一気に血液循環により、粘膜/皮膚の組織に押し寄せる。結果として、交感神経系緊張時、血液中の顆粒球数が増加する。交感神経緊張時、顆粒球が増加するメカニズムは、日中であり(概日リズムによる)(15)、肉体的ストレスの結果であり(10)、また、誕生時の肺呼吸開始による新生児顆粒球増加症によるもの(5)と同様である。

このような研究結果を考慮して、他医療機関において難病と診断された重症アトピー性皮膚炎患者の白血球分画の解析を行なった。このような患者において、顆粒球値が上昇し、リンパ球値が低下していた。すなわち、患者は免疫抑制性状態であった。重症アトピー性皮膚炎患者の中に認められる免疫抑制性状態については、他にも同様の報告がある(6,14,18,19)。

諸酸化物質(例えば、軟膏として使われるステロイドホルモン類から産生した酸化コレステロール)が、交感神経系優位を引き起こした(Fig. 4)と我々は仮定した。

実際、これらの若い患者のほぼ全員は頻脈、高血圧、不眠、不安、疲労感等の症状が見られた。この推論は尿検査の結果より確認できた。すなわち、遊離カテコールアミンおよびVMAが患者の尿では高値であった。17-KS値がなぜ患者において低値であったかは、不明である。患者において血清中、過酸化脂質(酸化コレステロールを含む)が高値であった。現時点では、何故、患者の血清総胆汁酸が減少したかは、不

Figure.3

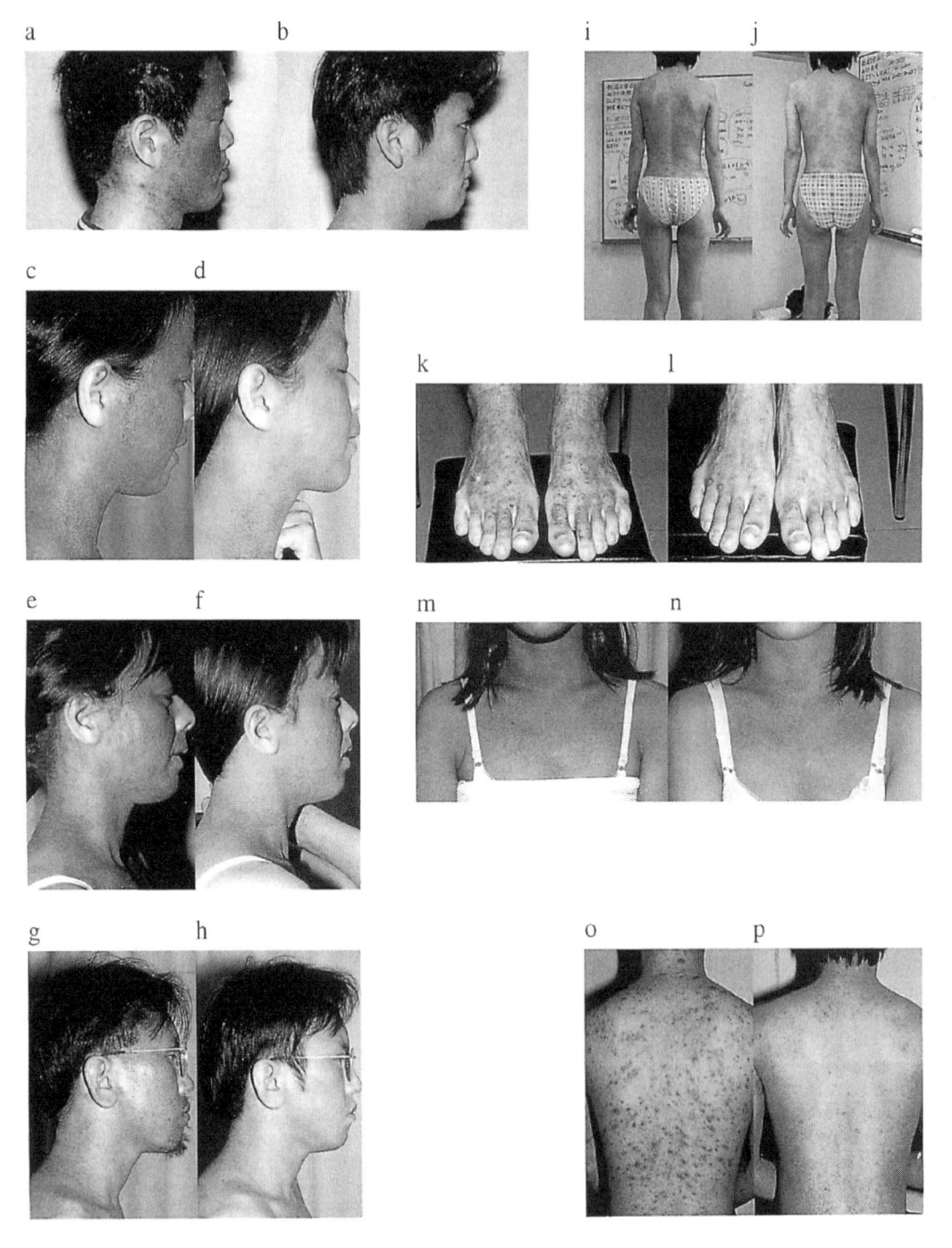

重症アトピー性皮膚炎の治療成功例
右：治療前（a, c, e, g, i, k, mおよびo）
左：治療後（a→b, c→d, e→f, g→h, i→j, k→l, m→nおよびo→p）
ステロイドホルモン含有軟膏使用中止後、患者は離脱症状に苦しむ。禁断症状に対し、鍼治療を行なったところ、1-数ヵ月で治療が成功した。

Figure.4

ステロイド投与における代謝の仮説

新鮮ステロイド　　　→　　17-OHCSとして
＜抗炎症性作用＞　　　　　尿中へ排泄
↓ 組織に停滞
酸化コレステロール　→　胆汁酸として肝臓から排泄
＜炎症作用＞
↓ 組織に沈着
＜アテローム性動脈硬化、老化＞

アトピー性皮膚炎患者に見られるステロイドの行方

明である。以下のように可能性の一つとして考えられるのは、患者においては胆汁酸の形で酸化コレステロール排出が加速されたことである。

以下は、仮説である。我々の治療では、ステロイドホルモンを含有する軟膏の使用を中断し、酸化されたコレステロールが皮膚から排出されたのではないかと考える。周知のように、代謝されたステロイドホルモン類を排出する通常の手段は、尿(17-OHCSとして)と胆汁(高酸化のため、胆汁酸として)である。しかし、ステロイド類は、長期間組織中に残留した場合、酸化コレステロールに変性し、顆粒球性の炎症を誘発すると推測される。最終的には、喘息や硬皮症のような自己免疫疾患により長期間、(数年間もしくはそれ以上)ステロイドホルモンを使用した患者の中には、全員というわけではないが、アテローム硬化症や老化を誘発する可能性がある。

重症アトピー性皮膚炎の治療に成功したことがこの仮説の根拠である。治療中、患者の皮膚から膿が排出された。ステロイドホルモンからの離脱症状克服のため精神的サポートとともに鍼治療を行なった。しかし、ステロイドホルモンを中断させずに鍼治療を行った場合の効果は限定的もしくは無効だった(未発表データ)。鍼治療により、副交感神経刺激反射がおこり、その結果、血液循環不全や他の疾患は治癒する(未発表データ)(11,16,21)

本研究のデータより、これらの患者の多くは、治療前後に好酸球が高値であり、アトピー性皮膚炎になりやすい傾向がみられる。患者のなかには再発に苦しんだ患者も存在した。しかし、おそらく年齢(16歳以上)が理由で、再発率はそれほど高くなかった(10%未満)。ステロイドホルモン含有軟膏未使用のアトピー性皮膚炎患者の場合は、2、3週間の鍼治療で、治癒に成功した。換言すると、アトピー性皮膚炎の重症例は、ステロイドホルモン長期使用の結果であると推測される。

このように考えれば、容易に理解できるのは、長期間ステロイドホルモンを使用した患者のステロイドホルモン投与量を減少させるのは困難だということである。困難であることからもステロイドホルモン依存症ともいえよう。ステロイドホルモンの量が増加した場合、必ず、停滞し、酸化物質を(一過性にせよ)中和する必要がある。

本仮説は、未だ推測の域を出ない、従って他の諸原因も考慮する必要がある。T細胞、IgEおよび、好酸球が、顆粒球同様、アトピー性皮膚炎の重症化に密接に関わっている可能性がある。このように、顆粒球増多はアトピー性皮膚炎の重症例と離脱症状と常に関連している。顆粒球増多の正確な基本メカニズムは未だ不明であるが、ひとつの可能性として交感神経緊張を誘発する停滞したステロイドホルモンを挙げられよう。

注

本研究で報告した患者データの収集後さらに500名の重症アトピー性皮膚炎患者治療に成功したことを付記する。

Stagnation of Steroid Hormones in Patients with Atopic Dermatitis and Unique Variation of Leukocyte Pattern during the Withdrawal Syndrome after Cessation of Steroid Ointment

Minoru Fukuda[1], Nobuaki Kawada[2], Nobuyo Katoh[3], Hiroki Kawamura[4] and Toru Abo[4]

[1] Fukuda-iin, Niigata, [2] Department of Obstetrics and Gynecology, Uhrin Hospital, Fukushima, [3] Department of Public Health, Juntendo University School of Medicine, Tokyo, and [4] Department of Immunology, Niigata University School of Medicine, Niigata, Japan

(Accepted 20 April 2003)

ABSTRACT

Patients with severe atopic dermatitis are sometimes seen even after 15–20 years of age, despite the fact that this is age when atopic dermatitis subsides in usual cases. We consider the possibility that steroid hormones administered as ointment stagnate in the skin and become oxidized cholesterols. Such substances may induce circulation failure and granulocyte-associated inflammation. We herein report the withdrawal of the above ointment in such patients, resulting in successful treatment within several months. Since they suffered from the withdrawal syndrome for the first two or three weeks, acupuncture was performed. Before therapy, these patients showed elevated levels of granulocytes and eosinophils, and an inverse decreased level of lymphocytes in the blood. The number and proportion of granulocytes are known to increase by sympathetic nerve stimulation. This, therefore, indicated that these patients were in a dominant state of the sympathetic nervous system. During the therapy, this leukocyte pattern became much worse due to the withdrawal syndrome. However, in parallel with the amelioration of inflammation, normalization of the leukocyte pattern was observed. These results revealed that, by some yet-undetermined reasons, patients with atopic dermatitis who had been treated by steroid ointment for long time, showed an unusual pattern of leukocytes (i.e., granulocytosis) and that this leukocyte pattern was normalized by the withdrawal of steroid hormones in parallel with the amelioration of the disease.

The onset of atopic dermatitis usually begins at infancy or childhood and some cases experience spontaneous cure before adolescence (3, 12). Primarily, people in childhood show a predominant state of the immune system (i.e., a high level of lymphocytes) (5). However, adults gradually show a decreased level of the immune system (9). The level of granulocytes surpasses that of lymphocytes at 15–20 years old in Japan (our unpublished observation). We speculate that this age-associated change of the immune system might be responsible for the spontaneous cure of atopic dermatitis. In other words, many cases of atopic dermatitis naturally subside due to an age-dependent decrease in the number of T cells.

In spite of the usual course described above, some patients with atopic dermatitis do not show spontaneous cure, but rather suffer from severe symptoms such as inflamed reddish facial skin (3, 12). Such patients have a long history of using topical ointment containing steroid hormones. Are these severe cases of atopic dermatitis inevitable because of their atopic nature or curable by some appropriate therapy? We speculate that if steroid hormones contained in ointment remain long in the dermal tissue of the skin, they become oxidized cholesterols. Ster-

Correspondence to: Dr. T. Abo, Department of Immunology, Niigata University School of Medicine, Asahimachi-dori 1, Niigata 951-8510, Japan
Fax: + 81-25-227-0766
E-mail: immunol2@med.niigata-u.ac.jp

oid hormones have a cholesterol structure, and the skin of patients with atopic dermatitis who use ointment containing such hormones smells bad. This would seem to indicate that the oxidized substance stimulates tissues and infiltration by granulocytes occurs. We confirmed this phenomenon in an animal model (7). Oxidized cholesterols directly induce the accumulation of granulocytes at the corresponding sites (our unpublished observation). Such granulocytes are further activated by many inflammatory cytokines, (e.g., TNFα, IFNγ, G-CSF, etc.), as well as by sympathetic nerve stimulation after the interaction with resident bacteria.

In the past four years, we have attempted to eliminate such oxidized substances from the skin of patients with severe atopic dermatitis and have been successful in almost all such cases (> 95%). Since our patients suffered from the withdrawal syndrome of steroid hormones during therapy, we applied acupuncture. If we knew the actual drug adverse reaction of steroid hormones, we, as well as other clinicians, would be able to successfully treat many patients with severe atopic dermatitis, even those addicted to steroid hormones. Although the precise reasons are not yet determined, granulocytosis seen in patients with severe atopic dermatitis and in the withdrawal syndrome during therapy is interesting. We have to consider the function of granulocytes as well as the functions of IgE, T cells, and eosinophils (1, 20), at least in severe cases of atopic dermatitis.

MATERIALS AND METHODS

Patients. Patients with severe atopic dermatitis (total n = 89, male n = 45, and female n = 44; ages 12 to 28, average 19.9 ± 6.0) were treated. The severity of the atopic dermatitis was estimated according to a previously reported system of grading (13). As indicated by the authors in that paper (13) and others (2), the measurement of disease activity in atopic dermatitis is not so easy. If we apply the simplest method to categorize such patients, "mild", "moderate" and "severe" atopic dermatitis groups can be classified (13). Since almost all patients (approximately 100%) in this study had used ointment containing steroid hormones for several years, at least 80% of patients with atopic dermatitis should be classified as "severe" cases. Age-matched healthy controls (n = 100) were also selected so as to compare their leukocyte pattern with that of the patients.

Leukocyte pattern. The number of white blood cells (total leukocytes) was enumerated in the blood of healthy controls and patients with severe atopic dermatitis. The proportions of granulocytes (including neutrophils and basophils), eosinophils, and lymphocytes were determined by May-Grünwald-Giemsa staining. These data were obtained for the blood of the controls and that of the patients during the therapy.

Measurement of free catecholamines, vanillylmandelic acid (VMA), 17-ketosteroids (17-KS), and 17-OH corticosteroids (17-OHCS) in urine. Urine was collected from 13 patients with atopic dermatitis (before therapy) and 20 age-matched healthy controls for 24 hrs, and the concentrations (/liter) of these substances were measured by the HPLC method (8).

Measurement of serum levels of lipids and cholesterols. All parameters was measured in the laboratory of SRL (Tokyo, Japan, http://www.SRL-inc.co.jp/).

Acupuncture. In addition to psychological support for the patients, we applied acupuncture. Briefly, fingers and toes were punctured with 26-gauge needles; more precisely, sites lateral to the nails were punctured, resulting in some bleeding. This stimulation induced parasympathetic nerve activation, e.g., recovery of peripheral circulation, a decrease in the blood pressure, relief from the itching, etc. In some cases, the severe withdrawal syndrome occurred during the therapy and some elevation of serum transaminases, indicating hepatic failure, was seen. In such severe cases (less than 10% of the patients treated), transfusion of physiological saline (500 ml containing a diuretic) was intravenously administered once a day (up to several times).

Statistical analysis. Differences between the results obtained from healthy control subjects and patients with atopic dermatitis were analyzed by using Student's *t*-test.

RESULTS

Immunoparameters in patients

To determine the immunologic states in patients with severe atopic dermatitis (n = 89), the number of leukocytes and the percentage of the leukocyte population were enumerated in the peripheral blood (Table 1). These patients suffered from severe atopic dermatitis of the face and other sites of the body. All patients had used ointment containing steroid hormones for several months to several years. Before visiting our hospital, they had been treated at several

Table 1 A comparison of the distribution of leukocytes between healthy subjects and patients with atopic dermatitis

Parameter	Healthy subjects (n = 100)	Patients with severe atopic dermatitis (n = 89)		
		Before therapy	2 wks after therapy	At discharge
Number of leukocytes	6,500 ± 1,180	7,700 ± 1,800*	8,500 ± 2,400*	7,500 ± 1,800*
% Granulocytes[a]	57.0 ± 9.2	59.5 ± 10.7	63.3 ± 10.9*	52.0 ± 10.3
% Eosinophils	1.8 ± 1.0	11.8 ± 8.4*	13.1 ± 8.1*	13.7 ± 8.5*
% Lymphocytes	38.9 ± 5.2	27.8 ± 8.6*	22.6 ± 8.8*	34.2 ± 9.4

[a] Neurophils and basophils (not including eosinophils)
* $p < 0.05$

other hospitals. For a comparison of the leukocyte pattern, age-matched healthy subjects (n = 100) were examined in parallel. Before our therapy, these patients showed elevated levels of the number of leukocytes and the proportion of eosinophils, and a decreased level of the proportion of lymphocytes ($P < 0.05$). As for the absolute number of leukocytes, it was estimated that the numbers of granulocytes and eosinophils, but not of lymphocytes, increased ($P < 0.05$).

Urine levels of catecholamines
We previously reported that predominance of the sympathetic nervous system induces an elevation of granulocytes in the peripheral blood and other tissues of humans (5, 8, 15) and mice (4, 10, 22). Since this is the case, it was speculated that the sympathetic nervous system of patients with severe atopic dermatitis who showed elevated levels of granulocytes might be predominant. This was obvious from the fact that the majority of the patients suffered from tachycardia and insomnia. We also examined the urine level of catecholamines as well as of metabolites of innate steroid hormones (Fig. 1). The patients showed elevated levels (per day) of free catecholamines and VMA (a metabolite of catecholamines) ($P < 0.05$). The level of 17-KS was low ($P < 0.05$) while that of 17-OHCS remained normal ($P > 0.05$).

Serum levels of lipids and cholesterols
To examine the possibility that sympathetic nerve activation was induced by oxidized cholesterols derived from stagnated steroids, we measured the serum levels of lipids and cholesterols (Fig. 2). Among tested parameters, the levels of total lipid, total cholesterol, β-lipoprotein, cholesterol ester, and free cholesterol were comparable between controls and the patients. However, the level of lipid peroxide (which is known to include oxidized cholesterols) increased but that of total bile acid decreased in the patients ($P < 0.01$).

Recovery from atopic dermatitis
According to our hypothesis (i.e., accumulation of oxidized cholesterols in the skin), we began the treatment of patients. It included 1) the cessation of ointment usage, 2) acupuncture, and 3) psychological support. Two weeks after commencement of the therapy, the leukocyte pattern (the increase in the number of granulocytes and eosinophils) seen in patients with severe atopic dermatitis became much more prominent (see Table 1). Namely, one of the major signs of the withdrawal syndrome was the worsening of the leukocyte pattern, as well as the worsening of inflammation. However, these symptoms gradually subsided (Table 1 and Fig. 3). At the time of discharge from the hospital (Table 1, right column), the leukocyte pattern had become almost normal, except for the value of eosinophils. As shown in Fig. 3, we were able to achieve a remarkable improvement of severe atopic dermatitis in all patients.

Time intervals before and after the present treatment ranged from one month to five months. However, at the beginning of therapy, some patients (approximately 5%) gave up the therapy, dropping out due to the severe withdrawal syndrome. Some patients (approximately 20%) showed a sporadic exacerbation of atopic dermatitis even after discharge. However, these symptoms gradually disappeared as a function of time. We recommended exercise for these patients since appropriate exercise seems to be very effective for eliminating the exacerbation.

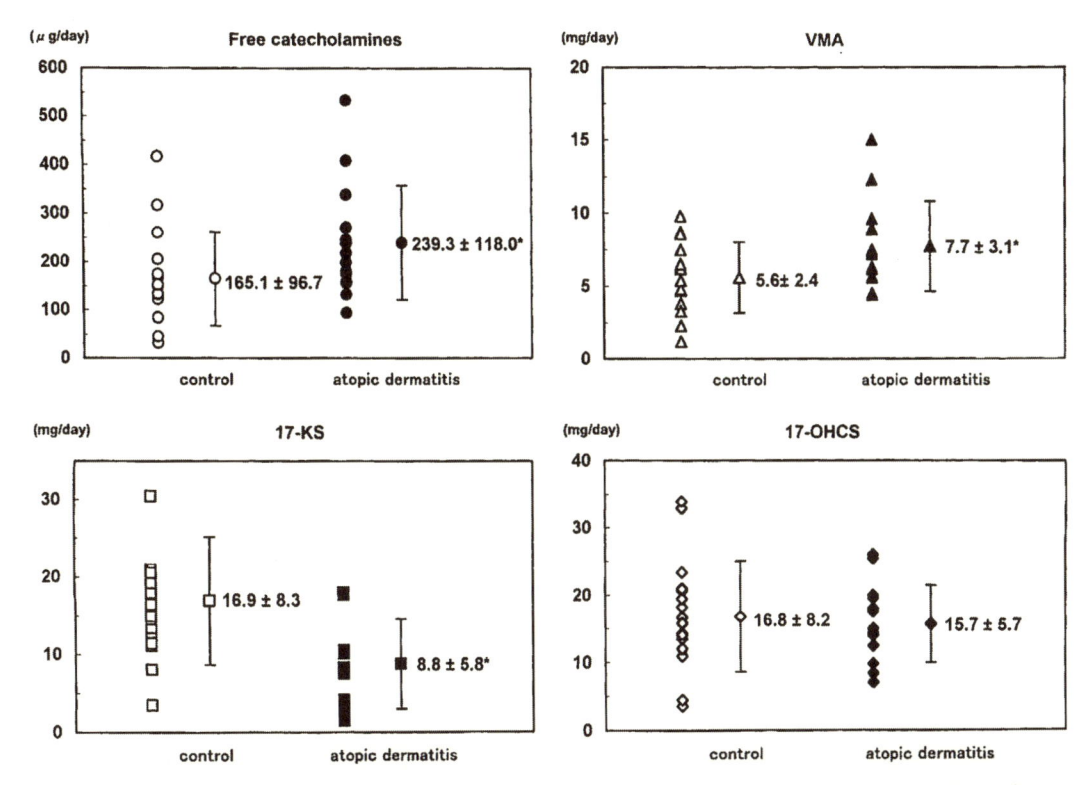

Fig. 1 Excretion of free catecholamines, VMA, 17-KS, and 17-OHCS into the urine (per day) in controls and the patients. Urine was collected from patients with severe atopic dermatitis (n = 13) and age-matched healthy controls (n = 20). * P < 0.05

DISCUSSION

In a series of recent studies, we reported that immunologic states are under the regulation of the autonomic nervous system (4, 5, 8, 10, 15, 17, 22). This is due to the fact that granulocytes carry surface adrenergic receptors (11) and lymphocytes carry surface cholinergic receptors (17). If the sympathetic nervous system is stimulated, granulocytes are activated in number and function. Inversely, if the parasympathetic nervous system is stimulated, lymphocytes such as T and B cells are activated in number and function. A rapid change in the distribution of leukocytes arises from the fact that the life span of leukocytes is very short, e.g., the life span of granulocytes being only 2 days after maturation (10). Moreover, sympathetic nerve stimulation induces the acceleration of granulocyte trafficking, i.e., the bone marrow (the pool organ of granulocytes) → the circulation → the mucosal/cutaneous tissues. As a consequence, sympathetic nervous system stimulation increases the number of granulocytes in the blood. This includes the granulocytosis seen in the daytime (the circadian rhythm) (15), that resulting from physical stress (10), and neonatal granulocytosis induced by commencement of pulmonary respiration at birth (5).

In light of these findings, we herein analyzed the leukocyte pattern in patients with severe atopic dermatitis, who had been diagnosed as suffering from an incurable disease (or state) at other hospitals. In contrast to our anticipation, the level of granulocytes was found to be elevated while that of lymphocytes was low in these patients. Namely, they were in an immunosuppressive state. The immunosuppressive state seen in patients with severe atopic dermatitis has been similarly reported by other investigators (6, 14, 18, 19).

We postulated that some oxidized substances (e.g., oxidized cholesterols resulting from steroid

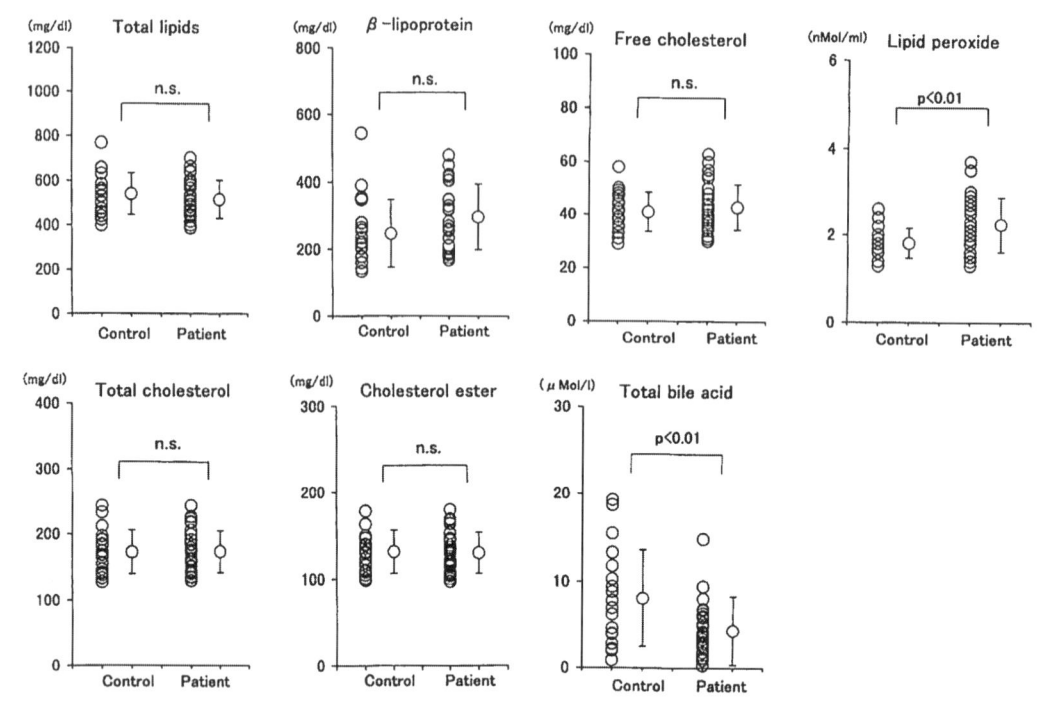

Fig. 2 A comparison of the serum levels of lipids and cholesterols between control and patients with severe atopic dermatitis. Blood samples were collected from severe atopic dermatitis (n = 29) and age-matched healthy controls (n = 19) and the serum levels of lipids and cholesterols were measured. The level of lipid peroxide increased but that of total bile acid decreased in the patients (P < 0.01).

hormones used as ointment) had induced sympathetic nervous system dominance (Fig. 4). Indeed, almost all of these young patients had symptoms such as tachycardia, hypertension, insomnia, anxiety, fatigue, etc. This postulation was confirmed by the results of urine analysis, namely, the levels of free catecholamines and VMA were elevated in the urine of the patients. We do not know why the level of 17-KS was low in these patients. The elevated serum level of lipid peroxide (which includes oxidized cholesterols) was also found to be elevated in the patients. At present, we do not know why the patients showed a decreased serum level of total bile acid. As mentioned below, one possibility is acceleration of the excretion of oxidized cholesterols as bile acid in the patients.

According to our hypothesis, we discontinued the use of the ointment containing steroid hormones and waited for the oxidized cholesterols to be excreted from the skin. As well established, the usual routes for the excretion of metabolized steroid hormones are the urine (as 17-OHCS) and the bile (as bile acid because of high oxidization). However, if they remain in the tissue for long, it is speculated that they become oxidized cholesterols which then induce granulocyte-associated inflammation. Finally, they may induce atherosclerosis and aging, as seen in some patients, if not all, with asthma and autoimmune diseases such as scleroderma, who have used steroid hormones for a long time (i.e., several years or longer).

Our successful treatment of severe atopic dermatitis supports our hypothesis. During the therapy, patients experienced the excretion of a purulent substance from the skin. To overcome the withdrawal syndrome from steroid hormones, we applied acupuncture as well as giving psychological support. However, when we applied acupuncture without the cessation of steroid hormones, the effects were limited or nil (our unpublished observation). Acupuncture induces the reflex of parasympathetic nerve stimulation (11, 16, 21) and results in the recovery

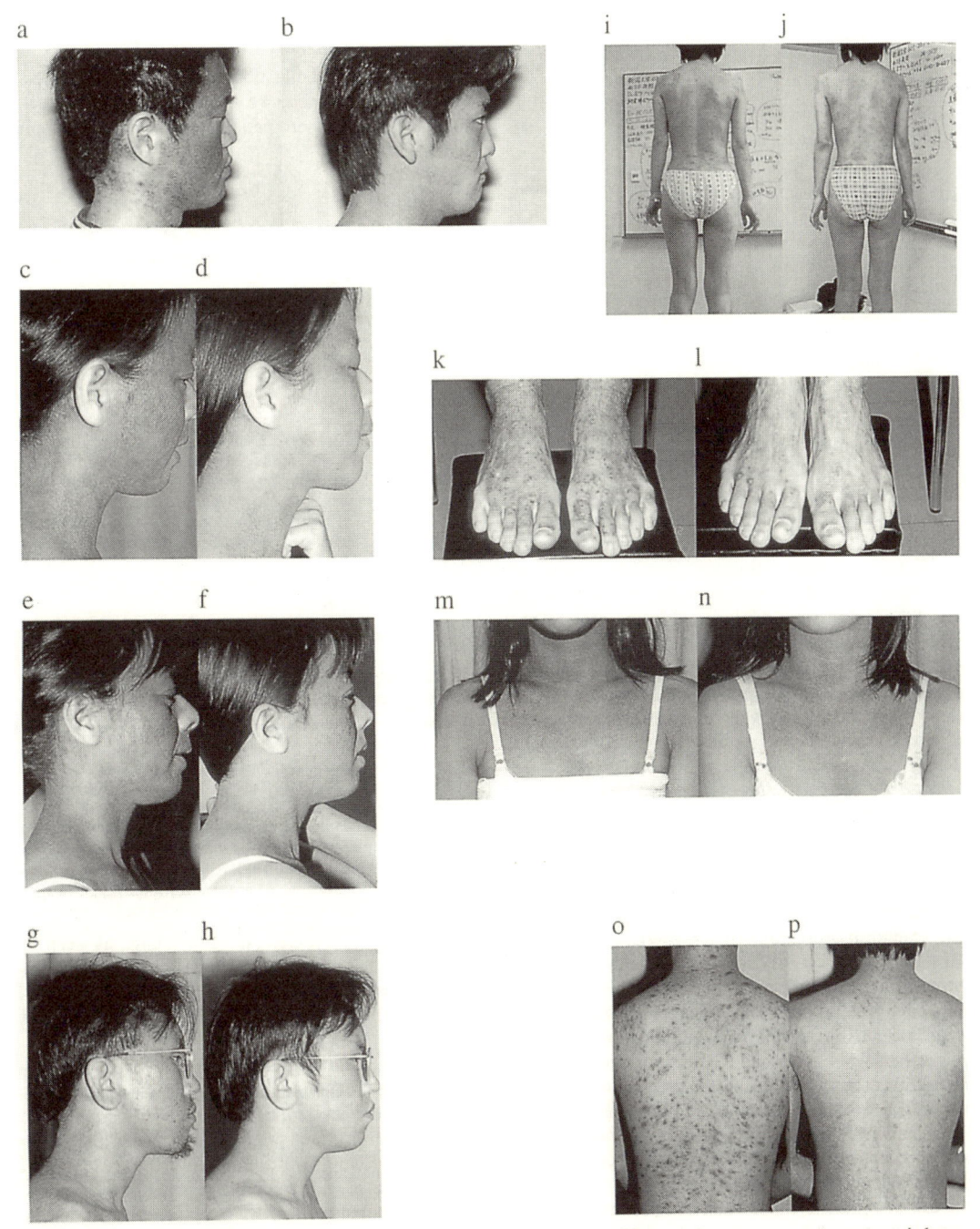

Fig. 3 Successful treatment of severe atopic dermatitis by acupuncture. Right: before treatment (a, c, e, g, i, k, m, and o), Left: after treatment (a → b, c → d, e → f, g → h, i → j, k → l, m → n, and o → p). After cessation of the use of ointment containing steroid hormones, the patients suffered from the withdrawal syndrome. This was, however, countered by acupuncture, resulting in successful treatment within one month to several months.

Possible metabolism of administered steroids

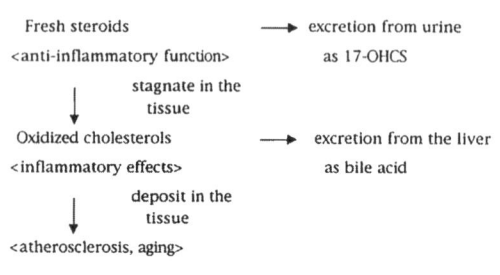

Fresh steroids → excretion from urine as 17-OHCS
<anti-inflammatory function>
↓ stagnate in the tissue
Oxidized cholesterols → excretion from the liver as bile acid
<inflammatory effects>
↓ deposit in the tissue
<atherosclerosis, aging>

Fig. 4 Fate of administered steroids in patients with atopic dermatitis

from circulation failure or other ailments (our unpublished observations).

As shown by the present data, many of these patients were genetically predisposed to atopy as reflected by the high level of eosinophils before and after therapy. In this regard, some patients suffered a recurrence of disease. However, possibly because of their ages (older than 16 years), the recurrence ratio was not so high (less than 10%). In the case of patients with atopic dermatitis who had not yet used ointment containing steroid hormones, two or three weeks were sufficient to achieve successful treatment by acupuncture. In other words, severe cases of atopic dermatitis might result from long use of steroid hormones.

With the present concept, we can easily understand the reason for the difficulty in reducing doses of steroid hormones in many diseased persons who have used such hormones for a long time. We call it steroid hormone addiction. Increased amounts of steroid hormones are always required for neutralization (but still temporary) of the stagnated, oxidized substance.

Our hypothesis still remains a speculation, and we also have to consider many other reasons. Not only T cells, IgE, and eosinophils but also granulocytes might be highly associated with severity of atopic dermatitis. Thus, granulocytosis was always accompanied with severe cases of atopic dermatitis and with the withdrawal syndrome. Although we do not yet know the precise mechanisms underlying granulocytosis, one of the candidates may be stagnated steroid hormones which then induce sympathetic nerve activation.

Note

Subsequent to collection of the data on the patients herein reported, we achieved successful treatment of 500 other patients with severe atopic dermatitis.

REFERENCES

1. Bos J. D., Van Leent E. J. M. and Smitt J. H. S. (1998) The millennium criteria for the diagnosis of atopic dermatitis. *Exp. Dermatol.* 7, 132-138.
2. Finlay A. Y. (1996) Measurement of disease activity and outcome in atopic dermatitis. *Br. J. Dermatol.* 135, 509-515.
3. Kaplan R. J. and Rosenberg E. W. (1978) Atopic dermatitis: clinical and immunologic aspects and treatment. *Postgrad. Med.* 64, 52-56.
4. Kawamura H., Kawamura T., Kokai Y., Mori M., Matsuura A., Oya H., Honda S., Suzuki S., Weerasinghe A., Watanabe H. and Abo T. (1999) Expansion of extrathymic T cells as well as granulocytes in the liver and other organs of G-CSF transgenic mice. Why they lost the ability of hybrid resistance. *J. Immunol.* 162, 5957-5964.
5. Kawamura T., Toyabe S., Moroda T., Iiai T., Takahashi-Iwanaga H., Fukuda M., Watanabe H., Sekikawa H., Seki S. and Abo T. (1997) Neonatal granulocytosis is a postpartum event which is seen in the liver as well as in the blood. *Hepatology* 26, 1567-1572.
6. Lesko M. J., Lever R. S., Mackie R. M. and Parrott D. M. (1989) The effect of topical steroid application on natural killer cell activity. *Clin. Exp. Allergy* 19, 633-636.
7. Maruyama S., Minagawa M., Shimizu T., Oya H., Yamamoto S., Musha N., Abo W., Weerasinghe A., Hatakeyama K. and Abo T. (1999) Administration of glucocorticoids markedly increases the numbers of granulocytes and extrathymic T cells in the bone marrow. *Cell. Immunol.* 194, 28-35.
8. Minagawa M., Narita J., Tada T., Maruyama S., Shimizu T., Bannai M., Oya H., Hatakeyama K. and Abo T. (1999) Mechanisms underlying immunologic states during pregnancy: possible association of the sympathetic nervous system. *Cell. Immunol.* 196, 1-13.
9. Miyaji C., Watanabe H., Minagawa M., Toma H., Nohara Y., Nozaki H., Sato Y. and Abo T. (1997) Numerical and functional characteristics of lymphocyte subsets in centenarians. *J. Clin. Immunol.* 17, 420-429.
10. Moroda T., Iiai T., Tsukahara A., Fukuda M., Suzuki S., Tada T., Hatakeyama K. and Abo T. (1997) Association of granulocytes with ulcer formation in the stomach of rodents exposed to restraint stress. *Biomed. Res.* 18, 423-437.
11. Nishijo K., Mori H., Yoshikawa K. and Yazawa K. (1997) Decreased heart rate by acupuncture stimulation in humans via facilitation of cardiac vagal activity and suppression of cardiac sympathetic nerve. *Neurosci. Lett.* 227, 165-168.
12. Rajka G. (1986) Natural history and clinical manifestations of atopic dermatitis. *Clin. Rev. Allergy* 4, 3-26.
13. Rajka G. and Langeland T. (1989) Grading of the severity of atopic dermatitis. *Acta Derm. Venereol.* 144, 13-14.
14. Rogge J. L. and Hanifin J. M. (1976) Immunodeficiencies in severe atopic dermatitis. *Arch. Dermatol.* 112, 1391-1396.
15. Suzuki S., Toyabe S., Moroda T., Tada T., Tsukahara A., Iiai T., Minagawa M., Maruyama S., Hatakeyama K., Endo K. and Abo T. (1997) Circadian rhythm of leukocytes and lymphocyte subsets and its possible correlation with the function

of autonomic nervous system. *Clin. Exp. Immunol.* **110**, 500–508.
16. Tam K. C. and Yiu H. H. (1975) The effect of acupuncture on essential hypertension. *Am. J. Chin. Med.* **3**, 369–375.
17. Toyabe S., Iiai T., Fukuda M., Kawamura T., Suzuki S., Uchiyama M. and Abo T. (1997) Identification of nicotinic acetylcholine receptors on lymphocytes in periphery as well as thymus in mice. *Immunology* **92**, 201–205.
18. Vandercam B., Lachapelle J. M., Janssens P., Tennstedt D. and Lambert M. (1997) Kaposi's sarcoma during immunosuppressive therapy for atopic dermatitis. *Dermatology* **194**, 180–182.
19. Walker C., Kagi M. K., Ingold P., Braun P., Blaser K., Bruijnzeel-Koomen C. A. and Wuthrich B. (1993) Atopic dermatitis: correlation of peripheral blood T cell activation, eosinophilia and serum factors with conical severity. *Clin. Exp. Allergy* **23**, 145–153.
20. Werfel T. and Kapp A. (1999) What do we know about the etiopathology of the intrinsic type of atopic dermatitis? *Curr. Probl. Dermatol.* **28**, 29–36.
21. Williams T., Mueller K. and Cornwall M. W. (1991) Effect of acupuncture-point stimulation on diastolic blood pressure in hypertensive subjects: a preliminary study. *Phys. Ther.* **71**, 523–529.
22. Yamamura S., Arai K., Toyabe S., Takahashi E. H. and Abo T. (1996) Simultaneous activation of granulocytes and extrathymic T cells in number and function by excessive administration of nonsteroidal anti-inflammatory drugs. *Cell. Immunol.* **173**, 303–311.

AGE-RELATED BIAS IN FUNCTION OF NATURAL KILLER T CELLS AND GRANULOCYTES AFTER STRESS: RECIPROCAL ASSOCIATION OF STEROID HORMONES AND SYMPATHETIC NERVES

ストレス後のナチュラル・キラーT細胞と顆粒球の機能は加齢に関連して変化する：
各ステロイドホルモンと交感神経との相互関係

Clinical Experimental Immunology, 135: 56-63, 2004

chapter 16

Age-related bias in function of natural killer T cells and granulocytes after stress:reciprocal association of steroid hormones and sympathetic nerves

ストレス後のナチュラル・キラーT細胞と顆粒球の機能は加齢に関連して変化する：各ステロイドホルモンと交感神経との相互関係

K. SAGIYAMA[*,†], M. TSUCHIDA[*], H. KAWAMURA[*], S. WANG[*], C. LI[*], X. BAI[*], T. NAGURA[*], S. NOZOE[†] &T. ABO[*]

[*]Department of Immunology, Niigata University School of Medicine, Niigata and [†]Department of Psychosomatic Medicine, Kagoshima University Faculty of Medicine, Kagoshima, Japan

【キーワード】

ストレス、ナチュラルキラーT細胞　顆粒球　ステロイドホルモン　交感神経

【要約】

ストレスに関連した免疫応答について若齢(8週齢)マウスと老齢(56週齢)マウスとで比較した。ストレスを受けると、新しい免疫系(T細胞やB細胞)の抑制が起こるが、反対に古い免疫系(胸腺外分化T細胞、NKT細胞および顆粒球)の活性化が起こる。そこで拘束ストレス実験(24時間)を行い、新しい免疫系と古い免疫系の各パラメータの解析を行った。加齢により胸腺が萎縮し、肝臓のリンパ球数の増加が見られた。ストレスを受けた後、胸腺と肝臓のリンパ球数の減少が見られたが、胸腺の方が顕著であった。ストレスに耐性があるリンパ球サブセットを特定するため肝臓と脾臓において二重免疫蛍光染色を行なったところ、若齢マウスの肝臓では、NKT細胞が該当することが明らかになった。一方、ストレスによる顆粒球浸潤は、若齢マウスよりも老齢マウスの肝臓において顕著であった。ストレスの結果としての肝障害は、若齢マウスにおいて顕著であった。NKT細胞と顆粒球の機能が加齢により異なることは、ストレスを受けた後、カテコラミン(老齢マウスで高い)とコルチコステロン(若齢マウスで高い)の反応の相違と関連があると考えられた。実際、アドレナリンを投与すると主に顆粒球浸潤が現れ、一方、コルチゾールを投与するとNKT細胞の活性化が見られた。これら結果が示すのは、NKT細胞や顆粒球の機能がストレスを受けた後、加齢により異なること、そして、このような相違は、顆粒球は若齢マウスと老齢マウスとで交感神経と諸ステロイドホルモンの反応が異なることが原因である可能性がある。

はじめに

最近の研究[1.5]において、ストレスを受けると胸腺におけるT細胞分化が停止し、結果として胸腺萎縮が現れることを明らかにした。この経路は胸腺のT細胞分化の主流と呼ばれ、従来型のTCRの発現が高い細胞(TCR^{high}細胞)が分化する[6,7]。ストレスのため胸腺のT細胞分化が低下する結果として、他の末梢免疫器官にも免疫抑制が出現する。一方胸腺内の代替経路(ナチュラル・キラーT(NKT)細胞を産生[8.10])および胸腺外である肝臓経路　(NK1.1$^-$ intermediateTCR細胞(TCR^{int}細胞)[11,12]を産生)がストレスを受けると活性化する。このような徴候は、加齢でも見られる(胸腺萎縮と胸腺外分化T細胞の活性化)。緊急事態の下に

出現した異常な自己細胞を処理するのは、古い性質を持つ自己応答性 T 細胞 (NKT 細胞と NK1.1⁻TCR^{int} 細胞)[13,14] および自己抗体産生 B 細胞 (B-1 細胞)[15] である可能性がある。

これらの結果を考慮して、さらに、若齢マウスと老齢マウスでストレスにより免疫系がどのように変化するか検証した。このように加齢に関連した検証は興味深い。というのは免疫系におけるこれらの異なる経路がストレスと関係なく、加齢を要因として変化するからである[16,18]。本研究の結果より、若齢マウスと老齢マウスでは拘束ストレスに若干異なる免疫応答を示すことが明らかになった。すなわち、ストレスを受けた後、NKT 細胞の機能活性化による肝障害は、老齢マウスよりも若齢マウスにおいて非常に顕著であった。若齢マウスにおいて NKT 細胞の機能がこのように独特の変化を示したことは、ストレス後、各ステロイドホルモン産生が上昇したことに関連があるようだ。対照的に、老齢マウスでは、ストレスを受けると、むしろ交感神経緊張が出現し、その結果、主として顆粒球の組織浸潤が現れた。従って、本研究では、免疫系の持つ二つの異なる面を報告する。つまり、ストレス後の免疫応答は加齢と関連して変化すること、交感神経系とステロイドホルモン分泌と密接に関連して変化することである。

最後に、我々はストレスを受けた際には、免疫応答反応には、二本の軸が存在することを提唱する。主として NKT 細胞を誘導する『副腎皮質軸』[1] と顆粒球を誘導する『交感神経軸』[2] である。この二本の軸は、ストレスとその後出現する組織損傷を結びつける。成熟した生体の場合、この二本の軸には密接な関係がある。しかし、老齢では『交感神経軸』が優位である一方、若齢では『副腎皮質軸』が優位である。

材料と方法

マウス

8、12 および 56 週齢の C57BL/6(B6) マウスを使用した。マウスは、新潟大学動物実験施設内、SPF(特定病原体未感染)下で飼育した。マウスに拘束ストレス(ステンレス・スチール・メッシュ固定、24 時間)を与えた。これまでの研究より、胃粘膜に顆粒球が増多し、結果として胃潰瘍が出現するのに充分な時間である [5]。

細胞分離

肝単核球 (MNC) を定法により分離した [19]。略述すると、摘出した肝臓を 200-ゲージ・ステンレス・スチール・メッシュで漉し、5mM の HEPES と 2% 非働化済仔牛血清を含んだ Eagle's MEM 培養液(日水製薬(株),東京,日本)に浮遊させた。培養液で一度洗浄した後、細胞を 15ml、35% パーコール溶液 (Amersham Pharmacia Biotech, Piscataway, NJ) の中に再浮遊させ、15 分間 2000rpm の比重遠心により肝細胞と単核球の分離を行なった。赤血球と単核球を含むペレットは赤血球溶血溶液 (155mm, NH_4Cl, 10mm $KHCO_3$, 1mm EDTA-Na および 170mm Tris., pH 7.3) の中に再浮遊させ赤血球を溶血させた。胸腺細胞と脾臓単核球は、胸腺と脾臓をそれぞれ 200-ゲージ・ステンレス・スチール・メッシュで漉して採取した。脾臓単核球採取には、溶血も行なった。

フローサイトメトリー解析

使用したモノクロナール抗体は、フルオレセイン・イソチオシアネート (FITC) 標識とフィコエリトリン (PE) 標識およびビオチン標識抗体である TRIcolor 標識ストレプトアビジン (Caltag Laboratory, San Francisco, CA) で発色させた [20]。本実験で使用したモノクロナール抗体は、抗 CD3(145-2C11)、抗 NK1.1(PK136)、抗 CD4(RM4-5)、抗 CD8α(Lyt-2)、抗マクロ

ファージ (M1/70) および抗顆粒球 (RB6-8C5) モノクロナール抗体 (BD PharMingen, San Diego, CA, USA) である。FACScan(BD Biosciences、Mountain View、CA、USA) を用い細胞の解析を行なった。モノクロナール抗体の非特異的結合を防ぐために、CD32/16(2.4G2 BD; PharMingen)にて前処理を行なった後、各種抗体を加えた。死細胞は、前方散乱、側方散乱とヨウ化プロピジウム・ゲーティングにより除外した。

トランスアミラーゼ測定

肝障害を調べるため、血清中アスパラギン酸アミノトランスフェラーゼ(AST)およびアラニンアミノトランスフェラーゼ(ALT)活性を測定した。それぞれの血清の活性をSTAテスト・キット(和光純薬(株),東京,日本)を用い測定した。

細胞傷害活性試験

YAC-1を標的細胞として用い、NK様細胞傷害活性を、4時間培養を行い、特異的^{51}Cr-遊離試験を用い検証した[21]。YAC-1細胞にクロム酸ナトリウム(^{51}Cr)(Amersham Int., Arlington Heights, IL, USA) で標識し、肝臓もしくは脾臓単核球をエフェクター細胞とした。細胞傷害活性率は、YAC-1細胞(10^4個/well)を標的細胞として用い、エフェクター細胞:標的細胞(E/T ratio)を3well測定した。4時間培養時、標的細胞の(^{51}Cr) 遊離量は10-15%であり、この値を実験値の遊離量より除外した。

血漿カテコラミン値およびコルチコステロン値測定

マウス4匹の血漿を用いて、カテコラミン(アドレナリン、ノルアドレナリンとドーパミン)値およびコルチコステロン値を測定した。血漿カテコラミン値の測定には、HPLC法を用いた。マウスの血漿コルチコステロン値は、標識免疫検定法を若干修正して測定した。マウス

Figure.1

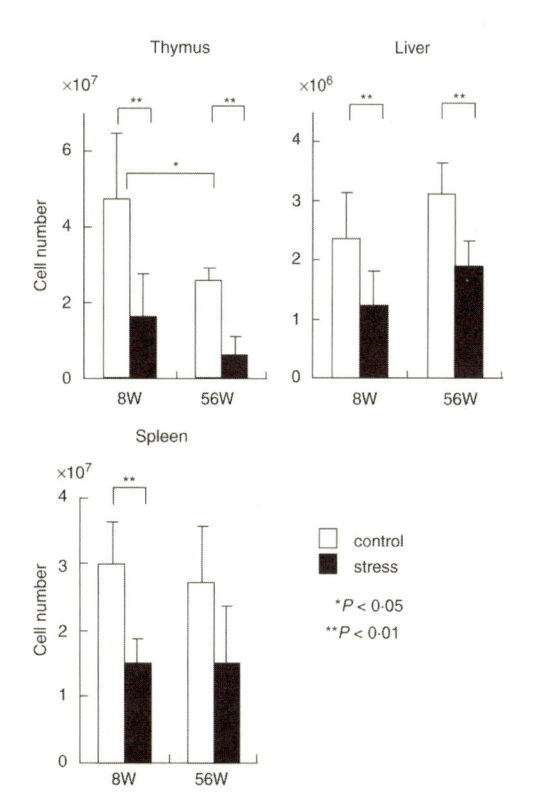

加齢とストレスに関連した胸腺、肝臓と脾臓における単核球数の変化。若齢(8週齢)マウスと老齢(56週齢)マウスとを用い、拘束ストレス(24時間)を与えた。MNC数、平均値±1SDは、4匹のマウスを用いて算出した。

の場合、コルチコステロンが主要なステロイドホルモンである。

アドレナリンおよびヒドロコルチゾン・コハク酸ナトリウム投与

カテコラミンの影響を検証するため、アドレナリン(Sigma Chemicals Co., St Louis, MO, USA) (100μg/匹)を腹腔内投与した。各ステロイドホルモンの影響を検証するため、ヒドロコルチゾン・コハク酸塩(ファルマシア(株),東京,日本) (10mg/匹)を腹腔内投与した。そして、投与24時間後の単核球を測定した。先行研究[2,5]より、これら試薬による最大の反応を測定する投与量と時間を決定した。

Figure.2

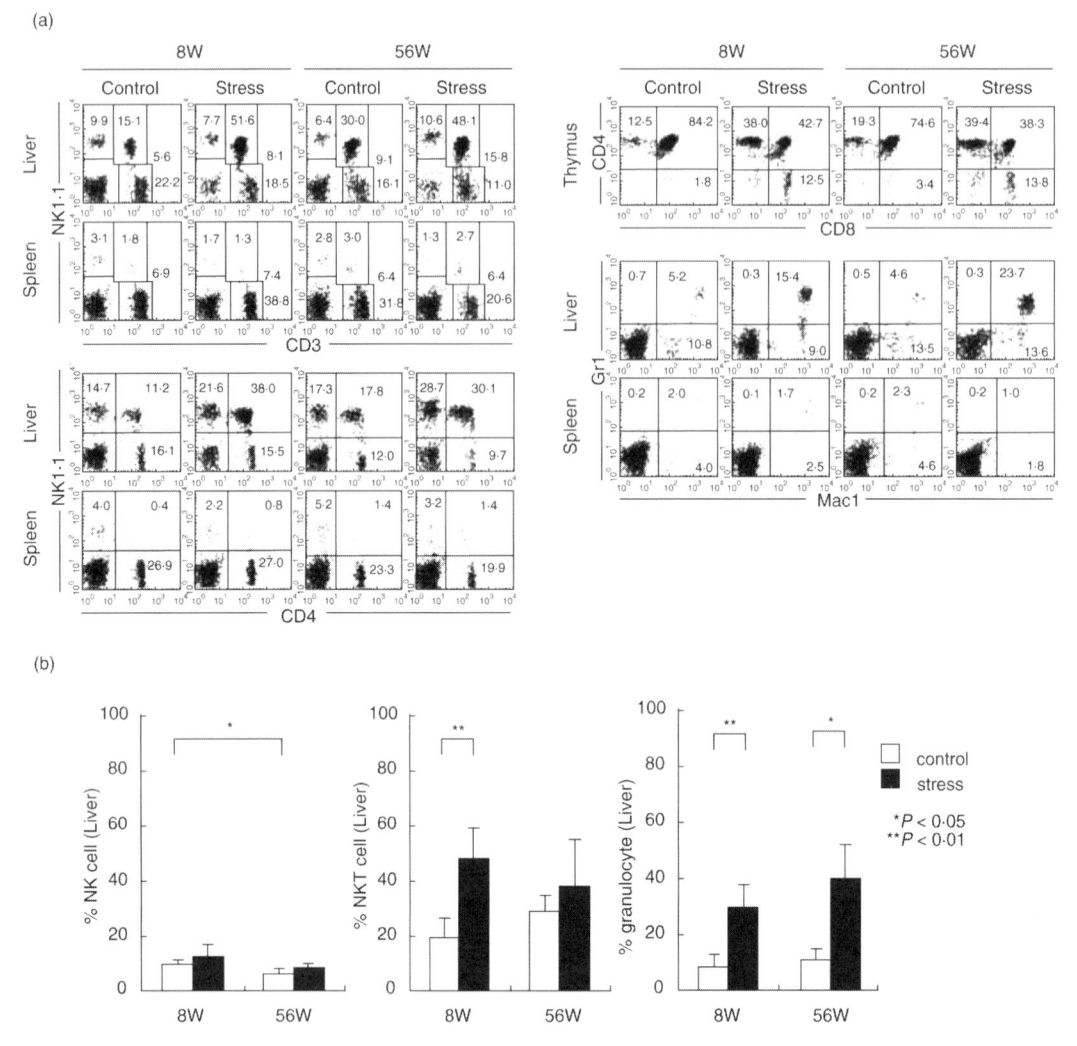

肝臓と脾臓におけるストレス耐性リンパ球サブセットの解析。(a)様々な組み合わせで、リンパ球の二重染色を行なった。(b)NKT細胞比率増加(若齢マウス)および顆粒球比率増加(老齢マウス)。単核球を若齢および老齢マウスのストレス前後で測定し、細胞のフェノタイプを免疫蛍光染色により確認した。NK細胞、NKT細胞と顆粒球比率は、4度実験を行い、平均値±1SDを4/匹のマウスを用いて算出した。

統計分析

有意差解析には、二元配置分散分析法を用いた。

結果

各免疫器官のリンパ球数と肝リンパ球のストレスに対する耐性は加齢により変化する

様々な免疫器官におけるストレスによる影響が加齢により変化することを検証するため、若齢および老齢マウスの胸腺、肝臓と脾臓においてまず計測を行なった (Fig. 1)。拘束ストレス(24時間)後、胸腺細胞数の減少において加齢による違いが見られた。つまり、老齢マウスでは若齢マウス50%の減少を示した。一方、肝リンパ球数は増加し、加齢との関連がみられた。しかし、脾臓リンパ球数には、ほとんど変化が見られなかった。若齢マウスでも老齢マウスで

Figure.3

老齢マウスおよび若齢マウスにおけるストレスの前後のNK様細胞傷害活性。リンパ球を肝臓と脾臓から分離し、YAC-1細胞に対するNK様細胞傷害活性を4時間培養した後にE/T比率を測定した。各実験には3wellを使用し、平均値±1SDを算出した。

Figure.4

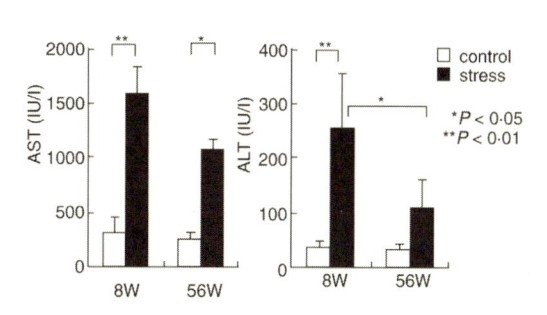

ストレス後の老齢マウスおよび若齢マウスの肝臓障害の程度比較。肝臓障害の程度を検証するため血清中ASTとALT値を測定した。平均値±1SDは、4匹マウスを用いて算出した。

Figure.5

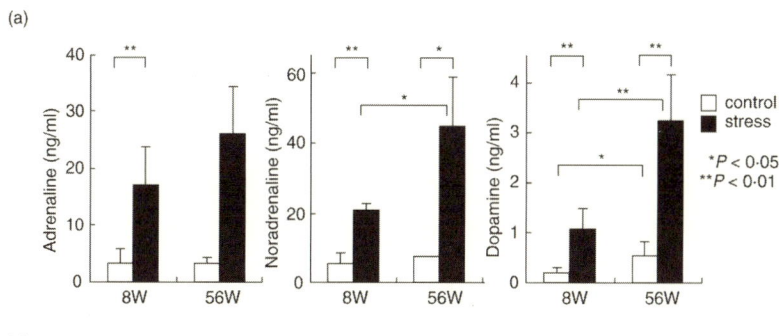

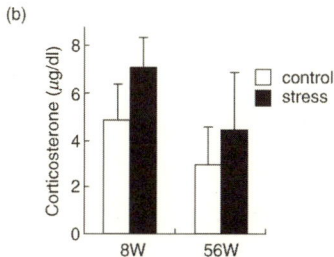

ストレス後の若齢マウスと老齢マウスの間における血清中カテコールアミン値と血清コルチコステロン値の比較。平均値±1SDは、マウス4匹の血漿を用いて算出した。

もストレスの影響で、胸腺細胞が減少した。拘束ストレスの結果、肝臓と脾臓においてリンパ球数減少が、若齢で老齢マウスでも見られた。しかし、胸腺では、肝臓、脾臓よりも、はるかに顕著な減少を示した。

肝臓におけるストレス耐性リンパ球サブセットの特定

リンパ球サブセットのうち、ストレスに強い耐性を持つサブセットを特定するため、肝臓と脾臓において様々な抗体の組み合わせでリンパ球の二重染色を行なった (Fig. 2a)。CD3

Figure.6

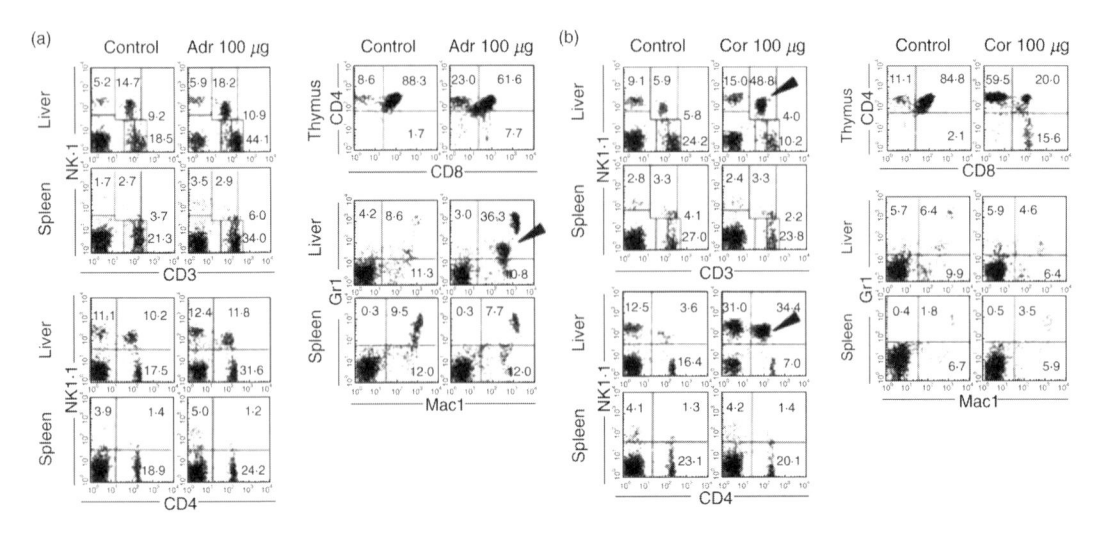

若年マウス（12週齢）に(a)アドレナリン（Adr）または(b)ヒドロコルチゾン（コルチゾール）(Cor)を投与した。肝臓、脾臓と胸腺の単核球を、各薬剤投与前と後（24h）に分離した。図示の組合せの二重染色を行なった。3度実験を行なった典型例を示す。

とNK1.1二重染色では、肝臓において最もストレスに耐性があるリンパ球サブセットは、$CD3^{int}NK1.1^+$細胞（NKT細胞）であった。CD4とNK1.1二重染色によりこれらの細胞の大部分は$CD4^+$ NKT細胞であった。脾臓では、検証したすべてのサブセットにおいて変化は最小限だった。

胸腺萎縮では、ダブルポジティブ細胞（DP細胞）$CD4^+8^+$細胞の比率が常に減少することが知られている[2]。胸腺萎縮の影響で、CD4とCD8二重染色では、DP($CD4^+CD8^+$)細胞の顕著な減少（若齢マウス；85.6 → 42.7%、老齢マウス；74.6 → 38.3%）が見られた。

本実験の最終段階では、Mac-1とGr-1二重染色を行い、顆粒球（Gr-1$^+$Mac-1$^+$）とマクロファージ（Gr-1$^-$Mac-1$^+$）を確認した。拘束ストレスの結果として肝臓における顆粒球の比率も増加を示した。この反応は、老齢マウスにおいて顕著であった。

実験は全て複数回（n=4）行い、リンパ球と顆粒球の平均値 ± 1SDは、4匹のマウスを用いて算出した（Fig. 2b）。NK細胞はほとんど変化を示さなかったが、NKT細胞と顆粒球の変化は統計的に有意であった（P<0.05またはP<0.01）。若齢マウスではNKT細胞の比率の増加が顕著であった。一方、老齢マウスでは顆粒球の増加が顕著であった。

細胞傷害活性と肝臓障害

NKT細胞が活性化すると、NK様の細胞傷害活性を有することが知られている。本実験では、肝臓と脾臓のリンパ球を用いてYAC-1細胞に対するNK様細胞傷害活性を検証した（Fig. 3）。ストレスを受けた後、若齢マウスと老齢マウスの肝臓において、NK様の細胞傷害活性の顕著な低下が見られた。NK細胞とNKT細胞の比率が若齢マウスよりも老齢マウスで高かったが、逆に、ストレスを受ける前の細胞傷害活性は、老齢マウスよりも若齢マウスで高かった。

Figure.7

```
                    Axis                          Activation
                  Adrenocortical axis*  ─────→  NKT cells
                 ↗                                        ↘
        Stress                                              Tissue injury
                 ↘                                        ↗
                  Sympathetic nerve axis+ ────→  Granulocytes
```

*dominance in young animals

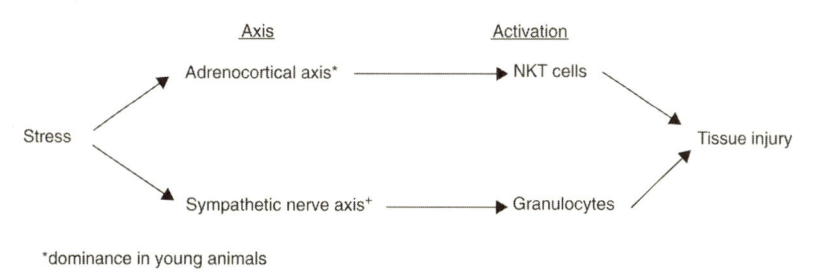

+dominance in old animals

（仮説）ストレスを組織損傷と繋ぐ二本の軸(1)NKT細胞活性化を伴う『副腎皮質軸』および(2)顆粒球活性化を伴う『交感神経軸』

これらの結果が示すのは、最初、NKT細胞数が増加するが、ストレスが長期化した結果、機能が不活化したことである。

そこで、ストレスの刺激を受けたNKT細胞が、肝臓傷害に関連した可能性を検証した（Fig. 4）。ストレスの前後にマウスにおける血清中トランスアミナーゼ（ASTおよびALT）値を検証した。ASTおよびALTの最高値が、ストレス後の若齢マウスで常に出現した。換言すると、特に若齢マウスでNKT細胞数の上昇と肝臓障害の程度には関連性があるようであった（Fig. 2）。

NKT細胞と顆粒球の活性化の根元的メカニズム

ストレスを受けると交感神経緊張とステロイドホルモン分泌が誘導されることはよく知られている[2,3]。本実験では、拘束ストレスの前後のマウスを用いて血清中カテコラミン値（アドレナリン、ノルアドレナリンとドーパミン）とコルチコステロン値を測定した（Fig. 5）。やはり、拘束ストレス後にカテコラミンとコルチコステロン値の顕著な上昇が観察された。カテコラミンの場合、老齢マウスにおいて、特にノルアドレナリンとドーパミンの高値が見られる傾向にあった。対照的に、若齢マウスでも老齢マウスでもコルチコステロン値の上昇は緩やかであった。しかしながら、老齢マウスに比べ若齢マウスにおいてコルチコステロンのベースラインは高値であった。

アドレナリン投与では顆粒球が、一方、ステロイドホルモン投与ではNKT細胞が誘導される

このように、本実験が示唆するのは、ストレスを受けた後、カテコラミンと顆粒球出現の関連およびコルチコステロンとNKT細胞出現誘導との関連についてである。この仮説を、マウスに薬剤を投与して確認した（Fig. 6）。若齢マウス(12週齢)にアドレナリン(100μg/匹)またはヒドロコルチゾン(コルチゾール)(10mg/匹)を若齢マウス(12週齢)に腹腔内投与し、24時間後に細胞のフェノタイプを解析した。アドレナリン投与は、NKT細胞の比率にほとんど影響を及ぼさなかった（Fig. 6a）。胸腺ではDP $CD4^+8^+$細胞が緩やかな減少(88.3→61.6%)を示したのみで、著明な胸腺萎縮は見られなかった。興味深いことに、特に肝臓において、顆粒球($Mac-1^+$ $Gr-1^+$)の比率が顕著に増加した(8.6→36.3% 矢印で示す)。ヒドロコルチゾン（コルチゾール）投与により、肝臓においてNKT細胞の比率が顕著

に増加した (Fig. 6b)。CD3^{int} NK1.1$^+$ 細胞は、CD4$^+$ であった (矢印で示す)。また、胸腺における DP CD4$^+$8$^+$ 細胞の比率は減少した (84.8 → 20.0%)。興味深いことに、ヒドロコルチゾン (コルチゾール) を投与しても顆粒球の比率は変化を示さなかった。

考察

本研究の結果より、ストレスを受けた後、免疫応答と続いて起こる組織障害の出現には2系統の軸が存在することとが示された (Fig.7)。一つの軸は、ストレスをコルチコステロン (ステロイドホルモン) 分泌および NKT 細胞の活性化とを結ぶ『副腎皮質軸』である。この時、胸腺萎縮が出現するが、これは、胸腺における T 細胞分化が停止したことを示す。もう一つの軸は、ストレスを交感神経刺激 (カテコラミンの分泌) および顆粒球の活性化とを結ぶ『交感神経軸』である。このことから考えられるのは、NKT 細胞が自分のもつ細胞傷害活性により組織障害を誘導する可能性、そして顆粒球の超酸化物産生により組織障害が誘導される可能性である。

第1に、ストレスと関連した免疫応答のこれらの2本の軸には、平時にも相互関係があるようである。しかし、これらの軸がそれぞれ、若齢マウスでも老齢マウスでも、一つの方向に偏ることが明らかになった。若齢マウスに拘束ストレスを与えると、胸腺萎縮と肝臓における NKT 細胞の活性化が顕著になった。老齢マウスに同様のストレスを与えた場合には、特に肝臓において、顆粒球増多が顕著であった。白血球がこのような反応を示していた時、主に若齢マウスにおいては血清コルチコステロン値が上昇した。一方、老齢マウスにおいては血清カテコラミン値が上昇した。換言すると、若齢マウスでも老齢マウスでもストレスを受けた後、肝障害が見られたが、その関連メカニズムは軸の一つの方向に偏るようであった。

最近の研究において、特にステロイドホルモンによって、胸腺における T 細胞分化と肝臓における胸腺外分化 T 細胞分化は相互的に調節されていることを報告した [2,3]。胸腺外経路の活性化の原因には、加齢 [16.18] 以外にもストレス [1.5]、悪性腫瘍 [22,23]、自己免疫疾患 [24.26]、妊娠 [27,28] および慢性 GVH(移植片対宿主) 病 [29,30] がある。本研究では、加齢とストレス二つの因子が存在する場合、顕著な相互反応が出現した (Fig. 1)。NKT 細胞は主として胸腺内の代替経路で産生された後、、肝臓に移動する [8.10]。しかし、肝臓における NKT 細胞は、成人後、胸腺からの供給が継続されないことが判明している [31]。換言すると、NKT 細胞の前駆細胞は新生児期には肝臓に移動し、その後肝臓内で補充が繰り返される。

本研究により「交感神経 - 顆粒球」の軸が加齢とともに顕著になることを明らかになった。交感神経と顆粒球が関連する理由は、顆粒球表面上にアドレナリン受容体が存在するためである [32]。多くのアドレナリン刺激を受けると、多くの場合、最終的に、末梢では顆粒球の機能が活性化し [33,34]、骨髄では顆粒球が増多する [35]。

本研究において、ストレスを受けた後、NKT 細胞の比率の増加が顕著であったが、NK 細胞の比率の増加は肝臓においてさほど顕著ではなかったことが明らかとなった。本研究では、NKT 細胞が NK 様細胞傷害活性を持つため [11,36]、NKT 細胞活性時における NK 様細胞傷害活性を測定した。NK 様細胞傷害活性の顕著な不活化が肝臓では見られたが、脾臓では見られなかった。特に若齢マウスにおいては、この細胞傷害活性は、ストレスによる肝障害と関係ある可能性がある。しかし、ストレ

スが長期化するにつれ、最後にはNKT細胞の細胞傷害活性の抑制が現れた。NKT細胞によるNK様細胞傷害活性は、Fasリガンド/Fas系[21]およびパーフォリン系[37]によるものであることを、以前報告した。α-Gal-Cer(α-galactosilceramide)などの刺激により活性化したNKT細胞が、自己応答による組織傷害を調節できることは広く知られている[34,38,39]。この場合でも、活性化されたNKT細胞の機能は、最終的に消耗する。

一方、顆粒球による肝障害に、超酸化物が関わっている可能性がある。顆粒球が超酸化物を産生する主な細胞であることはよく知られている[40,41]。活性化した顆粒球や好中球は、肝臓、肺など諸器官の組織傷害と密接に関連していることも知られている[42,44]。

最後に、この仮説(ストレス関連の反応には2本の軸が存在する)を検証するため、アドレナリンと糖質コルチコイドを若年マウスに投与した。アドレナリンを投与後、顕著な胸腺萎縮は現れなかったが、顆粒球は多量に出現した。糖質コルチコイド投与後、顕著な胸腺萎縮とNKT細胞の活性化が出現したが、顆粒球出現は最小限だった。これらの結果は、ストレス関連の免疫応答についての我々の仮説を裏打ちするものである。ストレス関連の免疫応答には2本の軸があるという概念は、ストレスを受けて起こる生理反応とそれに続いて起こる組織傷害を適切に理解することにとって大変重要であるようだ。この現象には、年齢による偏向があることも興味深い。

謝辞

本研究は、文部科学省科学研究費補助金によるものである。原稿浄書について渡辺正子氏に感謝する。

Age-related bias in function of natural killer T cells and granulocytes after stress: reciprocal association of steroid hormones and sympathetic nerves

K. SAGIYAMA*†, M. TSUCHIDA*, H. KAWAMURA*, S. WANG*, C. LI*, X. BAI*, T. NAGURA*, S. NOZOE† & T. ABO* *Department of Immunology, Niigata University School of Medicine, Niigata and †Department of Psychosomatic Medicine, Kagoshima University Faculty of Medicine, Kagoshima, Japan

(Accepted for publication 27 October 2003)

SUMMARY

Stress-associated immune responses were compared between young (8 weeks of age) and old (56 weeks) mice. Since stress suppresses the conventional immune system (i.e. T and B cells) but inversely activates the primordial immune system (i.e. extrathymic T cells, NKT cells, and granulocytes), these parameters were analysed after restraint stress for 24 h. The thymus became atrophic as a function of age, and an age-related increase in the number of lymphocytes was seen in the liver. Although the number of lymphocytes in both the thymus and liver decreased as the result of stress, the magnitude was much more prominent in the thymus. To determine stress-resistant lymphocyte subsets, two-colour immunofluorescence tests were conducted in the liver and spleen. NKT cells were found to be such cells in the liver of young mice. On the other hand, an infiltration of granulocytes due to stress was more prominent in the liver of old mice than in young mice. Liver injury as a result of stress was prominent in young mice. This age-related bias in the function of NKT cells and granulocytes seemed to be associated with a difference in the responses of catecholamines (high in old mice) and corticosterone (high in young mice) after stress. Indeed, an injection of adrenaline mainly induced the infiltration of granulocytes while that of cortisol activated NKT cells. The present results suggest the existence of age-related bias in the function of NKT cells and granulocytes after stress and that such bias might be produced by different responses of sympathetic nerves and steroid hormones between young and old mice.

Keywords stress natural killer T cells granulocytes steroid hormones sympathetic nerves

INTRODUCTION

In a series of recent studies [1–5], we have revealed that stress induces the arrest of T-cell differentiation in the thymus, resulting in thymic atrophy. This pathway is termed the mainstream of T-cell differentiation in the thymus, by which conventional high TCR cells (TCR[high] cells)[1] are generated [6,7]. The decreased level of T-cell differentiation in the thymus due to stress then results in immunosuppression in various peripheral immune organs. On the other hand, an alternative intrathymic pathway which produces natural killer T (NKT) cells [8–10] and an extrathymic, hepatic pathway which produces NK1·1 intermediate TCR cells (TCR[int] cells) [11,12] are inversely activated by stress. A similar phenomenon was also seen with ageing (i.e. thymic involution and the activation of extrathymic T cells) [6]. This reciprocal immune response after stress may be extremely important for adaptation of our body under emergency conditions. Abnormal self-cells which are generated by emergencies may be processed by autoreactive T cells with primordial properties (i.e. NKT cells and NK1·1 TCR[int] cells) [13,14] and auto antibody-producing B cells (i.e. B-1 cells) [15].

In light of these findings, we further investigated how the immune system was modulated by stress in young and old mice. This age-related examination is of interest because these different pathways of the immune system vary as a function of age apart from stress [16–18]. Our findings revealed that young and old mice had somewhat different immune responses to restraint stress. Namely, liver injury which was induced by the functional activation of NKT cells after stress was much more predominant in young mice than in old mice. This unique bias in the function of NKT cells seen in young mice seemed to be related to the higher production of steroid hormones after stress. In contrast, old mice rather deviated to sympathetic nerve activation after stress, which resulted mainly in an infiltration of granulocytes into tissues. Therefore, we report two different aspects of the immune system in this study, namely, age-related change of

Correspondence: Dr T. Abo, Department of Immunology, Niigata University School of Medicine, Asahimachi 1, Niigata 951–8510, Japan.
E-mail: immunol2@med.niigata-u.ac.jp

© 2004 Blackwell Publishing Ltd

immune responses after stress and an intimate association of change with the sympathetic nervous system and steroid hormone secretion.

Finally, we propose the existence of two axes of immune responses after stress, including [1] an 'adrenocortical axis' which induces mainly NKT cells and [2] a 'sympathetic nerve axis' which induces granulocytes. These axes connect stress with subsequent tissue injury. In adult animals, these two axes are interwined. However, the 'adrenocortical axis' is dominant in young animals while the 'sympathetic nerve axis' becomes predominant in old animals.

MATERIALS AND METHODS

Mice
C57BL/6 (B6) mice were used at the age of 8, 12 or 56 weeks. All mice were fed under specific pathogen-free conditions in the animal facility of Niigata University (Niigata, Japan).

Restraint stress
Mice were fixed in stainless steel mesh and kept for 24 h in a cage. As shown previously [5], these periods of stress are sufficient to induce granulocytosis in the gastric mucosa and result in gastric ulcers.

Cell preparations
Hepatic mononuclear cells (MNC) were isolated by a previously described method [19]. Briefly, the liver was removed, pressed through 200-gauge stainless steel mesh, and suspended in Eagle's MEM (Nissui Pharmaceutical, Tokyo, Japan) supplemented with 5 mm HEPES and 2% heat-inactivated newborn calf serum. After being washed once with medium, the cells were fractionated by centrifugation in 15 ml of 35% Percoll solution (Amersham Pharmacia Biotech, Piscataway, NJ) for 15 min at 2000 r.p.m. The pellet was resuspended in erythrocyte lysing solution (155 mm NH_4Cl, 10 mm $KHCO_3$, 1 mm EDTA-Na, and 170 mm Tris, pH 7·3).

Thymocytes and splenic MNC were obtained by forcing the thymus and spleen, respectively, through 200-gauge stainless steel mesh. Splenic MNC were also used after treatment with the erythrocyte lysing soulution.

Immunofluorescence tests
FITC-, PE- or biotin-conjugated reagents of mAbs were used and biotin-conjugated reagents were developed with Tricolor-conjugated streptavidin (Caltag Laboratories, San Francisco, CA, USA) [20]. The mAbs used here were anti-CD3 (145–2C11), anti-NK1·1 (PK136), anti-CD4 (RM4-5), anti-CD8α (Lyt-2), anti-macrophage (M1/70), and anti-granulocyte (RB6–8C5) mAbs (BD PharMingen, San Diego, CA, USA). Cells were analysed by FACScan (BD Biosciences, Mountain View, CA, USA). To prevent nonspecific binding of mAbs, CD16/32 (2·4G2; BD PharMingen) was added before staining with labelled mAb. Dead cells were excluded by forward scatter, side scatter, and propidium iodide gating.

Measurement of transaminases
Liver injury was used to estimate the activity of asparate aminotransferase (AST) and alanine aminotransferase (ALT) in sera. The activity in each supernatant was quantified with an STA TEST KIT (Wako Pure Industries, Tokyo, Japan).

Cytotoxic assay
Using YAC-1 targets, NK-like cytotoxicity was examined by specific ^{51}Cr-release assay with an incubation time of 4 h [21]. YAC-1 cells labelled with sodium chromate (^{51}Cr) (Amersham Int., Arlington Heights, IL, USA) were used, and effector cells were identified as hepatic or splenic MNC. Percent cytotoxicity was determined using 10^4 YAC-1 cells at the indicated target-to-effector ratios in triplicate cultures. During a 4-h incubation assay, spontaneous chromium release of targets ranged from 10 to 15%. This release was eliminated by calculation.

Measurement of plasma concentration of catecholamines and corticosterone
Plasma pooled from 4 mice was used to measure the concentration of adrenaline, noradrenaline, dopamine, and corticosterone. The plasma levels of these catecholamines were analysed by the HPLC method. Plasma corticosterone of mice was also detected by radioimmunoassay with minor modifications. In the case of mice, corticosterone is the major steroid hormone.

Administration of adrenaline and hydrocortisone sodium succinate
To investigate the effect of catecholamines, 100 μg (per mouse) of adrenaline (Sigma Chemicals Co., St Louis, MO, USA) was intraperitoneally injected. To investigate the effects of steroid hormones, 10 mg (per mouse) of hydrocortisone sodium succinate (Pharmacia Co., Tokyo, Japan) was intraperitoneally injected. MNC were then examined at 24 h after administration. In earlier experiments [2,5], we decided the maximum responses of these reagents in terms of doses of reagents and evaluation time.

Statistical analysis
Differences among the data were analysed by two-factor anova test.

RESULTS

Age-related change in the number of lymphocytes in various immune organs and resistance to stress of liver lymphocytes
To examine age-dependence of stress in various lymphoid organs, the numbers of lymphocytes were first enumerated in the thymus, liver, and spleen of young and old mice (Fig. 1). Restraint stress was conducted for 24 h. The number of thymocytes showed an age-associated decrease, namely, the number in old mice decreased up to 50% of the number in young mice. On the other hand, the number of liver lymphocytes increased as a function of age while that of splenic lymphocytes remained almost unchanged. Stress-associated decreases in the number of thymocytes was seen in both young and old mice. As a result of restraint stress, a decrease in the number of lymphocytes in the liver and spleen was also seen in both young and old mice but the magnitude of the decrease in these organs was not as prominent as that in the thymus.

Identification of stress-resistant lymphocyte subsets in the liver
To examine the level of stress-resistance among various lymphocyte subsets, two-colour stainings of lymphocytes for various combinations were conducted in the liver and spleen (Fig. 2a). Two-colour staining for CD3 and NK1·1 showed the most

Cytotoxic activity and liver injury

It is known that NKT cells mediate NK-like cytotoxicity when they are activated. In this experiment, such NK-like activity against YAC-1 cells was examined by using lymphocytes in the liver and spleen (Fig. 3). In the liver of both young and old mice, a prominent inactivation of NK-like cytotoxicity was demonstrated after stress. Although the proportion of NK and NKT cells was higher in old mice than that in young mice, the cytotoxicity was inversely high in young mice before stress. These results suggested that NKT cells were initially activated in number but that long-lasting stress finally induced functional inactivation.

The possibility that NKT cells stimulated by stress mediated liver injury was then investigated (Fig. 4). The serum levels of transaminases (AST and ALT) were examined in mice before and after stress. The highest levels of AST and ALT were always seen in young mice after stress. In other words, the activation of NKT cells in number (see Fig. 2) and the level of liver injury seemed to be correlated, especially in young mice.

Mechanisms underlying the activation of NKT cells and granulocytes

It is well established that stress induces the activation of the sympathetic nervous system and the secretion of steroid hormones [2,3]. In this experiment, the serum levels of catecholamines (i.e. adrenaline, noradrenaline and dopamine) and corticosterone were examined in mice before and after restraint stress (Fig. 5). As expected, a prominent elevation in the concentration of catecholamines and corticosterone was observed. In the case of catecholamines, old mice tended to show an elevated level, especially in the levels of noradrenaline and dopamine. In contrast, the increased level of corticosterone was moderate in both young and old mice, although the baseline of corticosterone was higher in young mice than in old mice.

Induction of granulocytes by the administration of adrenaline but induction of NKT cells by the administration of steriod hormone

The experiments thus far described indicated corticosterone to be related to the induction of NKT cells while catecholamines seemed to be related to the induction of granulocytes after stress. This hypothesis was confirmed by *in vivo* injections (Fig. 6). Adrenaline (100 µg/mouse) or hydrocortisone (10 mg/mouse) was intraperitoneally injected into adult mice (12 weeks of age) and the phenotype of cells was examined 24 h after the injection. When adrenaline was injected, the proportion of NKT cells remained almost unchanged (Fig. 6a). Thymic atrophy was not prominent, namely, there was only a moderate decrease of DP CD4$^+$8$^+$ cells in the thymus (88·3 to 61·6%). Interestingly, the proportion of granulocytes (Mac-1$^+$Gr-1$^+$) increased prominently, especially in the liver (8·6 to 36·3%, indicated by an arrowhead).

When hydrocortisone was injected, the proportion of NKT cells increased prominently in the liver (Fig. 6b). CD3^{int}NK1·1$^+$ cells belonged to the CD4$^+$ subset (indicated by arrowheads, respectively). At this time, the proportion of DP CD4$^+$8$^+$ cells decreased (84·8 to 20·0%) in the thymus. Interestingly, the proportion of granulocytes remained unchanged by this injection.

DISCUSSION

Findings of the present study indicate the existence of two axes which induce immune responses and subsequent tissue damage

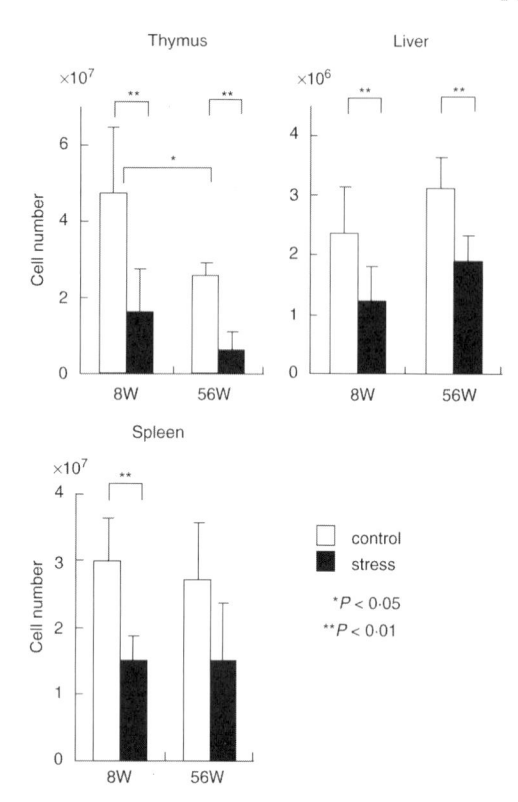

Fig. 1. Age-related and stress-associated changes in the number of MNC yielded by the thymus, liver and spleen. Young mice at the age of 8 weeks and old mice at the age of 56 weeks were used. Restraint stress was conducted for 24 h. The number of MNC was enumerated in 4 mice and the mean and one SD were produced.

stress-resistant lymphocyte subset to be CD3^{int}NK1·1$^+$ cells (i.e. NKT cells) in the liver. The majority of these cells were CD4$^+$ NKT cells as estimated by the staining of CD4 and NK1·1. In the spleen, the change was minimal in all tested subsets.

It is known that thymic atrophy is always accompanied by a decrease in the proportion of double-positive (DP) CD4$^+$8$^+$ cells [2]. Reflecting this situation, the proportion of DP cells decreased significantly as shown by the staining of CD4 and CD8 (i.e. 85·6 to 42·7% in young mice and 74·6 to 38·3% in old mice).

In a final portion of these experiments, two-colour staining for Mac-1 and Gr-1 was conducted to identify granulocytes (Gr-1$^+$Mac-1$^+$) and macrophages (Gr-1$^-$Mac-1$^+$). The proportion of granulocytes was also found to increase in the liver as the result of restraint stress. This response was prominent in old mice.

All these experiments were repeated ($n = 4$) and the mean and one SD in the populations of lymphocytes subsets and granulocytes were determined (Fig. 2b). The change of NK cells was minimal, but that of NKT cells and granulocytes was statistically significant ($P < 0.05$ or < 0.01). The increase in the proportion of NKT cells was prominent in young mice, whereas that of granulocytes was prominent in old mice.

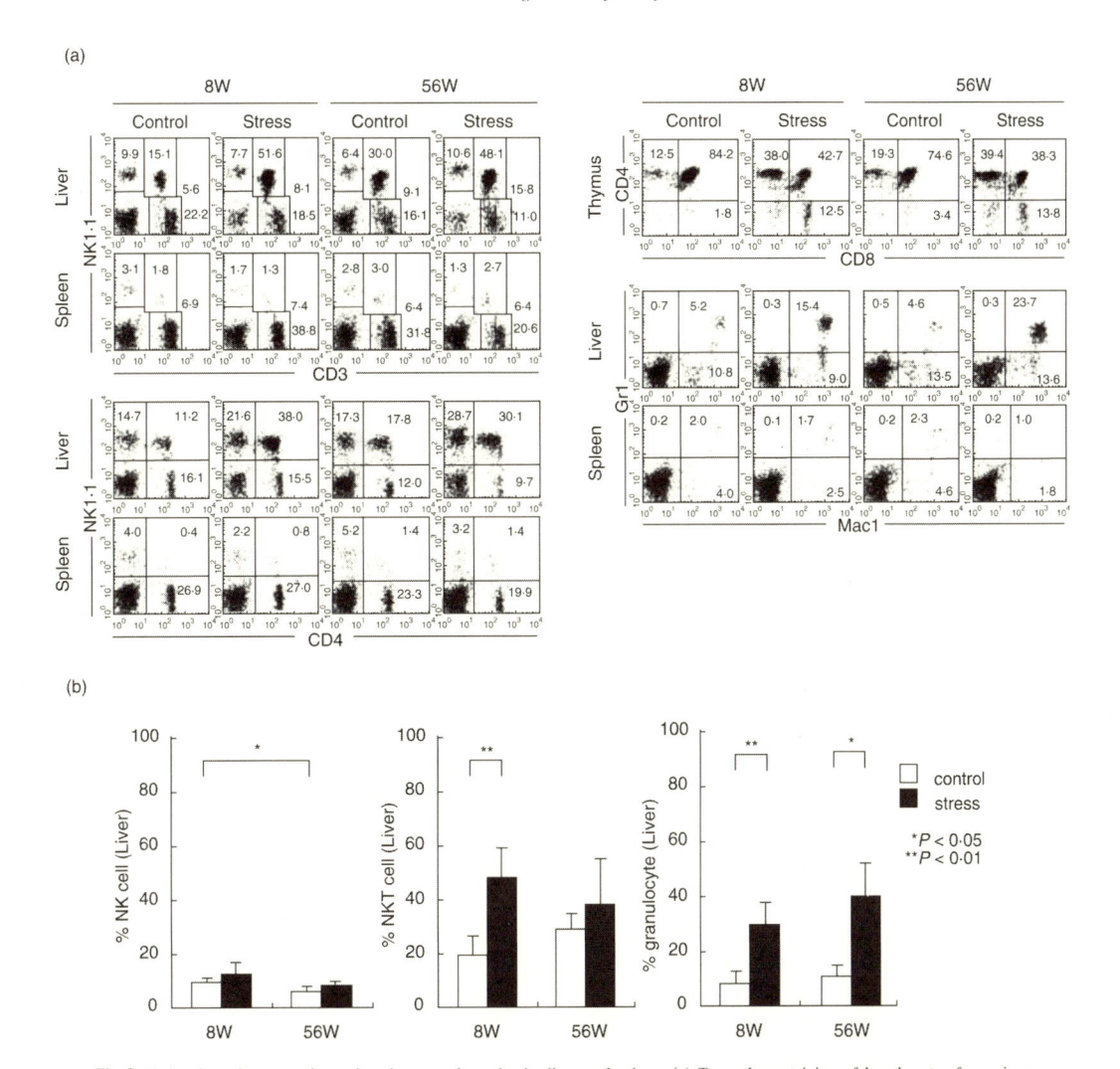

Fig. 2. Estimation of stress-resistant lymphocyte subsets in the liver and spleen. (a) Two-colour staining of lymphocytes for various combinations. (b) Increase in the proportion of NKT cells in young mice and of granulocytes in old mice. MNC were obtained before and after stress in young and old mice and the phenotype of cells was identified by immunofluorescence tests. Numbers in the figure indicate the percentages of fluorescence-positive cells in corresponding areas. The mean and one SD in the proportion of NK cells, NKT cells and granulocytes were produced by repeated experiments ($n = 4$).

after stress (Fig. 7). One axis was the 'adrenocortical axis' which connected stress with the secretion of corticosterone (i.e. steroid homones) and the activation of NKT cells. At such time, thymic atrophy, which suggested an arrest of the mainstream of T-cell differentiation in the thymus, occurred. Another axis was the 'sympathetic nerve axis' which connected stress with sympathetic nerve stimulation (i.e. the secretion of catecholamines) and the activation of granulocytes. It is conceivable that NKT cells may induce tissue damage *in vivo* by their cytotoxicity while granulocytes may induce tissue damage through the production of superoxides.

Primarily, these two axes of stress-associated immune responses seemed to be intertwined under usual conditions. However, these axes were found to be biased in one direction in young and old mice, respectively. When young mice were exposed to restraint stress, thymic atrophy and the activation of NKT cells in the liver became prominent. When old mice were exposed to the same stress, granulocytosis became prominent, especially in the liver. In parallel with these responses seen in leucocytes, the elevation in the serum level of corticosterone was mainly seen in young mice while the elevation in the serum level of catecholamines was mainly seen in old mice. In other words,

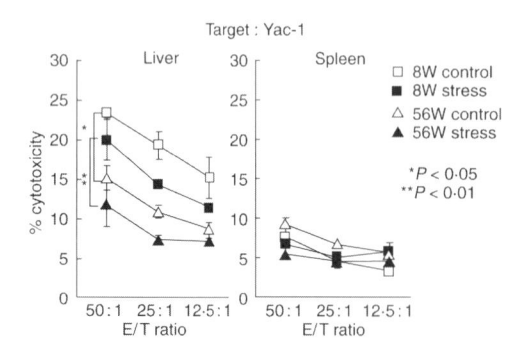

Fig. 3. NK-like cytotoxicity before and after stress in young and old mice. Lymphocytes were isolated from the liver and spleen, and NK-like cytotoxicity against YAC-1 cells was determined by 4 h-incubation at the indicated E/T ratios. The mean and one SD were produced in triplicate cultures.

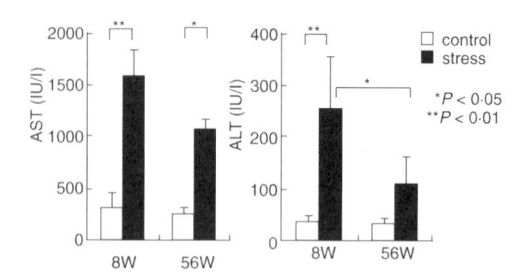

Fig. 4. A comparison of the magnitude of liver injury between young and old mice after stress. To determine the magnitude of liver injury, serum levels of AST and ALT were measured. The mean and one SD were produced from 4 mice.

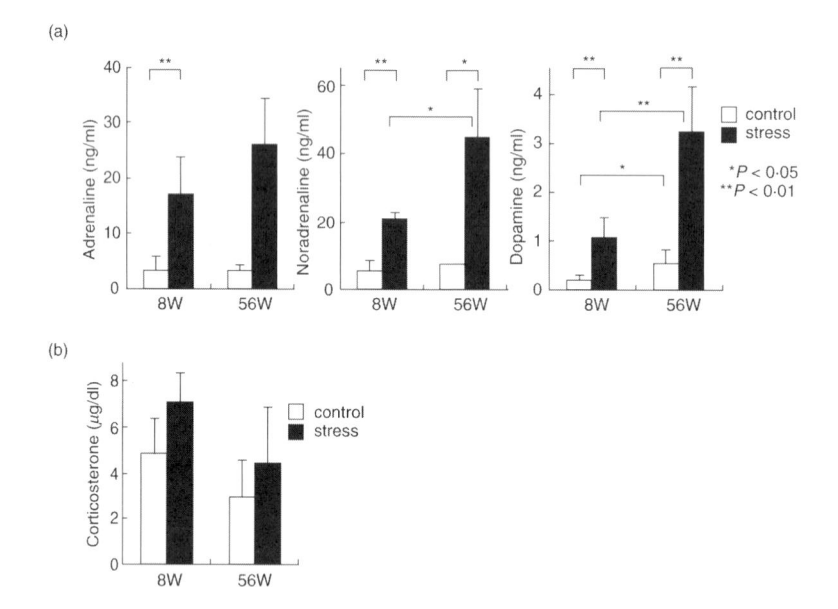

Fig. 5. Comparisons of serum levels of catecholamines and corticosterone between young and old mice after stress. Sera were obtained from 4 mice at each column to produce the mean and one SD.

although both young and old mice showed liver injury after stress, the associated mechanisms appeared to deviate toward one direction of the axes.

In recent studies [2,3], we have reported that the mainstream of T-cell differentiation in the thymus and the extrathymic pathway of T-cell differentiation in the liver are reciprocally regulated, especially by steroid hormones. In addition to ageing [16–18], an activation of the extrathymic pathway is induced by stress [1–5], malignancy [22,23], autoimmune diseases [24–26], pregnancy [27,28], and chronic GVH disease [29,30]. When ageing and stress were both present, a reciprocal response was prominently seen in the present study (see Fig. 1). NKT cells are primarily generated by an alternative intrathymic pathway and then home to the liver [8–10]. However, it has been found that the population of NKT cells in the liver is maintained without a continuous supply from the thymus during adult life [31]. In other words, their precursors home to the liver at the neonatal stage and are renewed *in situ* thereafter.

The present results also revealed that the axis of sympathetic nerves and granulocytes became prominent as a function of age. The connection between sympathetic nerves and granulocytes is due to the presence of surface adrenergic receptors on

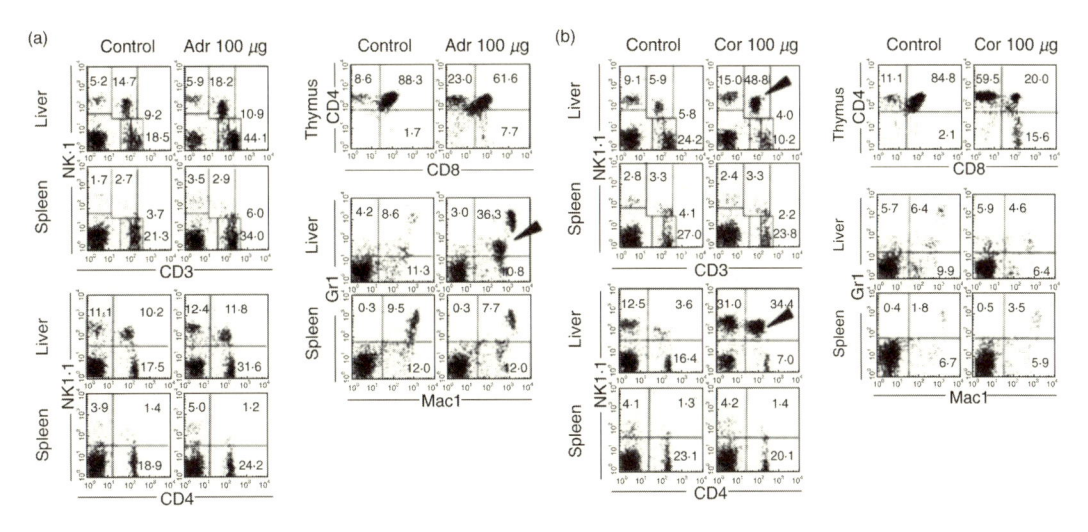

Fig. 6. *In vivo* injection of adult mice (12 weeks of age) with (a) adrenaline (Adr) or (b) hydrocrotisone (Cor). MNC were isolated from the liver, spleen and thymus before and after each injection (24 h). Two-colour stainings for the indicated combinations were conducted. Representative results of three experiments are depicted.

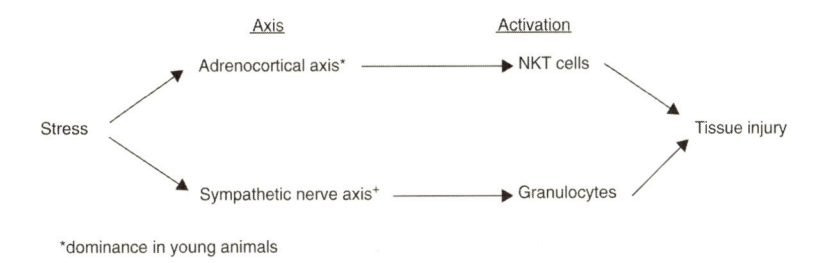

Fig. 7. Hypothesis on two axes which connect stress with tissue injury, including (1) the adrenocortical axis with the activation of NKT cells and (2) the sympathetic nerve axis with the activation of granulocytes.

granulocytes [32]. Many adrenergic stimulations eventually activate the function of granulocytes in the periphery [33,34] and the number of granulocytes in the bone marrow [35].

In the present study, it was found that the increase in the proportion of NKT cells was prominent or that the increase in the proportion of NK cells was not so prominent in the liver after stress. Since NKT cells mediate NK-like cytotoxicity when they are activated [11,36], the level of such cytoxicity was examined in this study. A prominent inactivation of NK-like cytotoxicity was demonstrated in the liver, but not in the spleen. This cytotoxicity might be associated with liver injury after stress, especially in young mice. However, long-lasting stress finally suppressed the cytotoxicity of NKT cells. We previously reported that NK-like cytotoxicity by NKT cells is mediated through both the Fas ligand/Fas system [21] and the perforin system [37]. It is well established that NKT cells activated by α-galactosilceramide and other stimuli can mediate tissue damage due to their autoreactivity [34,38,39]. Even in these cases, the function of activated NKT cells are finally exhausted *in vivo*.

On the other hand, liver injury induced by granulocytes might be mediated by superoxides. It is well established that granulocytes are the main source of cells for superoxide production [40,41]. It is also known that activated granulocytes or neutrophils are intimately related to tissue damage, including that of the liver, lung and other organs [42–44].

Finally, to confirm our hypothesis (i.e. the existence of two axes of stress-associated responses), we conducted *in vivo* injections of adult mice with adrenaline and glucocorticoid. By the injection of adrenaline, thymic atrophy was not so prominent, but the induction of granulocytes was. By the injection of glucocorticoid, thymic atrophy and the activation of NKT cells were prominent, but the induction of granulocytes was minimal. These results support our speculation about stress-associated immune responses. The concept of two axes of stress-associated immune responses seems to be extremely important for properly understanding the physiological responses after stress and subsequent tissue injury. Age-associated bias in this phenomenon is also interesting.

ACKNOWLEDGEMENTS

This work was supported by a Grant-in-Aid for Scientific Research from the Ministry of Education, Science and Culture, Japan. We wish to thank Mrs Masako Watanabe for preparation of the manuscript.

REFERENCES

1 Kawamura T, Toyabe S, Moroda T et al. Neonatal granulocytosis is a postpartum event which is seen in the liver as well as in the blood. Hepatology 1997; **26**:1567–72.
2 Maruyama S, Tsukahara A, Suzuki S, Tada T, Minagawa M, Watanabe H, Hatakeyama K, Abo T. Quick recovery in the generation of self-reactive CD4^{low} natural killer (NK) T cells by an alternative intrathymic pathway when restored from acute thymic atrophy. Clin Exp Immunol 1999; **117**:587–95.
3 Shimizu T, Kawamura T, Miyaji C et al. Resistance of extrathymic T cells to stress and a role of endogenous glucocorticoids in stress-associated immunosuppression. Scand J Immunol 2000; **51**:285–92.
4 Oya H, Kawamura T, Shimizu T et al. The differential effect of stress on natural killer T (NKT) and NK cell function. Clin Exp Immunol 2000; **121**:384–90.
5 Kawamura T, Miyaji C, Toyabe S, Fukuda M, Watanabe H, Abo T. Suppressive effect of anti-ulcer agents on granulocytes – A role for granulocytes in gastric ulcer formation. Dig Dis Sci 2000; **45**:1786–91.
6 Abo T, Kawamura T, Watanabe H. Physiological responses of extrathymic T cells in the liver. Immunol Rev 2000; **174**:135–49.
7 Abo T. Extrathymic pathways of T-cell differentiation and immunomodulation. Int Immunopharmacol 2001; **1**:1261–73.
8 Hammond K, Cain W, van Driel I, Godfrey D. Three day neonatal thymectomy selectively depletes NK1.1$^+$ T cells. Int Immunol 1998; **10**:1491–9.
9 Tilloy F, Di Santo JP, Bendelac A, Lantz O. Thymic dependence of invariant Vα14+ natural killer-T cell development. Eur J Immunol 1999; **29**:3313–8.
10 Coles MC, Raulet DH. NK1.1+ T cells in the liver arise in the thymus and are selected by interactions with class I molecules on CD4+CD8+ cells. J Immunol 2000; **164**:2412–8.
11 Halder RC, Kawamura T, Bannai M, Watanabe H, Kawamura H, Mannoor MDK, Morshed SRM, Abo T. Intensive generation of NK1.1- extrathymic T cells in the liver by injection of bone marrow cells isolated from mice with a mutation of polymorphic major histocompatibility complex antigens. Immunology 2001; **102**:450–9.
12 Miyakawa R, Miyaji C, Watanabe H, Yokoyama H, Tsukada C, Asakura H, Abo T. Unconventional NK1.1- intermediate TCR cells as major T lymphocytes expanding in chronic graft-versus-host disease. Eur J Immunol 2002; **32**:2521–31.
13 Kawachi Y, Watanabe H, Moroda T, Haga M, Iiai T, Hatakeyama K, Abo T. Self-reactive T cell clones in a restricted population of interleukin-2 receptor β$^+$ cells expressing intermediate levels of the T cell receptor in the liver and other immune organs. Eur J Immunol 1995; **25**:2272–8.
14 Naito T, Kawamura T, Bannai M et al. Simultaneous activation of natural killer T cells and autoantibody production in mice injected with denatured syngeneic liver tissue. Clin Exp Immunol 2002; **129**:397–404.
15 Morshed SR, Mannoor K, Halder RC, Kawamura H, Bannai M, Sekikawa H, Watanabe H, Abo T. Tissue-specific expansion of NKT and CD5+B cells at the onset of autoimmune diseases in (NZB–NZW) F1 mice. Eur J Immunol 2002; **32**:2551–61.
16 Iiai T, Watanabe H, Seki S et al. Ontogeny and development of extrathymic T cells in mouse liver. Immunology 1992; **77**:556–63.
17 Tsukahara A, Seki S, Iiai T et al. Mouse liver T cells. Their change with aging and in comparison with peripheral T cells. Hepatology 1997; **26**:301–9.
18 Miyaji C, Watanabe H, Minagawa M et al. Numerical and functional characteristics of lymphocyte subsets in centenarians. J Clin Immunol 1997; **17**:420–9.
19 Watanabe H, Miyaji C, Kawachi Y, Iiai T, Ohtsuka K, Iwanaga T, Takahashi-Iwanaga H, Abo T. Relationships between intermediate TCR cells and NK1.1$^+$T cells in various immune organs. NK1.1$^+$T cells are present within a population of intermediate TCR cells. J Immunol 1995; **155**:2972–83.
20 Watanabe H, Miyaji C, Seki S, Abo T. c-kit$^+$ stem cells and thymocyte precursors in the livers of adult mice. J Exp Med 1996; **184**:687–93.
21 Moroda T, Iiai T, Suzuki S et al. Autologous killing by a population of intermediate T cell receptor cells and its NK1.1$^+$ and NK1.1$^-$ subsets, using Fas ligand/Fas molecules. Immunology 1997; **91**:219–26.
22 Kawamura T, Kawachi Y, Moroda T et al. Cytotoxic activity against tumour cells mediated by intermediate TCR cells in the liver and spleen. Immunology 1996; **89**:68–75.
23 Kawamura T, Seki S, Takeda K, Narita J, Ebe Y, Naito M, Hiraide H, Abo T. Protective effect of NK1.1$^+$ T cells as well as NK cells against intraperitoneal tumors in mice. Cell Immunol 1999; **193**:219–25.
24 Yamagiwa S, Kuwano Y, Hasegawa K et al. Existence of a small population of IL-2Rβ^{hi} TCR^{int} cells in SCG and MRL-*lpr/lpr* mice which produce normal Fas mRNA and Fas molecules from the *lpr* gene. Eur J Immunol 1996; **26**:1409–16.
25 Arai K, Yamamura S, Hanyu T, Takahashi HE, Umezu H, Watanabe H, Abo T. Extrathymic differentiation of resident T cells in the joints of mice with collagen-induced arthritis. J Immunol 1996; **157**:5170–7.
26 Moroda T, Iiai T, Kawachi Y, Kawamura T, Hatakeyama K, Abo T. Restricted appearance of self-reactive clones into T cell receptor intermediate cells in neonatally thymectomized mice with autoimmune disease. Eur J Immunol 1996; **26**:3084–91.
27 Kimura M, Watanabe H, Sato S, Abo T. Female predominance of extrathymic T cells in mice: Statistical analysis. Immunol Lett 1994; **39**:259–67.
28 Minagawa M, Narita J, Tada T, Maruyama S, Shimizu T, Bannai M, Oya H, Hatakeyama K, Abo T. Mechanisms underlying immunologic states during pregnancy. possible association of the sympathetic nervous system. Cell Immunol 1999; **196**:1–13.
29 Watanabe T, Kawamura T, Kawamura H, Haga M, Shirai K, Watanabe H, Eguchi S, Abo T. Intermediate TCR cells in mouse lung. Their effector function to induce pneumonitis in mice with autoimmune-like graft-versus-host disease. J Immunol 1997; **158**:5805–14.
30 Weerasinghe A, Kawamura T, Moroda T, Seki S, Watanabe H, Abo T. Intermediate TCR cells can induce graft-versus-host disease after allogeneic bone marrow transplantation. Cell Immunol 1998; **185**:14–29.
31 Kameyama H, Kawamura T, Naito T, Bannai M, Shimamura K, Hatakeyama K, Abo T. Size of the population of CD4+ natural killer T cells in the liver is maintained without supply by the thymus during adult life. Immunology 2001; **104**:135–41.
32 Suzuki SS, Toyabe T, Moroda T et al. Abo. Circadian rhythm of leukocytes and lymphocytes subsets and its possible correlation with the function of autonomic nervous system. Clin Exp Immunol 1997; **110**:500–8.
33 Maruyama S, Minagawa M, Shimizu T et al. Administration of glucocorticoids markedly increases the numbers of granulocytes and extrathymic T cells in the bone marrow. Cell Immunol 1999; **194**:28–35.
34 Minagawa M, Oya H, Yamamoto S, Shimizu T, Bannai M, Kawamura H, Hatakeyama K, Abo T. Intensive expansion of natural killer T cells in the early phase of hepatocyte regeneration after partial hepatectomy in mice and its association with sympathetic nerve activation. Hepatology 2000; **31**:907–15.
35 Yamamura S, Arai K, Toyabe S, Takahashi HE, Abo T. Simultaneous activation of granulocytes and extrathymic T cells in number and

function by excessive administration of nonsteroidal anti-inflammatory drugs. Cell Immunol 1996; **173**:303–11.
36 Weerasinghe A, Sekikawa H, Watanabe H *et al.* Association of intermediate T cell receptor cells, mainly their NK1.1- subset, with protection from malaria. Cell Immunol 2001; **207**:28–35.
37 Bannai MH, Oya T, Kawamura T *et al.* Disparate effect of beige mutation on cytotoxic function between natural killer and natural killer T cells. Immunology 2000; **100**:165–9.
38 Eberl G, MacDonald HR. Rapid death and regeneration of NKT cells in anti-CD3e- or IL-12-treated mice: a major role for bone marrow in NKT cell homeostasis. Immunity 1998; **9**:345–53.
39 Osman Y, Kawamura T, Naito T, Takeda K, van Kaer L, Okumura K, Abo T. Activation of hepatic NKT cells and subsequent liver injury following administration of a-galactosylceramide. Eur J Immunol 2000; **30**:1919–28.
40 Suzuki M, Miura S, Mori M, Kai A, Suzuki H, Fukumura D, Suematsu M, Tsuchiya M. Rebamipide, a novel antiulcer agent, attenuates Helicobacter pylori induced gastric mucosal cell injury associated with neutrophil derived oxidants. Gut 1994; **35**:1375–8.
41 Takeda Y, Watanabe H, Yonehara S, Yamashita T, Saito S, Sendo F. Rapid acceleration of neutrophil apoptosis by tumor necrosis factor-α. Int Immunol 1993; **5**:691–4.
42 Brown AP, Schultze AE, Holdan WL, Buchueitz JP, Rot RA, Ganey PE. Lipopolysaccharide-induced hepatic injury is enhanced by polychlorinated biphenyls. Environ Health Perspect 1996; **104**:634–40.
43 Partrick DA, Moore FA, Moore EE Jr, Barnett CC, Silliman CC. Neutrophil priming and activation in the pathogenesis of postinjury multiple organ failure. New Horiz 1996; **4**:194–210.
44 Srinivasan RJP, Buchweitz PE. Ganey. Alteration by flutamide of neutrophil response to stimulation. Implications for tissue injury. Biochem Pharmacol 1997; **53**:1179–85.

No mixing of granulocytes and other lymphocytes in the inflamed joints of parabiosis mice with collagen-induced arthritis: possible in situ generation

コラーゲン誘導性関節炎のマウスとパラビオーゼ（並体結合）した
マウスの関節においてパートナーの顆粒球とリンパ球は混在しない：
顆粒球およびリンパ球の局所産生の可能性

Immunology, 114: 133-138, 2005

chapter **17**

No mixing of granulocytes and other lymphocytes in the inflamed joints of parabiosis mice with collagen-induced arthritis: possible in situ generation

コラーゲン誘導性関節炎のマウスとパラビオーゼ（並体結合）した
マウスの関節においてパートナーの顆粒球とリンパ球は混在しない：
顆粒球およびリンパ球の局所産生の可能性

Tetsuro Nishizawa,[1)2)] Toshihiko Kawamura,[1)] Nakao Izumi,[1)] Hiroki Kawamura,[1)] Katsuyuki Fujii,[2)] and Toru Abo[1)]

[1]Department of Immunology, Niigata University School of Medicine, Niigata, Japan, and
[2]Department of Orthopaedic Surgery, Jikei University School of Medicine, Tokyo, Japan

【キーワード】

コラーゲン誘導性関節炎、顆粒球、B細胞、並体結合（パラビオーゼ）

【要約】

リポ多糖体と抗Ⅱ型コラーゲン抗体を投与してコラーゲン誘導性関節炎モデルマウスを作成した。関節炎が発症すると、顆粒球（大型多顆粒性、フェノタイプは、Mac-1$^+$Gr-1$^+$）が、モデルマウスの関節で増大した。関節における主要なリンパ球サブセット（集団）は、疾患の有無にかかわらず、CD3$^-$B220$^+$フェノタイプのリンパ球（B220$^+$ B細胞）であった。関節やその他の器官の中の、この白血球集団の由来を特定するため、CBF$_1$Ly5.1とCBF$_1$Ly5.2マウスを用い、コラーゲン誘導性関節炎を発症したマウスとコラーゲン誘導性関節炎なしのマウスを結合させる（パラビオーゼ）実験を行なった。予想通り、肝臓と脾臓の白血球集団は、自己の細胞とパートナーの細胞（例えばLy5.2$^+$パートナー・マウス体内の〜45％がLy5.1$^+$マウス細胞）の半々が混在していた。しかし、関節炎のマウスの場合でも、関節や骨髄ではこのような自己とパートナーの細胞は長い期間、混在しなかった。これら結果が示唆することは以下のとおりである。関節では循環血液が交換されないために、顆粒球や他のリンパ球は、コラーゲン誘導性関節炎モデルマウスの炎症を起こしている関節で分化したか、もしくは骨髄から供給された可能性である。関節内の顆粒球が、関節滑膜で産生されなくとも増多したことは興味深い。

はじめに

関節リウマチは、なんらかの免疫学的要因が関節炎発症と関係する自己免疫疾患であることが知られている。他の自己免疫疾患と同様に、B-1細胞が産生する自己抗体が、発症と関連することが実証されている[1-3]。複数のエビデンスにより、胸腺外分化T細胞が炎症組織に浸潤することが、関節炎の原因であることも明らかになった[4-6]。これらの免疫学的要因に加えて、最

---

doi:10.1111/j.1365-2567.2004.01995.x
Received 21 October 2003; revised 20 August 2004; accepted 13 September 2004.
Correspondence: Dr T. Abo, Department of Immunology, Niigata University School of Medicine, Niigata 951–8510, Japan.
Email: immunol2@med.niigata-u.ac.jp

Abbreviations: CIA, collagen-induced arthritis; DN, double-negative; IL-2Rβ, interleukin-2 receptor β-chain; MNC, mononuclear cells; TCR^{int}, TCR^{high}, intermediate and high levels of T-cell receptor for antigens.

近の研究で、組織破壊的な顆粒球が、関節炎の悪化と直接関係することが明らかになった[7,8]。

関節リウマチに関するヒトと齧歯類の研究より、これまで多くの研究者が信じてきたのは、自己応答性によりリンパ球活性化が起こり、周囲のリンパ組織から組織を破壊する顆粒球が移動して来て、関節炎が起こるということである。しかし、他の可能性も存在する。すなわち、関節の中の各所には、固有のリンパ球が存在し、関節リウマチが起こると、何らかの自己抗原が、これまで知られていないメカニズムで、関節固有のリンパ球を刺激している可能性がある。

さらに、コラーゲン誘導性関節炎発症時の関節内には、常に、以下の独特のT細胞集団が存在した：インターロイキン2レセプター（IL-2R）$\alpha^-\beta^+$ T細胞、$\gamma\delta$ T細胞、$CD8\alpha^+\beta^-$ 細胞および$CD44^+$ L-セレクチン$^-$細胞である。これら細胞の性質は全て、体内の独特な場所における胸腺外分化T細胞の特性と一致する[9-11]。より正確に言うと、胸腺外分化T細胞が存在するのは、肝臓[12]、腸[13]、子宮[14]および外分泌腺[15]である。関節リウマチ患者やコラーゲン誘導性関節炎モデルマウスの関節における胸腺外分化T細胞の起源を知ることは興味深い。同様に、炎症を起こした関節内の主要な白血球集団である顆粒球の起源も考慮しなければならない。

本研究では、コラーゲン誘導性関節炎モデルマウス[4]を使用して、パラビオーゼの実験を行った[16,17]。$CBF_1Ly5.1$と$CBF_1Ly5.2$マウスとを並体結合（パラビオーゼ）した際、末梢の免疫器官の大多数のリンパ球は、2週以内にパートナーのリンパ球を受け入れた。その結果、受け入れた器官（例、脾臓やリンパ節）では、多くのリンパ球サブセットは、自己の細胞とパートナー細胞との半々の混在となった。全く対照的に、関節内の白血球集団（顆粒球や他のリンパ球）には、パートナーの細胞が見られないことが明らかになった。このことから、コラーゲン誘導性関節炎マウスにおいて、炎症中の関節の中にある白血球集団は、骨髄から供給されたものではなく、関節で分化したものである可能性が高まった。

材料と方法

マウス

（C57BL/6.Ly5.2 x BALB/c）F_1（$CBF_1Ly5.2$）および（C57BL/6.Ly5.1 x BALB/c）F_1（CBF1Ly5.1）8-12週齢雌マウスを使用した。マウスは、新潟大学動物施設内、SPF（特定病原体未感染）下で飼育した。

コラーゲン誘導性関節炎モデルマウス作製

（株）免疫生物研究所（群馬，日本）社製の関節炎抗体キットの添付プロトコルに従い[18]、関節炎モデルマウスを作製した[19]。略述すると、実験初日（day0）に4種の抗コラーゲン・モノクローナル抗体（mAb）（各2mg）の混和剤を腹腔内投与し、続いて3日後にリポ多糖体（LPS）（大腸菌，O111: B4（株）免疫生物研究所，群馬，日本）50μgを腹腔内投与した。マウスにおいて、投与3日後にコラーゲン誘導性関節炎発症が、そして7-10日後に重症期（劇症期）が出現し、その後、緩やかに軽症化した[20]。その後、マウスの関節炎発症を毎日観察し、関節炎を、以下のように臨床評価した: grade 0、腫脹なし; grade 1、単数の肢指腫脹; grade 2、複数の肢指腫脹; grade 3、高度腫脹および強直。四肢すべて臨床評価を行い、一匹あたり12点満点である。

パラビオーゼ

定法に従い、同じ体重の8週齢雌、CBF1Ly5.1マウスとCBF1Ly5.2マウスの並体結合（パラビオーゼ）を行なった[17]。麻酔下、剃毛後、皮膚をエタノール消毒し、耳後部よりマウス側面を一直線に尾部へ皮膚切開し、二

頭のマウスを一緒に縫合した。処置後一週間、ケージ内で飼育し、食餌、飲水を別個に与えた。ストレスにより胸腺萎縮を起こしたパラビオーゼのマウスは実験から排除した。

細胞分離

定法に従い、肝単核球（MNC）を分離した[21]。略述すると、エーテルで麻酔したマウスの腋窩動脈・静脈から脱血し、摘出した肝臓を、剪刀で細切し、ステンレス・スチール・メッシュで漉し、5mMのHEPES（日水製薬（株）、東京、日本）と2%非働化済仔牛血清（JRH Biosciences, Lenexa, KS）を含んだEagle's MEM培養液中に浮遊させた。一度洗浄した後、ペレットを100U/mlヘパリン（ニプロファーマ（株）、大阪、日本）を加えた35%パーコール溶液（Pharmacia Fine Chemicals, Piscataway, NJ）の中に再浮遊させ、15分間400gで比重遠心分離を行なった。単核球と赤血球を含むペレットは赤血球溶血溶液（155mM NH_4Cl, 10mM $KHCO_3$, 1mM EDTA, 170mM Tris-HCl, pH 7.3）の中に再浮遊させた。脾臓MNCは、脾臓を200-ゲージ・ステンレス・スチール・メッシュで漉し、溶血を行い採取したものを使用した。炎症を起こした関節よりMNCをWooleyらの方法に若干、技術的な修正を加えて分離した[22]。関節を足から切断し、皮膚を取り除き、剪刀で裁断したものを200-ゲージ・ステンレススチールメッシュで漉して、培養液に浮遊させた。骨髄細胞を、培養液で大腿骨をフラッシングによる、洗浄後、溶血を行い採取した。

フローサイトメトリー解析

顆粒球とリンパ球同定を側方散乱光（顆粒の存在）と前方散乱光（細胞サイズ）を用いて行なった。つまり、リンパ球のサイズは小型で、顆粒を含まない。フローサイトメトリーを用いリンパ球のフェノタイプを一重、二重、あるいは三重免疫蛍光試験を行い解析した[25]。フローサイトメトリー解析のため、抗CD3［145-2C11: マウス, 免疫グロブリンG1（IgG1）, κ］, 抗NK1: 1（PK136: マウス, IgG2a, κ）, 抗B220（RA3-6B2: ラット, IgG2a, κ）, 抗顆粒球（Gr-1; RB68C5: ラット, IgG2b, κ）, 抗マクロファージ（Mac-1. M1/70.15, ラット, IgG2b）, 抗Ly5.1（A20.1.7: マウス, IgG2a, κ）, および抗Ly5.2（ALI-4A2: マウス, IgG2a, κ）モノクロナール抗体をPharMingen（San Diego, CA）より購入した。顆粒球のサイズは大型で、顆粒を有するので、Gr-1 Mac-1モノクロナール抗体を用い染色した。これらモノクロナール抗体はいずれも、フルオレセイン・イソチオシアネート（FITC）標識とフィコエリトリン（PE）標識およびビオチン標識である。ビオチン標識抗体は、TRIColor標識ストレプトアビジン（Caltag Laboratory,San Francisco, CA）で発色させた。FACS（Becton Dickinson Co., Mountain View, CA）を用い細胞の解析を行なった。モノクロナール抗体の非特異的結合を防ぐために、CD32/16（2.4G2）にて前処理を行なった後、各種抗体を加えた。死細胞は、前方散乱光または側方散乱光により除外した。

結果

コラーゲン誘導性関節炎モデルマウス作製

本実験では、LPSと抗コラーゲン抗体を混和したものを、コラーゲン誘導性関節炎モデルマウス作製のため投与した（Fig. 1a）。LPSのみでは、関節炎は誘発されなかった。しかし、両剤を混和したものでは、重度の関節炎が出現し、炎症は最長1ヵ月間続いた。関節炎の劇症期（day 7）において、白血球を骨髄と関節より分離し、そして、フェノタイプ特徴を分析した（Fig. 1b）。散乱光解析では、大型で多顆粒性の細胞が骨髄と関節に豊富に存在することが

chapter 17　351

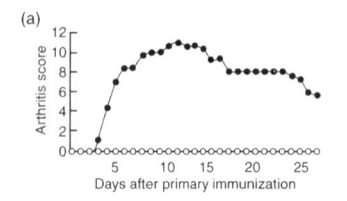

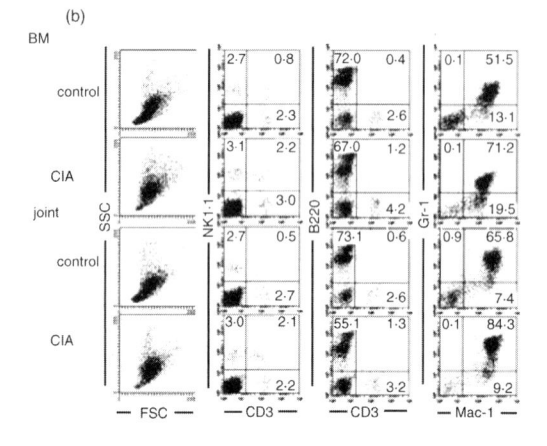

Figure.1

(a) CBF₁マウスの関節炎スコアの経時的変化。(b) コラーゲン誘導性関節炎モデルマウス骨髄と関節における白血球フェノタイプの特徴：LPS単剤を投与（○）またはLPSと抗II型コラーゲンの混和剤（●）を投与。白血球投与1週間後に分離し、図示の組み合わせで二重染色を行なった。各分画内の数値は蛍光陽性細胞の比率を示す。

Figure.2

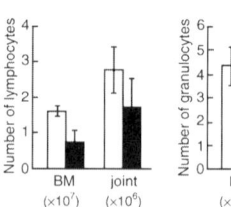

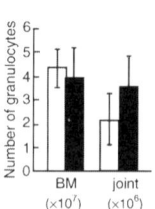

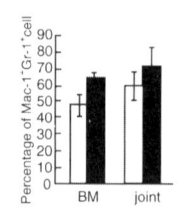

正常マウス（□）とコラーゲン誘導性関節炎（CIA）マウス（■）におけるリンパ球数と顆粒球数および骨髄と関節内の顆粒球比率の比較（各群ともn=4）。投与1週間後に、白血球を分離し、図示の組み合わせで二重染色を行なった。投与7日後に、CIAマウスから白血球を分離した。ノーマルマウス（□）とコラーゲン誘導性関節炎（CIA）の比較には、対応のないスチューデントのt検定を用いた。平均値±SEM *$P<0.05$。

示された。リンパ球のゲーティング解析を用いて行った後、CD3とNK1.1およびCD3とB220の二重染色を行なった。対照群マウスの骨髄や関節にあるリンパ球のほとんどは、B220⁺ B細胞であり、関節炎の発症後、若干減少した。一方、CD3⁺ T細胞の比率が、関節炎に関係なく少ないものの、NK1.1抗原の有無にかかわらず上昇した。大きく光散乱する貪食細胞にゲーティングを用いたところ、主要な集団は、顆粒球（Mac-1⁺ Gr-1⁺）であること；顆粒球の割合が、関節炎の発症後、増加したことが明らかになった。複数回実験を行ったデータより、リンパ球と顆粒球の数を算出した（Fig. 2）。ところが、リンパ球の数は、骨髄も関節も発症後、減少した。特に関節において減少した割合の変化を示す（Fig. 2）。これらの結果を総合的に考察すると、炎症を起こしている関節において、主要な白血球の集団は、顆粒球であったことが明らかになった。

正常マウス同士の並体結合（パラビオーゼ）

独特な性質を持つ胸腺外分化T細胞が関節炎のマウスの関節に存在したこと、そして、関節の胸腺外分化T細胞は、他の器官（肝臓や腸など）のものとは異なったことをこれまでの研究で報告した。従って、関節の白血球の中には、関節で分化するものもあると推察し、関節の顆粒球にその可能性があるか検証した（Fig. 3）。本実験では、CBF₁Ly5.1マウスとCBF₁Ly5.2マウスとのパラビオーゼを行い、Gr-1、Mac-1およびLy5.1の三重染色をパラビオーゼ2週後と4週後に行なった（Fig. 3a）。肝臓、脾臓、骨髄と関節のすべての白血球を分析したところ、CBF₁Ly5.2マウスの肝臓と脾臓の白血球中には、2週後でも4週後でも少なからぬ割合で

Figure.3

パートナーの細胞（Ly5.1$^+$）の存在することが明らかになった。肝臓と脾臓における顆粒球（Mac-1$^+$ Gr-1$^+$）にもこの傾向があった。

全く対照的に、Ly5.2マウスの骨髄と関節において、パートナー細胞（Ly5.1$^+$）が存在する割合は、顆粒球でもリンパ球でも著しく少なかった。これらの経時的変化を示す（Fig. 3(b)）。これらの結果が示すのは、肝臓と脾臓では、他の白血球（例、B220$^+$ B細胞）と同じく顆粒球の半数は他所から移動してくることである。ところが、骨髄と関節では、すべての顆粒球と他の白血球は、もともと骨髄と関節で分化したものだった。つまり、骨髄と関節では、他の器官で分化した白血球の混在が見られなかったのである。

パートナーの顆粒球は、炎症の部位へさえ流入しない

CBF$_1$Ly5.1マウスとCBF$_1$Ly5.2マウスのパラビオーゼを行い、LPSと抗コラーゲン抗体の混合物をそれぞれのパートナー投与した（Fig. 4）。各々のパートナーは、投与3-4日後に関節炎発症が見られた（Fig. 4a）。7日後に、白血球をそれぞれのパートナーの骨髄と関節から分離した（Fig. 4b）。CBF1Ly5.1パートナーでもCBF1Ly5.2パートナーでも、散乱光の大きな白血球数が増加したが、最大の増加を示したのは顆粒球（Mac-1$^+$ Gr-1$^+$）であった。

7日目にCBF$_1$Ly5.2パートナーより白血球を分離して、Mac-1、Gr-1とLy5.1の三重染色を行なった（Fig. 5）。Ly5.1$^+$パートナー細胞は、肝臓と脾臓のすべての顆粒球（Mac-1$^+$Gr-1$^+$）だけでなくすべての白血球の分画に見られた。一方、Ly5.1$^+$パートナー細胞は、骨髄と関節の白血球分画でも顆粒球の分画でも見つからなかった。

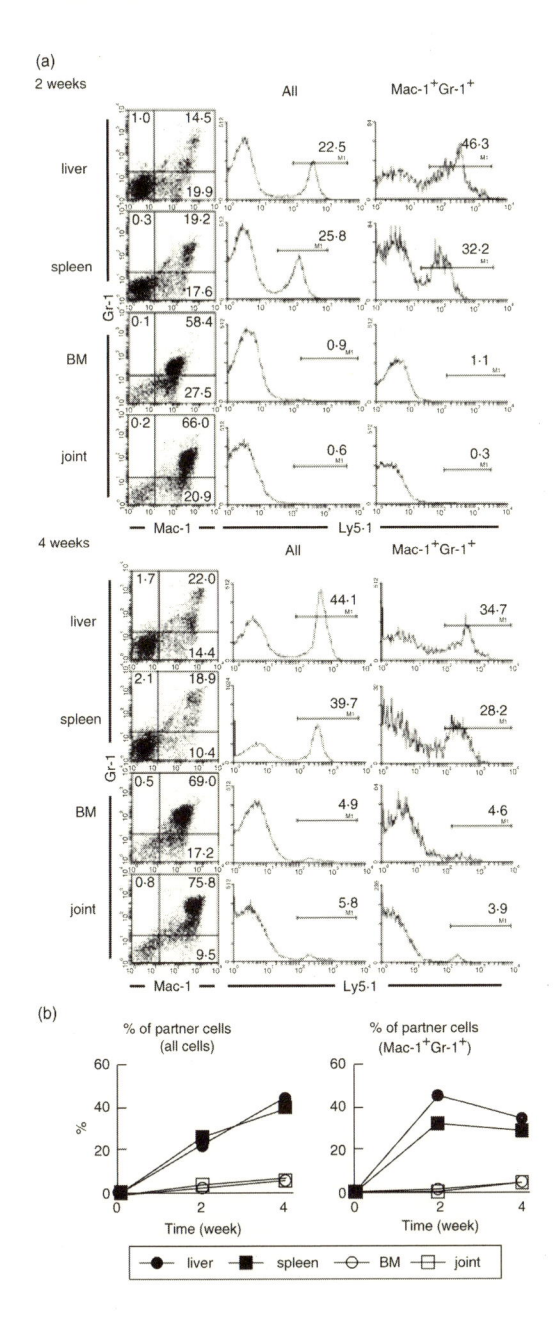

正常マウスの並体結合。(a) Mac-1, Gr-1 およびLy5.1の三重染色、(b) Ly5.1$^+$パートナー細胞の混在割合。CBF1Ly5.1とCBF1Ly5.2マウスの並体結合を行った。Ly5.1$^+$パートナー細胞の並体結合の2週後および4週後に、肝臓（●）、脾臓（■）、骨髄（○）および関節（□）より白血球を分離した。そして、三重染色を行なった。ゲーティングを行い、Ly5.1$^+$パートナー細胞の混在割合は、白血球総数と顆粒球（Mac-1$^+$ Gr-1$^+$）分画より算出した。

Figure.4

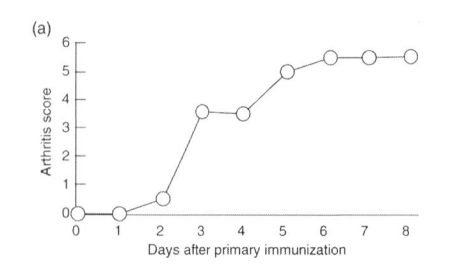

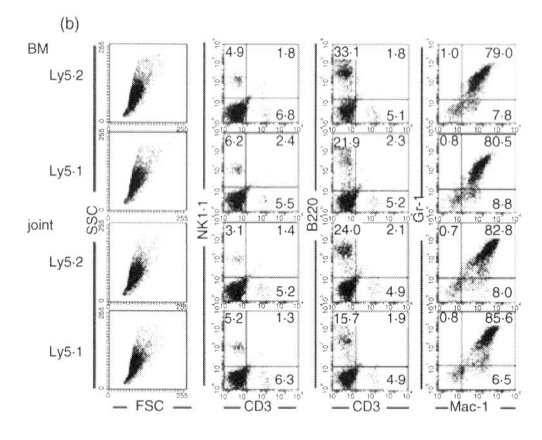

(a) Arthritis score / Days after primary immunization

(b) BM Ly5.2 / Ly5.1, joint Ly5.2 / Ly5.1
SSC—FSC, CD3—NK1.1, CD3—B220, Mac-1—Gr-1

コラーゲン誘導性関節炎（CIA）マウスの並体結合。(a) CBF1Ly5.2マウスの関節炎スコアの経時的変化。(b) コラーゲン誘導性関節炎モデルマウス（CIA）(day7）における骨髄と関節の白血球のフェノタイプの特徴。(b) の各分画内の数値は蛍光陽性細胞の比率を示す。

Figure.5

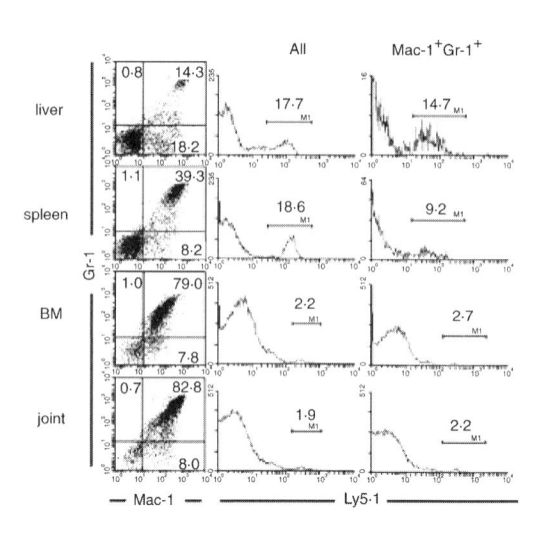

All / Mac-1⁺Gr-1⁺
liver, spleen, BM, joint
Mac-1 — Ly5.1

Ly5.1⁺パートナー細胞の流入を、並体結合の実験を行い示す。Mac-1、Gr-1およびLy5.1の三重染色を行なった。各分画内の数値は蛍光陽性細胞の比率を示す。ゲーティングを行い、Ly5.1⁺パートナー細胞の流入を、白血球総数と顆粒球（Mac-1⁺ Gr-1⁺）分画より算出した。4度実験を行った典型例を示す。

考察

本研究において、顆粒球が関節のコラーゲン誘導性関節炎の炎症に関係する主要な白血球集団であること示した。他の研究者たちも、そのような顆粒球が骨髄で産生され、炎症部位に移動するかもしれないと信じていた。しかし、この予想は、パラビオーゼ実験では証明されなかった。関節でも骨髄でも、白血球でも顆粒球でも、関節炎のマウスでも関節炎でないマウスでも、パラビオーゼしたマウスのパートナー細胞を受け入れることはなかった。全く対照的に、肝臓と脾臓の白血球は、パラビオーゼ後、速やかに（パラビオーゼ後の2週以内）、パートナー細胞を受け入れた。これら結果が示すのは、炎症に有無に関係なく、関節内に存在するすべての白血球は関節内で分化することである。

以前、胸腺外分化の性質を持つT細胞がコラーゲン誘導性関節炎でマウスの関節に存在すると報告した[4,5]。そのようなT細胞には、T細胞レセプター（TCR）-$\alpha\beta$またはTCR-$\gamma\delta$を有するIL-2R$\alpha^-\beta^+$ TCR^{int}細胞がある。胸腺外分化T細胞は、現在、腸、肝臓、子宮と骨髄を含む体のいろいろな場所に存在することが知られている[12-15]。

このことより、胸腺外分化T細胞に加えて、顆粒球が骨髄以外で分化する可能性が高まった。その一つが関節である。一方、肝臓と脾臓の顆粒球は、他の部位（おそらく骨髄）が由来である。骨髄と関節の部位は、密接に関連している。これらの状況でも、種類の違う顆粒球の交流が

存在しなかったことは、興味深い。もう一つの可能性は、骨髄で分化した顆粒球が、血液循環することなく、炎症している関節へ直行することである。現時点では、このような経路が存在するかは不明である。

関節では、炎症にかかわりなく、かなりの割合でB220$^+$ B細胞が存在した。他の研究者にも同様の報告がある。[24] コラーゲン誘導性関節炎の発症時には、自己抗体産生が見られることが多いが、そのようなB220$^+$ B細胞はおそらく自己抗体を産生するB-1細胞であろう[11]。B220$^+$ B細胞の中には、関節内で分化するものもある可能性も考慮する必要がある。骨髄も関節も系統学的に間葉由来の幹細胞が起源であるので、骨髄と関節の起源は密接に関連している。推測できることの一つは、骨髄にも関節にも、胸腺外分化T細胞、自己抗体産生B細胞（B-1細胞）と顆粒球を含む特定の白血球を生産する能力があることである。さらに、予備実験において、血清中炎症性サイトカイン値（TNF-α、インターロイキン-6）は、上昇していた。これらサイトカインは、炎症した関節における白血球産生を調整している可能性がある。[25] さらに、炎症を起こした関節において、このようなサイトカインを遮断して造血を抑制すれば、関節リウマチの新しい治療となるかもしれない。いずれにせよ、本実験で行なったパラビオーゼの結果より、関節は白血球分化増殖器官の1つであるという新しい可能性が高まった。

謝辞

本研究は、文部科学省科学研究費補助金によるものである。原稿浄書について渡辺正子氏に感謝する。

IMMUNOLOGY ORIGINAL ARTICLE

No mixing of granulocytes and other lymphocytes in the inflamed joints of parabiosis mice with collagen-induced arthritis: possible *in situ* generation

Tetsuro Nishizawa,[1,2] Toshihiko Kawamura,[1] Nakao Izumi,[1] Hiroki Kawamura,[1] Katsuyuki Fujii,[2] and Toru Abo[1]

[1]*Department of Immunology, Niigata University School of Medicine, Niigata, Japan, and* [2]*Department of Orthopaedic Surgery, Jikei University School of Medicine, Tokyo, Japan*

doi:10.1111/j.1365-2567.2004.01995.x
Received 21 October 2003; revised 20 August 2004; accepted 13 September 2004.
Correspondence: Dr T. Abo, Department of Immunology, Niigata University School of Medicine, Niigata 951–8510, Japan.
Email: immunol2@med.niigata-u.ac.jp

Summary

Collagen-induced arthritis was evoked by an injection of lipopolysaccharide and anti-type II collagen antibody in mice. In parallel with the onset of arthritis, granulocytes with large light scatter and a Mac-1$^+$ Gr-1$^+$ phenotype expanded in the joints of these mice. Lymphocytes with a CD3$^-$ B220$^+$ phenotype (i.e. B220$^+$ B cells) were the major population among lymphocyte subsets in the joints, irrespective of disease. To determine the origin of these leucocyte populations in the joints and other organs, parabiotic experiments using CBF$_1$Ly5.1 and CBF$_1$Ly5.2 mice were conducted in mice with and without collagen-induced arthritis. As expected, leucocyte populations in the liver and spleen became a half-and-half mixture of their own cells and partner cells (e.g. ~45% of Ly5.1$^+$ cells in Ly5.2$^+$ partner mice). However, such a mixture was extremely delayed in the joints and bone marrow, even in mice with arthritis. These results suggest that, because circulatory blood is not exchanged in the joints, granulocytes and other lymphocytes are generated *in situ* in the inflamed joints of mice with collagen-induced arthritis or are possibly supplied by the bone marrow. It is of interest that granulocytes in the joints expanded, even without a supply from another site, namely, the synovium.

Keywords: collagen-induced arthritis; granulocyte; B-cell parabiosis

Introduction

Rheumatoid arthritis is known to be an autoimmune diseases in which some immunological factors are associated with the onset of inflammation of the joints. Similar to other autoimmune diseases, it is well established that autoantibodies produced by B-1 cells are related to the onset of disease.[1–3] Cumulative evidence has also revealed that invasion of inflammatory tissue by extrathymic T cells causes inflammation of the joints.[4–6] In addition to these immunological factors, recent studies have found that tissue-destructive granulocytes are directly associated with the deterioration of inflamed joints.[7,8]

Based on human and murine studies of rheumatoid arthritis, many investigators have believed that some activated lymphocytes with autoreactivity and tissue-destructive granulocytes migrate from the surrounding lymphoid tissues and evoke arthritis. However, there is another possibility, namely, that resident lymphocytes in the joints exist at the respective sites and that, in the case of rheumatoid arthritis, some self-antigens stimulate such resident lympho-cytes by a yet unknown mechanism.

Furthermore, in the onset of collagen-induced arthritis, the joints always contain unique T-cell populations, including interleukin 2 receptor (IL-2R) $\alpha^-\beta^+$ T cells, $\gamma\delta$ T cells, CD8$\alpha^+\beta^-$ cells, and CD44$^+$ L-selectin$^-$ cells. All of these properties coincide with those of extrathymic T cells at unique sites in the body.[9–11] More precisely, extrathymic T cells are present in the liver,[12] intestine,[13] uterus[14] and glands of external secretion.[15] It is of interest to know the origin of extrathymic T cells in the joints of patients with rheumatoid arthritis or of mice with collagen-induced arthritis. Similarly, we have to consider the origin of granulocytes, which constitute the major leucocyte population in inflamed joints.

Abbreviations: CIA, collagen-induced arthritis; DN, double-negative; IL-2Rβ, interleukin-2 receptor β-chain; MNC, mononuclear cells; TCR^{int}, TCR^{high}, intermediate and high levels of T-cell receptor for antigens.

In the present study, we applied a mouse model of collagen-induced arthritis[4] and carried out parabiotic experiments.[16,17] When parabiosis of $CBF_1Ly5.1$ and $CBF_1Ly5.2$ mice was conducted, the majority of lymphocytes in the peripheral immune organs accepted partner lymphocytes within 2 weeks. As a result, various lymphocyte subsets in such organs (e.g. the spleen and lymph nodes) became a half-and-half mixture of their own cells and partner cells. In sharp contrast, the leucocyte population, including granulocytes and other lymphocytes, which existed in the joints were found not to accept partner cells. This raises the possibility that the leucocyte population in the inflamed joints of mice with collagen-induced arthritis is generated *in situ* without a supply from the bone marrow.

Materials and methods

Mice

(C57BL/6.Ly5.2 × BALB/c)F_1 (i.e. $CBF_1Ly5.2$) and (C57BL/6.Ly5.1 × BALB/c)F_1 (i.e. $CBF_1Ly5.1$) female mice were used at the age of 8–12 weeks. Mice were maintained under specific pathogen-free conditions in the animal facility of Niigata University.

Anti-collagen antibody-induced arthritis

Arthritis antibody kits were obtained from Immuno-Biological Laboratories (Gunma, Japan)[18] and arthritis was induced in the mice according to the manufacturer's instructions.[19] Briefly, mice were injected intraperitoneally with a mixture of four anti-type II collagen monoclonal antibodies (mAbs) (2 mg each) on day 0, followed by intraperitoneal injection with 50 μg lipoplysaccharide (LPS) (*Escherichia coli*, 0111:B4 Immuno-Biological Laboratories) 3 days later. The onset of collagen-induced arthritis was seen in mice 3 days after the primary immunization and the severe phase of the disease (fulminate stage) was noted between days 7 and 10, thereafter, the disease gradually weakened.[20] Mice were observed daily for the onset of arthritis. Clinical arthritis was assessed using a scoring system as follows: grade 0, no swelling; grade 1, paws with swelling in a single digit; grade 2, paws with swelling in multiple digits; grade 3, severe swelling and joint rigidity. The total score for clinical disease activity was based on all four paws, with a maximum score of 12 for each animal.

Parabiosis

Parabiosis of $CBF_1Ly5.1$ and $CBF_1Ly5.2$ mice at the age of 8 weeks was produced as described previously.[17] Briefly, weight-matched female mice were used. Under anaesthesia, hair was shaved and the skin was disinfected with ethanol. A skin incision was made on the lateral side of the mouse from the back of the ear straight down to the tail, and pairs of mice were then sutured together. For a week after the operation, feed was broken into pieces, soaked in water and placed on the bottom of the cage. A few individual parabiotic mice that suffered from stress which resulted in thymic atrophy were eliminated from the experiments.

Cell preparation

Hepatic mononuclear cells (MNC) were prepared as previously described.[21] Briefly, mice were anaesthetized with ether before being killed by total exsanguination from the incised axillary artery and vein. The liver was removed, cut into small pieces with scissors, pressed through stainless steel mesh, and suspended in Eagle's minimal essential medium containing 5 mm HEPES (Nissui Pharmaceutical Co., Tokyo, Japan) and 2% heat-inactivated newborn calf serum (JRH Biosciences, Lenexa, KS). After one washing, the pellet was resuspended in 35% Percoll solution (Pharmacia Fine Chemicals, Piscataway, NJ) containing 100 U/ml heparin (Nipro Pharma, Osaka, Japan) and centrifuged at 400 *g* for 15 min. The pellet was resuspended in erythrocyte-lysing solution (155 mm NH_4Cl, 10 mm $KHCO_3$, 1 mm sodium ethylene diaminetetraacetic acid, 170 mm Tris–HCl, pH 7·3).

Splenic MNC were obtained by forcing the spleen through 200-gauge stainless steel mesh. Splenic MNC were used after erythrocyte lysis. To prepare MNC from the inflamed joints, a minor modification of the technique previously described by Wooley *et al.*[22] was used. The joints were dissected away from the paws, the skin was removed, and the joints were cut into small pieces with scissors. The small pieces were pressed through 200-gauge stainless steel mesh and suspended in the medium.

Bone marrow cells were obtained by flushing femurs in the medium followed by erythrocyte lysis.

Immunofluorescence tests

Distinction of granulocytes and lymphocytes was performed using side scatter (existence of granules) and forward scatter (cell size). Namely, lymphocytes were small and contained no granules. Phenotypes of lymphocytes were identified by a single-, two-, or three-colour immunofluorescence test using flow cytometry.[23] For flow cytometric analysis, anti-CD3 [145-2C11: mouse, immuno-globulin G1 (IgG1), κ], anti-NK1.1 (PK136: mouse, IgG2a, κ), anti-B220 (RA3-6B2: rat, IgG2a, κ), anti-granulocyte (Gr-1; RB68C5: rat, IgG2b, κ), anti-macrophage (Mac-1; M1/70.15, rat, IgG2b), anti-Ly5.1 (A20.1.7: mouse, IgG2a, κ), and anti-Ly5.2 (ALI-4A2: mouse, IgG2a, κ) mAbs were purchased from PharMingen (San Diego, CA). Granulocytes were large, had granules and were dyed using Gr-1 and Mac-1 mAbs. All mAbs were used in a fluorescein isothiocyanate (FITC)-, phycoerythrin (PE)-, or biotin-conjugated form. Biotinylated reagents were developed with TRIColor-conjugated streptavidin (Caltag Laboratory, San Francisco, CA). Cells were analysed on a fluorescence-activated cell sorter (Becton Dickinson Co., Mountain View, CA). To prevent non-specific binding of mAbs, CD32/16 (2.4G2) was added before staining with the labelled mAbs. Dead cells were excluded by forward scatter or side scatter.

Results

Induction of collagen-induced arthritis

In this experiment, a mixture of LPS and anti-collagen antibody was injected to evoke collagen-induced arthritis (Fig. 1a). LPS alone did not induce arthritis. However, the mixture induced severe arthritis, and inflammation continued for up to 1 month. At the fulminant stage (day 7) of arthritis, leucocytes were isolated from the bone marrow and joints, and phenotypic characterization was conducted (Fig. 1b). Light scatter showed that cells with

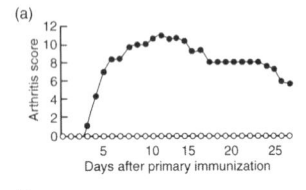

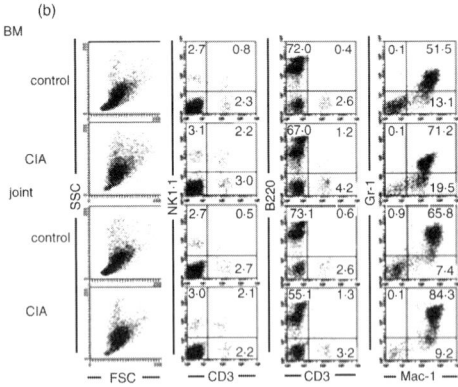

Figure 1. Collagen-induced arthritis. (a) Time-kinetics of arthritis score of a CBF_1 mouse; (b) phenotypic characterization of leucocytes in the bone marrow and joints of mice with collagen-induced arthritis. Mice were injected with LPS alone (○) or a mixture of LPS and anti-type II collagen (●). Leucocytes were isolated 1 week after the injection. Two-colour stainings were conducted for the indicated combinations. Numbers represent the percentage of fluorescence-positive cells in corresponding quadrants.

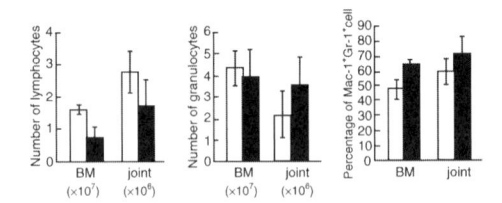

Figure 2. Comparisons of the numbers of lymphocytes and granulocytes and the percentages of granulocytes in the bone marrow and joint between normal mice (□) and mice with collagen-induced arthritis (CIA) (■) ($n = 4$ mice per group). Leucocytes were isolated from mice with CIA on day 7 after injection. Data are expressed as means ± SEM. *$P < 0.05$ for the difference between control and CIA mice. Comparisons of data between control and CIA mice were performed using Student's unpaired t-test.

large scatter were abundant in both the bone marrow and joints. Using gated analysis of lymphocytes, two-colour staining for CD3 and NK1.1 and for CD3 and B220 was then conducted. The majority of lymphocytes in the bone marrow and joints of control mice were $B220^+$ B cells. This population decreased somewhat after the onset of arthritis. Instead, the proportion of $CD3^+$ T cells. with or without NK1.1 antigens, increased, although the proportions were small irrespective of arthritis. Using gated analysis of phagocytes with larger light scatter, the major population was found to be granulocytes (i.e. $Mac-1^+$ $Gr-1^+$), and the proportion of this population increased after the onset of arthritis. The absolute number of lymphocytes and granulocytes was calculated from these data and from repeated experiments (Fig. 2). The number of lymphocytes decreased after the onset of disease in both organs, whereas that of granulocytes increased, especially in the joints. The change in the proportion of granulocytes ($Mac-1^+$ $Gr-1^+$) is also shown in Fig. 2. Taken together, these findings indicate that the major population of leucocytes in the inflamed joints was granulocytes.

Parabiosis between normal mice

In a previous study, we reported that extrathymic T cells with unique properties were present in the joints of mice with arthritis and that their properties were different from those of extrathymic T cells in other organs (e.g. the liver or intestine). We therefore speculated that some of the leucocytes in the joints were generated *in situ*. Such a possibility was examined for granulocytes in the joints (Fig. 3). In this experiment, parabiosis of $CBF_1Ly5.1$ and $CBF_1Ly5.2$ mice was conducted and three-colour staining for Gr-1, Mac-1 and Ly5.1 was carried out 2 and 4 weeks after initiation of parabiosis (Fig. 3a). When all the leucocytes in the liver, spleen, bone marrow and joints were analysed, those in the liver and spleen of $CBF_1Ly5.2$ mice were found to

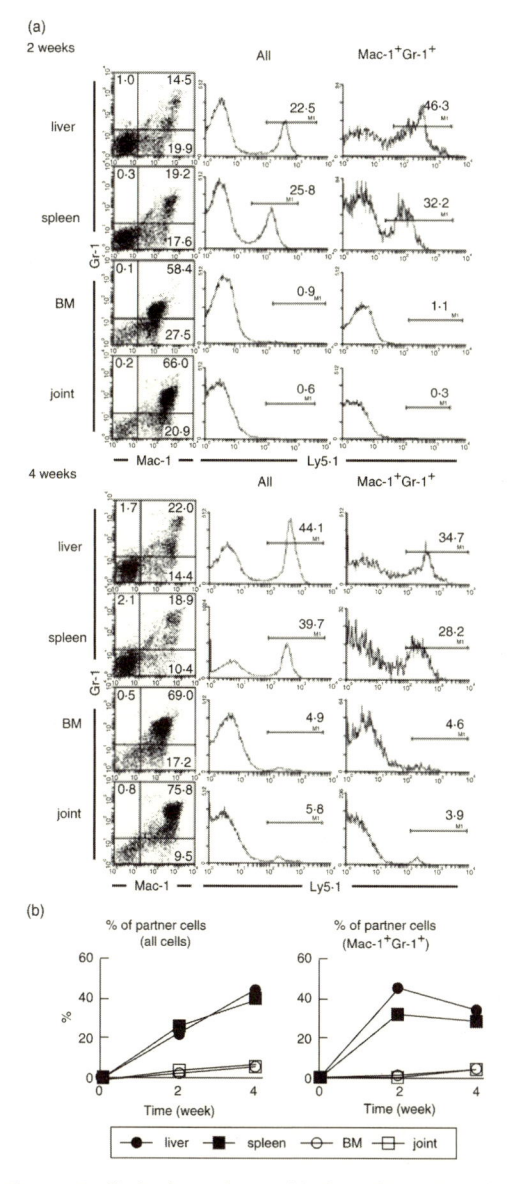

Figure 3. Parabiosis of normal mice. (a) Three-colour staining for Mac-1, Gr-1 and Ly5.1, (b) entrance of Ly5.1$^+$ partner cells. Parabiosis of CBF$_1$Ly5.1 and CBF$_1$Ly5.2 mice was conducted. Leucocytes were isolated from the liver (●), spleen (■), bone marrow (○) and joints (□) 2 and 4 weeks after parabiosis and three-colour staining was conducted. By gated analysis, the entrance of Ly5.1$^+$ partner cells was estimated in the fractions of all leucocytes and granulocytes (Mac-1$^+$ Gr-1$^+$).

include a large proportion of partner cells (Ly5.1$^+$) at both 2 and 4 weeks. This tendency was also observed for granulocytes (Mac-1$^+$ Gr-1$^+$) in the liver and spleen.

In sharp contrast, the presence of partner cells (Ly5.1$^+$) in the bone marrow and joints of Ly5.2 mice was extremely low for all leucocytes as well as for all granulocytes. These kinetics are shown in Fig. 3(b). These results suggested that half of the granulocytes, as well as other leucocytes (e.g. B220$^+$ B cells), in the liver and spleen came from other sites, whereas all the granulocytes and other leucocytes in the bone marrow and joints were generated *in situ*. Namely, there was no mixture of leucocytes in the bone marrow and joints from other organs.

No entrance of partner granulocytes, even into the site of inflammation

Parabiosis of CBF$_1$Ly5.1 and CBF$_1$Ly5.2 mice was conducted and a mixture of LPS and anti-collagen antibody was injected into each partner (Fig. 4). Each partner showed the onset of arthritis up to 3–4 days after the injection (Fig. 4a). On day 7, leucocytes were isolated from the bone marrow and joints of each partner (Fig. 4b). Both partners showed an increased number of leucocytes with large light scatter, the biggest increase being the granulocyte (Mac-1$^+$ Gr-1$^+$) population.

Leucocytes were isolated in the CBF$_1$Ly5.2 partner on day 7 and three-colour staining for Mac-1, Gr-1 and

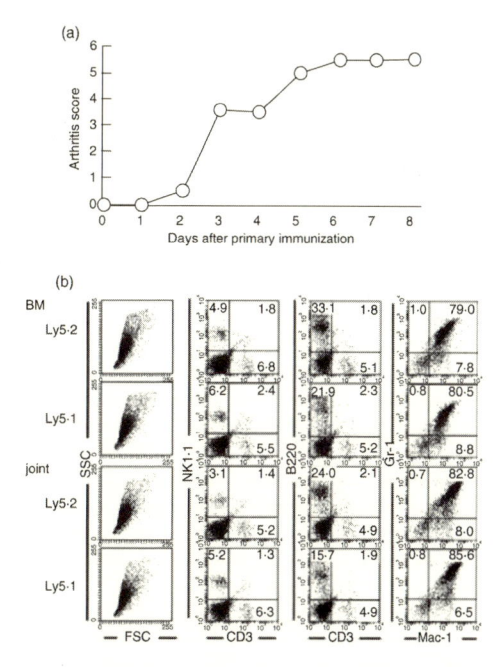

Figure 4. Parabiosis of mice with collagen-induced arthritis (CIA). (a) Time-kinetics of arthritis score of CBF1Ly5.2 mice. (b) Phenotypic characterization of leucocytes in the bone marrow and joints of mice with CIA (on day 7). Numbers in (b) represent the percentages of fluorescence-positive cells in corresponding quadrants.

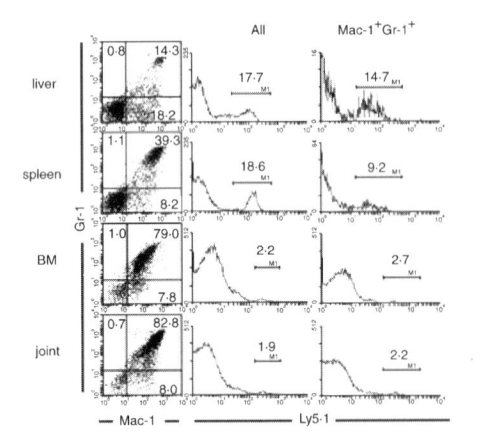

Figure 5. Entrance of Ly5.1⁺ partner cells indicated by parabiotic experiments. Three-colour staining for Mac-1, Gr-1 and Ly5.1 was conducted. Numbers in the quadrants represent the per cent of fluorescence positive cells. The entrance of Ly5.1⁺ partner cells was estimated in the fractions of all leucocytes and granulocytes (Mac-1⁺Gr-1⁺) by gated analysis. Representative results of four experiments are depicted.

Ly5.1 was conducted (Fig. 5). Ly5.1⁺ partner cells were found in the fractions of all leucocytes as well as all granulocytes (Mac-1⁺ Gr-1⁺) in the liver and spleen. On the other hand, Ly5.1⁺ partner cells were not found in the fractions of leucocytes or granulocytes in the bone marrow and joints.

Discussion

In the present study, we demonstrate that granulocytes are the major leucocyte population involved in the inflammation of collagen-induced arthritis in joints. We, and possibly other investigators, had believed that such granulocytes might be generated in the bone marrow and before migrating to the sites of inflammation. However, this expectation was not borne out by the parabiosis experiments. None of the leucocytes and granulocytes in the joints, nor those in the bone marrow, of mice with or without arthritis, accepted the partner cells in parabiotic mice. In sharp contrast, leucocytes in the liver and spleen immediately accepted partner cells after parabiosis (within 2 weeks after parabiosis). These results suggest that all the leucocytes which exist in the joints are generated *in situ*, irrespective of inflammation.

We previously reported that T cells with extrathymic properties were present in the joints of mice with collagen-induced arthritis.[4,5] Such T cells included IL-2Rα⁻β⁺ TCR^{int} cells with T-cell receptor (TCR)-αβ or TCR-γδ. Extrathymic T cells are now known to be present at various sites in the body, including the intestine, liver, uterus and bone marrow.[12–15] This raises the possibility that in addition to extrathymic T cells, granulocytes might be generated outside the bone marrow. One such site is the joint. On the other hand, granulocytes in the liver and spleen were derived from other sites, possibly the bone marrow. The sites of the bone marrow and joints are closely related. Even under these conditions, it is of interest that there was no communication with regard to the entrance of granulocytes. Another possibility is that the leucocyte population moves directly from the bone marrow to the inflamed joints without entering the circulation. At present, we do not know whether such a route exists.

In the case of joints, a considerable proportion of B220⁺ B cells were present, irrespective of the inflammation. A similar observation has been reported by other investigators.[24] Since the onset of collagen-induced arthritis often accompanies the production of autoantibodies, such B220⁺ B cells might possibly be B-1 cells, which produce autoantibodies.[11] We also have to consider the possibility that some B220⁺ B cells are generated *in situ* in the joints. The origins of bone marrow and joints are closely related because both organs are derived phylogenetically from stem cells of mesenchymal origin. One speculation is that both the bone marrow and joints have the ability to produce certain leucocytes, including extrathymic T cells, autoantibody-producing B cells (i.e. B-1 cells) and granulocytes. Moreover serum levels of inflammatory cytokines (tumour necrosis factor-α, interleukin-6) were elevated in a preliminary experiment. Such cytokines may regulate leucopoiesis in inflamed joints.[25] Furthermore, in inflamed joints, suppression of haematopoiesis by blocking such cytokines may become a new medical treatment for rheumatoid arthritis. In any case, the present results from parabiotic experiments raise the unique possibility that the joints are one of the organs of leucopoiesis.

Acknowledgements

We wish to thank Mrs Masako Watanabe for here preparation of the manuscript. This work was supported by a Grant-in-Aid for Scientific Research and Cancer Research from the Ministry of Education, Science and Culture, Japan.

References

1 Cambridge G, Leandro MJ, Edwards JC, Ehrenstein MR, Salden M, Bodman-Smith M, Webster AD. Serologic changes following B lymphocyte depletion therapy for rheumatoid arthritis. *Arthritis Rheum* 2003; **48**:2146–54.

2 Scofield RH. Autoantibodies as predictors of disease. *Lancet* 2004; **363**:1544–6.

3 Mantovani L, Wilder RL, Casali P. Human rheumatoid B-1a (CD5+ B) cells make somatically hypermutated high affinity IgM rheumatoid factors. *J Immunol* 1993; **151**:473–88.

4 Arai K, Yamamura S, Hanyu T, Takahashi HE, Umezu H, Watanabe H, Abo T. Extrathymic differentiation of resident T cells in the joints of mice with collagen-induced arthritis. *J Immunol* 1996; **157**:5170–7.
5 Arai K, Yamamura S, Seki S, Hanyu T, Takahashi HE, Abo T. Increase of CD57$^+$ T cells in knee joints and adjacent bone marrow of rheumatoid arthritis (RA) patients: implication for an anti-inflammatory role. *Clin Exp Immunol* 1998; **111**:345–52.
6 Chiba A, Oki S, Miyamoto K, Hashimoto H, Yamamura T, Miyake S. Suppression of collagen-induced arthritis by natural killer T cell activation with OCH, a sphingosine-truncated analog of alpha-galactosylceramide. *Arthritis Rheum* 2004; **50**:305–13.
7 Wipke BT, Allen PM. Essential role of neutrophils in the initiation and progression of a murine model of rheumatoid arthritis. *J Immunol* 2001; **167**:1601–8.
8 Campbell IK, Rich MJ, Bischof RJ, Dunn AR, Grail D, Hamilton JA. Protection from collagen-induced arthritis in granulocyte-macrophage colony-stimulating factor-deficient mice. *J Immunol* 1998; **161**:3639–44.
9 Naito T, Kawamura T, Bannai M, Kosaka T, Kameyama H, Shimamura O, Hoshi K, Ushiki T, Hatakeyama K, Abo T. Simultaneous activation of natural killer T cells and autoantibody production in mice injected with denatured syngeneic liver tissue. *Clin Exp Immunol* 2002; **129**:397–404.
10 Miyakawa R, Miyaji C, Watanabe H, Yokoyama H, Tsukada C, Asakura H, Abo T. Unconventional NK1.1$^-$ intermediate TCR cells as major T lymphocytes expanding in chronic graft-versus-host disease. *Eur J Immunol* 2002; **32**:2521–31.
11 Morshed SRM, Mannoor K, Halder RC, Kawamura H, Bannai M, Sekikawa H, Watanabe H, Abo T. Tissue-specific expansion of NKT and CD5$^+$ B cells at the onset of autoimmune disease in (NZB × NZW) F$_1$ mice. *Eur J Immunol* 2002; **32**:2551–61.
12 Mannoor MK, Halder RC, Morshed SRM *et al.* Essential role of extrathymic T cells in protection against malaria. *J Immunol* 2002; **169**:301–6.
13 Bannai M, Kawamura T, Naito T *et al.* Abundance of unconventional CD8$^+$ natural killer T cells in the large intestine. *Eur J Immunol* 2001; **31**:3361–9.
14 Wang S, Li C, Kawamura H, Watanabe H, Abo T. Unique sensitivity to α-galactosylceramide of NKT cells in the uterus. *Cell Immunol* 2002; **215**:98–105.
15 Narita J, Kawamura T, Miyaji C, Watanabe H, Honda S, Koya T, Arakawa M, Abo T. Abundance of NKT cells in the salivary glands but absence thereof in the liver and thymus of *aly/aly* mice with Sjögren syndrome. *Cell Immunol* 1999; **192**:149–58.
16 Scheid MP, Triglia D. Further description of the Ly-5 system. *Immunogenetics* 1979; **9**:423–33.
17 Donskoyt E, Goldschneider I. Thymocytopoiesis is maintained by blood-borne precursors throughout postnatal life: a study in parabiotic mice. *J Immunol* 1992; **148**:1604–12.
18 Terato K, Harper DS, Griffiths MM, Hasty DL, Ye XJ, Cremer MA, Seyer JM. Collagen-induced arthritis in mice. Synergistic effect of *E. coli* lipopolysaccharide bypasses epitope specificity in the induction of arthritis with monoclonal antibodies to type II collagen. *Autoimmunity* 1995; **22**:137–47.
19 Wallace PM, MacMaster JF, Rouleau KA, Brown TJ, Loy JK, Donaldson KL, Wahl AF. Regulation of inflammatory responses by oncostatin M. *J Immunol* 1999; **162**:5547–55.
20 Yumoto K, Ishijima M, Rittling S *et al.* Osteopontin deficiency protects joints against destruction in anti-type II collagen antibody-induced arthritis in mice. *Proc Natl Acad Sci USA* 2002; **99**:4556–61.
21 Watanabe H, Miyaji C, Kawachi Y, Iiai T, Ohtsuka K, Iwanaga T, Takahashi-Iwanaga H, Abo T. Relationships between intermediate TCR cells and NK1.1$^+$T cells in various immune organs. NK1.1$^+$T cells are present within a population of intermediate TCR cells. *J Immunol* 1995; **155**:2972–83.
22 Wooley PH, Whalen JD, Chapdelaine JM. Collagen-induced arthritis in mice. VI. Synovial cells from collagen arthritic mice activate autologous lymphocytes *in vitro*. *Cell Immunol* 1989; **124**:227–38.
23 Sato K, Ohtsuka K, Hasegawa K, Yamagiwa S, Watanabe H, Asakura H, Abo T. Evidence for extrathymic generation of intermediate T cell receptor cells in the liver revealed in thymectomized, irradiated mice subjected to bone marrow transplantation. *J Exp Med* 1995; **182**:759–67.
24 Manabe N, Kawaguchi H, Chikuda H *et al.* Connection between B lymphocyte and osteoclast differentiation pathways. *J Immunol* 2001; **167**:2625–31.
25 Matthys P, Vermeire K, Billiau A. Mac-1$^+$ myelopoiesis induced by CFA. a clue to the paradoxical effects of IFN-γ in autoimmune disease models. *Trends Immunol* 2001; **22**:367–72.

Immunologic States of Autoimmune Diseases

自己免疫疾患における免疫学的状態

Immunologic Research, 33: 23-34, 2005

chapter 18

Immunologic States of autoimmune Diseases
自己免疫疾患における免疫学的状態

Toru Abo[1] Toshihiko Kawamura[1] Hisami Watanabe[2]

[1]Department of Immunology, Niigata University School of Medicine, Niigata
[2]Division of Cellular and Molecular Immunology, Center of Molecular Biosciences, University of Ryukyus, Okinawa, Japan

【キーワード】
　自己免疫疾患、胸腺外分化T細胞、自己応答、B-1細胞、免疫抑制

【要約】
　自己免疫疾患の病因や疫学的状態を論ずる際、これまで大概、胸腺外分化T細胞を考慮することはなかった。胸腺外分化T細胞は、肝臓、腸と外分泌腺の中に存在する。胸腺外分化T細胞は自己応答性があると同時に、自己抗体産生B-1細胞とともに活性化されることが多い。従って、自己免疫疾患における免疫学的状態を考慮する際には、この胸腺外分化T細胞やB-1細胞も考慮する必要がある。自己免疫疾患における免疫学的状態は、加齢、慢性移植片対宿主（GVH）病やマラリア感染時の免疫学的状態に似ている。すなわち、こういったすべての状況下では、（胸腺内で分化した）T細胞とB細胞は、胸腺萎縮・退縮と同時にむしろ抑制が起こる。対照的に、胸腺外分化T細胞とB-1細胞は、この時に逆に活性化する。これらの事実より、自己免疫疾患における免疫学的状態を、系統発生途上の原始リンパ球である可能性がある胸腺外分化T細胞や自己抗体産生B-1細胞の概念を考慮して再評価する必要があることが示唆される。

はじめに

　胸腺内分化するT細胞およびB（B-2）細胞以外に、胸腺外分化T細胞および自己抗体産生B（B-1）細胞について、20年間にわたり研究を行った（1-4）。系統発生学的には、（胸腺内分化した）T細胞およびB細胞は、生物の上陸以降、外来抗原を処理するため発生したと考えられる。実際、（胸腺内分化した）T細胞は、胸腺で自己応答性禁止クローンを除くために、システムの一部として発達した（5-7）。一方、胸腺外分化T細胞は、より初期の（もしくは原始的な）免疫系を構成するものである可能性があり、禁止クローン排除というよりは、むしろ異常もしくは変性した自己細胞を攻撃する（8, 9）。しかし、これら胸腺外分化T細胞と自己抗体産生B細胞が過度に拡大すると、自己免疫疾患が発症する可能性がある（10, 11）。あるいは、胸腺外分化T細胞が適度な拡大は、マラリアのような細胞内病原体に対する防御に重要である可能性がある（12）。胸腺外分化T細胞や自己抗体産生B細胞の概念を考慮しなければ、自己免疫疾患、マラリア感染、慢性移植片対宿主（GVH）病および悪性腫瘍など多くの疾患同

---

*Correspondence to : Dr. Toru Abo, Department of immunology, Niigata 951-8510, Japan. E-mail: immunol2@med.niigata-u.ac.jp

様、妊娠免疫もきちんと理解することはできない。

胸腺外分化T細胞とB-1細胞

胸腺外分化T細胞が存在する場所は、腸（1, 2）、肝臓（3, 4）、子宮（13）、関節（14）および分泌腺（15）である。脾臓やリンパ節には、この胸腺外分化T細胞はあまり見られない。脾臓やリンパ節に主として存在するのは、胸腺内分化T細胞とB細胞である。（従来型）T細胞は胸腺で発生する、一方（従来型）B細胞は骨髄で発生する。胸腺と骨髄が発達したのは、生物上陸以降であることから、それ以前の免疫臓器は、腸、肝臓（腸から発達したもの）および分泌腺（例、唾液腺、下顎腺や涙腺）であったと簡単に推測できる。もう一つ原始的な免疫の場所は、腹膜腔でありB-1細胞が最も豊富であるのはここである（16, 17）。いずれにせよ、胸腺外分化T細胞とB-1細胞の自己応答性は、原始リンパ球の特性の1つである可能性がある。最も原始的なリンパ球はNK細胞であり、NK細胞は、T細胞レセプター（TCR）、主要組織適合抗原（MHC）や免疫グロブリン（Ig）を利用しない。

マウスにおいては、T細胞中の自己応答性禁止クローンを、特定のVβ（内因性スーパー抗原Mlsに対して）を用いて同定可能である。実際、自己応答性禁止クローンは、胸腺内でT細胞が分化する際に負の選択のプロセス以前に排除される（5-7）。このような自己応答性Vβは、主として（胸腺内で分化した）T細胞でなく、胸腺外分化T細胞に存在することを明らかにした報告もある（8, 9）。胸腺外分化T細胞と自己抗体産生また、B-1細胞は、しばしば同時に活性化するという報告もある（10-12）。例えば、変性した肝臓組織をマウスに移入した際、胸腺外分化T細胞とB-1細胞は、それぞれ、肝臓および腹膜腔で活性化する。このようなリンパ球は変性した自己細胞を排除するのに重要である可能性があり、このような時はいつも胸腺萎縮が見られる。換言すると、胸腺由来のT細胞と胸腺外分化T細胞は、相互に活性化すると言える。この免疫抑制には、しばしば顆粒球増多が起こる。

T細胞分化における胸腺内代替経路

T細胞分化経路の主流は、胸腺内に存在する（Fig. 1）。この経路において分化がおこるのは主に胸腺皮質である、前駆細胞（TCR$^-$CD4$^-$8$^-$）から、大量にダブルポジティブな未熟T細胞（TCR^{dull}CD4$^+$8$^+$）が生まれ、アポトーシスにより消滅する。一方、この時残った少量の細胞のみが、成熟T細胞（TCR^{high}CD4$^+$またはTCR^{high}CD8$^+$）となる。アポトーシスの際、自己抗原とMHCの複合体の相互作用により、自己応答性禁止クローンを排除する。成熟後、T細胞は、末梢にある免疫器官に向かう。

主なT細胞分化の経路以外にも、もう一つT細胞分化胸腺内経路が胸腺に存在することが明らかになった（Fig. 1）。このもう一つの経路が主に胸腺髄質に存在する（8, 9）。図のように、この細胞集団の前駆細胞は、直接、CD4^{low}NK1.1$^+$TCR^{int}細胞（NKT細胞）となる。細胞集団の残り半分が、ダブルネガティブ（CD4$^-$8$^-$）NK1.1-TCR^{int}細胞となる。通常、若いマウスでは、この代替経路を経由するリンパ球（TCR^{int}IL-2Rβ^+）は、胸腺リンパ球の総数のわずか1.2%にすぎない。しかし、TCR^{int}IL-2Rβ^+細胞がストレス耐性であるため、胸腺萎縮の際には、この細胞の割合が増加する（8）。

TCR^{int}IL-2Rβ^+（NK1.1$^+$またはNK1.1-）細胞のフェノタイプは、代替胸腺内経路を経由して発生する。これは、肝臓内に存在する胸腺外分化T細胞のフェノタイプに酷似している。胸腺および肝臓内におけるTCR^{int}細胞は、系統発生

Figure.1

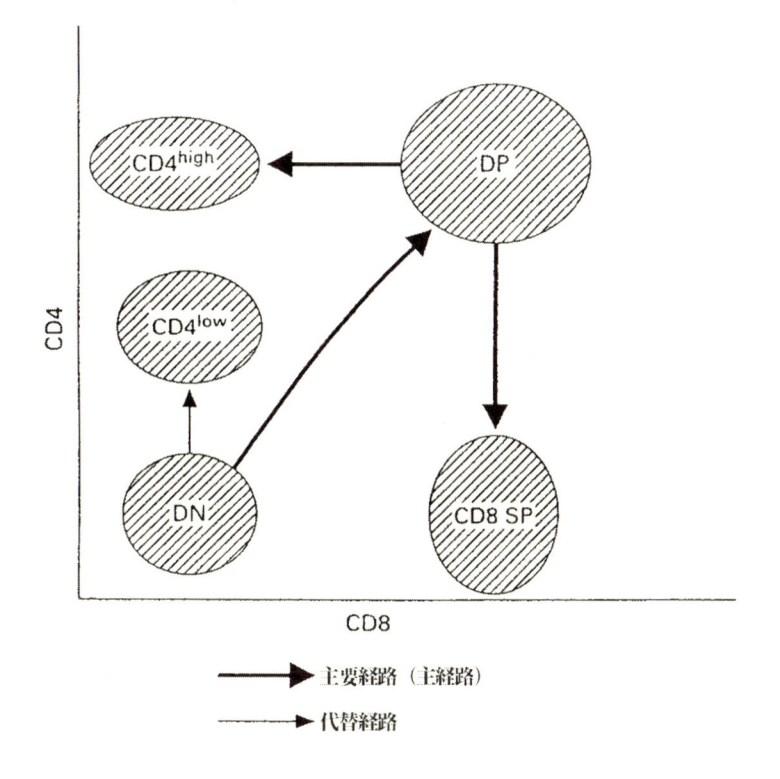

胸腺内T細胞分化主要経路（主流）と代替経路。胸腺には、T細胞分化の主要な経路（主流）と代替経路がある。

学における原始T細胞であると推測される。胸腺髄質は、起源が鰓孔であるため外胚葉上皮細胞を含む。その一方、胸腺皮質は、起源がえらであるので、内皮上皮細胞を含む (18)。鰓孔には、皮膚 (外胚葉) に存在する原始リンパ球がある可能性がある。従って、胸腺髄質は原始リンパ球が残っていて、腸や肝臓の場合に似ている。

NK1.1⁻TCR^{int}細胞とNK1.1⁺TCR^{int}細胞の関係

TCR^{int}IL-2Rβ^+細胞は肝臓と胸腺の中に存在し、NK1.1⁺とNK1.1の二種類のサブセットがある (小集団) (19)。換言すると、TCR^{int}IL-2Rβ^+細胞は、NK1.1⁺TCR^{int}サブセットとNK1.1⁻TCR^{int}サブセットの半々の混成である。興味深いことに、先天的に胸腺が欠損しているヌードマウスには、NK1.1⁻TCR^{int}細胞だけがある (Fig. 2)。TCR^{int}IL-2Rβ^+細胞は、加齢やIL-12投与で増加する。しかしながら、これらT細胞は、すべてNK1.1⁻TCR^{int}細胞である。IL-12を投与した胸腺欠損マウスにおけるNK1.1⁺TCR^{int}細胞は少数である。このNKT細胞はすべてCD8⁺である、すなわち、CD4⁺フェノタイプやVα14Jα281を持つ従来型NKT細胞ではない (20)。その後の研究により、NK1.1⁺TCR^{int}細胞 (NKT細胞) およびその前駆細胞は胸腺で発生することが明らかになった (21-24)。しかし、成人の胸腺を摘出した際、肝臓においてNKT細胞数減少は見られなかった (25)。それは、NKT細胞の前駆細胞は、新生児期に肝臓に存在すること、および、この前駆細胞から成人期に肝臓においてNKT細胞が発生することが考えられる。

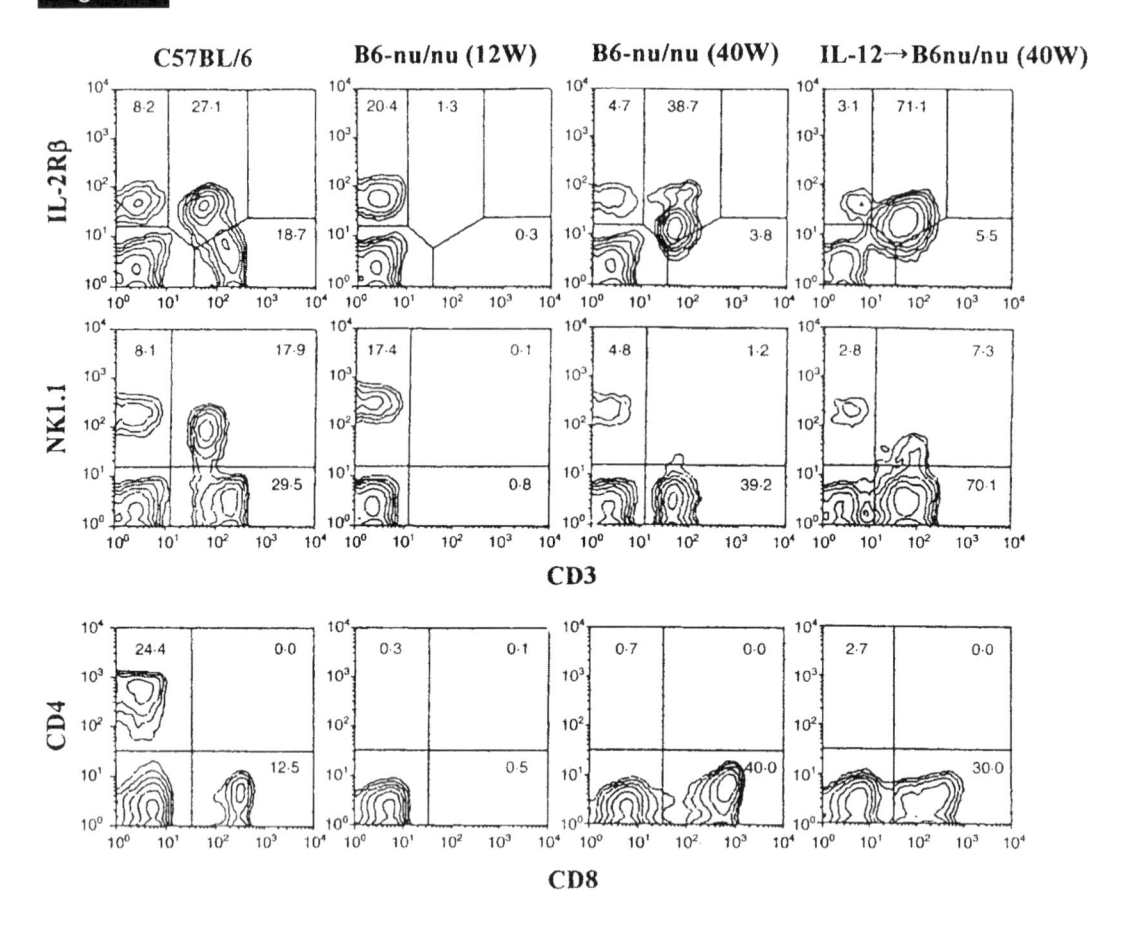

Figure.2

胸腺欠損ヌードマウスで見られるT細胞は、NK1.1⁻TCR^int細胞である。IL-2Rβ⁺CD3^int細胞はすべてNK1.1⁻CD8⁺であった。IL-12を投与すると、少数のNK1.1⁺CD3^int細胞が、肝臓に出現した。しかし、これらのT細胞は、CD8を発現している従来型ではないNKT細胞であった。

すべてのNK細胞、NKT細胞およびNK1.1⁻TCR^int細胞は、悪性腫瘍（26, 27）、マラリア原虫感染肝細胞（12, 28, 29）と変性した自己細胞（10）に対して自己応答性である。NK細胞は、MHC-自己細胞（missing self）に対して自己応答性の反応をする。NKT細胞が特定の糖脂質抗原（α-ガラクトシルセラミドなど）を認識することが知られている（30-32）。他方、NK1.1⁻TCR^int細胞は、再生肝細胞と自己（由来の）胸腺細胞（33, 34）に対して細胞傷害性を発揮する。この原始リンパ球すべてが「自然免疫」として異常な自己細胞や再生自己細胞を除去する

のに重要であると推測される。NKT細胞が増殖している従来型T細胞と相互に作用するならば、そのようなNKT細胞は特定の自己免疫疾患モデルに見られる調節性リンパ球として作用する可能性がある（35-40）。

腸管内T細胞

もともと、原始リンパ球は、系統学的には消化管と皮膚で発生したと考えられる（18）。上部消化管（えら）で分化したリンパ球は胸腺で従来型T細胞になり、下部消化管（腸管と肝臓）で成長したリンパ球は、腸管内T細胞と肝内T細胞になった。両方とも胸腺外分化T細胞であ

るが、腸管内T細胞と肝内T細胞の間に、類似点も相違点も実在する。マウスの腸管内T細胞は、TCR^{high}であり、NK1.1抗原はなく（41-47）、IL-2Rβ^+とIL-2Rβ^-の混成である。マウスの小腸において、IL-2Rβ^+T細胞の大多数は$\gamma\delta$T細胞である、一方、IL-2Rβ^-T細胞の大多数は、$\alpha\beta$T細胞である。

マウス胸腺外分化T細胞のサブセットは、大腸（48）および虫垂（49）では独特である。大腸にはNK1.1$^+$CD8$^+$T細胞など特殊なNKT細胞が存在する。（NK1.1$^+$CD8$^+$T細胞は、従来型NKT細胞に見られるVα14Jα281は利用されない。虫垂には、B220$^+$T細胞が存在する。ヒトの胸腺外分化T細胞は、CD56$^+$T細胞、CD57$^+$T細胞およびCD161$^+$T細胞として同定できる（50-57）。換言すると、胸腺外分化T細胞は、細胞表面にNKマーカーを発現している。ヒトのCD56$^+$T細胞は肝臓に多数存在（56, 57）し、CD57$^+$T細胞は骨髄（58-60）や関節（14）に多く存在する、また、CD161$^+$T細胞は腸管に多く存在する（54）。

自己免疫疾患

自己免疫疾患では、血清中における自己抗体価が高値であるという特徴が知られている。自己抗体に加えて、この時、胸腺外分化T細胞（CD57$^+$T細胞）もヒトにおいて増加する（52）。マウスでは、胸腺外分化T細胞（ここではNKT細胞）およびB-1細胞が活性化する（Fig. 3）。発症（蛋白尿出現）後、NKT細胞の割合と絶対数が、肝臓において増加した（矢印）。この時、胸腺萎縮あるいは胸腺退縮が見られた（Fig. 4）。全く対照的に、原始リンパ球の数は、肝臓、脾臓および腹膜腔（PEC）（ここでは、B-1細胞）において増加を示した。これらすべての結果より、自己免疫疾患の場合には、原始T細胞および原始B細胞は活性化状態にあるが、その反対に、従来型T細胞およびB細胞は抑制

Figure.3

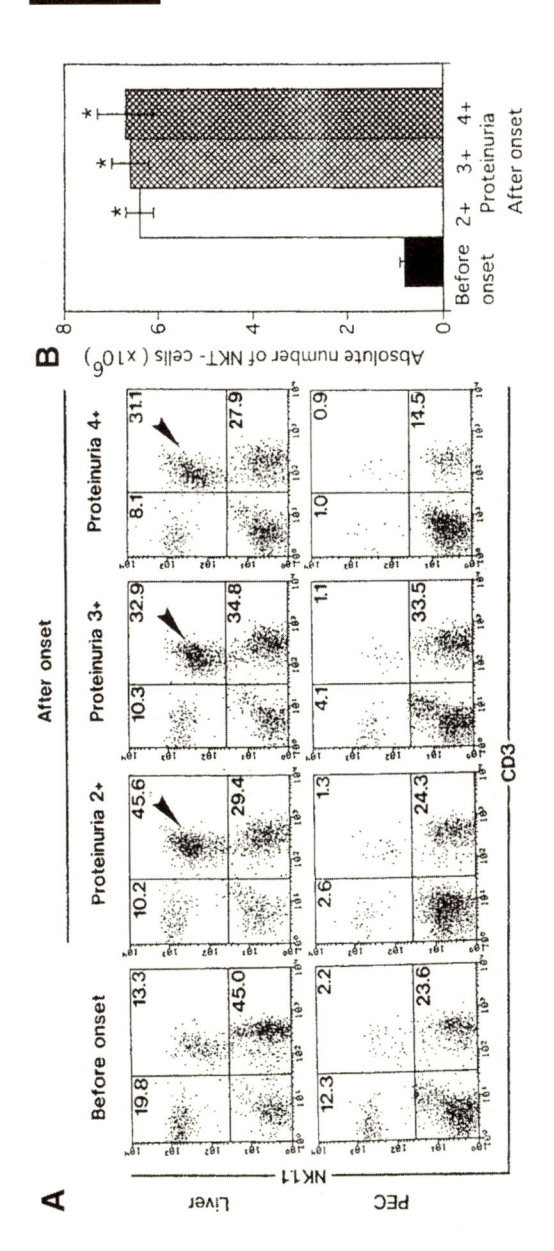

自己免疫モデルNZB/W F$_1$マウスの肝臓におけるNKT細胞の増多。(A) CD3およびNK1.1二重染色；(B) NKT細胞の絶対数。発症後、肝臓ではNKT細胞（CD4$^+$Vα14Jα281$^+$）が増大した。

Figure.4

発症後、自己免疫NZB/W F₁マウスに胸腺萎縮が出現した。発症後、肝臓や腹膜腔においてリンパ球数が増加した。全く対照的に、胸腺の細胞数は、顕著な減少を示した。

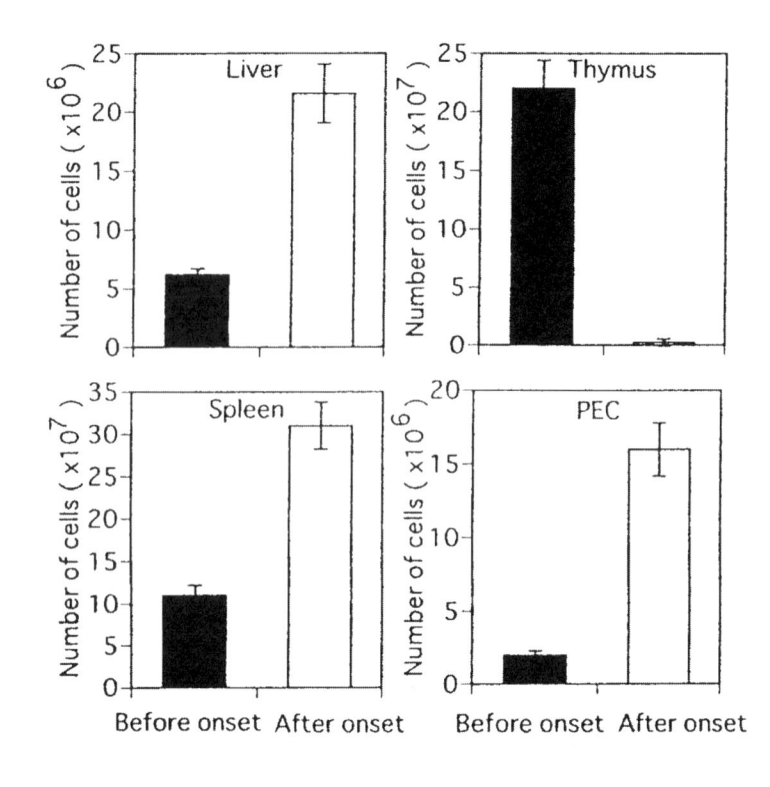

状態にあることが示される (11)。

問題は、胸腺過形成が、なぜ自己免疫疾患において見られるかということである。例えば、ヒトにおける重症筋無力症（MG）やマウスにおけるMRL-*lpr/lpr*自己免疫疾患である。理由は、MG患者（61）およびMRL-*lpr/lpr*マウス（62）の胸腺においては原始T細胞が増多するからである。いずれの場合でも、外胚葉由来上皮細胞が内在する胸腺髄質の過形成や原始T細胞（$NK1.1^-TCR^{int}$細胞）が見られる (63, 64)。胸腺皮質（従来型T細胞分化が起こる）は、自己免疫疾患では、むしろ萎縮する。これらのことから、自己免疫疾患の免疫学状態は、従来型T細胞およびB細胞は免疫抑制性状態であるといえる。

自己抗体産生の他の状況

高齢者において、血清中の自己抗体価が高値を示すことが知られている (65-70)。そこで、百寿者において一本鎖DNA（抗核抗体）に対する血清中の自己抗体価を測定した (Fig. 5)。

Figure.5

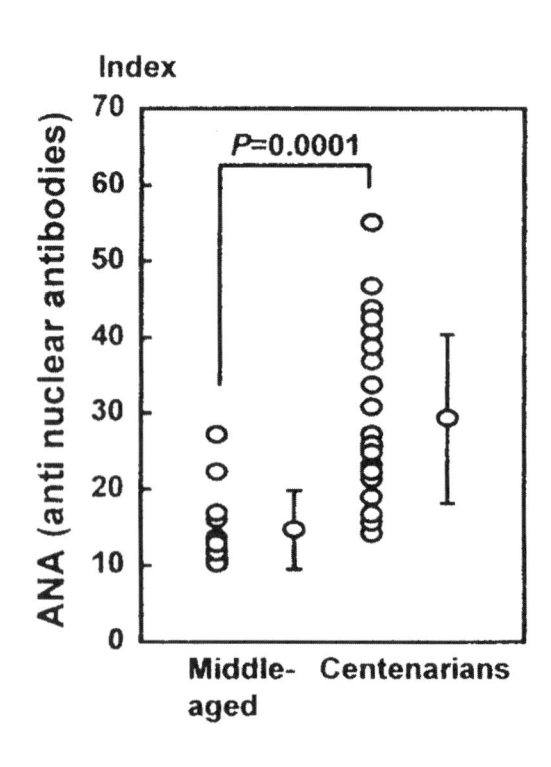

百寿者の血清中の変性DNAに対する自己抗体価が上昇した。百寿者（n=20）と壮年（n=8）を測定した。

百寿者において、DNAに対する自己抗体の高値が見られた。百寿者の末梢血でも胸腺外分化T細胞（CD56$^+$TとCD57$^+$T細胞）は高値を示した（71）。胸腺退縮した高齢者では、胸腺外分化T細胞と自己抗体産生B-1細胞の値の増加がその理由と結論づけられた。この状態は、自己免疫疾患の場合によく似ている。

慢性GVH病では、血清中の自己抗体高値が見られることも知られている（72-75）。そのうえ、胸腺外分化T細胞が、骨髄移植（BMT）を施した慢性GVH病マウスで増加することが明らかになった（11, 76, 77）。

この時、胸腺萎縮も、慢性GVH病のマウスでも見られた。ヒトにおいて、慢性GVH病の症状として、下痢、肝炎および分泌腺の炎症が見られることは知られている。これらの部所はすべて、胸腺外分化T細胞が主に存在する部所である。類似した症状が、自己免疫疾患において見られる。これらの事実はすべて、自己免疫疾患だけでなく慢性GVH病も自己応答性胸腺外分化T細胞の活性化が誘発していることを示す。

マラリア感染では、患者の多くに血清中の自己抗体価が高いという報告がある（78-82）。この事実を、マラリア感染したマウスを研究して確認した。胸腺外分化T細胞の活性化は、マラリア感染のマウスでも見られる（12, 28, 29）。これらの結果は、マラリア感染には、胸腺外分化T細胞と自己抗体産生B-1細胞が関連していることを示唆する。これらの原始リンパ球の自己応答性が、マラリア感染肝細胞や赤血球と相互に作用した結果、マラリアから身を守ると結論できる。ここでは、自己応答は、細胞内感染の防御に有益である。

激しいストレスと感染症による免疫抑制

一連の最近の研究において、従来型TとB細胞における免疫抑制と原始型T細胞とB細胞の相互免疫増強が、マウスとヒトにおいてどのように出現するか検証を行なった（83-88）。拘束ストレスを与えたマウスは激しい胸腺萎縮が誘導されると同時に、末梢で従来型のT細胞やB細胞の抑制が見られた（89）。このようなマウスでは、胸腺外分化T細胞の活性化や自己抗体産生が起こることも多い（90）。

この場合を考慮するならば、上述した免疫抑制により、ウイルス感染（例えば単純疱疹ウイルス、帯状疱疹ウイルス、EBウイルス、ヒトパピローマウイルスやパルボウイルス等の常在ウイルス）が出現する可能性がある。自己免疫疾患発症時に、強いストレスや感冒様の感染症を経験する患者は多い。

重要な証拠は他にもある。ストレスを与えたマウスでも自己免疫疾患患者［（関節リウマチ患者（RA）］でも末梢血中の顆粒球高値（顆粒急増多症）が出現した（Table I）。本表で示すように、顆粒球増多症だけのみならずリン

Table.I

RA患者の血液中の顆粒球増多とリンパ球減少 WBC＝白血球；RA＝関節リウマチ。

	n	No. of WBC (per mm^3)	Percentage	
			Granulocytes	Lymphocytes
Control	20	5620.0±423.3	58.0±3.4	33.2±3.1
RA：CRP$^+$	15	7707.7±621.4	71.7±2.7	20.9±2.2
RA：CRP$^-$	20	6228.6±550.3	60.4±3.8	31.2±4.5

WBC = White blood cells; RA = rheumatoid arthritis.

パ球減少症（主に従来型TとB細胞数の低下）も、RA患者の末梢血に見られた。活性が亢進した顆粒球は、スーパーオキシドを産生して組織や細胞を傷害することができる（91, 92）。このように炎症が起こっている時には、顆粒球だけでなくマクロファージが炎症性サイトカイン（IFNγ、TNFα、IL-1およびIL-6）を産生することが知られている。すべてのこれらの反応を、自己免疫疾患モデルマウスおよび自己免疫疾患もしくは膠原病患者において認めることができる。

最後に、ストレスと感染症が原因で、交感神経緊張とコルチゾール分泌が出現することを強調する必要がある。交感神経緊張と副腎皮質系の活性化により従来型T細胞とB細胞の免疫抑制や原始的T細胞とB細胞の相互の活性化が起こることは、広く知られている（93）。近年、SchwarzとCohenは以下のような推測を報告した。自己免疫応答そのものが、ストレスや感染症が原因である異常な自己細胞や異常な組織を排除する体にとって有益な反応である可能性がある（94）。さらに、原始T細胞およびB細胞が介在する適度な自己応答性が、生物をストレス、感染、細胞内感染症等の生体防御に重要である場面は多いと考えられる。

結論

自己免疫疾患における免疫学的状態は、系統発生の原始リンパ球である胸腺外分化T細胞の自己抗体産生B細胞の働きによるものである。強いストレスとストレスを受けたあとに起こる（ウイルス）感染が、原始リンパ球を活性化させ、自己免疫疾患の発症に関与していると考えられる。発症時、顆粒球は活性化状態である。顆粒球は組織傷害に関連する可能性があるが、組織傷害が起こった後に、自己応答する胸腺外分化T細胞や自己抗体産生B細胞の活性化が起こ

る可能性がある。従来型T細胞およびB細胞は、胸腺萎縮または退縮を伴う免疫抑制下で起こる。このような現象は、自己免疫疾患だけでなく加齢、慢性GVH病、マラリア感染等に見られる。

謝辞

本研究は、文部科学省科学研究費補助金によるものである。原稿浄書について金子裕子氏に感謝する。

Immunologic States of Autoimmune Diseases

Toru Abo[1]
Toshihiko Kawamura[1]
Hisami Watanabe[2]

[1]Department of Immunology, Niigata University School of Medicine, Niigata

[2]Division of Cellular and Molecular Immunology, Center of Molecular Biosciences, University of Ryukyus, Okinawa, Japan

Abstract

The etiology and immunologic states of autoimmune diseases have mainly been discussed without consideration of extrathymic T cells, which exist in the liver, intestine, and excretion glands. Because extrathymic T cells are autoreactive and are often simultaneously activated along with autoantibody-producing B-1 cells, these extrathymic T cells and B-1 cells should be introduced when considering the immunologic states of autoimmune diseases. The immunologic states of autoimmune diseases resemble those of aging, chronic GVH disease, and malarial infection. Namely, under all these conditions, conventional T and B cells are rather suppressed concomitant with thymic atrophy or involution. In contrast, extrathymic T cells and B-1 cells are inversely activated at this time. These facts suggest that the immunologic states of autoimmune diseases should be revaluated by introducing the concept of extrathymic T cells and autoantibody-producing B-1 cells, which might be primordial lymphocytes in phylogeny.

Key Words

Autoimmune disease
Extrathymic T cells
Autoreactivity
B-1 cells
Immunosuppression

Introduction

In addition to conventional T and B (B-2) cells, extrathymic T cells and autoantibody-producing B (B-1) cells have been studied in the past two decades *(1–4)*. In terms of phylogeny, conventional T and B cells are considered to have been generated for processing foreign antigens after living beings emerged onto land. Indeed, conventional T cells developed as part of a system to eliminate self-reactive forbidden clones in the thymus *(5–7)*. On the other hand, extrathymic T cells might constitute a more primitive (or primordial) immune system,

Correspondence to: Dr. T. Abo,
Department of Immunology,
Niigata University School of Medicine,
Niigata, 951-8510, Japan.
E-mail: immunol2@med.niigata-u.ac.jp

© 2005
Humana Press Inc.
0257–277X/05/
33/1:23–34/$30.00

which does not eliminate forbidden clones, but rather attacks abnormal or denatured self-cells *(8,9)*. However, too great an expansion of these extrathymic T cells and autoantibody-producing B cells may lead to the onset of certain autoimmune diseases *(10,11)*. Alternatively, appropriate expansion of extrathymic T cells may be important for protection against intracellular pathogens such as malaria *(12)*. Without introducing the concept of extrathymic T cells and autoantibody-producing B cells, the immunologic states during pregnancy, as well as those of many diseases such as autoimmune diseases, malarial infection, chronic graft versus host (GVH) disease, and malignancy cannot be properly understood.

Extrathymic T Cells and B-1 Cells

Major sites where extrathymic T cells exist are the intestine *(1,2)*, liver *(3,4)*, uterus *(13)*, joints *(14)*, and excretion glands *(15)*. These T cells are extremely few in the spleen and lymph nodes, where conventional T and B cells mainly exist. Conventional T cells are generated in the thymus, whereas conventional B cells are generated in the bone marrow. Because the thymus and bone marrow developed after living beings emerged onto land, it is easily speculated that more primordial sites for immune organs were the intestine, liver (which was developed from the intestine), and excretion glands (for example, the salivary glands, mandibular glands, and lacrimal glands). Another primordial site of the immune system is the peritoneal cavity, where B-1 cells are most abundant *(16,17)*. In any case, the autoreactive nature of extrathymic T cells and B-1 cells might be one of the properties of primordial lymphocytes. The most primordial lymphocytes are NK cells, which do not use T cell receptors (TCR), major histocompatibility complex (MHC) antigens, or immunoglobulins (Ig).

In the case of mice, self-reactive forbidden clones among T cells can be identified by the use of specific Vβs (against the endogenous superantigen Mls). Indeed, self-reactive forbidden clones are eliminated by a process of negative selection in the mainstream of T-cell differentiation in the thymus *(5–7)*. Other studies have revealed that such autoreactive Vβs are mainly present on extrathymic T cells but not on conventional T cells *(8,9)*. Other evidence is that extrathymic T cells and autoantibody-producing B-1 cells are often activated simultaneously *(10–12)*. For example, when denatured liver tissues are injected into mice, both extrathymic T cells and B-1 cells are activated in the liver and peritoneal cavity, respectively. These lymphocytes might be important for the elimination of denatured self-cells, at which time, thymic atrophy always occurs. In other words, conventional T cells and extrathymic T cells are reciprocally activated. This immunosuppression is often accompanied by granulocytosis.

An Alternative Intrathymic Pathway of T Cell Differentiation

The mainstream of T cell differentiation pathway lies in the thymus (Fig. 1). The major differentiation area of this pathway is the cortex, and many immature T cells with double-positive phenotype (TCR^{dull}CD4$^+$8$^+$), which are derived from precursors (TCR$^-$CD4$^-$8$^-$), undergo apoptosis, while only a small proportion of such cells become mature T cells (TCR^{high}CD4$^+$ or TCR^{high}CD8$^+$). During apoptosis, self-reactive forbidden clones are eliminated by interaction with the complex of self-antigens and MHC. Mature T cells are then distributed to the peripheral immune organs.

In addition to the mainstream of T-cell differentiation, it was found that there is an alternative intrathymic pathway of T cell dif-

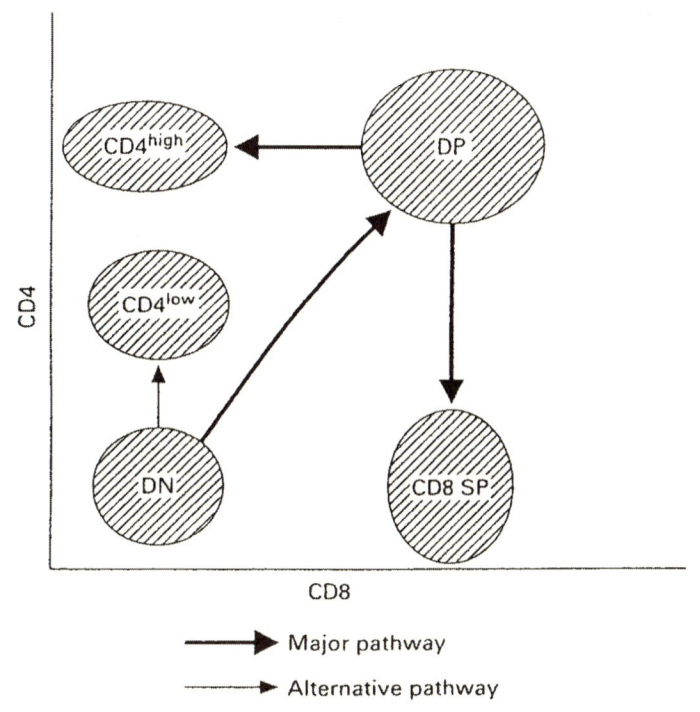

Fig. 1. Schema of the major pathway (mainstream) and alternative pathway of T cell differentiation in the thymus. The thymus comprises both the major pathway (the mainstream) and an alternative pathway of T cell differentiation.

ferentiation in the thymus (Fig. 1). The major area of this alternative pathway is the medulla (8,9). As shown in this figure, the precursors of this population directly become CD4^{low}NK1.1$^+$TCR^{int} cells (i.e., NKT cells). The other half population becomes double-negative (CD4$^-$8$^-$) NK1.1$^-$TCR^{int} cells. Under normal conditions in young mice, lymphocytes (TCR^{int}IL-2Rβ^+) belonging to this alternative pathway constitute only 1–2% of the total number of thymic lymphocytes. However, this proportion increases when the thymus becomes atrophic because TCR^{int}IL-2Rβ^+ cells are stress-resistant (8).

The phenotype of TCR^{int}IL-2Rβ^+ (NK1.1$^+$ or NK1.1$^-$) cells generated through the alternative intrathymic pathway resembles that of extrathymic T cells that exist in the liver. It is speculated that TCR^{int} cells in both the thymus and liver are primordial T cells in phylogeny. The thymic medulla contains ectodermal epithelial cells because of their origin in the gill cleft, whereas the thymic cortex contains endodermal epithelial cells because of their origin in the gill itself (18). The gill cleft might carry primordial lymphocytes which exist in the skin (ectoderm). Therefore, the thymic medulla still contains primordial lymphocytes, similar to the case of the liver as well as the intestine.

Relationships between NK1.1$^-$TCR^{int} Cells and NK1.1$^+$TCR^{int} Cells

TCR^{int}IL-2Rβ^+ cells that exist in both the liver and the thymus contain the subsets NK1.1$^+$

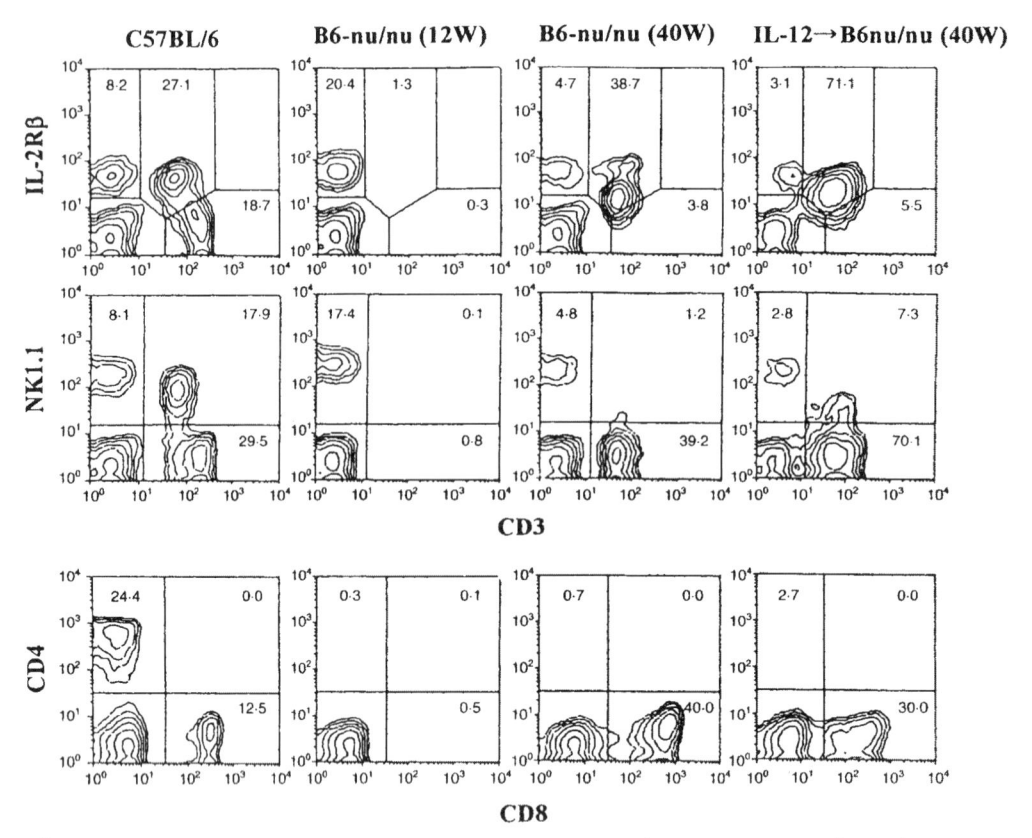

Fig. 2. T cells seen in athymic nude mice are NK1.1⁻TCR^{int} cells. All IL-2Rβ⁺CD3^{int} cells were NK1.1⁻CD8⁺. By IL-12 injection, a small proportion of NK1.1⁺CD3^{int} cells appeared in the liver. However, these T cells were unconventional NKT cells expressing CD8.

and NK1.1⁻ *(19)*. In other words, TCR^{int}IL-2Rβ⁺ cells are a half-and-half mixture of NK1.1⁺TCR^{int} subsets and NK1.1⁻TCR^{int} subsets. Interestingly, congenitally athymic nude mice carry only NK1.1⁻TCR^{int} cells (Fig. 2). TCR^{int}IL-2Rβ⁺ cells expand with aging or by IL-12 injection. However, all these T cells are NK1.1⁻TCR^{int} cells. There is a small population of NK1.1⁺TCR^{int} cells in athymic mice injected with IL-12. These NKT cells are all CD8⁺, namely, they are not conventional NKT cells with CD4⁺ phenotype and usage of Vα14Jα281 *(20)*. Subsequent study has revealed that NK1.1⁺TCR^{int} cells (i.e., NKT cells) and their precursors are generated in the thymus *(21–24)*. However, adult thymectomy was not found to decrease the number of NKT cells in the liver *(25)*. It is conceivable that the precursors of NKT cells home to the liver at the neonatal stage and that NKT cells are generated from such precursors in the liver at the adult stage.

All NK cells, NKT cells, and NK1.1⁻TCR^{int} cells are autoreactive against malignant tumors *(26,27)*, malarial-infected hepatocytes *(12,28, 29)*, and denatured self-cells *(10)*. NK cells mediate autoreactivity against MHC⁻ self-cells (or missing self). NKT cells are known to recognize certain glycolipid antigens (e.g., α-glactosylceramide) *(30–32)*. On the other hand, NK1.1⁻TCR^{int} cells mediate their cytotoxicity regenerating hepatocytes and autologous thymocytes *(33, 34)*. It is speculated that all these primordial lymphocytes are important for the elimination of abnormal self-cells or regenerating self-cells as "innate immunity." If NKT cells interact with proliferating conventional T cells, such NKT cells may act as regulatory lymphocytes as shown in certain autoimmune disease models *(35–40)*.

Intestinal T Cells

Primarily, primordial lymphocytes are considered to have been phylogenetically generated in the digestive tract and the skin *(18)*. Lymphocytes that developed in the upper digestive tract (i.e., the gills) became conventional T cells in the thymus, while those which developed in the lower digestive tract (i.e., the intestine and liver) became intestinal T cells and hepatic T cells. There are similarities and also differences in nature between intestinal T cells and hepatic T cells, despite both being extrathymic T cells. In mice, intestinal T cells carry TCR^{high} and lack NK1.1 antigen *(41–47)*. They are a mixture of IL-2Rβ⁺ and IL-2Rβ⁻. In the small intestine of mice, the majority of IL-2Rβ⁺T cells are γδT cells, while the majority of IL-2Rβ⁻T cells are αβT cells.

The large intestine *(48)* and appendix *(49)* carry unique subsets of extrathymic T cells in mice. There are unconventional NKT cells in the large intestine, including NK1.1⁺CD8⁺T cells (they lack the usage of Vα14Jα281 seen in conventional NKT cells). There are B220⁺T cells in the appendix. In the case of humans, extrathymic T cells can be identified as CD56⁺T cells, CD57⁺T cells, or CD161⁺T cells *(50–57)*. In other words, extrathymic T cells express an NK marker on the cell surface. CD56⁺T cells are abundant in the liver *(56,57)*, CD57⁺T cells are abundant in the bone marrow *(58–60)* and joints *(14)*, and CD161⁺T cells are abundant in the intestine *(54)* of humans.

Autoimmune Diseases

Autoimmune diseases are known to be characterized by an elevated level of autoantibodies in sera. In addition to autoantibodies, extrathymic T cells (e.g., CD57⁺T cells) are simultaneously elevated in humans *(52)*. In the case of mice, extrathymic T cells (NKT cells in this case) and B-1 cells are also activated as shown in a model of autoimmune NZB/W F$_1$ mice (Fig. 3). After the onset of disease (i.e., proteinuria), the proportion and absolute number of NKT cells expanded in the liver (indicated by arrowheads). At this time, thymic atrophy or thymic involution occurred (Fig. 4). In sharp contrast, the number of primordial lymphocytes expanded in the liver, spleen, and peritoneal cavity (PEC) (B-1 cells in this site). All these findings suggest that primordial T and B cells are under activated conditions but that conventional T and B cells are inversely under suppressive conditions in autoimmune diseases *(11)*.

A question is raised as to why thymic hyperplasia is seen in certain autoimmune diseases such as myasthenia gravis (MG) (in humans) and MRL-*lpr/lpr* autoimmune diseases in mice (in mice). This is due to the expansion of primordial T cells in the thymus in patients with MG *(61)* and in MRL-*lpr/lpr* mice *(62)*. In both cases, there is hyperplasia of the thymic medulla, where ectodermal epithelial cells exist, and primordial T cells (e.g., NK1.1⁻TCR^{int} cells) are expanding *(63,64)*. The cortex area, where the differentiations of conventional T cells occur, becomes rather atrophic in these diseases. Taken together, the

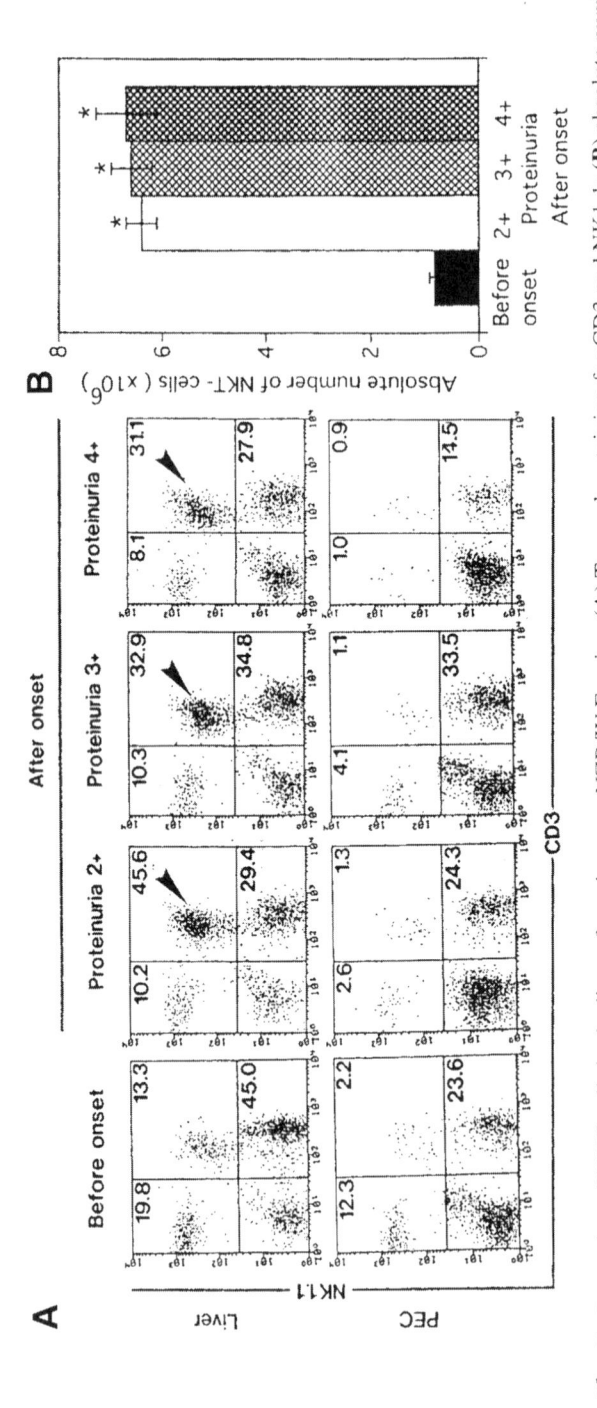

Fig. 3. Expansion of NKT cells in the liver of autoimmune NZB/W F_1 mice. **(A)** Two-color staining for CD3 and NK1.1; **(B)** absolute number of NKT cells. After the onset of disease, NKT cells (CD4$^+$Vα14Jα281$^+$) expanded in the liver.

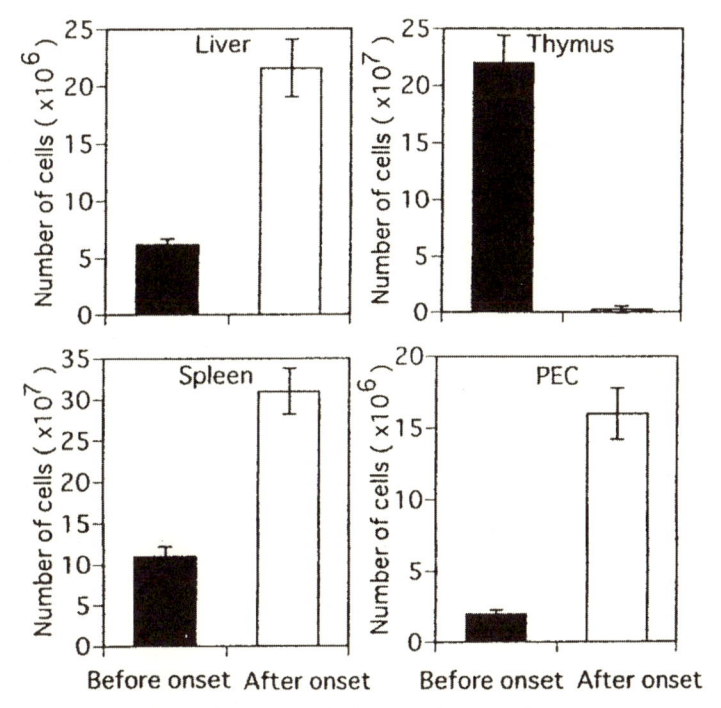

Fig. 4. Thymic atrophy seen in autoimmune NZB/W F_1 mice after the onset of disease. After the onset of disease, the number of lymphocytes in the liver and peritoneal cavity increased. In sharp contrast, the number of thymocytes decreased prominently.

immunologic states of autoimmune diseases are under immunosuppressive conditions of conventional T and B cells.

Other Conditions of Autoantibody Production

It is known that elderly people show elevated levels of autoantibodies in sera *(65–70)*. In this regard, the serum level of autoantibody against single-stranded DNA (i.e., anti-nuclear antibody) was measured in centenarians (Fig. 5). The elevated level of autoantibodies against DNA was demonstrated in centenarians. As already reported, centenarians also show the elevated level of extrathymic T cells (CD56$^+$T and CD57$^+$T cells) in the peripheral blood *(71)*. It is concluded that elderly people with thymic involution have elevated levels of

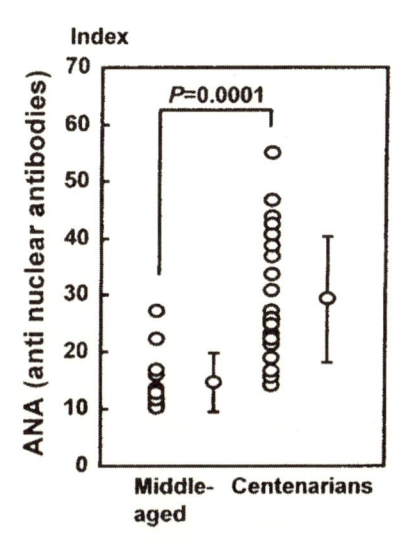

Fig. 5. Increased levels of autoantibodies against denatured DNA in sera of centenarian. Centenarians (*n*=20) and middle-aged persons (*n*=8) were examined.

extrathymic T cells and autoantibody-producing B-1 cells. This condition is quite similar to that of autoimmune diseases.

Chronic GVH disease is also known to show an elevated level of autoantibodies in sera *(72–75)*. In addition, extrathymic T cells have been found to expand in mice with chronic GVH disease after bone marrow transplantation (BMT) *(11,76,77)*. At such time, thymic atrophy was also seen in mice with chronic GVH disease. In humans, symptoms of chronic GVH disease are known to include diarrhea, hepatitis, and inflammation of excretion glands. All these sites are areas where extrathymic T cells are primarily present. Similar symptoms are observed in the case of autoimmune diseases. All these facts indicate that not only autoimmune diseases but also chronic GVH diseases are induced by the activation of autoreactive extrathymic T cells.

In the case of malarial infection, it has been reported that many patients show an elevated level of autoantibodies in sera *(78–82)*. This fact was confirmed in mice infected with malaria in our studies. The activation of extrathymic T cells is also found in mice with malarial infection *(12,28,29)*. These results suggest that malarial infection is also an event involving extrathymic T cells and autoantibody-producing B-1 cells. It is concluded that the autoreactivity of these primordial lymphocytes interacts with malaria-infected hepatocytes and erythrocytes and results in protection from malaria. Autoreactivity is beneficial for protection against intracellular infection in this case.

Immunosuppression by Severe Stress and Infections

In a series of recent studies *(83–88)*, we have investigated how the immunosuppression of conventional T and B cells and the reciprocal immunopotentiation of primordial T and B cells are induced in mice and humans. Restriction stress of mice induces severe thymic atrophy and simultaneous suppression of conventional T and B cells in the periphery *(89)*. At such time, the activation of extrathymic T cells and autoantibody production often occur in these mice *(90)*.

If we consider the case of humans, the above-mentioned immunosuppression might result in viral infections (possibly, resident viruses such as Herpes simplex virus, Hepes zoster virus, EB virus, human papilloma virus, or parvovirus). Many patients with autoimmune diseases experience severe stress and common cold-like infections at the onset of disease.

Other important evidence is that mice exposed to stress and many patients with autoimmune diseases show elevated levels of granulocytes (i.e., granulocytosis) in the peripheral blood [e.g., patients with rheumatoid arthritis (RA)] (Table 1). As shown in this table, lymphocytopenia (namely, decreased levels of conventional T and B cells) as well as granulocytosis were seen in the peripheral blood of RA patients. The overactivated granulocytes have the ability to damage tissues or cells via their production of superoxides *(91,92)*. Under these inflammatory conditions, macrophages as well as granulocytes are known to produce inflammatory cytokines such as IFNγ, TNFα, IL-1, and IL-6. All these responses are seen in autoimmune-prone mice and patients with autoimmune diseases or collagen diseases.

Finally, it should be emphasized that stress and infections induce sympathetic nerve activation and the secretion of cortisols. It is well-established that these autonomic nervous conditions and the activation of the adrenocortical axis accompany the immunosuppression of conventional T and B cells and the reciprocal activation of primordial T and B cells *(93)*. In a recent report, Schwarz and Cohen speculate that the autoimmune response itself may be

Table 1. Granulocytosis and Lymphocytopenia in the Blood of RA Patients

	n	No. of WBC (per mm³)	Percentage Granulocytes	Lymphocytes
Control	20	5620.0±423.3	58.0±3.4	33.2±3.1
RA:CRP⁺	15	7707.7±621.4	71.7±2.7	20.9±2.2
RA:CRP⁻	20	6228.6±550.3	60.4±3.8	31.2±4.5

WBC = white blood cells; RA = rheumatoid arthritis.

a beneficial reaction in the body to eliminate abnormal self-cells or abnormal tissues, which are induced by stress and infections (94). We also consider that an appropriate level of autoreactivity mediated by primordial T and B cells is often essential to protect living beings from stress, infection, intracellular infections, and so on.

Conclusions

The immunologic states of autoimmune diseases are events of extrathymic T cells and autoantibody-producing B cells that may be primordial lymphocytes in phylogeny. It is conceivable that severe stress and subsequent (viral) infections are associated with the onset of autoimmune diseases via the activation of primordial lymphocytes. At such time, granulocytes are also in an activated state. Granulocytes may be related to tissue damage and such damaged tissues may then induce the activation of autoreactive extrathymic T cells and autoantibody-producing B cells. Conventional T and B cells are under conditions of immunosuppression accompanying thymic atrophy or involution. Similar phenomena are seen in not only autoimmune diseases but also aging, chronic GVH disease, malarial infection, and so on.

Acknowledgments

This work was supported by a Grant-in-Aid for Scientific Research from the Ministry of Education, Science and Culture, Japan. The authors wish to thank Mrs. Yuko Kaneko for preparation of the manuscript.

References

1. Guy-Grand D, Cerf-Bensussan N, Malissen B, Malassis-Seris M, Briottet C, Vassalli P: Two gut intraepithelial CD8⁺ lymphocyte populations with different T cell receptors: a role for the gut epithelium in T cell differentiation. J Exp Med 1991;173:471.
2. Rocha B, Vassalli P, Guy-Grand D: The V beta repertoire of mouse gut homodimeric alpha CD8⁺ intraepithelial T cell receptor alpha/beta + lymphocytes reveals a major extrathymic pathway of T cell differentiation. J Exp Med 1991;173:483.
3. Abo T, Ohteki T, Seki S, et al.: The appearance of T cells bearing self-reactive T cell receptor in the livers of mice injected with bacteria. J Exp Med 1991;174:417.
4. Sato K, Ohtsuka K, Hasegawa K, et al.: Evidence for extrathymic generation of intermediate T cell receptor cells in the liver revealed in thymectomized, irradiated mice subjected to bone marrow transplantation. J Exp Med 1995;182:759.
5. Kappler JW, Roehm N, Marrack P: T cell tolerance by clonal elimination in the thymus. Cell 1987;49:273–280.
6. MacDonald HR, Schneider R, Lees RK, et al.: T-cell receptor V beta use predicts reactivity and tolerance to Mlsa-encoded antigens. Nature 1988;332:40.
7. Finkel TH, Cambier JC, Kubo RT, Born WK, Marrack P, Kappler JW: The thymus has two functionally distinct populations of immature alpha beta⁺ T cells: one popu-

lation is deleted by ligation of alpha beta TCR. Cell 1989;58:1047.
8. Kawachi Y, Watanabe H, Moroda T, et al.: Self-reactive T cell clones in a restricted population of interleukin-2 receptor β^+ cells expressing intermediate levels of the T cell receptor in the liver and other immune organs. Eur J Immunol 1995;25:2272.
9. Moroda T, Iiai T, Kawachi Y, Kawamura T, Hatakeyama K, Abo T: Restricted appearance of self-reactive clones into intermediate T cell receptor cells in neonatally thymectomized mice with autoimmune disease. Eur J Immunol 1996;26:3084.
10. Naito T, Kawamura T, Bannai M, et al.: Simultaneous activation of natural killer T cells and autoantibody production in mice injected with denatured syngeneic liver tissue. Clin Exp Immunol 2002;129:397.
11. Morshed SRM, Mannoor K, Halder RC, et al.: Tissue-specific expansion of NKT and CD5$^+$B cells at the onset of autoimmune disease in (NZB × NZW)F$_1$ mice. Eur J Immunol 2002;32:2551.
12. Mannoor MK, Halder RC, Morshed SRM, et al.: Essential role of extrathymic T cells in protection against malaria. J Immunol 2002;169:301.
13. Wang S, Li C, Kawamura H, Watanabe H, Abo T: Unique sensitivity to α-galactosylceramide of NKT cells in the uterus. Cell Immunol 2002;215:98.
14. Arai K, Yamamura S, Hanyu T, et al.: Extrathymic differentiation of resident T cells in the joints of mice with collagen-induced arthritis. J Immunol 1996;157:5170.
15. Narita J, Kawamura T, Miyaji C, et al.: Abundance of NKT cells in the salivary glands but absence thereof in the liver and thymus of *aly/aly* mice with Sjögren syndrome. Cell Immunol 1999;192:149.
16. Kantor AB, Merrill CE, Herzenberg LA, Hillson JL: An unbiased analysis of V[H]-D-J[H] sequences from B-1a, B-1b, and conventional B cells. J Immunol 1997;158:1175.
17. Ochi H, Takeshita H, Suda T, Nisitani S, Honjo T, Watanabe T: Regulation of B-1 cell activation and its autoantibody production by Lyn kinase-regulated signallings. Immunology 1999;98:595.
18. Abo T, Watanabe H, Sato K, et al.: Extrathymic T cells stand at an intermediate phylogenetic position between natural killer cells and thymus-derived T cells. Nat Immun 1995;14:173.
19. Watanabe H, Miyaji C, Kawachi Y, et al.: Relationships between intermediate TCR cells and NK1.1$^+$T cells in various immune organs. NK1.1$^+$T cells are present within a population of intermediate TCR cells. J Immunol 1995;155:2972.
20. Maruyama S, Tsukahara A, Suzuki S, et al.: Quick recovery in the generation of self-reactive CD4^{low} NKT cells by an alternative intrathymic pathway when restored from acute thymic atrophy. Clin Exp Immunol 1999;117:587.
21. Emoto M, Mittrücker H-W, Schmits R, Mak TW, Kaufmann SHE: Critical role of leukocyte function-associated antigen-1 in liver accumulation of CD4$^+$NKT cells. J Immunol 1995;162:5094.
22. Hammond K, Cain W, Van Driel I, Godfrey D: Three day neonatal thymectomy selectively depletes NK1.1$^+$T cells. Int Immunol 1998;10:1491.
23. Tilloy F, Di Santo JP, Bendelac A, Lantz O: Thymic dependence of invariant Vα14$^+$ natural killer-T cell development. Eur J Immunol 1999;29:3313.
24. Coles MC, Raulet DH: NK1.1$^+$T cells in the liver arise in the thymus and are selected by interactions with class I molecules on CD4$^+$CD8$^+$ cells. J Immunol 2000;164:2412.
25. Kameyama H, Kawamura T, Naito T, et al.: Size of the population of CD4$^+$ natural killer T cells in the liver is maintained without supply by the thymus during adult life. Immunology 2001;104:135.
26. Minagawa M, Oya H, Yamamoto S, et al.: Intensive expansion of natural killer T cells in the early phase of hepatocyte regeneration after partial hepatectomy in mice and its association with sympathetic nerve activation. Hepatology 2000;31:907.
27. Miyaji C, Watanabe H, Miyakawa R, et al.: Identification of effector cells for TNFα-mediated cytotoxicity against WEHI164S cells. Cell Immunol 2002;216:43.
28. Weerasinghe A, Sekikawa H, Watanabe H, et al.: Association of intermediate T cell receptor cells, mainly their NK1.1$^-$ subset, with protection from malaria. Cell Immunol 2001;207:28.
29. Mannoor MK, Weerasinghe A, Halder RC, et al.: Resistance to malarial infection is achieved by the cooperation of NK1.1$^+$ and NK1.1$^-$ subsets of intermediate TCR cells which are constituents of innate immunity. Cell Immunol 2001;211:96.
30. Kawano T, Junqing C, Koezuka Y, et al.: CD1d-restricted and TCR-mediated activation of Vα14 NKT cells by glycosylceramides. Science 1997;278:1626.
31. Burdin N, Brossary L, Koezuka Y, et al.: Selective ability of mouse CD1 to present glycolipids: α-Galactosylceramide specifically stimulates Vα14$^+$NK T lymphocytes. J Immunol 1998;161:3271.
32. Brossary L, Naidenko O, Burdin N, Matsuda J, Sakai T, Kronenberg M: Structural requirements for galactosylceramide recognition by CD1-restricted NK T cells. J Immunol 1998;161:5124.
33. Osman Y, Kawamura T, Naito T, et al.: Activation of hepatic NKT cells and subsequent liver injury following administration of α-galactosylceramide. Eur J Immunol 2000;30:1919.
34. Kawabe S, Abe T, Kawamura H, Gejyo F, Abo T: Generation of B220^{low} B cells and production of autoantibodies in mice with experimental amyloidosis: association of primordial T cells with this phenomenon. Clin Exp Immunol 2004;135:200.
35. Segal BM, Shevach EM: IL-12 unmasks latent autoimmune disease in resistant mice. J Exp Med 1996;184:771.
36. Takeda K, Dennert G: The development of autoimmunity in C57BL/6 1pr mice correlated with the disappearance of natural killer type 1-positive cells: evidence of their suppressive action on bone marrow stem cell proliferation, B cell immunoglobulin secretion, and autoimmune symptoms. J Exp Med 1993;177:155.

37. Wilson SB, Kent SC, Patton KT, et al.: Extreme Th1 bias of invariant Valpha24JalphaQ T cells in type 1 diabetes. Nature 1998;391:177.
38. Godfrey DI, Kinder SJ, Silvera P, Baxter AG: Flow cytometric study of T cell development in NOD mice reveals a deficiency in αβTCR$^+$CD4$^-$CD8$^-$ thymocytes. J Autoimmun 1997;10:279.
39. Baxter AG, Kinder SJ, Hammond KJ, Scollay R, Godfrey DI: Association between αβTCR$^+$CD4$^-$CD8$^-$ T-cell deficiency and IDDM in NOD/Lt mice. Diabetes 1997;46:572.
40. Lehuen A, Lantz O, Beaudoin L, et al.: Overexpression of natural killer T cells protects Vα14-Jα281 transgenic nonobese diabetic mice against diabetes. J Exp Med 1998;188:1831.
41. Ferguson A: Intraepithelial lymphocytes of the small intestine. Gut 1977;18:921.
42. Guy-Grand D, Griscelli C, Vassalli P: The mouse gut T lymphocyte, a novel type of T cell. J Exp Med 1978;148:1661.
43. De Geus B, Van den Enden M, Coolen C, Nagelkerken L, Van der Heijden P, Rozing J: Phenotype of intraepithelial lymphocytes in euthymic and athymic mice: implications for differentiation of cells bearing a CD3-associated γδ T cell receptor. Eur J Immunol 1990;20:291.
44. Bandeira A, Itohara S, Bonneville M, et al.: Extrathymic origin of intestinal intraepithelial lymphocytes bearing T-cell antigen receptor γδ. Proc Natl Acad Sci USA 1991;88:43.
45. Rocha B, Vassali P, Guy-Grand D: The extrathymic T-cell development pathway. Immunol Today 1992;13:449.
46. Ohtsuka K, Iiai T, Watanabe H, et al.: Similarities and differences between extrathymic T cells residing in mouse liver and intestine. Cell Immunol 1994;153:52.
47. Ohtsuka K, Hasegawa K, Yamagiwa S, et al.: Intraepithelial lymphocytes in colon have similar properties to intraepithelial lymphocytes in small intestine and hepatic intermediate TCR cells. Digest Dis Sci 1996;41:902.
48. Bannai M, Kawamura T, Naito T, et al.: Abundance of unconventional CD8$^+$ natural killer T cells in the large intestine. Eur J Immunol 2001;31:3361.
49. Yamagiwa S, Sugahara S, Shimizu T, et al.: The primary site of CD4$^-$8$^-$B220$^+$ T cells in lpr mice: the appendix in normal mice. J Immunol 1998;160:2665.
50. Takii Y, Hashimoto S, Iiai T, Watanabe H, Hatakeyama K, Abo T: Increase in the proportion of granulated CD56$^+$T cells in patients with malignancy. Clin Exp Immunol 1994;97:522.
51. Okada T, Iiai T, Kawachi Y, et al.: Origin of CD57$^+$ T cells which increase at tumour sites in patients with colorectal cancer. Clin Exp Immunol 1995;102:159.
52. Arai K, Yamamura S, Seki S, Hanyu T, Takahashi HE, Abo T: Increase of CD57$^+$ T cells in knee joints and adjacent bone marrow of rheumatoid arthritis (RA) patients: implication for an anti-inflammatory role. Clin Exp Immunol 1998;111:345.
53. Miyaji C, Watanabe H, Toma H, et al.: Functional alteration of granulocytes, NK cells, and natural killer T cells in centenarians. Human Immunol 2000;61:908.
54. Iiai T, Watanabe H, Suda T, Okamoto H, Abo T, Hatakeyama K: CD161$^+$ T (NT) cells exist predominantly in human intestinal epithelium as well as in liver. Clin Exp Immunol 2002;129:92.
55. Watanabe H, Weerasinghe A, Miyaji C, et al.: Expansion of unconventional T cells with natural killer markers in malaria patients. Parasitol Int 2003;52:61.
56. Norris S, Collins C, Doherty DG, et al.: Resident hepatic lymphocytes are phenotypically different from circulating lymphocytes. J Hepatol 1998;28:84.
57. Doherty DG, Norris S, Madrigal-Estebas L, et al.: The human liver contains multiple populations of NK cells, T cells, and CD3$^+$CD56$^+$ natural T cells with distinct cytotoxic activities and Th1, Th2, and Th0 cytokine secretion patterns. J Immunol 1999;163:2314.
58. Hilbe W, Eisterer W, Schmid C, et al.: Bone marrow lymphocyte subsets in myelodysplastic syndromes. J Clin Pathol 1994;47:505.
59. Gorochov G, Debre P, Leblond V, Sadat-Sowti B, Sigaux F, Autran B: Oligoclonal expansion of CD8$^+$CD57$^+$ T cells with restricted T-cell receptor β chain variability after bone marrow transplantation. Blood 1994;83:587.
60. Autran B, Leblond V, Sadat-Sowti B, et al.: A soluble factor released by CD8$^+$CD57$^+$ lymphocytes from bone marrow transplanted patients inhibits cell-mediated cytolysis. Blood 1991;77:2237.
61. Tsuchida M, Hashimoto M, Abo T, Miyamura H, Hirano T, Eguchi S: CD5$^+$B cells in the thymus of patients with myasthenia gravis. Biomed Res 1993;14:19.
62. Ohteki T, Seki S, Abo T, Kumagai K: Liver is a possible site for the proliferation of abnormal CD3$^+$4$^-$8$^-$ double-negative lymphocytes in autoimmune MRL-lpr/lpr mice. J Exp Med 1990;172:7.
63. Iiai T, Kimura M, Kawachi Y, et al.: Characterization of intermediate T-cell-receptor cells expanding in the liver, thymus and other organs in autoimmune lpr mice: parallel analysis with their normal counterparts. Immunology 1995;85:601.
64. Yamagiwa S, Kuwano Y, Hasegawa K, et al.: Existence of a small population of IL-2Rβ^{hi} TCR^{int}cells in SCG and MRL-lpr/lpr mice which produce normal Fas mRNA and Fas molecules from the lpr gene. Eur J Immunol 1996;26:1409.
65. Xavier RM, Yamauchi Y, Nakamura M, et al.: Antinuclear antibodies in healthy aging people: a prospective study. Mech Ageing Dev 1995;78:145.
66. Tomer Y, Shoenfeld Y: Ageing and autoantibodies. Autoimmunity 1988;1:141.
67. Rose NR: Thymus function, ageing and autoimmunity. Immunol Lett 1994;40:225.
68. Brill S, Globerson A: Autoimmunity and aging. Isr J Med Sci 1988;24:732.
69. Kay MM: Autoimmunity and aging. Concepts Immunopathol 1988;6:166.
70. Tomer Y, Shoenfeld Y: The significance of natural autoantibodies. Immunol Invest 1988;17:389.
71. Miyaji C, Watanabe H, Toma H, et al.: Functional alteration of granulocytes, NK cells, and natural killer T cells in centenarians. Human Immunol 2000;61:908.

72. Gleichmann E, Pals ST, Rolink AG, Radaszkiewicz T, Gleichmann H: Graft-versus-host reactions: clues to the etiopathology of a spectrum of immunological diseases. Immunol Today 1984;5:324.
73. Via CS, Shearer GM: T-cell interactions in autoimmunity: insights from a murine model of graft-versus-host disease. Immunol Today 1988;9:207.
74. Meyers CM, Tomaszewski JE, Glass JD, Chen CW: The nephritogenic T cell response in murine chronic graft-versus-host disease. J Immunol 1998;161:5321.
75. Okamoto I, Kohno K, Tanimoto T, et al.: IL-18 prevents the development of chronic graft-versus-host disease in mice. J Immunol 2000;164:6067.
76. Kawamura T, Kawachi Y, Kuwano Y, et al.: Mechanisms involved in Graft-versus-Host disease induced by the disparity of minor histocompatibility Mls antigens. Scand J Immunol 1999;49:258.
77. Halder RC, Kawamura T, Bannai M, et al.: Intensive generation of NK1.1⁻ extrathymic T cells in the liver by injection of bone marrow cells isolated from mice with a mutation of polymorphic major histocompatiblity complex antigens. Immunology 2001;102:450.
78. Wenisch C, Wenisch H, Bankl HC, et al.: Detection of anti-neutrophil cytoplasmic antibodies after acute *Plasmodium falciparum* malaria. Clin Diagn Lab Immunol 1996;3:132.
79. Lloyd CM, Collins I, Belcher AJ, Manuelpillai N, Wozencraft AO, Staines NA: Characterization and pathological significance of monoclonal DNA-binding antibodies from mice with experimental malaria infection. Infect Immun 1994;62:1982.
80. Ribeiro CD, Alfred C, Monjour L, Gentilini M: Normal frequency of anti-thyroglobulin antibodies in hyperendemic areas of malaria: relevance to the understanding of autoantibody formation in malaria. Trop Geogr Med 1984;36:323.
81. Kataaha PK, Facer CA, Mortazavi-Milani SM, Stierle H, Holborow EJ: Stimulation of autoantibody production in normal blood lymphocytes by malaria culture supernatants. Parasite Immunol 1984;6:481.
82. Ribeiro CT, De Roquefeuil S, Druilhe P, Monjour L, Homberg JC, Gentilini M: Abnormal anti-single stranded (ss) DNA activity in sera from *Plasmodium falciparum* infected individuals. Trans R Soc Trop Med Hyg 1984;78:742.
83. Kawamura T, Toyabe S, Moroda T, et al.: Neonatal granulocytosis is a postpartum event which is seen in the liver as well as in the blood. Hepatology 1997;26:1567.
84. Maruyama S, Minagawa M, Shimizu T, et al.: Administration of glucocorticoids markedly increases the numbers of granulocytes and extrathymic T cells in the bone marrow. Cell Immunol 1999;194:28.
85. Shimizu T, Kawamura T, Miyaji T, et al.: Resistance of extrathymic T cells to stress and the role of endogenous glucocorticoids in stress associated immuno suppression. Scand J Immunol 2000;51:285.
86. Abo T, Kawamura T, Watanabe H: Physiological responses of extrathymic T cells in the liver. Immunol Rev 2000;174:135.
87. Minagawa M, Oya H, Yamamoto S, et al.: Intensive expansion of natural killer T cells in the early phase of hepatocyte regeneration after partial hepatectomy in mice and its association with sympathetic nerve activation. Hepatology 2000;31:907.
88. Oya H, Kawamura T, Shimizu T, et al.: The differential effect of stress on natural killer T and NK cell function. Clin Exp Immunol 2000;121:384.
89. Kato T, Sato Y, Takahashi S, Kawamura H, Hatakeyama K, Abo T: Involvement of natural killer T cells and granulocytes in the inflammation induced by partial hepatectomy. J Hepatol 2004;40:285.
90. Kawabe S, Abe T, Kawamura H, Gejyo F, Abo T: Generation of B220^{low} B cells and production of autoantibodies in mice with experimental amyloidosis: association of primordial T cells with this phenomenon. Clin Exp Immunol 2004;135:200.
91. Tsukahara A, Tada T, Suzuki S, et al.: Adrenergic stimulation simultaneously induces the expansion of granulocytes and extrathymic T cells in mice. Biomed Res 1997;18:237.
92. Kawamura T, Miyaji C, Toyabe S, Fukuda M, Watanabe H, Abo T: Suppressive effect of anti ulcer agents on granulocytes—a role for granulocytes in gastric ulcer formation. Digest Dis Sci 2000;45:1786.
93. Kato T, Sato Y, Takahashi S, Kawamura H, Hatakeyama K, Abo T: Involvement of natural killer T cells and granulocytes in the inflammation induced by partial hepatectomy. J Hepatol 2004;40:285.
94. Schwartz M, Cohen IR: Autoimmunity can benefit self-maintenance. Immunol Today 2000;21:265.

PROTECTION AGAINST MALARIA DUE TO INNATE IMMUNITY ENHANCED BY LOW-PROTEIN DIET

低蛋白餌が自然免疫による
マラリア防御を強化する

Journal of Parasitology, 92: 531-538, 2006

chapter **19**

PROTECTION AGAINST MALARIA DUE TO INNATE IMMUNITY ENHANCED BY LOW-PROTEIN DIET

低蛋白餌が自然免疫によるマラリア防御を強化する

Anoja Ariyasinghe, Sufi Reza M. Morshed, M. Kaiissar Mannoor, Hanaa Y. Bakir, Hiroki Kawamura, Chikako Miyaji, Toru Nagura, Toshihiko Kawamura, Hisami Watanabe*, Hiroho Sekikawa, and Toru Abo[†]

Department of Immunology, Niigata University School of Medicine, Niigata.

【要約】

マウスに1週間、通常餌（25%の蛋白質）または低蛋白餌（蛋白質0 - 12.5%）を随時摂取させ、赤血球相の非致死株または、致死株Plasmodium yoelii（P. yoelii）に感染させた。マラリア感染から回復するまで、餌の種類は変更しなかった。通常餌群に非致死株を感染させた場合、重度のパラジテミアを呈したが、感染では死ぬことはなかった。致死株感染の場合、2週間以内に死亡した。しかし、低蛋白餌群では、致死株でも非致死株でも、顕著なパラジテミア（パラジテミアの小規模なピークはあった）を示すことなく、死亡することもなかった。死ななかったマウスは、マラリア感染中強力な自然免疫を獲得したことが明らかとなった。この時、NK1.1⁻TCR^{int}細胞と自己抗体産生の増強が見られた。低蛋白餌群でも、重症複合免疫不全（scid）マウス（TCR^{high}細胞とTCR^{int}細胞が欠損）は、P. yoelii致死株の感染後、生き残ることはなかった。これらの結果は、低蛋白餌が自然免疫を強化した一方、従来型免疫が低下したこと、これらの免疫学的変化により、マラリアに対する抵抗力をマウスが得たことを示唆する。本研究の結果とマラリア現地調査の経験とを照合すると、現地では一部の住民は、その後、再感染しなかったことが想起される。

最近の一連の研究（Mannoor et al., 2001; Weerasinghe et al., 2001; Mannoor et al., 2002）、において、我々は、自然免疫がマラリアを防御することを明らかにした。そして、自然免疫は、原始的T細胞（NK1.1⁻ TCR^{int}細胞）、胸腺外分化T細胞や自己抗体産生B-1細胞で構成される。主に炎症が起こるのは、肝臓と脾臓髄質（マラリア肝脾腫）であり、感染中、自己抗体が出現する。換言すると、マラリアに対する防御は、従来型の獲得免疫の免疫学的作用ではない可能性があり、そのとき働くのは、従来型T細胞（胸腺由来T細胞と従来型B（B-2）細胞）である。マラリア原虫の細胞内病原体は従来型リンパ球の攻撃を避けられるが、自己応答性T細胞または自己抗体の標的になる可能性が考えられる。この場合、変性した標的（例えば、マラリア感染した肝細胞や赤血球）は、脾臓のマクロファージや肝臓のクッパー細胞により最終的に処理される（Abo et al., 2000）。

我々は低蛋白餌（蛋白質0-12.5%）により胸腺萎縮が促進され、T細胞分化の主流に抑制が起こる一方、肝臓における自然免疫が活性化することが明らかにした。これら結果を考慮して、低蛋白餌をマラリア感染マウスに与えた。本

Received 28 December 2004; revised 24 August 2005, 4 November 2005; accepted 4 November 2005.

* Division of Cellular and Molecular Immunology, Center of Molecular Biosciences, University of Ryukyus, Okinawa, Japan.

[†] To whom correspondence should be addressed.

研究では、低蛋白餌を与えた後、*Plasmodium yoelii* 非致死株、さらには致死株に感染したマウスにおいて完全にマラリアを防御したことを報告する。これらマウスには、顕著なパラジテミアは見られず、感染中、マラリアに対する強力な自然免疫が見られた。

本研究は、今後、継続して研究すべきマラリアに対する防御手段が存在する可能性に光を投げかけるものである。

材料と方法

マウスと給餌

C57BL/6（B6）マウス（8-20週齢）を使用した。マウスは、新潟大学動物施設でSPF（specific pathogen-free）下で飼育した。

マウスには、以下の4種の食餌より1種を与えた：通常餌（蛋白質25％）、無蛋白質餌、低蛋白質餌（蛋白質5％または12.5％）（TEST Diet）（PMI Feeds Inc.、ミズリー州、セントルイス）。栄養、ミネラル、ビタミンおよびカロリーは、動物食餌製造会社開示の通りである。実験開始時点（Day0）より、マラリア感染マウスにもマラリア非感染マウスにも継続して給餌した。同様の実験を重症複合免疫不全（scid）マウス（TCR^{int}細胞およびTCR^{high}細胞欠損）を用い行なった。

マラリア感染

マラリア感染には、*P. yoelii* 非致死株（17XNL）または致死株 *P. yoelii*（17XL）に感染した赤血球10^4個（赤血球相）を腹腔内移入した（Weerasinghe et al., 2001）。

細胞分離

肝単核細胞を定法に従い分離した（Mannoor et al., 2001）。略述すると、摘出した肝臓を、200-ゲージ・ステンレ・スチール・メッシュで濾し、5mM HEPESおよび2％非働化済仔牛血清を含むEagleのMEM（日水製薬、日本東京）培養液中に浮遊させた。培養液で一度洗浄した後、細胞を35％のPercoll溶液15ml（Amersham Pharmacia Biotech, Piscataway, New Jersey）に浮遊させ、2,000rpm（15分）比重遠心分離を行った。その分離した細胞塊に、赤血球溶血用溶液（155mM NH_4Cl, 10mM $KHCO_3$, 1 mM EDTA-Naおよび170mM Tris [PH 7.3]）中に再懸濁し赤血球を除去した。脾臓と胸腺をステンレス・スチール・メッシュで濾過して脾臓細胞と胸腺細胞を得た。脾臓細胞を得るため、NH_4Clにて溶血させた。

フローサイトメトリー解析

フローサイトメトリー解析を用い、細胞のフェノタイプを検討した（Mannoor et al., 2002）。FITC-、PE-、または、ビオチン標識したモノクロナール抗体を使用し、ビオチン標識抗体は、TRI-COLOR標識ストレプトアビジン（Caltag Laboratory, San Francisco, California）を用いて発色させた。本実験で使用したモノクロナール抗体を以下記す。抗CD3（145-2C11）、抗IL-2Rβ（TM-β1）、抗NK1.1（PK136）と抗CD4（RM4-5）モノクロナール抗体（PharMingen, San Diego, California）。細胞をフローサイトメトリー（FACScan）（Becton-Dickinson Co., Mountain View, California）を用い解析した。モノクロナール抗体の非特異的結合を防ぐため、標識モノクロナール抗体による染色の前にCD16/32（2.4G2）（PharMingen）による前処理を行なった。死細胞をヨウ化プロピジウムで染色し、前方散乱、側方散乱でのゲーティングを行い除外した。

血清（グルタミン酸ピルビン酸トランスアミナーゼ（GPT）値

血清グルタミン酸ピルビン酸トランスアミナーゼ（GPT）値を、分光測光法を利用して市販キット（Wako Chemical Inc., 日本, 大阪）による標準酵素法を用いて測定した。

自己抗体測定

ELISA方法を用いssDNA抗体のIgGとIgM型について定法に従い測定した（Ito et al., 1992）。基準とする血清をMRL-*lpr/lpr*マウス（発症後）から採取し、それを抗DNA抗体100U/mlとした。各テストの測定値は、基準としたMRL-*lpr/lpr*マウス血清と比較した割合を示す。陽性対照（発症後の自己免疫モデルMRL-*lpr/lpr*マウス）を、100U/mlとした。

肝臓組織切片

組織検査ための組織を、10%リン酸緩衝ホルマリン固定し、パラフィン封埋を行なった。切片（厚さ4mm）をヘマトキシリン・エオシン染色した。

ソーティングおよび細胞移入

二重染色（IL-2Rβ と CD3）後、TCR^{high}細胞およびTCR^{int}細胞をセルソーター（FACS Vantage. Becton-Dickinson Co.）を用い肝臓リンパ球から選別して分離した。このように選別して分離した細胞も肝臓すべてのリンパ球も、5%低蛋白質餌群（マラリア免疫あり）より採取した。細胞移入するマウスには、細胞移入実験前に放射線照射を行なった（6.5Gy）。照射したレシピエントマウスは、マラリア免疫がないマウスであった。

統計分析

二群間の統計分析には、一元配置分散分析法、またはスチューデントt検定を用いた（p<0.05）。

結果

低蛋白餌によるマラリア感染防御

マラリア感染前、マウスに通常餌（蛋白質25%）、無蛋白質餌、5%低蛋白質餌または12.5%低蛋白質餌を一週間与えた。それぞれの食餌に適応させた後マウスに*P. yoelii*（17XNL非致死株）感染赤血球（10^4/匹）を移入し、マ

Figure.1

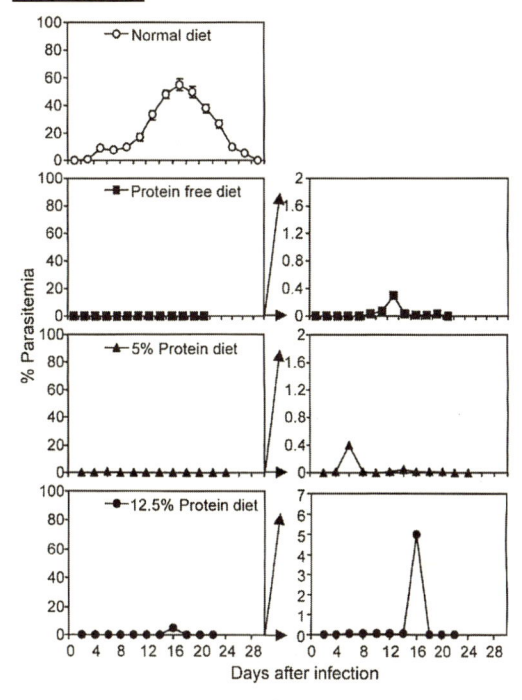

マラリア感染前後のマウスのパラジテミアの経時的変化。マウスに、通常餌（蛋白質25%）と低蛋白餌（0、5または12.5%）を一週間与えた。実験開始時（Day0）より、マラリア感染マウスにもマラリア非感染マウスにも給餌した。マラリア感染には、非致死株*P. yoelii*（17XNL）感染赤血球10^{4}個（赤血球相）を移入した。感染後、一ヶ月間パラジテミアを計測した。パラジテミアの平均値±SDを通常餌を与えた4匹のマウスを用い算出した。その他の群では、マウス3匹を用いた独立した実験を3度行った典型例を用いた。

ラリア感染させ、回復まで同じ餌を継続して与えた。通常餌群では、マラリア感染後18日にパラジテミアのピークを呈した（Fig. 1）。興味深いのは、このようなパラジテミアが、無蛋白質餌群、低蛋白質（5%）群、低蛋白質（12.5%）群には出現しなかったことである。パラジテミアの数値変化を示したが（右側）、これら三群では、パラジテミアの程度は低く、結局、すべてのマウスが生き残った。

低蛋白質餌による免疫の変化

マウスに、通常餌、5%蛋白質餌、無蛋白質餌を一週間与えた（Day0=食餌投与1週間後）。その後も、4週間同じ食餌を継続して与えた後、肝臓、脾臓と胸腺からリンパ球を採取して計測した（Fig. 2.左図）。肝臓と脾臓におけるリン

Figure.2

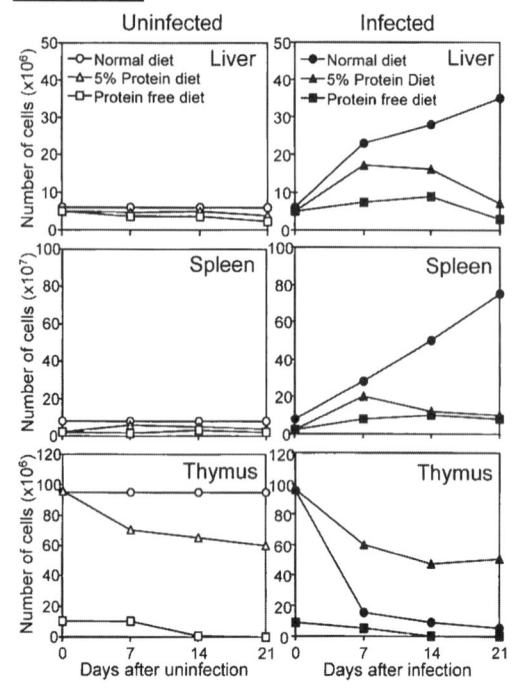

Uninfected / Infected — Liver, Spleen, Thymus における Number of cells (x10⁶ / x10⁷ / x10⁶) の経時的変化 (Days after uninfection / infection, 0, 7, 14, 21)。Normal diet (○/●), 5% Protein diet (△/▲), Protein free diet (□/■)。

マラリア感染前後のマウスのリンパ球数の経時的変化。マウスに、通常餌(蛋白質25％)と低蛋白餌(0、5または12.5％)を一週間与えた。実験開始時(Day0)より、マラリア感染マウスにもマラリア非感染マウスにも給餌した。マラリア感染には、非致死株 P. yoelii (17XNL) 感染赤血球 10^4 個(赤血球相)を移入した。リンパ球を、肝臓、脾臓および胸腺より採取した。その他の群についてはマウス3匹を用いた独立した実験を3度行った典型例を用いた。

パ球数は、全食餌群、全時点においてほぼ同じであった(非感染時)。一方、非感染であっても胸腺細胞数には、差異を認められた。胸腺細胞数は、通常餌群では変わらなかったが、5％蛋白質餌群では、徐々に減少した。無蛋白質餌群の胸腺細胞数は、Day 0 (実験開始1週間後)において、他の食餌群よりも低値で、その後も低値であった。

各食餌投与開始1週間後、マウスをマラリア感染させた(Fig. 2, 右図)。通常餌群では、肝臓および脾臓のリンパ球数は、感染後21日頃に顕著に増加した。対照的に、肝臓と脾臓のリンパ球数の増加は、5％の蛋白質餌群および無蛋白質餌群ではそれほどではなかった。食餌群により、胸腺細胞数に、独特の差異が見られた。胸腺細胞数の減少は通常餌群では顕著であった

Figure.3

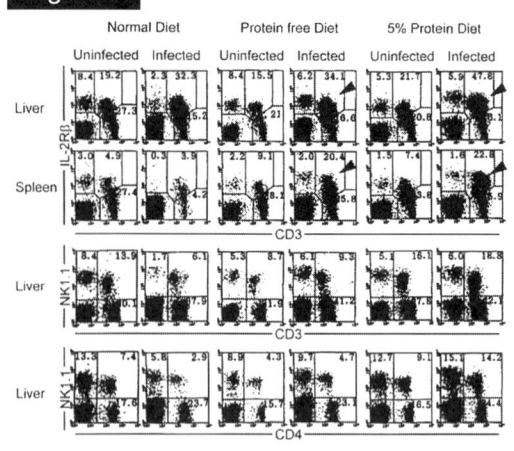

Normal Diet / Protein free Diet / 5% Protein Diet, Uninfected と Infected 条件における Liver・Spleen のフローサイトメトリー解析 (IL-2Rβ vs CD3, NK1.1 vs CD3, NK1.1 vs CD4)。

マラリア感染マウスのリンパ球フェノタイプの特徴。肝臓と脾臓リンパ球のCD3およびIL-2Rβの二重染色を行ない、CD3⁻IL-2Rβ⁺細胞(NK細胞)、CD3^{int}IL-2Rβ⁺細胞(intermediate CD3細胞)およびCD3highIL-2Rβ⁻細胞(従来型T細胞)を調べた。肝臓リンパ球を用いCD3およびNK1.1の二重染色を行い、NK1.1⁺CD3^{int}細胞(NKT細胞)とNK1.1⁻CD3^{int}細胞を調べた。肝臓リンパ球を用いCD4およびNK1.1の二重染色を行い、NK1.1⁺CD4⁺細胞(大多数のNKT細胞)を調べた。本実験では、マウスに通常餌と低蛋白餌(0または5％)を与えた。各分画内の数値は、その分画の蛍光陽性細胞の比率を示す。本図では、マウス3匹を用いた独立した実験を3度行った典型例を用いた。

が、5％蛋白質餌群ではそれほど顕著な減少を認めなかった。無蛋白質餌群における胸腺細胞数は、もともと低値であったが、これは感染と関係なく萎縮によるものであった。12.5％蛋白質餌群のデータは、5％蛋白質餌群とほぼ同じであった(非表示データ)。

肝臓で増多したリンパ球のフェノタイプの特徴

マラリア感染時、肝臓において主に増大しているリンパ球はNK1.1⁻TCR^{int}細胞(NK1.1⁻ intermediate TCR細胞)であるという報告を以前行なった(Mannoor et al., 2001; Weerasinghe et al., 2001; Mannoor et al., 2002)。我々は、同様の免疫反応が無蛋白質餌群や5％蛋白質餌群のマラリア感染マウスに現れるかについて検証を行なった(Fig. 3)。通常餌群の場合と同様、無蛋白質餌群でも5％蛋白質餌群でも肝臓および脾臓おいて、マラリア感染(感染14日後)時、CD3^{int}IL-2Rβ⁺の増大が認められた(Fig. 3上

段、矢印）。CD3^{int}細胞の中でのNK1.1-サブセットもNK1.1$^+$サブセット（NKT細胞）も増大を認めた。因みに、CD3^{int}細胞には、NK1.1$^-$CD3^{int}とNK1.1$^+$CD3^{int}の二つのサブセットがある（Fig.3, 中央および下）。5%蛋白質餌群では、他の食餌群に比して肝臓のNKT細胞はより顕著な増大を示した（例18.8%）。本実験におけるマラリア感染のデータは、感染後14日のものである。

組織標本とその他指標

マラリア感染時の、炎症の規模を測定するために、ヘマトクリット値と肝臓の組織標本を検証した（Fig.4）。通常餌群では、大きくヘマトクリット値が減少（60→20%）を示した（Fig.4A）。全く対照的に、無蛋白質餌（PF）、5%蛋白質餌群や12.5%蛋白質餌群では、マラリア感染に関係なくそのような現象は見られなかった。大変興味深いのは、無蛋白質餌群と5%の蛋白質餌群では、感染前に、1週間の食餌の影響で若干ヘマトクリットの減少が見られた事であった。

非感染時の肝臓（Fig.4B, 上）と対照的に、通常餌群（感染後21日）の肝臓でリンパ球や網状赤血球の集団が沢山肝臓で見られた（Fig.4B, 中央）。対照的に、5%蛋白質餌群の肝臓は、マラリア感染後（21日）でも、ほぼ正常だった（Fig.4B, 下）。この結果に対応して、通常餌群には血清GPT高値が見られ、肝障害が観察された（Fig. 4C）（p<0.05）。GPT高値は、5%蛋白質餌群には見られなかった。

マラリア感染時、自己抗体産生と胸腺外分化T細胞の増多が同時に起こると以前報告した（Mannoor et al., 2001; Mannoor et al., 2002）。他の研究者も同様の報告をしている（Kataaha et al., 1984; Alfred et al., 1984; Ribeiro, De Roquefeuil et al.,1984; Lloyd et al.,1994; Wenische et al.,1996）。ELISA法を用いて、無蛋白質餌群、5%蛋白

Figure.4

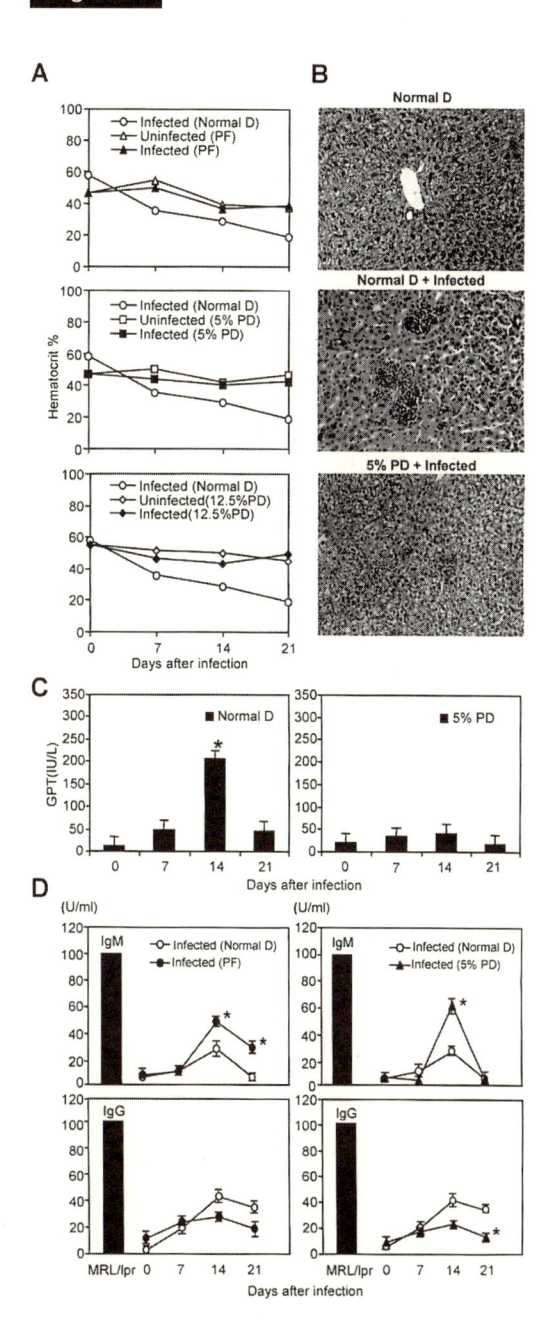

その他医学的指標の特徴。(A)ヘマトクリット値の経時間的変化、(B)肝臓組織切片、(C)血清中GPT値、(D)自己抗体価。実験A-Dにおいて、マラリア感染後7、14および21日の、各種食餌を与えたマウスを用いて、ヘマトクリットと変成したDNAに対する血清中自己抗体価を測定した。肝臓組織を、マラリア感染21日後において、通常餌と5%蛋白質餌の間で比較した。変性したDNAに対する自己抗体のIgM型およびIgG型についてELISA法にて測定した。実験AとBでは、3匹のマウスが、各々の実験で使われた。実験CおよびDでは、各時点において平均値±1SDを3匹のマウスを用い算出した。*P<0.05.

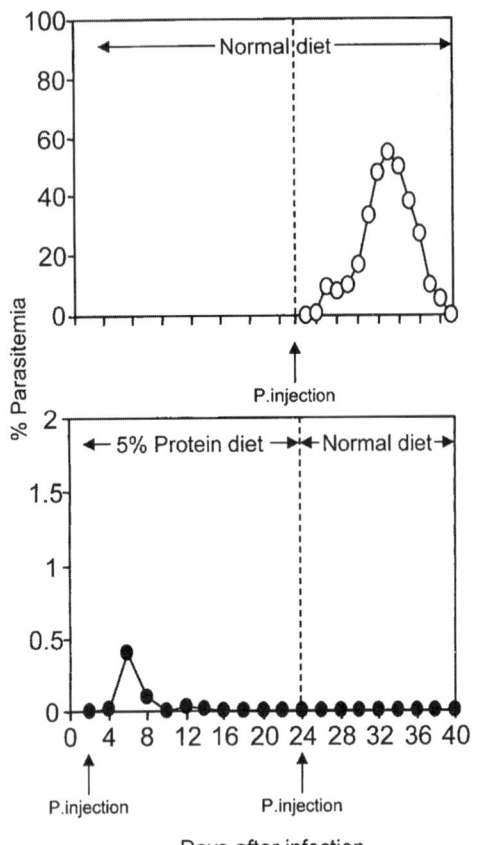

Figure.5

低蛋白餌(5%)を与えたマウスにおけるマラリア感染後の獲得した免疫　通常餌を与えた後でさえ、マウスは非致死株の再感染後におけるパラジテミアを回避することができた。マウス3匹を用いた中の典型例を示した。

Figure.6

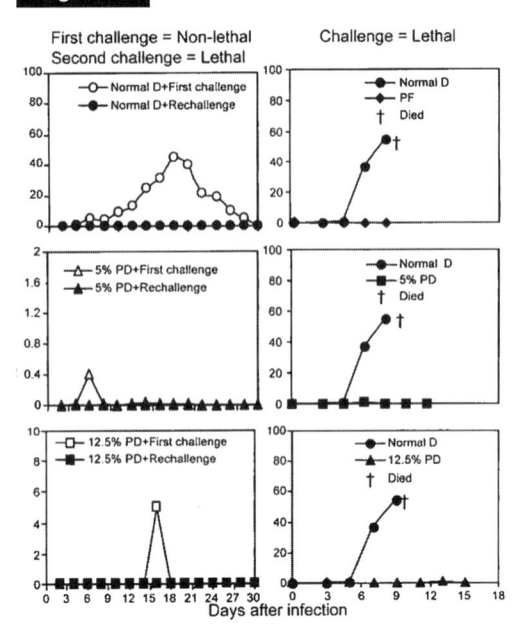

各種食餌を与えたマウスのパラジテミアの経時的変化　本実験では、マウスに予め通常餌もしくは低蛋白餌を与え、非致死株接種の後、致死株再接種(左側)、もしくは、最初から致死株 P. yoelii 移入を行った(右側)。パラジテミアの平均値±SDを4匹のマウスを用い算出した(左図)、また実験の典型例を示す(左側)。本実験では、Figure 1において回復したマウスを使用した。再移入の間隔は、2-4ヵ月であった。

質餌群において変性DNAに対してどのように自己抗体を産生するか検証した(Fig.4D)。すべての群で血清中に自己抗体が産生されたが、IgM型自己抗体は、通常餌群より5%蛋白質餌群の方が高値であった ($p < 0.05$)。しかし、IgG型自己抗体の結果は真逆で、5%蛋白質餌群が低値であった。

低蛋白食餌群における
マラリアに対する免疫獲得

5%蛋白質餌群でマラリア感染より回復したマウスを用いP. yoelii非致死株を再感染させる実験を行なった(Fig.5, 下)。回復したマウスに通常餌を与えた後、非致死株を感染させた。再感染させても、パラジテミアの徴候は見られなかった。実験時、通常餌を与えたマラリア初感染マウス(陽性対照)は顕著なパラジテミアを示した(Fig.5,上)。換言すると、低蛋白餌群は、マラリア感染の間、完全な免疫を獲得したのであった。

マラリア非致死株と
致死株を使った感染防御実験

我々は、マラリア致死株(17XL)を使って再感染実験を行った(Fig.6)。通常餌のマウスにP. yoelii非致死株を初感染させた場合、パラジテミアを示したが(Fig.6左図)、回復後に致死株を再感染させた場合、パラジテミアが出現しなかった。通常餌を摂取したマウスの場合と同様で、5%の蛋白質餌のすべてのマウスが再感染させてもパラジテミアが出現しなかった(Fig.6左列中段)。この現象は、12.5%の蛋白餌

Figure.7

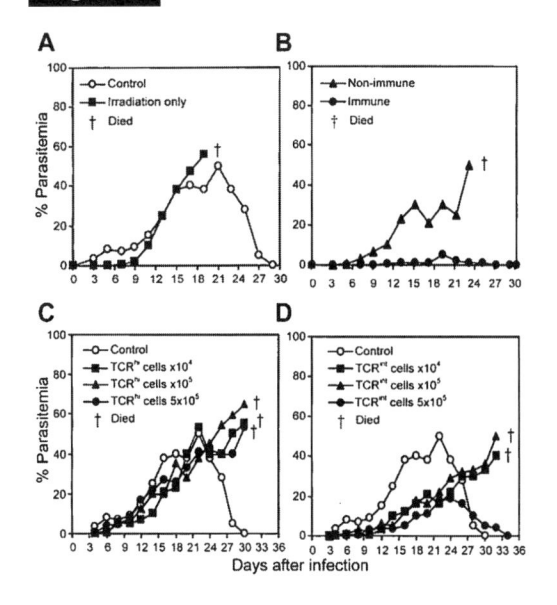

6.5Gy放射線照射したマウスに分離したTCR^{high}およびTCR^{int}細胞を細胞移植した実験 (A) 対照群マウス（未感作、非照射マウス）と放射線照射のみ。(B)未感作マウスと免疫されたマウスから得た分離していないリンパ球を移入。(C) TCR^{high}細胞移入 (D) TCR^{int}細胞移入。TCR^{high}細胞とTCR^{int}細胞を、セルソーターを用いて分離し、静脈注射した。マウス3匹を用いた中の典型例を示した。

のマウスにもみられた（Fig. 6 左列下段）。換言すると、低蛋白餌を摂取したマウスは最初の感染のマラリア非致死株と同様に致死株に対しても感染防御を獲得していた。

より著しい証拠として、無蛋白、5%及び12.5%の蛋白質餌（Fig.6右列）を摂取したマウスへの P. yoelii 致死株（17XL）の初感染でも感染防御が見られた事であった。すべてのこれらのマウスは、非常に低いパラジテミアで致死株の最初の感染でさえ生き残った。ここ（Fig. 6右列対照）で示されるように、通常餌を摂取したマウスではマラリア致死株の感染で生き延びることはできなかった。

TCR^{int}細胞のマラリア感染に対する防御作用

セルソーターを用いて、TCR^{int}細胞とTCR^{high}細胞を分離し、P. yoelii に対する防御効果を検証した（Fig. 7）。分離していない全リンパ球と分離したT細胞サブセットは、5%蛋白質餌群と P. yoelii 感染（致死株）回復群から採取した。これらのリンパ球を、放射線照射（6.5Gy）した通常餌群の静脈より移入した。放射線照射のみの群ではパラジテミアの発症は遅かったが、最後に全てのマウスが死亡した（Fig. 7A）。しかし、マラリア感染回復したマウスから分離した 2×10^6 個の肝リンパ球を移入した群では、完全にマラリアを防御できた。対照的に、この防御は、マラリアの免疫がないマウスから採取した肝臓リンパ球を移入してもマラリア感染防御はできなかった（Fig. 7B）。

TCR^{high}とTCR^{int}細胞を放射線照射したレシピエントマウスに移入したところ、TCR^{high}細胞にはマラリア感染を防御する能力のないことが明らかになった（Fig. 7C）。TCR^{int}細胞を移入した場合の感染防御力は、移入した細胞数に比例した（Fig. 7D）。5×10^5 個のTCR^{int}細胞をマウスに移入した場合、マラリアを防御する能力があったが、若干パラジテミアを認めた。1×10^5 個もしくは 1×10^4 個のTCR^{int}細胞をレシピエントマウスに移入したところ若干、パラジテミアの値が抑制されたもの、最終的には、高率のパラジテミアを呈し全滅した。図7は、マウス3匹を用いた実験を複数回行なった典型例を示している。

低蛋白質餌を与えたscidマウスにおけるマラリア感染防御不全

本研究の最終段階では、TCR^{high}細胞と同様にTCR^{int}細胞も先天的に欠損しているscidマウスを使用し実験を行った（Fig. 8）。

通常マウス（B6マウス）同様、scidマウスに通常餌、12.5%蛋白質餌、5%蛋白質餌または無蛋白質餌を与えたのち、P. yoelii 致死株を感染させた。通常餌群のscidマウスは、重症のパラジテミアを呈し感染後6日で死亡した。これに対し、無蛋白質餌群のscidマウスでは、パラジ

Figure.8

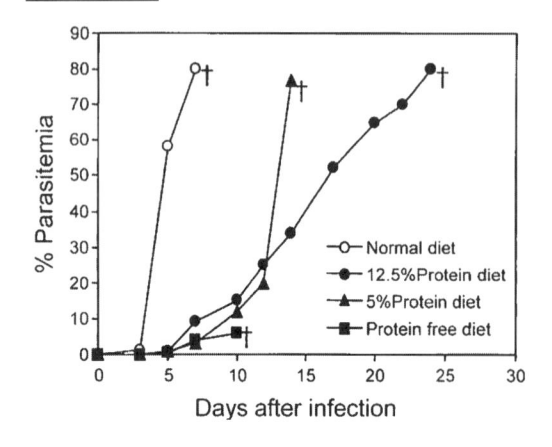

低蛋白餌の重症複合免疫不全マウス(scid)におけるマラリア防御欠如。TCR^{high}およびTCR^{int}細胞が欠損したscidマウスを使用した。マラリア感染(致死株 *P. yoelii*) 前、scidマウスには通常餌または低蛋白餌を2週間与え、感染後も同じ餌を与えた。マウス3匹を用いた中の典型例を示した。

テミアの発症は遅れたが、感染後10日で結局死亡した。12.5%蛋白質餌群と5%蛋白質餌群のscidマウスでは、パラジテミア発症は遅れたが、最終的に高率のパラジテミアを呈して死亡した。換言すると、低蛋白餌を与えても、scidマウスは、マラリア感染後生存不能であった。

考察

本研究において、低蛋白餌により完全にマラリア感染を防御できることが明らかになった。驚くべきことに、低蛋白餌群では、致死株マラリア感染でさえパラジテミアの低値を示し、生き残ることができた。これは、自然免疫の増強によるものである可能性が考えられた。本実験では、マラリア感染から完全に回復するまで、無蛋白質餌または低蛋白餌(5%または2.5%)を与えた。

低(無)蛋白餌実験期間中のマラリア感染後、マウスにおいて胸腺委縮と肝臓のIL-2Rβ^+TCR^{int}細胞比率増加が常に出現していた。

マラリア感染防御は、自然免疫、特にNK1.1抗原の発現が欠如したIL-2Rβ^+TCR^{int}細胞によるものであることを明らかにした報告を以前行なった(Mannoor et al.,2001; Weerasinghe et al., 2001; Mannoor et al., 2002)。このIL-2Rβ^+NKl.1$^-$TCR^{int}細胞は、実際、胸腺外由来であり、胸腺が欠損しているヌードマウスで見られるT細胞はすべて、この集団に含まれる(Halder et al., 2001; Kameyama et al., 2001)。全体として、本研究の結果より以下のことが示唆される。低蛋白餌により、胸腺退縮と同時に胸腺外分化T細胞増多が促進され、この増強した自然免疫によりマラリア感染を完全に防御する結果となった。

当初は、低蛋白餌群は、マラリア感染に対し脆弱であろうと考えられた。しかし、結果は正反対で、マウスはマラリアに抵抗力を示すようになった。この段階では、栄養状態が悪いこと自体は*P. yoelii*感染には不利な条件であろうと考えられたが、またも、予想は覆された。無蛋白質餌や低蛋白質餌群のマウスは全て、*P. yoelii*を移入すると、マラリアに対する強力な免疫を獲得した。興味深いことに、このようにして免疫を獲得したマウスに、後日、通常餌を与えてもマラリアに対する強い免疫は失われなかった。この結果からも、初回感染時に、強化された自然免疫を獲得した可能性が示唆される。少食や栄養失調がマウスとヒトにおけるパラジテミアの程度を軽減させるという類似した報告はされてきたものの、胸腺外分化T細胞の概念はまだ認識されない、または、検討されなかった(Fagnenro-Beyioku et al., 1990; Levander et al., 1990; Bhatia et al., 1991; Shankar, 2000; Takakura et al., 2001 ; Kicska et al., 2003)。

本研究中に、低蛋白餌群における免疫反応が、ストレス関連応答に似ていることに気がついた。以前、拘束ストレスにより自然免疫(胸腺外分化T細胞等)が増強され、その逆に胸腺におけるT細胞分化は抑制されることを以前報告

した（Maruyama et al., 1999; Oya et al., 2000; Shimizu et al., 2000）。ストレスにより従来型の免疫抑制と関連するとともに胸腺委縮が起こることも広く知られている（Bryant et al., 1987; O'Leary 1990; Tagoh et al., 1995; Lewin 1998）。特に無蛋白質餌群では、一週間以内に健康状態が悪くなり、体重減少や衰弱が見られた。マラリア感染の完全防御には、健康であるうちに5-12.5%の低蛋白餌を選択する必要がある。

これまでの研究の中で、マラリアを防御するのは、自然免疫の免疫学的作用の結果であると強調してきた（Mannoor et al, 2001; Weerasinghe et al., 2001; Mannoor et al., 2002）。このように：(1) 主にマラリア感染を防御するリンパ球は、肝臓に存在するCD8$^+$NK1.1$^-$TCR^{int}細胞である；(2) 自己抗体は常に存在し、自己抗体産生B-1細胞の活性化が局所で起こる；(3) 胸腺のT細胞分化は、激しい胸腺萎縮で示されるように抑制される；そして、(4) マラリアに対して獲得した免疫は、感染後1年以内に消滅する。本研究の結果は、これら事実と矛盾しない。

さらに、本研究の結果は、マラリアの現地調査の経験を説明するのに役立ちそうである。現地調査では多くの住民は、最終的に、マラリア感染後では再感染しなかった。本研究では、TCR^{high}細胞とTCR^{int}細胞を分離して、細胞移入実験を行った。レシピエントマウスの体内で、移入した細胞数が減少しないように、マウスに6.5 Gyの放射線照射を行なった。マラリア免疫を持たないマウスから分離した肝リンパ球（2×10^6／匹）を移入しても、レシピエントマウスのマラリア感染（非致死株）を防御できないことが確認できた。正反対に、5%蛋白質餌（非致死株免疫あり）群から分離した肝リンパ球を移入すると完全に防御できた。同様の実験を行なったところ、TCR^{high}細胞（5×10^5／匹）では防御できなかったが、TCR^{int}細胞（5×10^5／匹）、マラリア（非致死株）からマウスを防御することができた。TCR^{int}細胞のみを分離して移入した場合、肝臓リンパ球全部を移入した場合よりも、マラリア防御力は弱かったように思える。B細胞（B-1細胞）の中にもTCR^{int}細胞と同時にマラリア防御を行なっている可能性がある。TCR^{int}細胞とB-1細胞は、どちらも自然免疫の基本である（Miyakawa et al., 2002; Morshed et al., 2002）。

低蛋白餌群では、マラリア原虫の増殖が抑制され、結果としてマラリア感染を抑制した可能性がある。この考えを完全に否定することはできないが、自然免疫の役割を考慮する必要がある。このように、低蛋白餌群では、マラリア感染より回復したが、パラジテミアの低値でマラリアに対する強力な免疫を得た。本研究より、TCR^{int}細胞がマラリア感染防御に深く関与していることが示唆される。本研究におけるTCR^{int}細胞の重要性を裏打ちするために、T細胞（TCR^{int}細胞を含む）が全て欠損しているscidマウスを使用して実験を行った。低蛋白餌群のscidマウスに*P. yoelii*致死株を感染させたとき、これらのマウスは全て死亡した。このscidマウスの実験の結果が示唆するのは、低蛋白餌群（B6マウス）が回復後、マラリアに対する免疫を獲得したのと同様のことである。つまり、マラリア致死株や非致死株を完全に防御するには、TCR^{int}細胞が重要な役割果たしていることである。しかし、低蛋白餌群のscidマウスでは、死亡前になってパラジテミアが高値となっていたので、低蛋白餌がマクロファージやNK細胞の活性化をさせた可能性や、低蛋白餌がマラリア原虫の増殖を抑制させた可能性も考慮する必要がある。いずれにせよ、scidマウスを用いた実験の結果より、TCR^{int}細胞は、低蛋白餌がマラリアを完全に防御するには不可欠で

あることを示唆するものである。

　最近、5%蛋白質餌をマウスに与えたところ、自然免疫が増強され、腫瘍の肺転移に抵抗する免疫を獲得したと報告した（Li et aL, 2004）。換言すると、低蛋白餌（食）の宿主における自然免疫の状態の変化を考慮する必要がある。

　5-12.5%蛋白質餌を与えたマウスは、致死株 *P. yoelii*（本研究）および *P. berghei*（未発表データ）にさえ抵抗力を示した。従って、本研究は、マラリア防御手段の可能性に光を投げ掛けるものである。

謝辞

　本研究は、文部科学省科学研究費補助金によるものである。原稿浄書について渡辺正子氏に感謝する。

PROTECTION AGAINST MALARIA DUE TO INNATE IMMUNITY ENHANCED BY LOW-PROTEIN DIET

Anoja Ariyasinghe, Sufi Reza M. Morshed, M. Kaiissar Mannoor, Hanaa Y. Bakir, Hiroki Kawamura, Chikako Miyaji, Toru Nagura, Toshihiko Kawamura, Hisami Watanabe*, Hiroho Sekikawa, and Toru Abo†

Department of Immunology, Niigata University School of Medicine, Niigata 951-8510, Japan. e-mail: immunol2@med.niigata-u.ac.jp

ABSTRACT: Mice were fed ad libitum with a normal diet (25% protein) or low-protein diets (0–12.5% protein) for a wk and then infected with a nonlethal or lethal strain of *Plasmodium yoelii*, that is, blood stage infection. The same diet was continued until recovery. Mice fed with a normal diet showed severe parasitemia during nonlethal infection, but survived the infection. They died within 2 wk in the case of lethal infection. However, all mice fed with low-protein diets survived without apparent parasitemia (there were small peaks of parasitemia) in cases of both nonlethal and lethal strains. These surviving mice were found to have acquired potent innate immunity, showing the expansion of NK1.1$^-$TCR^{int} cells and the production of autoantibodies during malarial infection. Severe combined immunodeficiency (scid) mice, which lack TCR^{int} cells as well as TCR^{high} cells, did not survive after malarial infection of lethal strain of *P. yoelii*, even when low-protein diets were given. These results suggest that low-protein diets enhanced innate immunity and inversely decreased conventional immunity, and that these immunological deviations rendered mice resistant against malaria. The present outcome also reminds us of our experience in the field study of malaria, in which some inhabitants eventually avoided contracting malaria even after apparent malarial infection.

In a series of recent studies (Mannoor et al., 2001; Weerasinghe et al., 2001; Mannoor et al., 2002), we revealed that malarial protection is achieved by innate immunity, the constituents of which are primordial T cells (NK1.1$^-$TCR^{int} cells, or T cells of extrathymic origin) and autoantibody-producing B-1 cells. The major inflammatory sites are the liver and the splenic medulla, that is, hepatosplenomegaly in malaria, and autoantibodies appear during infection. In other words, protection against malaria may not be an immunological event of conventional acquired immunity, the constituents of which are conventional T cells, that is, T cells of thymic origin, and conventional B (B-2) cells. It is conceivable that an intracellular pathogen of the malaria protozoan can avoid the attack by conventional lymphocytes, but possibly becomes the target of autoreactive T cells or autoantibodies. In this case, such denatured targets, for example, malaria-infected hepatocytes or erythrocytes, would be finally processed by macrophages in the spleen and Kupffer cells in the liver (Abo et al., 2000).

We have also found that low-protein diets (0–12.5% protein) accelerate thymic atrophy, which indicates the suppression of the mainstream of T-cell differentiation, and inversely activates innate immunity in the liver. In light of these findings, we provided low-protein diets to mice infected with malaria. We herein report that complete protection against malaria was achieved in mice that were fed with low-protein diets and then infected with nonlethal and even lethal strains of *Plasmodium yoelii*. Without apparent parasitemia, these mice exhibited potent innate immunity against malaria during infection. The present study sheds light on possible preventative measures against malaria that should be examined by future studies.

MATERIALS AND METHODS

Mice and feeding

C57BL/6 (B6) mice were used at the age of 8–20 wk. These mice were fed under specific pathogen-free conditions in the animal faculty of Niigata University. Mice were fed 1 of 4 diets, namely, a normal diet (25% protein) and low-protein diets (0, 5, and 12.5%) (TEST Diet) (PMI Feeds Inc., St. Louis, Missouri) for 1 wk. Contents of nutrients, minerals, vitamins, and calories were indicated by the animal diet guide of this company. From this point of time (day 0), mice continued to be fed with or without malarial infection. A similar experiment was conducted using severe combined immunodeficiency (scid) mice, which primarily lack TCR^{int} cells, as well as TCR^{high} cells.

Malarial infection

For malarial infection, 10^4 erythrocytes infected with a nonlethal strain (17XNL) or a lethal strain (17XL) of *P. yoelii* were injected, that is, a blood-stage infection of malaria (Weerasinghe et al., 2001).

Cell preparations

Hepatic lymphocytes were isolated by a previously described method (Mannoor et al., 2001). Briefly, the liver was removed, pressed through 200-gauge stainless-steel mesh, and suspended in Eagle's MEM (Nissui Pharmaceutical, Tokyo, Japan), supplemented with 5 mM HEPES and 2% heat-inactivated newborn calf serum. After being washed once with medium, the cells were fractionated by centrifugation in 15 ml of 35% Percoll solution (Amersham Pharmacia Biotech, Piscataway, New Jersey) for 15 min at 2,000 rpm. The pellet was resuspended in erythrocyte lysing solution (155 mM NH$_4$Cl, 10 mM KHCO$_3$, 1 mM EDTA-Na, and 170 mM Tris [pH 7.3]). Splenocytes and thymocytes were obtained by forcing the spleen and thymus through stainless steel mesh. Splenocytes were used after the treatment with NH$_4$Cl erythrocyte lysing buffer. In some experiments, liver lymphocytes were also used after the treatment with erythrocyte lysing buffer.

Immunofluorescence tests

Immunofluorescence tests were used to identify cell phenotype (Mannoor et al., 2002). FITC-, PE-, or biotin-conjugated reagents of mAbs were used and biotin-conjugated reagents were developed with TRI-COLOR-conjugated streptavidin (Caltag Laboratory, San Francisco, California). The mAbs used here included anti-CD3 (145-2C11), anti-IL-2Rβ (TM-β1), anti-NK1.1 (PK136), and anti-CD4 (RM4-5) mAbs (PharMingen, San Diego, California). Cells were analyzed by FACScan (Becton-Dickinson Co., Mountain View, California). To prevent non-specific binding of mAbs, CD16/32 (2.4G2) (PharMingen) was added before staining with labeled mAb. Dead cells were excluded by forward scatter, side scatter, and propidium iodide gating.

Serum level of glutamic pyruvic transaminase (GPT)

Serum glutamic pyruvic transaminase (GPT) levels were measured spectrophotometrically by a standard enzymatic method with a commercial kit (Wako Chemical Inc., Osaka, Japan).

Measurement of autoantibody

Measurements of the reaction of IgG and IgM Abs with ssDNA by the ELISA method were modified as previously described (Ito et al.,

---

Received 28 December 2004; revised 24 August 2005, 4 November 2005; accepted 4 November 2005.

* Division of Cellular and Molecular Immunology, Center of Molecular Biosciences, University of Ryukyus, Okinawa, Japan.

† To whom correspondence should be addressed.

1992). Standard sera were obtained from MRL-*lpr/lpr* mice (after the onset of disease) and arbitrarily determined to contain 100 U of anti-DNA Ab. In each test, the titer was expressed as a percentage in comparison with the standard sera. A positive control (sera of autoimmune prone MRL-*lpr/lpr* mice after the onset of disease) was used as 100 U/ml.

Histology of the liver

Tissues for histology were fixed in 10% phosphate-buffered formalin and embedded in paraffin. Sections at 4 μm in thickness were stained with hematoxylin and eosin.

Cell sorting and cell transfer

TCR[high] and TCR[int] cells were purified from liver lymphocytes by a cell sorter (FACS Vantage, Becton-Dickinson Co.) after 2-color staining for IL-2Rβ and CD3. These purified fractions as well as whole liver lymphocytes were isolated from immune mice fed with the 5% protein diet. Cell-transfer recipients were irradiated (6.5 Gy) before cell transfer experiments. These irradiated recipient mice were nonimmune mice.

Statistical analysis

Significant differences between 2 groups were determined by the 1-factor ANOVA test or Student's *t*-test. P values less than 0.05 were considered to be statistically significant.

RESULTS

Malarial protection by low-protein diets

Prior to infection, mice were fed a normal diet (25% protein), a protein-free diet, a 5% protein diet or a 12.5% protein diet for 1 wk. After this diet-adaptation period, mice were injected with *P. yoelii* (17XNL nonlethal strain)-infected erythrocytes (10^4/mouse). The same diets were continued until recovery. In the case of mice fed with the normal diet, prominent parasitemia peaked 18 days postinfection (PI) (Fig. 1). Interestingly, there was no such parasitemia in mice with the protein-free diet, the 5% protein diet, or the 12.5% protein diet. Magnification of figures (right column) showed only a small peak of parasitemia in these mice. All recovered mice eventually survived.

Immunomodulation by low-protein diets

Mice were fed a normal diet, a 5% protein diet, or a protein-free diet for 1 wk (Day 0 = 1 wk after diet adaptation); thereafter, the same diet was continued up to 4 wk and the numbers of lymphocytes yielded by the liver, spleen, and thymus were enumerated (Fig. 2, left column). The numbers of lymphocytes in the liver and spleen were almost the same at all points of time in all tested mice (uninfected). On the other hand, variation in the number of thymocytes was observed without infection. The number of thymocytes remained unchanged in mice that received the normal diet, but decreased gradually in mice fed with the 5% protein diet. The number of thymocytes in mice given the protein-free diet reached its lowest level at Day 0 (1 wk after diet adaptation) and continued at that level thereafter.

After 1 wk of diet adaptation, mice were infected with malaria (Fig. 2, right column). In mice on the normal diet, the numbers of lymphocytes in the liver and spleen increased prominently toward 21 days after infection. In contrast, the increase in the numbers of lymphocytes in the liver and spleen was limited in mice on the 5% protein diet and mice on the protein-free diet. Variation in the number of thymocytes was unique, depending on each group of mice. A decrease in the number of thymocytes was prominent in mice on the normal diet, but such

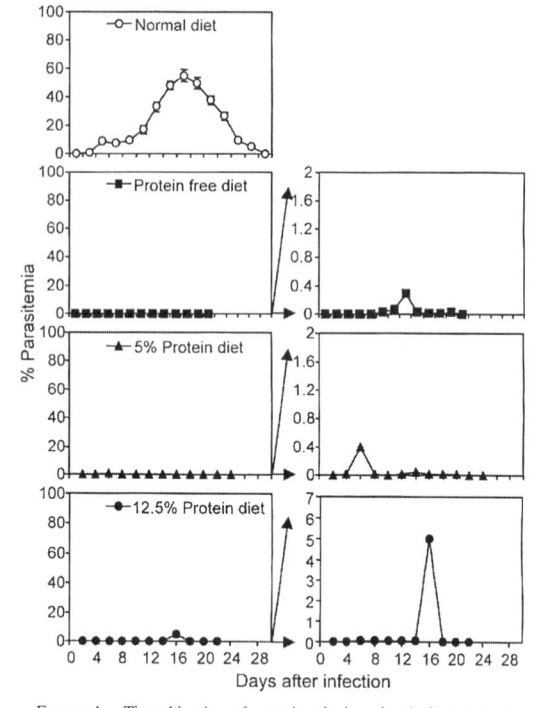

FIGURE 1. Time kinetics of parasitemia in mice before and after malarial infection. Mice were fed with a normal diet (25% protein) and low-protein diets (0, 5, and 12.5%) for a week. From this point of time (Day 0), mice were fed further with or without malarial infection. For malarial infection, 10^4 erythrocytes infected with a nonlethal strain (17XNL) of *P. yoelii* were injected, that is, a blood-stage infection of malaria. Parasitemia was enumerated up to 1 mo after infection. The mean and 1 SD of parasitemia were produced from 4 mice receiving a normal diet. In other cases, a typical sample is represented from 3 independent experiments, each of 3 mice.

a decrease was not so prominent in mice on the 5% protein diet. In mice on the protein-free diet, the number of thymocytes was primarily low, that is, atrophic, irrespective of infection. The data from mice on the 12.5% protein diet were almost the same as those from mice on the 5% protein diet (data not shown).

Phenotypic characterization of expanding lymphocytes in the liver

We have previously reported that the major expanding lymphocytes during malarial infection were NK1.1⁻TCR[int] cells (NK1.1⁻ intermediate TCR cells) in the liver (Mannoor et al., 2001; Weerasinghe et al., 2001; Mannoor et al., 2002). We examined whether or not a similar immune response was induced in malaria-infected mice fed with the protein-free diet or the 5% protein diet (Fig. 3). Mice fed with the normal diet were examined in parallel. It was found that, similar to the case of mice on the normal diet, malarial infection (Day 14 PI) induced the expansion of CD3[int]IL-2Rβ⁺ cells (indicated by arrowheads

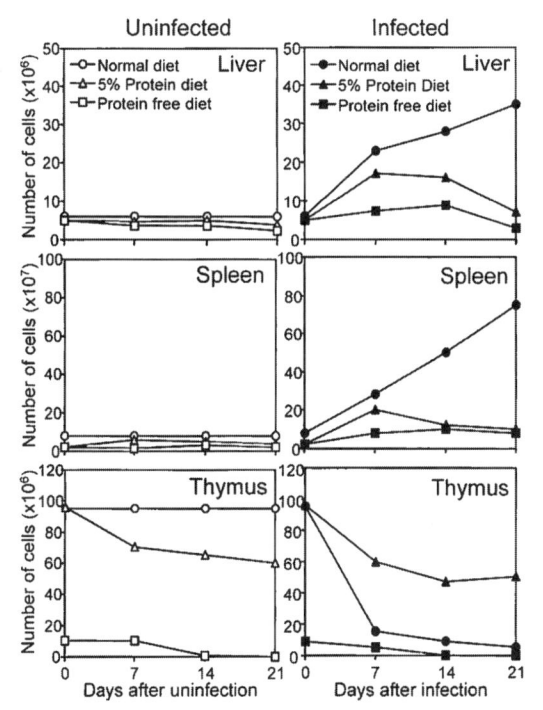

FIGURE 2. Time kinetics of the number of lymphocytes in mice before and after malarial infection. Mice were fed with a normal diet (25% protein) and low-protein diets (0 and 5%) for a week. From this point of time (Day 0), mice continued to be fed with or without malarial infection. For malarial infection, 10^4 erythrocytes infected with a nonlethal strain of *P. yoelii* were injected. Lymphocytes were isolated from the liver, spleen, and thymus. A typical sample is represented from 3 independent experiments, each of 3 mice.

in Fig. 3) in both the liver and spleen of mice on the protein-free diet and those on the 5% protein diet (Fig. 3, top). The expansion of the NK1.1$^-$ subset, as well as the NK1.1$^+$ subset (NKT cells) among CD3^{int} cells (namely, this population includes both NK1.1$^-$CD3^{int} and NK1.1$^+$CD3^{int} subsets), was seen by subsequent stainings (Fig. 3, center and bottom). In mice fed with the 5% protein diet, the expansion of NKT cells was much more prominent, for example, 18.8% CD3^{int}NK1.1$^+$ cells in the liver, than in mice fed with the other diets. In all these experiments, the data of malarial infection were produced on Day 14.

Histological study and other parameters

To determine the magnitude of inflammation during malarial infection, the hematocrits and histology of the livers were examined (Fig. 4). Mice on the normal diet showed a severe decrease (60→20%) in the hematocrit (Fig. 4A). In sharp contrast, none of the mice fed with the protein-free diet (PF), the 5% protein diet, and the 12.5% protein diet, showed such a decrease, irrespective malarial infection. It was very interesting that mice fed with the protein-free diet and those fed with the 5% protein diet showed a somewhat decreased level of hematocrit before infection, that is, dietary effects for 1 wk.

Histology of the liver explained the above-mentioned situation. In contrast to the normal liver (Fig. 4B, top), many clusters of lymphocytes and reticulocytes were seen in the livers of mice receiving the normal diet (Day 21 PI) (Fig. 4B, middle). In contrast, the livers of mice receiving the 5% protein-free diet were almost normal even after malarial infection (Day 21) (Fig. 4B, bottom). Reflecting these results, an elevation of GPT in sera that showed liver damage was observed in mice fed with normal diet (Fig. 4C) ($P < 0.05$). Such an elevation was not seen in mice fed with the 5% protein diet.

We previously reported that autoantibody production always accompanies the expansion of extrathymic T cells during malarial infection (Mannoor et al., 2001; Mannoor et al., 2002). Similar observations have been reported by other investigators (Kataaha et al., 1984; Ribeiro, Alfred et al., 1984; Ribeiro, De Roquefeuil et al., 1984; Lloyd et al., 1994; Wenisch et al., 1996). Using the ELISA method, we examined how mice fed with the protein-free or 5% protein diets produced autoantibodies against denatured DNA (Fig. 4D). Although all mice produced autoantibodies in sera, the IgM type of autoantibodies showed a higher titer in mice receiving the protein-free and 5% protein diets than in mice receiving the normal diet ($P < 0.05$). However, the IgG type deviated in the opposite direction, that is, it decreased, in these mice.

Acquisition of immunity against malaria in mice fed with low protein diets

In this experiment, rechallenge of the nonlethal strain of *P. yoelii* was conducted in mice that were fed with a 5% protein diet and that had recovered from malarial infection (Fig. 5, bottom). After recovery, these mice were fed with a normal diet again and were then injected with the nonlethal strain. No signs of parasitemia were induced after the rechallenge. At this time, nonimmune mice fed with normal diet (a positive control) showed prominent parasitemia (Fig. 5, top). In other words, mice fed with low-protein diets acquired complete immunity during the infection.

Protection with the use of nonlethal and lethal strains of malaria

We then conducted re-challenge experiments using lethal-strain (17XL) injection (Fig. 6). The first challenge of the nonlethal strain of *P. yoelii* showed parasitemia in the case of the normal diet (left column), but the rechallenge with the lethal strain did not show such parasitemia. Similar to the case of mice fed with the normal diet, all mice on the 5% protein diet did not show parasitemia by the rechallenge (left column middle). This was also the case in mice on the 12.5% protein diet (left column bottom). In other words, mice fed with low-protein diets acquired immunity against malaria of lethal strain as well as nonlethal strain by the first challenge.

More striking evidence was produced with the use of the lethal strain (17XL) of *P. yoelii* (as the first challenge) in mice fed with the protein-free, 5%, and 12.5% protein diets (Fig. 6, right column). All these mice survived the first challenge of even the lethal strain with very low parasitemia. Of course,

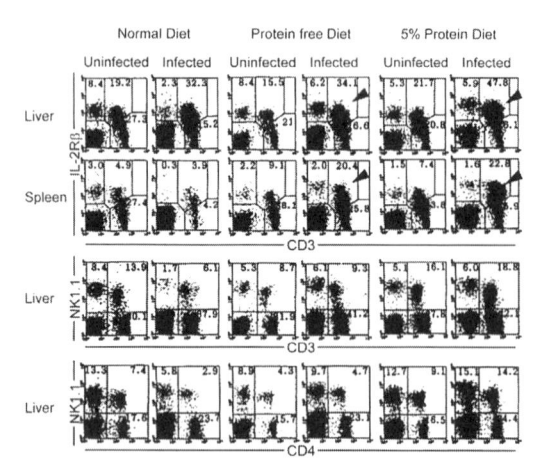

FIGURE 3. Phenotypic characterization of lymphocytes in mice after malarial infection. Two-color staining for CD3 and IL-2Rβ was conducted with the use of liver and splenic lymphocytes to detect CD3⁻IL-2Rβ⁺ cells (NK cells), CD3^{int}IL-2Rβ⁺ cells (intermediate CD3 cells), and CD3^{high}IL-2Rβ⁻ cells (conventional T cells). Two-color staining of CD3 and NK1.1 was also conducted with the use of liver lymphocytes to detect NK1.1⁺CD3^{int} cells (NKT cells) and NK1.1⁻CD3^{int} cells. Two-color staining of CD4 and NK1.1 was also conducted with the use of liver lymphocytes to detect NK1.1⁺CD4⁺ cells (majority of NKT cells). In these experiments, mice were fed with a normal diet and low-protein diets (0 and 5% protein). Numbers in the figure show the percentages of fluorescence-positive cells in corresponding areas. The data shown here are representative of 3 independent experiments, each of 3 mice.

none of the mice receiving the normal diet survived lethal-strain infection, as shown here (right column control).

Protective effect of purified TCR^{int} cells on malarial infection

We examined whether TCR^{int} cells or TCR^{high} cells purified by a cell sorter exerted a protective effect against *P. yoelii* (Fig. 7). Unpurified lymphocytes or purified T-cell subsets were isolated from mice that were fed with a 5% protein diet and that recovered from *P. yoelii* infection (lethal strain). These lymphocytes were intravenously injected into 6.5 Gy-irradiated mice fed with a normal diet. As shown in Figure 7A, mice with only irradiation showed a retarded onset of parasitemia, but parasitemia finally appeared and the mice died. However, the injection of 2×10^6 liver lymphocytes that were isolated from recovered mice protected recipient mice completely. In contrast, this capability was absent in the case of liver lymphocytes that were isolated from nonimmune mice (Fig. 7B).

TCR^{high} and TCR^{int} cells were then injected into irradiated recipient mice. It was found that TCR^{high} cells did not have the

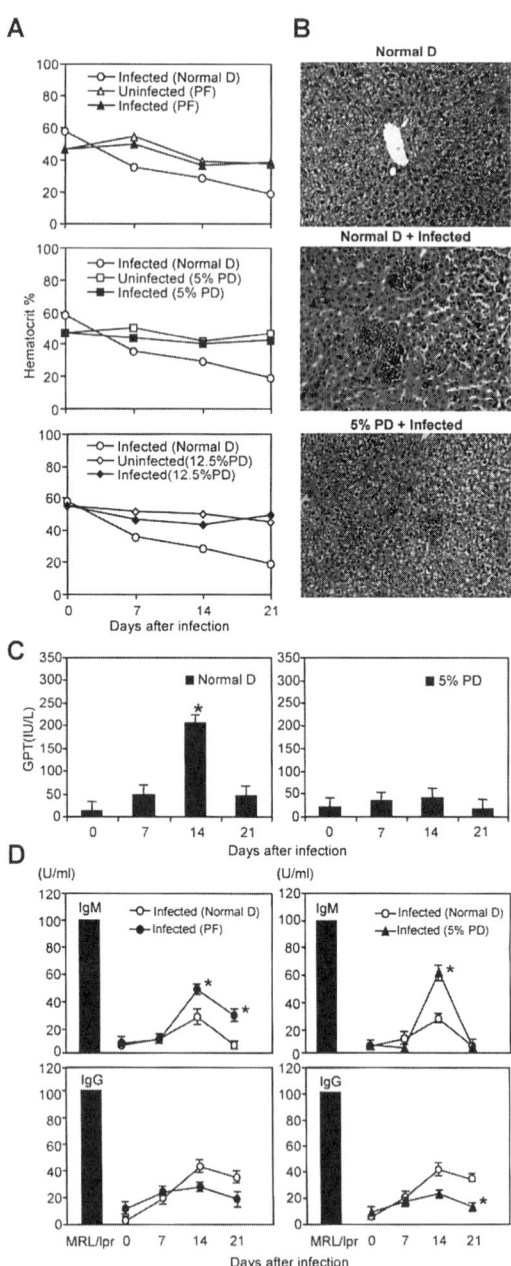

FIGURE 4. Further characterization of medical parameters. (**A**) Time-kinetics of hematocrit. (**B**) Histology of the liver. (**C**) Serum levels of GPT. (**D**) Serum titer of autoantibodies. In Experiments A–D, mice fed with various diets were killed at 7, 14, and 21 days after malarial infection. Hematocrit and serum titer of autoantibodies against denatured DNA were measured. Histology of the liver was compared between mice fed with the normal diet and those on the 5% protein diet at Day 21 after malarial infection. IgM and IgG types of autoantibodies against denatured DNA were measured by the ELISA method. In Experiments A and B, 3 mice were used in each experiment. In Experiments C and D, 3 mice were used to produce the mean and 1 SD at each point of time; *$P < 0.05$.

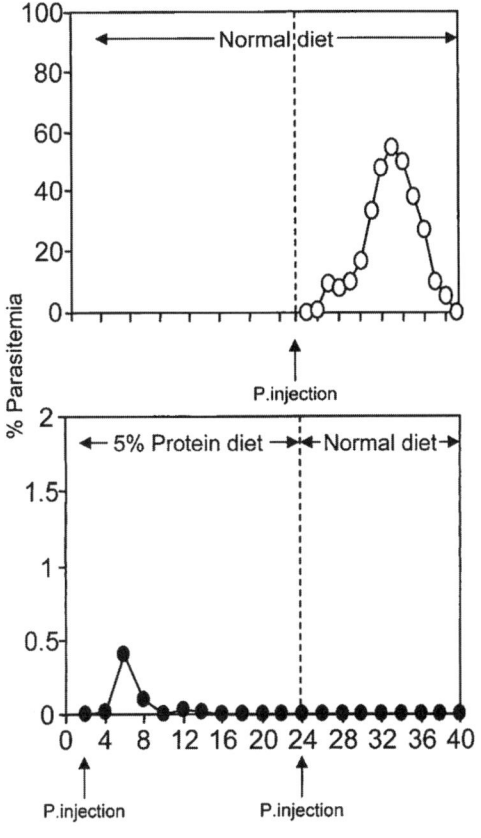

FIGURE 5. Acquisition of immunity after malarial infection in mice fed with the 5% protein diet. Even after being fed with the normal diet, mice were able to escape from parasitemia after rechallenge (nonlethal strain). Representative data of three mice are depicted.

ability to protect against malaria (Fig. 7C). In the case of TCR^{int} cells, the results were dependent on the number of cells injected (Fig. 7D). The injection of 5×10^5 TCR^{int} cells into mice had the ability to protect against malaria, although some levels of parasitemia appeared. The injection of 1×10^5 or 1×10^4 TCR^{int} cells into recipient mice resulted in a somewhat suppressed level of parasitemia, but these mice finally died, showing an elevated level of parasitemia. Representative data of repeated experiments (n = 3) are shown in Figure 7.

Failure of malaria protection in scid mice fed with low-protein diets

In a final portion of these experiments, we used scid mice that primarily lack TCR^{int} cells, as well as TCR^{high} cells (Fig. 8). Similar to the case of normal mice, scid mice were fed with the normal diet, 12.5% protein diet, 5% protein diet, and pro-

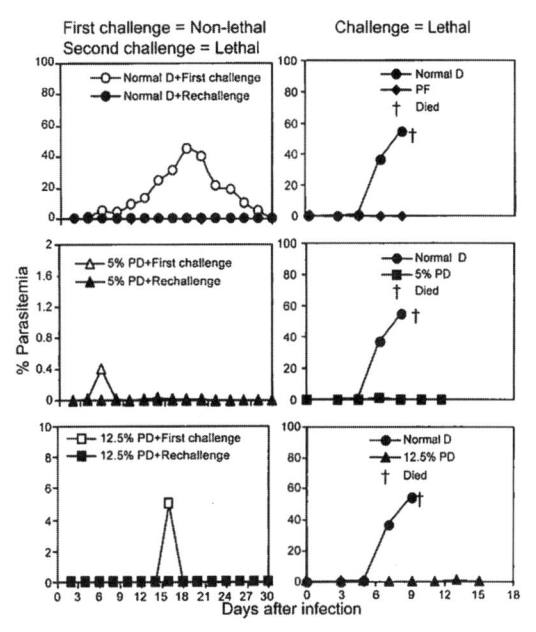

FIGURE 6. Time kinetics of parasitemia in mice fed with various diets. In these experiments, mice were first fed with a normal diet or low-protein diet and were then infected with either the nonlethal strain and rechallenged with lethal strain after recovery (left column) or primarily challenged with the lethal strain (right column) of *P. yoelii*. The mean and 1 SD of parasitemia were produced from 4 mice (left column), while a typical case is represented for some experiments (right column). In this experiment, recovered mice in Figure 1 were used. Interval for rechallenge was 2–4 mo.

tein-free diet, and then were infected with the lethal strain of *P. yoelii*. In the case of scid mice fed with a normal diet, they showed severe parasitemia and died on Day 6. In contrast, scid mice fed with the protein-free diet showed a delayed onset of parasitemia, but they finally died after Day 10. In the case of scid mice fed with 12.5% and 5% protein diets, there was a delayed onset of parasitemia, but they finally died with high levels of parasitemia. In other words, scid mice could not survive after malarial infection, despite low-protein diets.

DISCUSSION

In the present study, we demonstrated that complete protection against malaria was achieved by low-protein diets. Surprisingly, mice fed with low-protein diets could survive after malarial infection of even the lethal strain, showing low levels of parasitemia. This might be due to enhanced innate immunity. In these experiments, mice were fed with a protein-free diet or low-protein diets (5 and 12.5%) until complete recovery. During this period and after malarial infection, we always encountered thymic involution and an increase in the proportion of IL-2Rβ$^+$TCR^{int} cells in the livers of these mice. In previous reports, we revealed that protection against malaria was an immunological event of innate immunity, especially with IL-2Rβ$^+$TCR^{int} cells lacking the expression of NK1.1 antigens (Mannoor et al.,

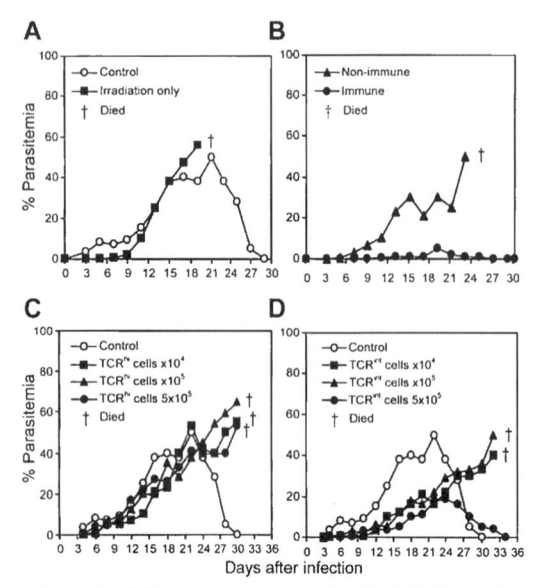

FIGURE 7. Cell-transfer experiments of purified TCR^{high} or TCR^{int} cells injected into 6.5 Gy-irradiated mice. (A) Control mice (nonimmune, nonirradiated mice) and irradiation only. (B) Transfer of unpurified lymphocytes obtained from nonimmune mice and immune mice. (C) Transfer of TCR^{high} cells. (D) Transfer of TCR^{int} cells. TCR^{high} and TCR^{int} cells were purified by a cell sorter and were intravenously injected. Representative data of 3 mice are depicted.

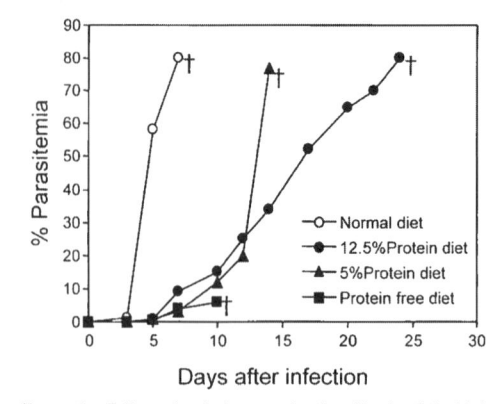

FIGURE 8. Failure of malaria protection in scid mice fed with low-protein diets. Scid mice that lack TCR^{int} cells as well as TCR^{high} cells were used. Before malarial infection of lethal strain of *P. yoelii*, scid mice were fed with the normal diet or low-protein diets for 2 wk and were continued corresponding diets even after infection. Representative data of 3 experiments of 3 mice each are depicted.

2001; Weerasinghe et al., 2001; Mannoor et al., 2002). These IL-2Rβ$^+$NK1.1$^-$TCR^{int} cells are truly of extrathymic origin and all T cells seen in athymic nude mice belong to this population (Halder et al., 2001; Kameyama et al., 2001). Overall, our present findings indicate that low-protein diets accelerated the expansion of extrathymic T cells in parallel with thymic involution and resulted in complete protection against malaria by this enhanced innate immunity.

Initially, we considered the possibility that low-protein diets would render mice sensitive to malarial infection. However, the result was the opposite and mice became resistant to malaria. At this stage, we had to consider the possibility that malnutrition itself was not a good condition for mice to survive *P. yoelii* infection. However, again, this was not the case. All mice fed with the protein-free diet or low-protein diets that were injected with *P. yoelii* acquired potent immunity against the parasite. Interestingly, some of these mice were then put on a normal diet and still retained potent immunity against malaria. These results also suggest that enhanced innate immunity may be acquired at the point of the first challenge. Although there have been similar studies in which a decreased dietary level or malnutrition diminished the level of parasitemia in mice and humans (Fagnenro-Beyioku et al., 1990; Levander et al., 1990; Bhatia et al., 1991; Shankar, 2000; Takakura et al., 2001; Kicska et al., 2003), the concept of extrathymic T cells was not yet known or had not been examined.

During the course of this study, we noticed that immune responses in mice fed with low-protein diets resembled stress-associated immune responses. We previously reported that restraint stress induces the enhancement of innate immunity, for example, extrathymic T cells, and inversely the arrest of the mainstream of T-cell differentiation in the thymus (Maruyama et al., 1999; Oya et al., 2000; Shimizu et al., 2000). It is also widely known that stress induces thymic atrophy, which is associated with the suppression of conventional immunity (Bryant et al., 1987; O'Leary 1990; Tagoh et al., 1995; Lewin 1998). Such mice became unhealthy within a week, especially in the case of a protein-free diet, showing weight loss and spontaneous debilitation. To achieve complete protection against malaria while still maintaining healthy conditions, 5–12.5% low-protein diets should be selected.

In a series of previous studies (Mannoor et al., 2001; Weerasinghe et al., 2001; Mannoor et al., 2002), we emphasized that malarial protection is the result of immunological events of innate immunity. Thus: (1) the major protective lymphocytes are CD8$^+$NK1.1$^-$TCR^{int} cells, which exist in the liver; (2) autoantibodies are always present and the activation of autoantibody-producing B-1 cells takes place; (3) the main stream of T-cell differentiation in the thymus is arrested as shown by severe thymic atrophy; and (4) acquired immunity against malaria disappears within 1 yr after infection. The present data did not contradict these facts. Moreover, the present results seem to somewhat explain our experience in a field study of malaria, in which many inhabitants eventually avoided contracting malaria even after apparent infection.

In the present study, we conducted cell-transfer experiments using purified TCR^{high} cells and TCR^{int} cells. To avoid cell dilution in the body, we used 6.5 Gy-irradiated mice as recipients. It was confirmed that liver lymphocytes (2 × 10^6/mouse) isolated from nonimmune mice could not protect recipient mice from malarial infection by the nonlethal strain. In sharp contrast, liver lymphocytes isolated from immune mice fed with the 5% protein diet (nonlethal strain) were able to protect mice completely. Similarly, TCR^{int} cells (5 × 10^5/mouse), but not TCR^{high} cells (5 × 10^5/mouse), were also able to protect mice from malarial infection of nonlethal strain. We feel that purified TCR^{int} cells had less ability to protect mice from malarial infection than did whole liver lymphocytes. There is a possibility that some B cells, e.g., B-1 cells, may also act to protect against malaria in parallel with TCR^{int} cells. TCR^{int} cells and B-1 cells are both primordial components of innate immunity (Miyakawa et al., 2002; Morshed et al., 2002).

There is a possibility that low-protein diets suppressed the growth of malaria parasites in the mice, which resulted in the suppression of malarial infection. We cannot deny such an effect completely. However, we must consider the role of innate immunity. Thus, the mice that were fed on a low-protein diet recovered from infection and showed low levels of parasitemia and also acquired the potent anti-malaria immunity. This study shows that TCR^{int} cells are important mediators against malaria. To support the importance of TCR^{int} cells in the present phenomenon, we conducted the experiments using scid mice that lack all T cells (including TCR^{int} cells). These mice fed with low-protein diets could not survive when lethal strain of *P. yoelii* was used. This result for scid mice, as well as the acquisition of immunity after recovery in normal mice fed with low-protein diets, suggest that TCR^{int} cells play essential roles for complete protection against both lethal and nonlethal strains of malaria. However, because scid mice fed with low-protein diet showed retarded parasitemia (high levels) before death, the activation of macrophages and NK cells by low-protein diets or the growth suppression of malaria parasites by low-protein diets should be considered as well. In any case, the results from scid mice suggest that TCR^{int} cells are essential for the complete protection against malaria induced by low-protein diets in the present situation.

In a recent study, we reported that mice fed with the 5% protein diet showed increased levels of innate immunity and these mice acquired immunity against tumor resistance on lung metastasis (Li et al., 2004). In other words, we must also consider a change in the level of innate immunity in hosts fed with low-protein diets.

The present study shed light on possible preventative measures against malaria, because 5–12.5% protein diets rendered mice resistant to lethal strains of *P. yoelii* (in the present study) and even those of *P. berghei* (data not shown).

ACKNOWLEDGMENTS

This work was supported by a Grant-in-Aid for Scientific Research and Cancer Research from the Ministry of Education, Science and Culture, Japan. The authors wish to thank Mrs. Masako Watanabe for manuscript preparation.

LITERATURE CITED

ABO, T., T. KAWAMURA, AND H. WATANABE. 2000. Physiological responses of extrathymic T cells in the liver. Immunological Reviews **174**: 135–149.

BHATIA, A., AND V. K. VINAYAK. 1991. Dietary modulation of malaria infection in rats. Indian Journal of Malariology **28**: 237–242.

BRYANT, H. U., E. W. BERNTON, AND J. W. HOLADAY. 1987. Immunosuppressive effects of chronic morphine treatment in mice. Life Sciences **41**: 1731–1738.

FAGNENRO-BEYIOKU, A. F., AND J. P. OYERNINDE. 1990. Effect of host-diet inadequacy on the course of infection of *Plasmodium yoelii nigeriensis*. West African Journal of Medicine **9**: 124–128.

HALDER, K. C., I. KAWAMURA, M. BANNAI, H. WATANABE, H. KAWAMURA, M. D. K. MANNOOR, S. R. M. MORSHED, AND T. ABO. 2001. Intensive generation of NK1.1$^-$ extrathymic T cells in the liver by injection of bone marrow cells isolated from mice with a mutation of polymorphic MHC antigens. Immunology **102**: 450–459.

ITO, S., M. UENO, S. NISHI, M. ARAKAWA, Y. IKARASHI, T. SAITOH, AND M. FUJIWARA. 1992. Histological characteristics of lupus nephritis in F$_1$ mice with chronic graft-versus-host reaction across MHC class II difference. Autoimmunity **12**: 79–87.

KAMEYAMA, H., T. KAWAMURA, T. NAITO, M. BANNAI, K. SHIMAMURA, K. HATAKEYAMA, AND T. ABO. 2001. Size of the population of CD4$^+$ natural killer T cells in the liver is maintained without supply by the thymus during adult life. Immunology **104**: 135–141.

KATAAHA, P. K., C. A. FACER, S. M. MORTAZAVI-ORTAZAVI-MILIANI, H. STIERLE, AND E. J. HOLBOROW. 1984. Stimulation of autoantibody production in normal blood lymphocytes by malaria culture supernatants. Parasite Immunology **6**: 481–492.

KICSKA, G. A., L. M. TING, V. L. SCHRAMM, AND K. KIM. 2003. Effect of dietary p-aminobenzoic acid on murine *Plasmodium yoelii* infection. Journal of Infectious Diseases **188**: 1776–1781.

LEVANDER, O. A., A. L. AGER, V. C. MORRIS, JR., AND R. G. MAY. 1990. *Plasmodium yoelii*: Comparative antimalarial activities of dietary fish oils and fish oil concentrates in vitamin E-deficient mice. Experimental Parasitology **70**: 323–329.

LEWIN, R. 1988. Stress proteins: Are links in disease. Science **240**: 1732–1733.

LI, C., X. BAI, C. TOMIYAMA-MIYAJI, T. NAGURA, T. KAWAMURA, AND T. ABO. 2004. Immunopotentiation of NKT cells by low-protein diet and the suppressive effect on tumor metastasis. Cellular Immunology **231**: 96–102.

LLOYD, C. M., I. COLLINS, A. J. BELCHER, N. MANUEELPILLAI, A. O. WOZENCRAFT, AND N. A. STAINES. 1994. Characterization and pathological significance of monoclonal DNA-binding antibodies from mice with experimental malaria infection. Infection and Immunity **62**: 1982–1988.

MANNOOR, M. K., R. C. HALDER, S. R. M. MORSHED, A. ARIYASHINGHE, H. Y. BAKIR, H. KAWAMURA, H. WATANABE, H. SEKIKAWA, AND T. ABO. 2002. Essential role of extrathymic T cells in protection against malaria. Journal of Immunology **169**: 301–306.

———, A. WEERASINGHE, R. C. HALDER, S. R. M. MORSHED, A. ARIYASHINGHE, H. WATANABE, H. SEKIKAWA, AND T. ABO. 2001. Resistance to malarial infection is achieved by the cooperation of NK1.1$^+$ and NK1.1$^-$ subsets of intermediate TCR cells which are constituents of the innate immunity. Cellular Immunology **211**: 96–104.

MARUYAMA, S., A. TSUKAHARA, S. SUZUKI, T. TADA, M. MINAGAWA, H. WATANABE, K. HATAKEYAMA, AND T. ABO. 1999. Quick recovery in the generation of self-reactive CD4^{low} NKT cells by an alternative intrathymic pathway when restored from acute thymic atrophy. Clinical Experimental Immunology **117**: 587–595.

MIYAKAWA, R., C. MIYAJI, H. WATANABE, H. YOKOYAMA, C. TSUKADA, H. ASAKURA, AND T. ABO. 2002. Unconventional NK1.1$^-$ intermediate TCR cells as major T lymphocytes expanding in chronic graft-versus-host disease. European Journal of Immunology **32**: 2521–2531.

MORSHED, S. R. M., K. MANNOOR, R. C. HALDER, H. KAWAMURA, M. BANNAI, H. SEKIKAWA, H. WATANABE, AND T. ABO. 2002. Tissue-specific expansion of NKT and CD5$^+$B cells at the onset of autoimmune disease in (NZB × NZW)F$_1$ mice. European Journal of Immunology **32**: 2551–2561.

O'LEARY, A. 1990. Stress, emotion, and human immune function. Psychological Bulletin **108**: 363–382.

OYA, H., T. KAWAMURA, T. SHIMIZU, M. BANNAI, H. KAWAMURA, M. MINAGAWA, H. WATANABE, K. HATAKEYAMA, AND T. ABO. 2000. The differential effect of stress on NKT and NK cell function. Clinical Experimental Immunology **121**: 384–390.

RIBEIRO, C. D., C. ALFRED, L. MONJOUR, AND M. GENTILINI. 1984. Normal frequency of anti-thyroglobulin antibodies in hyperendemic areas of malaria: Relevance to the understanding of autoantibody formation in malaria. Tropical and Geographical Medicine **36**: 323–328.

———, S. DE ROQUEFEUIL, P. DRUILHE, L. MONJOUR, J. C. HOMBERG, AND M. GENTILINI. 1984. Abnormal anti-single stranded (ss) DNA activity in sera from *Plasmodium falciparum* infected individuals. Transaction of the Royal Society of Tropical Medicine and Hygiene **78:** 742–746.

SHANKAR, A. H. 2000. Nutritional modulation of malaria morbidity and mortality. Infectious Diseases **182:** S37–S53.

SHIMIZU, T., T. KAWAMURA, C. MIYAJI, H. OYA, M. BANNAI, S. YAMAMOTO, A. WEERASINGHE, R. C. HALDER, H. WATANABE, K. HATAKEYAMA, AND T. ABO. 2000. Resistance of extrathymic T cells to stress and a role of endogenous glucocorticoids in stress-associated immunosuppression. Scandinavian Journal of Immunology **51:** 285–292.

TAGOH, H., H. NISHIJO, T. UWANO, H. KISHI, T. ONO, AND A. MURAGUCHI. 1995. Reciprocal IL-1 beta gene expression in medial and lateral hypothalamic areas in SART-stressed mice. Neuroscience Letters **184:** 17–20.

TAKAKURA, M., M. UZA, Y. SASAKI, N. NAGAHAMA, S. PHOMMPIDA, S. BOUNYADETH, J. KOBAYASHI, T. TOMA, AND I. MIYAGI. 2001. The relationship between anthropometric indicators of nutritional status and malaria infection among youths in Khammouane Province, Laos PDR. The Southeast Asian Journal of Tropical Medicine and Public Health **32:** 262–267.

WEERASINGHE, A., H. SEKIKAWA, H. WATANABE, M. K. MANNOOR, S. R. M. KAWAMURA, S. SEKI, AND T. ABO. 2001. Association of intermediate T cell receptor cells, mainly their NK1.1$^-$ subset, with protection from malaria. Cellular Immunology **207:** 28–35.

WENISCH, C., H. WENISCH, H. C. BANKL, M. EXNER, W. GRANINGER, S. LOOAREESUWAN, AND H. RUMPOLD. 1996. Detection of anti-neutrophil cytoplasmic antibodies after acute *Plasmodium falciparum* malaria. Clinical and Diagnostic Laboratory Immunology **3:** 132–134.

Role of α-adrenergic stimulus in stress-induced modulation of body temperature, blood glucose and innate immunity

αアドレナリン刺激が、
体温、血糖、自然免疫におけるストレス適応反応に与える影響

chapter 20

Role of α-adrenergic stimulus in stress-induced modulation of body temperature, blood glucose and innate immunity

αアドレナリン刺激が、体温、血糖、自然免疫におけるストレス適応反応に与える影響

Mayumi Watanabe[a], Chikako Tomiyama-Miyaji[a,c], Eisuke Kainuma[a], Masashi Inoue[a], Hongwei Ren[a], Jiwei Shen[a,b], Toru Aboa,*

[a] Department of Immunology, Niigata University School of Medicine, Niigata 951-8510, Japan
[b] First Department of Surgery, Niigata University School of Medicine, Niigata 951-8510, Japan
[c] School of Health Sciences, Faculty of Medicine, Niigata University, Niigata 951-8518, Japan
Received 31 July 2007; received in revised form 28 September 2007; accepted 28 September 2007
Available online 23 October 2007

【キーワード】

ストレス； アドレナリン刺激； 高血糖； 低体温； 自然免疫

【要約】

　マウスに、3時間の拘束ストレスを与えた。この間、低体温（39℃→37℃未満）と高血糖（150mg/dl→220mg/dl）が同時に出現した。ストレス応答反応として、カテコラミンの血中濃度が上昇した。アドレナリン（α刺激）を投与したところ、ストレスに類似した体温・血糖の変化が出現した。一方、ノルアドレナリン（アドレナリンほど強力ではないα刺激）投与やイソプロテレノール（β）投与では、このような変化は見られなかった。このαアドレナリン刺激について、アドレナリンα受容体遮断薬とβ受容体遮断薬を使用してアドレナリンが誘発した低体温・高血糖について確認を行なった。さらに、α刺激により免疫学的指標がどのように変化するかを検証した。特に肝臓においては、ストレスに耐性があるリンパ球集団は、NK細胞、胸腺外分化T細胞およびNKT細胞が出現した。これらリンパ球の機能を解析したところ、アドレナリンα刺激によりNK細胞傷害活性とNKT細胞傷害活性増強を示した。これら結果から、アドレナリンα刺激は、ストレスが生体に影響する要因の1つであり、その結果、時として、ストレスを受けると低体温・高血糖・自然免疫活性化が誘導されることが明らかになった。

1. はじめに

　ストレスを受けると胸腺萎縮が起こると共に、特に末梢のTリンパ球とBリンパ球の免疫抑制が起こることが知られている［1-3］。この免疫抑制には、ステロイドホルモン分泌だけでなく、アドレナリン刺激（カテコラミン）の影響も関与する［4-6］。ストレスによる免疫調節（免疫抑制だけでなく免疫増強も含む）について多数の研究者が報告している［7-11］。最近、我々の予備研究により、マウスに拘束ストレスを与えると低体温・高血糖が誘導されることが明らかになった。ストレスにより低体温・高血糖が出現したことは、免疫抑制同様、非常に重要である可能性がある。というのは、ストレスに苦しむ患者には、血液循環不全（例えば、激しい血管収縮が原因）による低体温と高血糖（糖尿病の一因）が見られることが多いためである。［12-14］

　本研究では、上述の観察を考慮して、アドレナリン刺激がどのようにストレス適応反応（例えば免疫抑制、低体温と高血糖）に影響を及ぼ

すか検証した。我々は、以前、拘束ストレスを与えると、Tリンパ球やBリンパ球が介在する獲得免疫では免疫は抑制される一方、NK細胞とNKT細胞が介在する自然免疫はむしろ増強されることを報告してきた [15,16]。そこで、アドレナリン刺激（α刺激またはβ刺激）を与えた場合、同様の状況が出現するかどうか検証を行なった。

2. 材料と方法

2.1 マウス

C57BL/6（B6）マウスを、日本チャールズ・リバー株式会社（横浜）より購入した。本実験において使用したマウス全ては8-12週齢雄であった。マウスは、新潟大学動物飼育施設の室内で、一定温度（25±2℃）一定湿度（50-70%）、12時間 明/暗サイクル（点灯時間08:00 - 20:00）、SPF（特定病原体未感染）環境下にて飼育した。

2.2 拘束ストレス

実験群マウスに、ステンレス製メッシュを用いて3時間（09:00 - 12:00）拘束ストレスを与えた [5]。本実験は、新潟大学動物実験倫理委員会の承認を得て行なった。

2.3 体温と血糖の測定

マウスの直腸温度をTHERMAC SENSOR（芝浦電子、東京）を用いて、血糖をPrecision XtraTM（アボットジャパン、千葉）測定した。

2.4 カテコラミンおよびアドレナリン遮断薬の投与

アドレナリン（ボスミン,第一三共（株）,東京）、ノルアドレナリン（ノルアドレナリン,第一三共（株）,東京）および イソプロテレノール（プロタノール,興和（株）,東京）を用いた。上記薬物（0.2ml）を25.0、12.5または6.25μg/匹量マウスに腹腔内投与した。フェントラミン、α受容体遮断薬（レギチーン,ノバルティスファーマ（株）,東京）およびプロプラノロール、β受容体遮断薬（インデラル,アストラゼネカ（株）,大阪）も使用した。上記遮断薬（0.2ml）を12.5または6.25μg/匹量マウスに腹腔内投与した。

2.5 細胞分離

イソフルラン麻酔したマウスの鎖骨下動脈と静脈より脱血し、肝臓と脾臓を摘出し、肝単核細胞を定法に従い分離した [17]。略述すると、摘出した肝臓を200-ゲージ・ステンレス・スチール・メッシュで濾し、5mMのHEPESおよび2%非働化仔牛血清を添加したEagle MEM培養液中に浮遊させた。培養液で一度洗浄した後、この細胞に100U/ml ヘパリンを加え、35%パーコール溶液中に再懸濁させ、回転速度2000rpm（424 x g）で15分間比重遠心分離を行なった。分離した細胞塊を溶血溶液（155mM NH_4Cl, 10mM $KHCO_3$, 10mM EDTAおよび17mM Tris, pH 7.3）で赤血球（RBC）を溶血させ、培養液で二度洗浄した。脾臓と胸腺をステンレス・スチール・メッシュで濾過して、それぞれ脾臓細胞あるいは胸腺細胞を得た。脾臓細胞を得るため0.2% NaCl溶液を用いRBC除去を行なった。

2.6 フローサイトメトリー解析

リンパ球の表現型の解析には二重免疫蛍光染色を用いた [18]。本実験で用いたモノクローナル抗体を以下記す（BD PharMingen、San Diego、CA）；抗CD3ε（145-2C11）、抗IL-2Rβ（TM-β1）、抗NK1.1（PK136）、抗CD4（RM4-5）、抗CD8α（53-6.7）および抗B220（RA3-6B2）。これらは、いずれもイソチオシアン酸フルオレセイン（FITC）標識とフィコエリトリン（PE）標識されたモノクローナル抗体である。モノクローナル抗体の非特異的結合を防ぐため、抗CD16/CD32

（2.4G2）モノクロナール抗体にて前処理を行った後、各種標識抗体を加えた。懸濁させたリンパ球（5 x 10^5 – 2 x 10^6/tube）をモノクロナール抗体で染色し、染色したリンパ球をフローサイトメトリー（FACScan）（Becton-Dickinson社, Mountain View, CA）を用い解析した。死細胞は、ヨウ化プロピジウムで染色し、前方散乱と側方散乱でのゲーティングを行い除外した。

2.7 血漿中カテコラミン値測定

マウス4頭の血漿を用い、カテコラミン（アドレナリン、ノルアドレナリンとドーパミン）値測定を行なった。血漿中カテコラミン値はHPLC方法を用い測定した [19]。

2.8 細胞傷害性試験

定法に従い細胞傷害性試験を行なった [20]。YAC-1細胞（NK細胞傷害性）とB6マウス胸腺細胞（NKT細胞傷害性）を標的細胞として、細胞傷害活性測定を行なった。YAC-1細胞に対する細胞傷害活性の最低量は、NKT細胞にも関与するが、その影響は最低限である。標的細胞には、2時間 [^{51}Cr] ナトリウムクロム酸塩（NEN Life Science Products, Boston, MA, USA）で標識した後、RPMI-1640培養液で三度洗浄した。濃度を変えて希釈した各濃度のエフェクター細胞を、９６穴U底マイクロ培養テストプレートに入れ、[^{51}Cr] 標識した標的細胞（1 x 10^4 または2 x 10^4 ）と混和した。遠心分離した後、テストプレートを4時間37°C、培養を行なった。培養終了後、上清を100μl回収し、ガンマカウンターを用いて計測した。

2.9 統計分析

実験群間の有意差検定には、スチューデントのt検定と一元配置ANOVA検定を用いた。

Figure.1

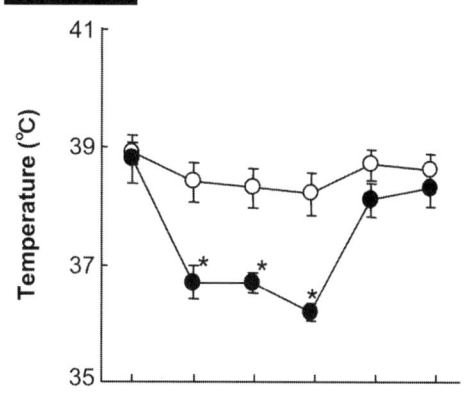

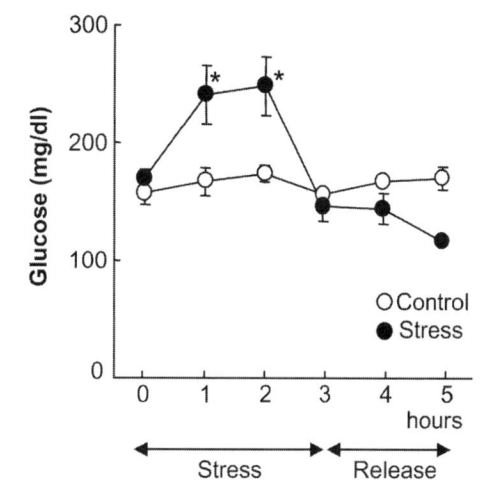

拘束ストレスの体温と血糖値の経時的変化　マウスに３時間の拘束ストレスを与えた後、開放した。各時点において体温と血糖を計測した。平均値±１SDは、３匹のマウスを用いて算出した。* $P<0.05$.

3. 結果

3.1 ストレス適応反応

マウスに3時間拘束ストレスを与えた後、開放した。各時点において体温と血糖を計測した（Fig. 1）。第1に、対照群の体温は高かったが（38.9 ± 0.5°C）、一方、ストレス実験群では低体温（36.0-37.0°C）が出現した（$P < 0.05$）。ストレスから開放した後、低体温は実験前の体温に回復した。

血糖値は、対照群では150mg/dlであったが、ストレス実験群では、高血糖（220-240mg/dl）

Figure.2

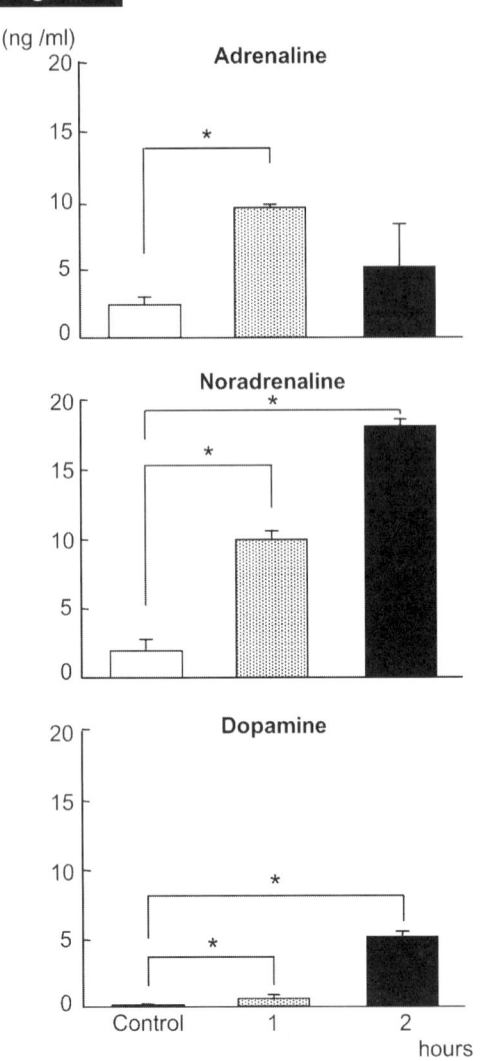

(グラフ: Adrenaline, Noradrenaline, Dopamine の Control、1時間後、2時間後の値)

拘束ストレス時の血漿中カテコールアミン値 実験開始時、一時間後、二時間後における血漿中カテコールアミン（アドレナリン、ノルアドレナリンおよびとドーパミン）値を測定した。平均値±SDは、実験を3度行い算出した。* $P<0.05$.

が出現した。ストレスから開放した後、高血糖は、実験前の値に回復した。

ストレスによる緊急反応において、血清中カテコラミン値が変化することが知られている[4]。そこで、ストレス前後における、血清中カテコラミン値を測定した（Fig. 2）。拘束ストレス実験開始後、アドレナリン、ノルアドレナリンおよびドーパミンの血漿濃度のすべてが上昇した（1, 2 h, $P < 0.05$）。この結果より、カテコラミンのいずれかが、Fig.1で観察されたストレス適応反応と関係している可能性があることが明らかになった。

3.2 アドレナリンα刺激

どの種類のカテコラミンが拘束ストレス実験時に見られた低体温・高血糖を誘発したか検証した（Fig. 3A）。予備実験を行った。そして、アドレナリン（α刺激）、ノルアドレナリン（アドレナリンほど強力ではないα刺激）投与でもイソプロテレノール（β）を投与しても、マウスに死亡や障害が出現しない最大投与量を決定した。アドレナリン投与時には、低体温・高血糖が同時に出現したが、ノルアドレナリン投与でもイソプロテレノール投与でもこのような変化は出現しなかった。アドレナリン投与量（25.0, 12.5 または 6.25μg/匹）による影響の変化のグラフを示した（Fig. 3B）。最も顕著な低体温と高血糖が25.0（μg/匹）投与した場合に観察された。

3.3 α受容体遮断薬とβ受容体遮断薬の使用

アドレナリンα刺激が、低体温・高血糖の原因であることを更に確認するため、アドレナリンα受容体遮断薬（フェントラミン）とアドレナリンβ受容体遮断薬（プロプラノロール）を、アドレナリンを投与して低体温と高血糖が出現した実験で使用した（Fig. 4）。

アドレナリン（25.0μg/匹）投与10分前にα受容体遮断薬またはβ受容体遮断薬（6.25μgまたは12.5μg/匹）を腹腔内投与した。事前実験を同じ投与量を用いて行なったところ、α受容体遮断薬のみもしくは、β受容体遮断薬のみでは、体温と血糖には全く影響しなかった（未発表データ）。特に、投与後期（2-3h）において、α受容体遮断薬投与により若干、低体温が軽減されることが明らかになった。さらに顕著であったのは、β受容体遮断薬投与により、アド

Figure.3

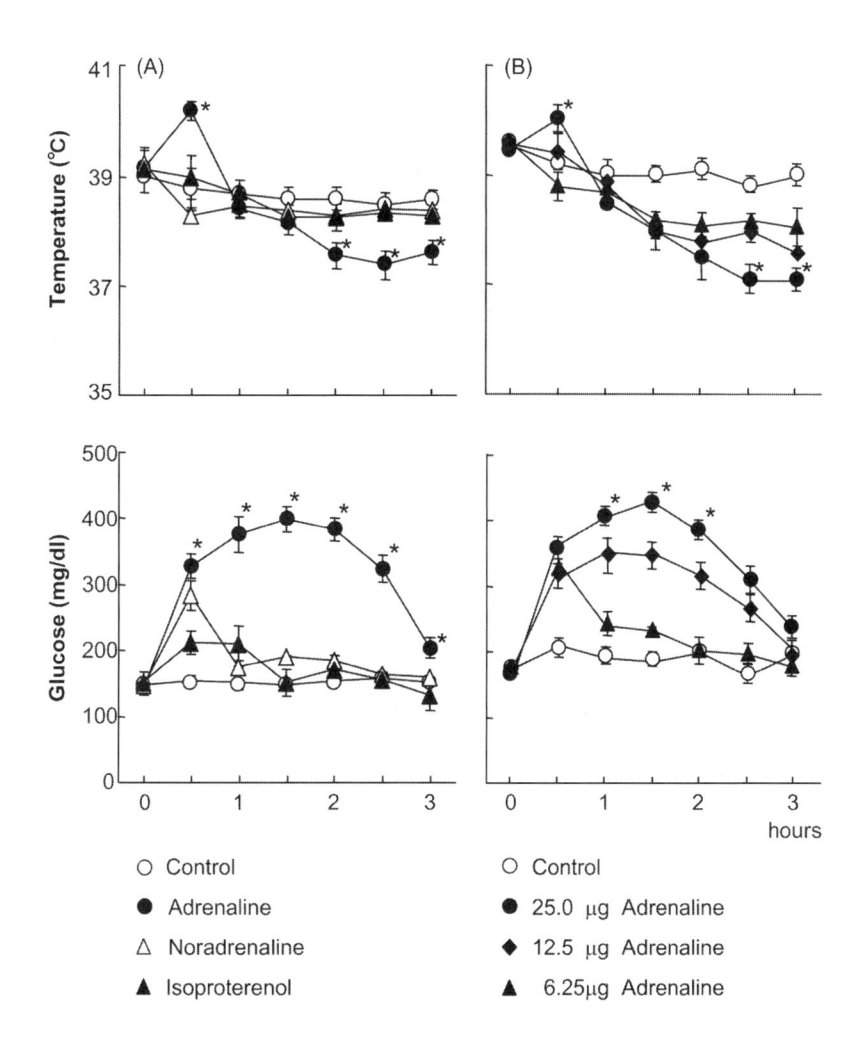

カテコールアミン投与が体温と血糖に与える影響（A）アドレナリン、ノルアドレナリンおよびとイソプロテレノールの投与（B）アドレナリン投与量による影響の変化（A）では、マウスにアドレナリン、ノルアドレナリンまたはイソプロテレノール25.0μgを腹腔内投与した。各時点において体温と血糖を計測した。（B）では、アドレナリン投与量による影響の変化を検証した。平均値±1 SDは、3匹のマウスを用いて算出した。* $P<0.05$.

Figure.4

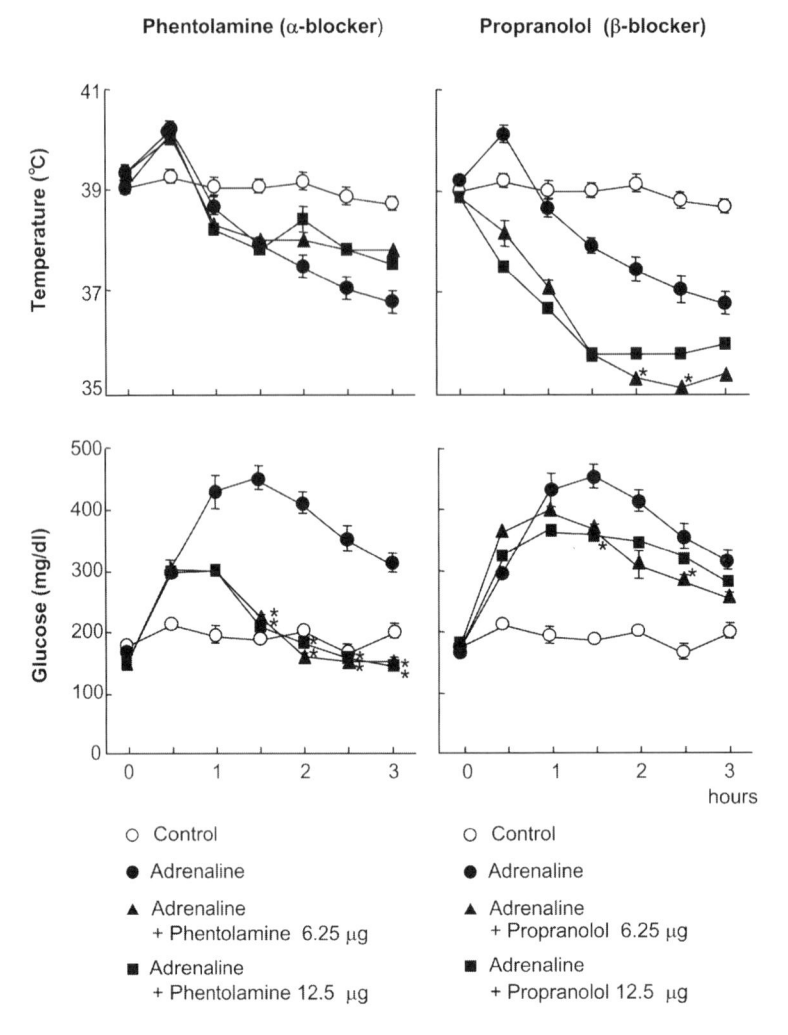

Phentolamine (α-blocker) / **Propranolol (β-blocker)**

縦軸: Temperature (°C), Glucose (mg/dl)
横軸: hours

凡例:
- ○ Control
- ● Adrenaline
- ▲ Adrenaline + Phentolamine 6.25 μg / Adrenaline + Propranolol 6.25 μg
- ■ Adrenaline + Phentolamine 12.5 μg / Adrenaline + Propranolol 12.5 μg

ストレス由来のαアドレナリン刺激が、低体温、高血糖に対するα遮断薬またはβ受容体遮断薬の影響 アドレナリン投与時、α遮断薬とβ受容体遮断薬も同時に皮下投与した。平均値±SDは、3頭のマウスを用いて算出した。* $P<0.05$.

レナリン投与時に出現する低体温が増強されていたことである。考えられるのは、βアドレナリン刺激は低体温を軽減する可能性である。血糖値では、α受容体遮断薬が高血糖の軽減効果があったが、β受容体遮断薬にはいずれの投与量でも、α受容体遮断薬のような顕著な効果は見られなかった。

3.4 アドレナリンα刺激による免疫調節

マウスに拘束ストレスを与えると、獲得免疫は抑制され、その反対に自然免疫が増強されると以前報告した [5、6]。そこで、アドレナリンα刺激を与えることで、拘束ストレスを与えた時に類似した状況を再現することが可能かを検証した（Fig. 5）。その結果、肝臓と胸腺のリンパ球の数は減少したが、脾臓のリンパ球は変化しなかった。

各臓器においてリンパ球サブセットの分布を特定するために、フローサイトメトリーによる解析を行なった（Fig. 6）。肝臓および脾臓において二重染色（CD3とIL-2Rβ、CD3と

Figure.5

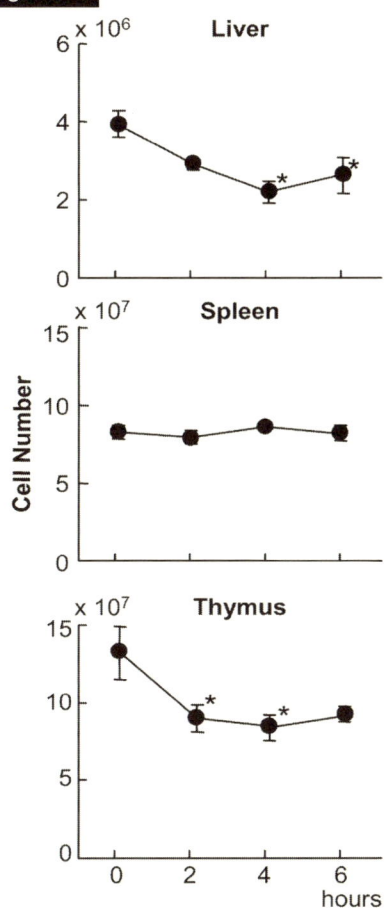

Figure.6

アドレナリンの投与後のリンパ球数 リンパ球は、肝臓、脾臓と胸腺より採取した。平均値±1 SDは、3匹のマウスを用いて算出した。* $P<0.05$.

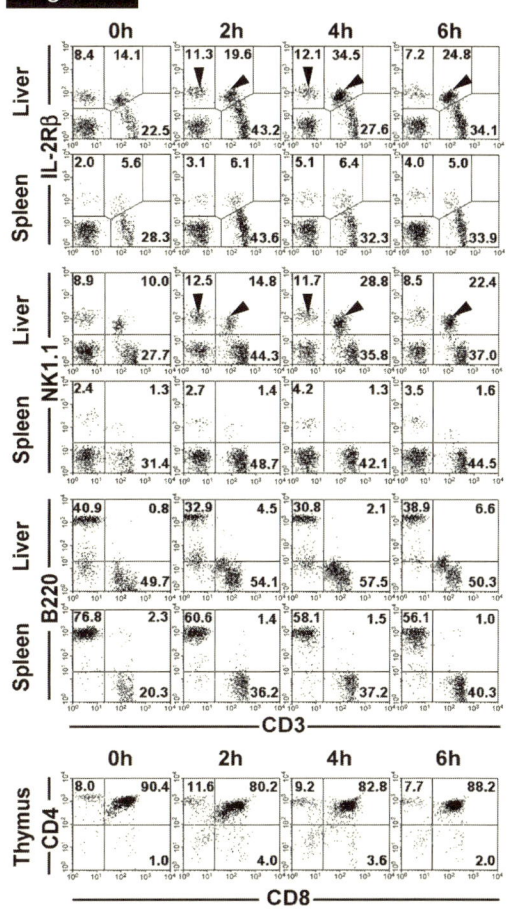

アドレナリン投与後の各臓器リンパ球の二重染色 各時点におけるリンパ球を採取し、リンパ球サブセットをフローサイトメトリーにより解析した。リンパ球の二重染色（CD3とIL-2Rβ、CD3とNK1.1もしくはCD3とB220）および胸腺細胞の二重染色（CD4とCD8）を行なった。3度実験を行った典型例を示す。各分画内の数値は蛍光陽性細胞の比率を示す。

NK1.1もしくはCD3とB220）を行なった。最も顕著な変化は、肝臓におけるNK細胞、胸腺外分化T細胞およびNKT細胞に見られた。2-6h時点において以下のように増加が見られた。NK細胞（IL-2Rβ$^+$またはNK1.1$^+$）（8.4→12.1%,4h)、胸腺外分化T細胞（IL-2Rβ$^+$CD3^{int}）（14.1→34.5%,4h）とNK1.1$^+$CD3^{int} NKT細胞（10.0→28.8%,4h）であった。比率が最も増加したのは4h時点であった。B220$^+$ B細胞とIL-2Rβ$^-$CD3^{high} T細胞の比率においてストレスよる変化は見られなかった。

胸腺においてCD4とCD8の二重染色を行なったところ、アドレナリンα刺激により若干CD4$^+$8$^+$ダブルポジティブ細胞の比率の低下が示された（90.4→80.2%,2h）(Fig. 6,下)。換言すると、本実験で投与したアドレナリンα刺激は、拘束ストレスほど強力ではなかった。

アドレナリンα刺激により肝臓におけるNK細胞とNKT細胞の比率が増加した。そこで、更に、機能活性に変化が起こったかを検証した（Fig. 7）。本実験では、肝臓と脾臓よりリンパ球を採取した。肝臓において、YAC-1細

Figure.5

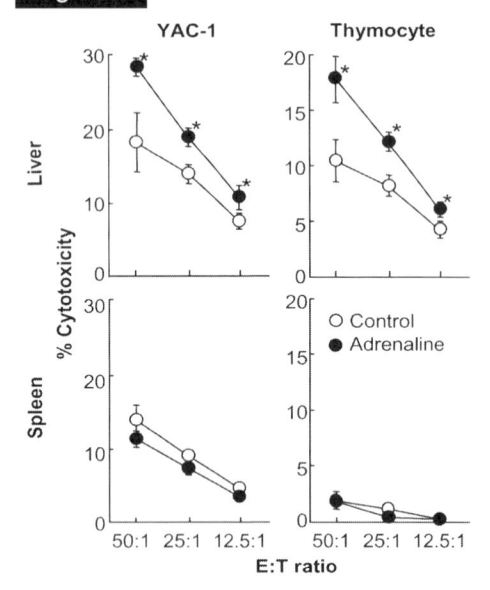

細胞傷害活性試験 YAC-1細胞に対するNK細胞傷害活性とB6マウスの胸腺細胞に対するNKT細胞傷害活性を（エフェクター細胞/ターゲット細胞（E/T）率）を検証した。平均値±1SDは、実験を3度行い算出した。* $P<0.05$。

胞に対するNK活性およびB6マウスの胸腺細胞に対するNKT細胞の活性が、アドレナリンα刺激により増強されることが明らかになった（$P<0.05$）。脾臓ではこのような増強は確認できなかった。

4. 考察

本研究では、アドレナリンα刺激をマウスに与えると、低体温、高血糖と自然免疫の活性といった、拘束ストレスにおける応答反応に類似した状況が誘導されることを証明した。拘束ストレスを与えると、カテコラミン、各種ステロイドホルモンや炎症性サイトカインの分泌が同時に起こることを報告した [4-6]。本研究では、これらホルモンのうち、カテコラミンに注目した。拘束ストレスを与えると、アドレナリン、ノルアドレナリンおよびドーパミンが分泌されることを確認できた。そこで、どの種類のアドレナリン刺激を与えると、ストレス応答反応に類似した反応が見られるか検証した。アドレナリンアドレナリン（α刺激）、ノルアドレナリン（アドレナリンほど強力ではないα刺激）、イソプロテレノール（β）投与を行った。薬剤投与してβ受容体刺激ではなく、α受容体刺激を行った場合、特に体温、血糖、免疫機能についてストレス関連反応が現れた。

そこで、アドレナリンα刺激が、低体温・高血糖の原因であるのか、アドレナリンα受容体遮断薬とβ受容体遮断薬を用いて確認した。アドレナリン投与により低体温が出現したが、α受容体遮断薬を投与すると、体温低下は若干、軽減された。しかしβ受容体遮断薬を投与したところ体温は更に低下した。β受容体刺激には、アドレナリン刺激を抑制する作用も含まれているようである。アドレナリン投与による高血糖は、α受容体遮断薬により、血糖値を上昇させない効果が見られた。一方、β受容体遮断薬を投与した場合では、このような効果は確認できなかった。

ストレスによる主な免疫抑制性反応について、末梢におけるTリンパ球とBリンパ球の免疫抑制および急性胸腺萎縮を含む報告を、これまで多数行なってきた [1-3]。この場合、各種ステロイドホルモンが、ストレス関連反応における免疫抑制では重要な役割を果たす。一方、アドレナリンα刺激を行なった結果出現したのは、肝臓と胸腺におけるリンパ球減少を伴う、マイルドな免疫抑制だけであった。さらに、アドレナリンα刺激によるダブルポジティブ$CD4^+8^+$細胞数の減少に対する影響は、顕著ではなかった（図5下）。これらの結果は、免疫抑制性反応は、複数のホルモンの要因が影響した結果であることを示唆する。

ストレスを与えた場合、T細胞とB細胞の免疫抑制が見られたのとは対照的に、NK細胞（$NK1.1^+CD3^-$）、胸腺外分化T細胞（IL-

$2R\beta^+CD3^{int}$) およびNKT細胞（NK1.1$^+$CD3^{int}）が関与する自然免疫は増加を示した。アドレナリン（α受容体刺激）投与によりこの反応も再現することができた。アドレナリンα刺激による機能活性を、NK細胞とNKT細胞傷害活性により確認した。本研究では、NK細胞傷害活性性にはYAC-1細胞を用い、NKT細胞傷害活性にはB6マウスの胸腺細胞（自己組織の細胞傷害活性）を用いて測定した [20]。

本来、交感神経刺激により代謝が亢進する結果、体温が上昇する。一方、副交感神経刺激により代謝が低下する結果、体温が低下する [21-23]。しかし、本研究の拘束ストレスのような強い交感神経刺激を受けると、おそらく血管収縮（循環不全）が出現し、低体温が出現する。緩徐でも強力でも、交感神経を刺激すると、必ず、高血糖が出現する [24、25]。ストレスにより低体温と高血糖が起きる可能性があるとこれまで沢山報告されてきた [12-14]。アドレナリンを投与してアドレナリンα刺激を行い、ストレス時に類似した低体温と高血糖が出現した。この時、同時に、自然免疫の活性化も現れた。アドレナリンβ刺激を行なっても、低体温と高血糖が出現することが知られているが [26]。しかし、本研究で示したように、アドレナリンβ刺激は、アドレナリンα刺激よりもマイルドであると思われる。

低体温と高血糖が同時に出現したことに加えて、自然免疫の活性化が見られたのは興味深い。本研究では、拘束ストレスのみならず [5, 6]、アドレナリンα刺激を行った場合でも同様に、T細胞とB細胞の免疫抑制がされた状況において自然免疫の活性化を確認されたのである。

謝辞

本研究は、文部科学省科学研究費補助金による。原稿浄書について金子裕子氏に感謝する。

Role of α-adrenergic stimulus in stress-induced modulation of body temperature, blood glucose and innate immunity

Mayumi Watanabe [a], Chikako Tomiyama-Miyaji [a,c], Eisuke Kainuma [a], Masashi Inoue [a], Yuh Kuwano [a], Hongwei Ren [a], Jiwei Shen [a,b], Toru Abo [a,*]

[a] *Department of Immunology, Niigata University School of Medicine, Niigata 951-8510, Japan*
[b] *First Department of Surgery, Niigata University School of Medicine, Niigata 951-8510, Japan*
[c] *School of Health Sciences, Faculty of Medicine, Niigata University, Niigata 951-8518, Japan*

Received 31 July 2007; received in revised form 28 September 2007; accepted 28 September 2007
Available online 23 October 2007

Abstract

Mice were exposed to restraint stress for 3 h. During this period, low body temperature (hypothermia, 39 °C → less than 37 °C) and high blood glucose levels (hyperglycemia, 150 mg/dl → up to 220 mg/dl) were simultaneously induced. Reflecting a stress-induced phenomenon, blood levels of catecholamines increased at that time. Administration of adrenaline (α-stimulus), but neither noradrenaline (α but less than adrenaline) nor isoproterenol (β), induced a similar stress-induced pattern of body temperature and blood glucose variations. This α-adrenergic effect was confirmed using α- and β-blockers in adrenaline-induced hypothermia and hyperglycemia. By applying this α-stimulus, the effect on immunoparameters was then investigated. Stress-resistant lymphocyte populations were found to be NK cells, extrathymic T cells and NKT cells, especially in the liver. Functional assays showed that both NK-cell cytotoxicity and NKT-cell cytotoxicity were augmented by α-stimulus. These results suggest that α-stimulus is one of the important factors in the stress-induced phenomenon and that it eventually produces hypothermia, hyperglycemia and innate-immunity activation seen during stress.
© 2007 Elsevier B.V. All rights reserved.

Keywords: Stress; Adrenergic stimuli; Hyperglycemia; Hypothermia; Innate immunity

1. Introduction

It is widely known that stress induces immunosuppression, especially against T and B lymphocytes in the periphery, accompanied by thymic atrophy [1–3]. Such immunosuppression is mediated by not only steroid hormones but also adrenergic stimuli (i.e., catecholamines) which are secreted due to stress [4–6]. Immunomodulations, including immunopotentiaion as well as immunosuppression, by stress were also reported by many investigators [7–11]. In a recent preliminary study, we noticed that restraint stress also induced hypothermia and hyperglycemia in mice. This observation as well as the immunosuppression might be very important because many patients suffering from stress show hypothermia derived from circulation failure (i.e., due to severe constriction of vessels) and hyperglycemia (i.e., one of the causes of diabetes mellitus) [12–14].

In light of the above-mentioned observation, in the present study, we investigated how adrenergic stimuli are associated with stress-induced responses such as the immunosuppression, hypothermia and hyperglycemia. In our previous study [15,16], we reported that innate immunity mediated by NK and NKT cells was rather augmented by restraint stress in parallel with the immunosuppression of acquired immunity mediated by T and B lymphocytes. It was therefore investigated whether adrenergic stimuli (α- or β-stimulus) were able to induce a similar phenomenon.

2. Material and methods

2.1. Mice

C57BL/6 (B6) mice were purchased from Charles River Japan (Yokohama, Japan). All mice were used at 8–12 weeks of age in these experiments. The mice were kept in a room under constant temperature (25 ± 2 °C) and humidity (50–70%) with a

---

* Corresponding author. Tel.: +81 25 227 2133; fax: +81 25 227 0766.
E-mail address: immunol2@med.niigata-u.ac.jp (T. Abo).

12 h light/dark cycle (light on from 8:00 to 20:00 h). They were fed under specific pathogen-free conditions in the animal facility of Niigata University (Niigata, Japan).

2.2. Restraint stress

Mice were exposed to restraint stress using stainless steel mesh for 3 h (from 9:00 to 12:00 h) [5]. All of the present experiments were done with the approval of the Animal Ethics Committee of Niigata University.

2.3. Measurement of body temperature and blood glucose

Body temperature was determined by using THERMAC SENSOR (Shibaura Denki Co., Tokyo) and blood glucose was measured by Precision Xtra TM (Abott Japan Co., Ltd., Chiba, Japan).

2.4. Administration of catecholamines and adrenergic blockers

Adrenaline (Bosmin, Daiichi Sankyo Co., Ltd., Tokyo), noradrenaline (NOR-ADRENALIN, Daiichi Sankyo Co., Ltd., Tokyo) and isoprotenolol (PROTERNOL, Nikken Chemicals, Co., Tokyo) were used. Each of these agents (0.2 ml) was i.p. administered into a mouse at a concentration of 25.0 (or 12.5 or 6.25) μg/mouse. Phentolamine, α-blocker (Regitin, NOVARTIS Pharma Co., Ltd., Tokyo) and Propranolol, β-blocker (Inderal, AstraZeneca Co., Ltd., Osaka) were also used. These agents (0.2 ml) were administered i.p. into a mouse at concentrations of 6.25 μg/mouse or 12.5 μg/mouse.

2.5. Cell preparation

Mice anaesthetized with isoflurane were sacrificed by exsanguination from the subclavian artery and vein, and the liver and spleen were removed. Hepatic lymphocytes were prepared as previously described [17]. Briefly, the liver was pressed through 200-gauge stainless steel mesh and suspended in Eagle's MEM medium supplemented with 5 mM HEPES and 2% FCS. After one washing, the pellet was resuspended in 35% Percoll solution containing 100 U/ml heparin and centrifuged

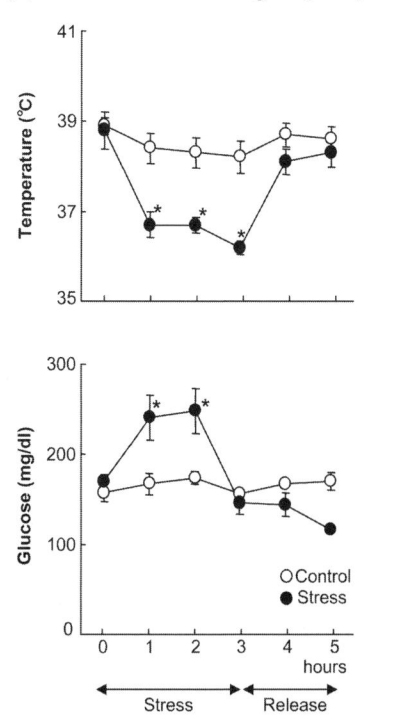

Fig. 1. Time-kinetic study on body temperature and blood glucose after restraint stress. Mice were exposed to restraint stress for 3 h and were then released. Body temperature and blood glucose were measured at the indicated points of time. Three mice were used to produce the mean and one S.D. $^*P<0.05$.

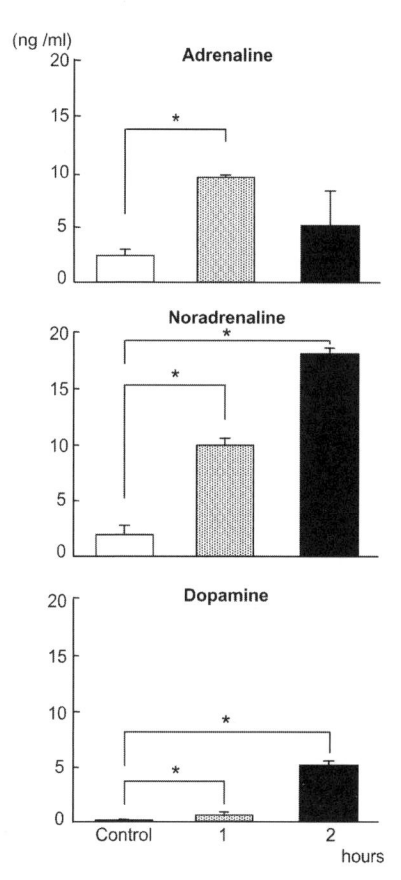

Fig. 2. Serum levels of catecholamines during restraint stress. Serum levels of adrenaline, noradrenaline and dopamine were measured at 1 and 2 h from an initial time. Three experiments were done to produce the mean and one S.D. $^*P<0.05$.

at 2000 rpm (424 × g) for 15 min. The pellet was resuspended in red blood cell (RBC) lysis solution (155 mM NH_4Cl, 10 mM $KHCO_3$, 1 mM EDTA, and 17 mM Tris, pH 7.3) and then washed twice with the medium. Splenocytes and thymocytes were obtained by forcing the spleen and thymus, respectively, through stainless steel mesh. Splenocytes were treated with 0.2% NaCl solution to remove RBC.

2.6. Immunofluorescence tests

The phenotype of lymphocytes was identified by two-color immunofluorescence tests [18]. The reagents used for this included anti-CD3ε (145-2C11), anti-IL-2Rβ (TM-β1), anti-NK1.1 (PK136), anti-CD4 (RM4-5), anti-CD8α (53-6.7), and anti-B220 (RA3-6B2) mAbs (BD PharMingen, San Diego, CA). All mAbs were used in fluorescein isothiocyanate (FITC)- and phycoerythrin (PE) conjugated-forms. To prevent non-specific binding of mAb, anti-CD16/CD32 (2.4 G2) mAb was added before staining with labeled mAbs. The suspended lymphocytes ($5 \times 10^5 - 2 \times 10^6$/tube) were stained with mAbs and stained lymphocytes were analyzed with a FACScan (Becton–Dickinson). Dead cells were excluded by forward scatter, side scatter and propidium iodide gating.

2.7. Measurement of plasma concentration of catecholamines

Plasma pooled from four mice was used to measure the concentration of adrenaline, noradrenaline and dopamine. The plasma levels of these catecholamines were analyzed by the HPLC method [19].

2.8. Cytotoxicity assays

Cytotoxicity assay was performed as previously described [20]. YAC-1 cells (NK cytotoxicity) and syngeneic thymocytes (NKT cytotoxicity) were used as target cells for each cytotoxicity. A low magnitude of cytotoxicity against YAC-1 cells is also mediated by NKT cells, but it is minimum. These targets were labelled with sodium [^{51}Cr] chromate (NEN Life Science

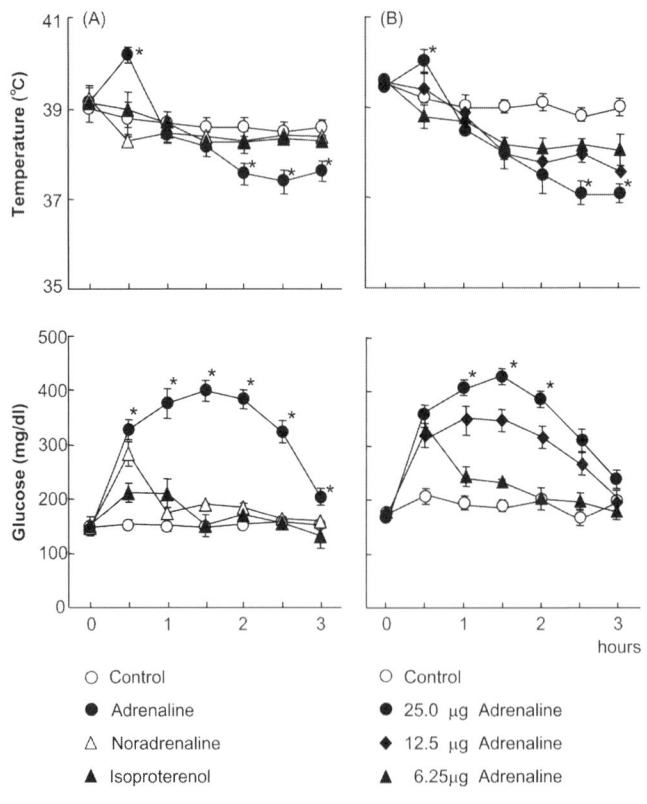

Fig. 3. Effect of the administration of catecholamines on body temperature and blood glucose. (A) Administration of adrenaline, noradrenaline and isoproterenol, (B) dose-dependent effects of adrenaline. Mice were i.p. administered with 25.0 μg of adrenaline, noradrenaline or isoproterenol in Exp. A. Body temperature and blood glucose were measured at the indicated points of time. In Exp. B, dose-dependent effects of adrenaline was examined. Three mice were used to produce the mean and one S.D. *$P < 0.05$.

Products, Boston, MA, USA) for 2 h and washed three times with RPMI-1640 medium. Effector cells were serially diluted and mixed with [^{51}Cr]-labelled target cells (1×10^4, or 2×10^4 cells) in a 96-well U-bottomed microculture plate. The plates were centrifuged and incubated for 4 h at 37 °C. At the end of the culture, 100 μl supernatant was counted in a gamma counter.

2.9. Statistical analysis

The difference between the values was determined by Student's *t*-test and one-factor ANOVA.

3. Results

3.1. Stress-induced responses

Mice were exposed to restraint stress for 3 h and were then released. Body temperature and blood glucose were examined at each point of time (Fig. 1). Primarily, control mice had a high body temperature of around 38.9 ± 0.5 °C, whereas mice exposed to stress showed decreased levels of body temperature between 36.0 and 37.0 °C ($P<0.05$). After release from stress, such body temperature returned to the control level.

In the case of blood glucose, control mice had a level of 150 mg/dl. However, mice exposed to stress showed elevated levels of blood glucose (220–240 mg/dl). These levels returned to the control level after the release from stress.

In an acute response to stress [4], plasma levels of catecholamines are known to vary. Therefore, the plasma levels of catecholamines were examined before and during stress (Fig. 2). The plasma levels of adrenaline, noradrenaline and dopamine were all elevated after stress (1 or 2 h, $P<0.05$). This raises the possibility that some catecholamines may be associated with the observed stress-induced responses.

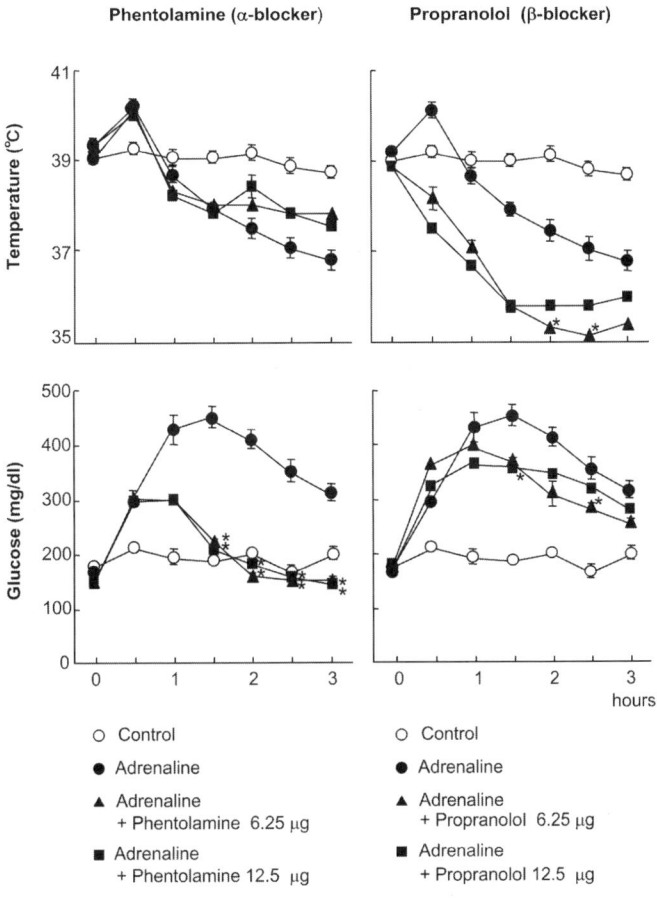

Fig. 4. Effect of α- or β-blockers on adrenaline-induced hypothermia and hyperglycemia. α- and β-blockers was subcutaneously administered at the same time when adrenaline was administered. Three mice were used to produce the mean and one S.D. $^*P<0.05$.

3.2. α-Adrenergic stimulus

We examined which types of catechalamines were able to induce both hypothermia and hyperglycemia seen in restraint stress (Fig. 3A). In preliminary experiments, the maximum doses of adrenaline (α-stimulus), noradrenaline (α but less than adrenaline) and isoproterenol (β) were determined to avoid the death or unhealthy conditions of mice. Adrenaline, but neither noradrenaline nor isoproterenol, was found to simultaneously induce hypothermia and hyperglycemia. In Fig. 3B, dose-dependent curve of adrenaline (25.0, 12.5 and 6.25 μg/mouse) was shown. Prominent effects of hypothermia and hyperglycemia were obtained at the dose of 25.0 μg/mouse.

3.3. Use of α- and β-blockers

To further confirm that α-adrenergic stimulus was responsible for the present phenomena, α-blocker (phentolamine) and β-blocker (propranolol) were used in the experiments of adrenaline-induced hypothermia and hyperglycemia (Fig. 4). Adrenaline (25.0 μg/mouse) was administered intraperitoneally while α- or β-blocker (6.25 μg or 12.5 μg/mouse) was administered intraperitoneally 10 min before adrenaline injection. In a preliminary experiment, α-blocker alone or β-blocker alone did not induce any effects on body temperature and blood glucose at the applied doses (data not shown). It was found that α-blocker suppressed partially hypothermia, especially at late phase (2–3 h). More prominently, β-blocker enhanced hypothermia induced by adrenaline. It is conceivable that β-adrenergic stimulus had a potential to suppress hypothermia. In the case of blood glucose, α-blocker had a potential to suppress hyperglycemia but β-blocker did not such a prominent potential at the both doses.

3.4. Immunomodulation by α-adrenergic stimulus

We previously reported that restraint stress in mice induced the suppression of acquired immunity but inversely augmented the innate immunity [5,6]. It was therefore investigated whether an α-stimulus was able to induce a phenomenon similar to that of restraint stress (Fig. 5). The number of lymphocytes in the liver and thymus decreased whereas that in the spleen remained unchanged.

To identify the distribution of lymphocyte subsets in various organs, immunofluorescence tests were conducted (Fig. 6). Two-color staining for CD3 and IL-2Rβ (or NK1.1 or B220) was conduced in the liver and spleen. The most prominent change was in NK cells, extrathymic T cells and NKT cells in the liver. At 2–6 h, the proportions of IL-2Rβ+ (or NK1.1+) NK cells (e.g., 8.4 → 12.1%, 4 h), IL-2Rβ+CD3^{int} extrathymic T cells (e.g., 14.1 → 34.5%, 4 h) and NK1.1+CD3^{int} NKT cells (e.g., 10.0 → 28.8%, 4 h) were found to increase. A peak time of elevation was seen at 4 h. B220+ B cells and IL-2Rβ−CD3^{high} T cells remained unchanged in proportion by stress.

Two-color staining for CD4 and CD8 in the thymus showed that the α-stimulus slightly reduced the proportion of CD4+8+ double-positive cells (e.g., 90.4 → 80.2%, 2 h) (bottom of

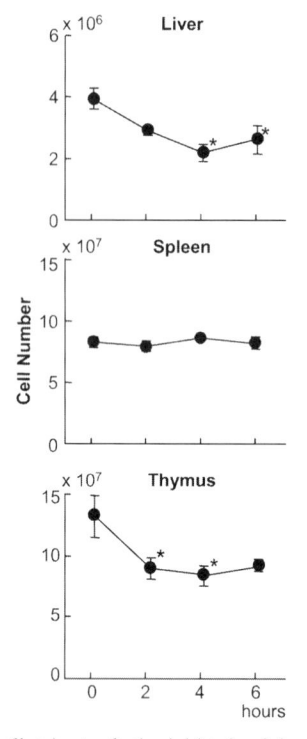

Fig. 5. Number of lymphocytes after the administration of adrenaline. Lymphocytes were isolated from the liver, spleen and thymus. Three mice were used to produce the mean and one S.D. $^*P<0.05$.

Fig. 6). In other words, the α-stimulus applied here as stress was not as severe as restraint stress.

Since the proportion of NK cells and NKT cells increased in the liver by the α-stimulus, it was examined whether there were any accompanying functional activities (Fig. 7). In this experiment, lymphocytes were isolated from both the liver and spleen. In the liver, but not the spleen, NK activity against YAC-1 cells and NKT activity against syngeneic thymocytes were found to be augmented by the α-stimulus ($P<0.05$).

4. Discussion

In the present study, we demonstrated that an α-adrenergic stimulus induced hypothermia, hyperglycemia and innate-immunity activation in mice, a phenomenon resembling stress-induced responses. In the case of restraint stress, it has been reported that the secretion of catecholamines, steroid hormones and inflammatory cytokines simultaneously occurs [4–6]. Among these humoral factors, attention was focused on catecholamines in this study. Since restraint stress was confirmed to induce adrenaline, noradrenaline and dopamine, we then examined which types of adrenergic stimuli could induce similar stress-associated responses. We administrated adrenaline

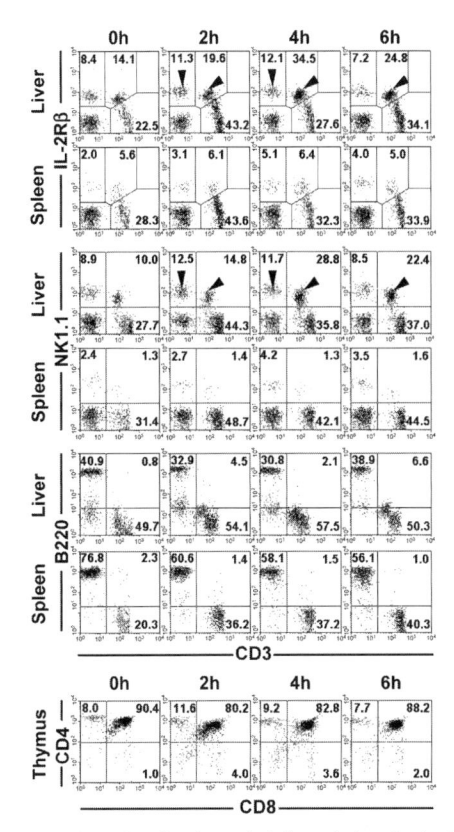

Fig. 6. Two-color staining of lymphocytes in the liver and spleen after the administration of adrenaline. Lymphocytes were isolated at the indicated points of time and immunofluorescence tests were conducted to identify lymphocyte subsets. Two-color staining of lymphocytes for CD3 and IL-2Rβ (or NK1.1 or B220) and that of thymocytes for CD4 and CD8 were conducted. Representative results of three experiments are depicted. Numbers in the figure represent the percentages of fluorescence-positive cells in corresponding areas.

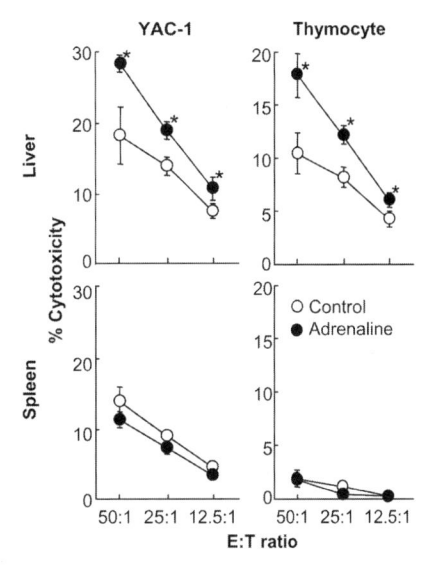

Fig. 7. Cytotoxicity assays. NK cytotoxicity against YAC-1 cells and NKT cytotoxicity against syngeneic thymocytes were examined at the indicated effector to target (E/T) ratios. Three experiments were done to produce the mean and one S.D. $^*P < 0.05$.

(α-stimulus), nonadrenaline (α but less than adrenaline) and isoproterenol (β-). The administration of α-stimulant but not that of β-stimulant seemed to induce stress-associated responses, especially with regard to body temperature, blood glucose and immune function.

The association of α-adrenergic effect with hypothermia and hyperglycemia was confirmed using α- and β-blockers. Adrenaline-induced hypothermia was partially suppressed by α-blockers but that was enhanced by β-blocker. Some suppressive effects of β-stimulus seemed to be included in adrenergic stimuli. In the case of adrenaline-induced hyperglycemia, α-blocker, but not β-blocker, was effective to eliminate this effect.

Many studies on stress to date have mainly dealt with immunosuppressive responses, including the immunosuppression of T and B lymphocytes in the periphery and in acute thymic atrophy [1–3]. In this case, steroid hormones play an important role in stress-associated immunosuppression. On the other hand, the α-adrenergic stimulus resulted in only mild immunosuppression, with a decreased number of lymphocytes in the liver and thymus. Moreover, the effect of the α-stimulus on the decrease in the number of double-positive CD4$^+$8$^+$ cells was limited (the bottom of Fig. 5). These results suggest that immunosuppressive responses may be the result of multiple effects of humoral factors.

In contrast to the immunosuppression of T and B cells during stress, the innate immunity mediated by NK cells (NK1.1$^+$CD3$^-$), extrathymic T cells (IL-2Rβ$^+$CD3^{int}) and NKT cells (NK1.1$^+$CD3^{int}) was augmented inversely. This response was also reproduced by the administration of adrenaline (α-stimulus). The functional activation by the α-stimulus was confirmed in NK and NKT cytotoxicities. In this study, NK cytotoxicity was determined using YAC-1 cells whereas NKT cytotoxicity was investigated using syngeneic thymocytes (i.e., autologous cytotoxicity) [20].

Primarily, sympathetic nerve stimulation increases body metabolism and results in the elevation of body temperature, whereas parasympathetic nerve stimulation inversely affects body metabolism and results in the decrease of body temperature [21–23]. However, severe sympathetic nerve stimulation, such as restraint stress in the present study, induces hypothermia, possibly due to the constriction of vessels (i.e., circulation failure). Mild or severe sympathetic nerve stimulation consistently leads to hyperglycemia [24,25]. There have been many reports that stress has a potential to induce hypothermia and hyperglycemia [12–14]. An α-adrenergic stimulus by the administration of adrenaline induced a similar pattern of hypothermia and hyperglycemia. At that time, the activation of innate immunity was also induced simultaneously. Although β-adrenergic stimulation is also known to induce hypothermia and hyperglycemia [26], such stimulation seems to be milder than an α-stimulus as shown in this study.

In addition to the simultaneous induction of hypothermia and hyperglycemia, the induction of innate-immunity activation might be of interest. The activation of innate immunity under conditions of immunosuppression of T and B cells was demonstrated by not only restraint stress [5,6], as well as by an α-adrenergic stimulus in this study.

Acknowledgements

This work was supported by a Grant-in-Aid for Scientific Research from the Ministry of Education, Science and Culture, Japan. The authors wish to thank Mrs. Yuko Kaneko for preparation of the manuscript.

References

[1] Kawamura T, Toyabe S, Moroda T, Iiai T, Takahashi-Iwanaga H, Fukuda M, et al. Neonatal granulocytosis is a postpartum event which is seen in the liver as well as in the blood. Hepatology 1997;26:1567–72.

[2] Maruyama S, Tsukahara A, Suzuki S, Tada T, Minagawa M, Watanabe H, et al. Quick recovery in the generation of self-reactive $CD4^{low}$ NKT cells by an alternative intrathymic pathway when restored from acute thymic atrophy. Clin Exp Immunol 1999;117:587–95.

[3] Maruyama S, Minagawa M, Shimizu T, Oya H, Yamamoto Y, Musha N, et al. Administration of glucocorticoids markedly increases the numbers of granulocytes and extrathymic T cells in the bone marrow. Cell Immunol 1999;194:28–35.

[4] Minagawa M, Narita J, Tada T, Maruyama S, Shimizu T, Bannai M, et al. Mechanisms underlying immunologic states during pregnancy: possible association of the sympathetic nervous system. Cell Immunol 1999;196:1–13.

[5] Shimizu T, Kawamura T, Miyaji C, Oya H, Bannai M, Yamamoto S, et al. Resistance of extrathymic T cells to stress and the role of endogenous glucocorticoids in stress associated immuno-suppression. Scand J Immunol 2000;51:285–92.

[6] Sagiyama K, Tsuchida M, Kawamura H, Wang S, Li C, Bai X, et al. Age-related bias in function of natural killer T cells and granulocytes after stress: reciprocal association of steroid hormones and sympathetic nerves. Clin Exp Immunol 2004;135:56–63.

[7] Cao L, Hudson CA, Lawrenece DA. Immune changes during acute cold/restraint stress-indced inhibition of host resistance to listeria. Toxicol Sci 2003;74:325–34.

[8] Kanemi O, Zhang X, Sakamoto Y, Ebina M, Nagatomi R. Acute stress reduces intraparechymal lung natural killer cells via beta-adrenergic stimulation. Clin Exp Immunol 2005;139:25–34.

[9] Starkie RL, Hargreaves M, Rolland J, Febbraio MA. Heat stress, cytokines, and the immune response to exercise. Brain Behav Immun 2005;19:404–12.

[10] Viswanathan K, Dhabhar FS. Stress-induced enhancement of leukocyte trafficking into sites of surgery or immune activation. PNAS 2005;102:5808–19.

[11] Eijkelkamp N, Engeland CG, Gajendrareddy PK, Marucha PT. Restraint stress impairs early wound healing in mice via α-adrenergic but not β-adrenergic receptors. Brain Behav Immun 2007;21:409–12.

[12] Welle SL, Thompson DA, Campbell RG. Beta-adrenergic blockade inhibits thermogenesis and lipolysis during glucoprivation in humans. Am J Physiol 1982;243:379–82.

[13] Haller EW, Wittmers Jr LE. Ethanol-induced hypothermia and hyperglycemia in genetically obese mice. Life Sci 1989;44:1377–85.

[14] Atrens DM, van der Reest A, Balleine BW, Menendez JA, Siviy SM. Effects of ethanol and tertiary butanol on blood glucose levels and body temperature of rats. Alcohol 1989;6:183–7.

[15] Minagawa M, Oya H, Yamamoto S, Shimizu T, Bannai M, Kawamura H, et al. Intensive expansion of natural killer T cells in the early phase of hepatocyte regeneration after partial hepatectomy in mice and its association with sympathetic nerve activation. Hepatology 2000;31:907–15.

[16] Oya H, Kawamura T, Shimizu T, Bannai M, Kawamura H, Minagawa M, et al. The differential effect of stress on natural killer T and NK cell function. Clin Exp Immunol 2000;121:384–90.

[17] Miyakawa R, Miyaji C, Watanabe H, Yokoyama H, Tsukada C, Asakura H, et al. Unconventional $NK1.1^-$ intermediate TCR cells as major T lymphocytes expanding in chronic graft-versus-host disease. Eur J Immunol 2002;32:2521–31.

[18] Morshed SRM, Mannoor K, Halder RC, Kawamura H, Bannai M, Sekikawa H, et al. Tissue-specific expansion of NKT and $CD5^+B$ cells at the onset of autoimmune disease in $(NZB \times NZW)F_1$ mice. Eur J Immunol 2002;32:2551–61.

[19] Yamagiwa S, Yoshida Y, Halder RC, Weerasinghe A, Sugahara S, Asakura H, et al. Mechanisms involved in enteropathy induced by administration of nonsteroidal anti inflammatory drugs (NSAIDs). Digest Dis Sci 2001;46:192–9.

[20] Miyaji C, Miyakawa R, Watanabe H, Kawamura H, Abo T. Mechanisms underlying the activation of cytotoxic function mediated by hepatic lymphocytes following the administration of glycyrrhizin. Int Immunopharmacol 2002;2:1079–86.

[21] Groenink L, van der Gugten J, Zethof T, van der Heyden J, Olivier B. Stress-induced hyperthermia in mice: hormonal correlates. Physiol Behav 1994;56:747–9.

[22] Valerio G, Franzese A, Carlin E, Pecile P, Perini R, Tenore A. High prevalence of stress hyperglycaemia in children with febrile seizures and traumatic injuries. Acta Paediatr 2001;90:618–22.

[23] Szekely M. The vagus nerve in thermoregulation and energy metabolism. Auton Neurosci 2000;85:26–38.

[24] Arai I, Hirose H, Muramatsu M, Aihara H. Effects of restraint and water-immersion stress and insulin on gastric acid secretion in rats. Physiol Behav 1987;40:357–61.

[25] Kappel M, Gyhrs A, Galbo H, Pedersen BK. The response on glucoregulatory hormones of in vivo whole body hyperthermia. Int J Hyperthermia 1997;13:413–21.

[26] Freeman BM, Manning AC. Short-term stressor effects of propranolol. Br Poult Sci 1980;21:55–9.

PROPOSAL OF ALTERNATIVE MECHANISM RESPONSIBLE FOR THE FUNCTION OF HIGH-SPEED SWIMSUITS

高速水着の着用効果に関するもう一つの重要なメカニズム

Biomedical Research, 30: 69-70, 2009

chapter 21

Proposal of alternative mechanism responsible for the function of high-speed swimsuits

高速水着の着用効果に関するもう一つの重要なメカニズム

Eisuke KAINUMA[1], Mayumi WATANABE[1], Chikako TOMIYAMA-MIYAJI[2], Masahi INOUE[1], Yoh KUWANO[1], HongWei REN[1] and Toru ABO[1]

[1] Department of Immunology, Niigata University School of Medicine, Niigata 951-8510 and
[2] School of Health Sciences, Faculty of Medicine, Niigata University, Niigata, 951-8518, Japan
(Received 12 December 2008; and accepted 17 December 2008)

【要約】

　スピード社製の水着（LZR Racer）を着用したトップの水泳選手が、次々と世界記録を破った。その理由は、この水着がしなやかな水泳選手の動きをコルセットのようにサポートし、水の抵抗力が減少するからだと考えられている。本論文では、もう一つのメカニズムを用いて解明を試みたい。スピード社の水着は、体にピタリと密着し、水泳選手の血液循環を抑制する。その結果、嫌気性解糖系が働き始める。反対に、好気性ミトコンドリア系が抑制される。特に短距離競技では、水泳選手の骨格筋（特に白筋）が利用する瞬発力は、解糖系が迅速に産生するATPである。

　スピード社製の水着LZR Racer（スピード・インターナショナル社, イギリス, ノッテインガム）を着用したトップの水泳選手が、次々と、世界記録を破った。今のところ、水着の開発者当人も、他の研究者も、LZR Racerの特徴は、下記のようなものだと信じている：水着が、コルセットのようにしっかりと締め付けて身体を包むおかげで、運動時に必要な柔軟性を失うことはない。従って、水泳選手は、水中で最適のボデイ・ポジションを維持することができる。さらに、この高速水着を着用すると、水泳選手の体表は、極めて平坦でスムースになり、水の抵抗が減少する。LZR Racerを着用した水泳選手が新記録を樹立できる理由は、上記のようなものだと信じられてきた。これらの意見に加えて、本論文では、もう一つのメカニズムに着目しLZR Racerの特徴を提唱する。着目したのは、この水着は、とてもぴったりしてきつく引き締め、水泳選手の血液循環を抑制する点である。

　ヒトおよび他の生物は、次の二つの系（システム）を用いてエネルギーを産生する（Table.1）：嫌気性解糖系（酸素非依存性のアデノシン三リン酸（ATP）産生）と好気性ミトコンドリア系（酸素依存性のATP産生）(5)。解糖系は、ミトコンドリア系よりもATPの産生効率が低いことが一般に知られている。しかし、解糖系はミトコンドリア系よりもATP産生速度がはるかに迅速である。この二種類系のATP産生速度を比較すると、解糖系はミトコンドリア系の約100倍速い速度でATPを産生できる (5)。

　解糖系は、骨格筋の白筋（タイプII繊維、速筋）に瞬間力を供給する。一方、ミトコンドリア系は、神経、心筋および骨格筋の赤筋（タイプI繊維、遅筋）に持続力を供給する (2,3)。LZR Racerは、体を締めつける。この時、血流の抑制が起こる。その結果、解糖系が起動し、瞬発力を得ることができる (1)。

chapter 21

Table 1 ヒトにおけるエネルギー生成

	解糖系	ミトコンドリア系
体温	低体温（32-36℃）	高体温（>37℃）
酸素	−	＋
高血糖	＋	−
ATP生成	速い（x 100） 効率低く、瞬発的	遅い（x 1） 効率高く、持続的
エネルギーを使うのは	白筋 分裂する細胞 （精子） （上皮細胞） （粘膜細胞） （骨髄細胞）	赤筋 分裂しない細胞 （卵子） （脳細胞） （心筋）

　実際、LZR Racerを着用した水泳選手が、世界新記録を樹立したのは、主に50mや100mのレースといった400m未満の短距離競技である。

　LZR Racerの着用効果が、水の抵抗を減らすことや水をはじく点にあるならば、400m以上の長距離競技でも、更なる新世界記録が樹立されていたはずである。しかし、今のところ、長距離競技では新記録はない。

　加圧トレーニングも、瞬発力を意識したトレーニング法として有名である（4, 6）。加圧トレーニングのメカニズムは、LZR Racer水着のメカニズムによく似ている。加圧トレーニングでは、体を締め付け、血流を抑制する。例えば、上腕筋や大腿筋をゴム製のカフで締付ける。そして、ミトコンドリア内呼吸の抑制し、反対に嫌気性の解糖を促進するのである。カフには、100-300mmHg（頻度が高いのは200mmHg）の加圧を与える。加圧トレーニングは、短時間（5-15分間）しか行わない。

　このように、高速水着で記録が伸びる秘密を理解するには、上述の二つのエネルギー産生系の特徴の理解と考慮をせざるを得ない。この二つのエネルギー産生系の理解が、スポーツ医学や一般医学の更なる発展に貢献できる可能性もある。

謝辞

金子裕子氏の浄書に感謝する。

Proposal of alternative mechanism responsible for the function of high-speed swimsuits

Eisuke KAINUMA[1], Mayumi WATANABE[1], Chikako TOMIYAMA-MIYAJI[2], Masashi INOUE[1], Yuh KUWANO[1], HongWei REN[1] and Toru ABO[1]

[1] Department of Immunology, Niigata University School of Medicine, Niigata 951-8510 and [2] School of Health Sciences, Faculty of Medicine, Niigata University, Niigata 951-8518, Japan

(Received 12 December 2008; and accepted 17 December 2008)

ABSTRACT

Since many top swimmers wearing Speedo LZR Racer swimsuits have broken world records, it is considered that the corset-like grip of suit supports the swimmers to maintain flexibility of movement and reducing water resistance. We propose an alternative mechanism to explain this phenomenon. The suits are so tight that the blood circulation of swimmers is suppressed. This effect accelerates the anaerobic glycolysis system but rather suppresses the aerobic mitochondrial respiration system. Because of the prompt production of ATP in the glycolysis system, the swimmers, especially in short distance competitions, obtain instantaneous force in white fibers of the skeletal muscles.

Many top swimmers wearing Speedo LZR Racer swimsuits (Speedo International Limited, Nottingham, England) have broken world records. Both swimsuit manufacture personnel and other researchers believe the characteristics of LZR Racer to be as follows: the corset-like grip of the suit supports and holds the swimmers so they can maintain the best body position in the water without losing flexibility of movement. Furthermore, this high-speed swimsuit makes the surface of swimmer's body very flat and smooth, thus reducing water resistance. These are believed to be the reasons why swimmers wearing the LZR Racer can set new records. In addition to these conventional opinions, we propose an alternative mechanism to explain the characteristics of LZR Racer suits, namely, that LZR Racer suits are so tight that the blood circulation of the swimmers is suppressed.

Humans and other living beings produce energy through the following two systems (Table 1): the anaerobic glycolysis system (oxgen-independent adenosine triphosphate (ATP) synthesis) and the aerobic mitochondrial respiration system (oxgen-dependent ATP synthesis) (5). It is known that the former system does not produce ATP as effectively as the latter system. However, the former produces ATP much more quickly than the later. Comparing the speed of the two types of ATP production, the glycolysis system is known to be almost 100 times faster than the mitochondrial system (5).

The glycolysis system is for obtaining instantaneous force in white fibers (fast-twitch type II fiber) of skeletal muscles, while the mitochondrial system is for realization of sustainable force in neurons, cardiac muscle and red fibers (slow-twitch type I fiber) of skeletal muscles (2, 3). LZR Racer suits tighten the body, which suppresses the bloodstream. This results in activation of the glycolysis system and induces instantaneous force in the body (1).

In fact, swimmers wearing LZR Racer suits have established new world records mainly in short distance competitions such as 50 m or 100 m races, new records being found in the races of no more than 400 m. If low drag and water repellency were the main factors, more new world records in longer distance races should have been established by

Address correspondence to: Dr. Toru Abo, Department of Immunology, Niigata University School of Medicine, Niigata 951-8510, Japan
Tel: +81-25-227-2133, Fax: +81-25-227-0766
E-mail: immunol2@med.niigata-u.ac.jp

Table 1 Energy production in our body

	Anaerobic glycolysis system	Aerobic mitochondria system
Body temperature	Low (32 to 36°C)	High (>37°C)
Oxygen	−	+
Hyperglycemia	+	−
ATP synthesis	Prompt (×100)	Slow (×1)
	Less effective and short-span	Effective and continuous
Supply of energy for:	White fiber muscle cells	Red fiber muscle cells
	Dividing cells	Non-dividing cells
	(Sperm)	(Ovum cells)
	(Epidermal cells)	(Brain cells)
	(Mucosal cells)	(Cardiac muscles)
	(Bone marrow cells)	

swimmers wearing LZR Race suits. So far, there have been no new records in long distance races.

KAATSU training is also well-known as a training method for realizing instantaneous force (4, 6). The mechanism of this training is similar to that of LZR Racer swimsuits. KAATSU training constricts the body (brachialis and femur muscles) to suppress bloodstream by rubber cuff, resulting in suppression of mitochondrial internal respiration, but inversely stimulating anaerobic glycolysis. The cuff pressue used is 100 to 300 mmHg (a most popular pressue is 200 mmHg). KAATSU training is done only for short periods of time (*i.e.*, 5 to 15 min).

In this way, the reason for the efficacy of LZR swimsuits cannot be known without understanding and considering the characteristics of the two energy production systems. Such understanding would also contribute to further development of sports medicine and general medical science.

Acknowledgments

We wish to thank Mrs. Yuko Kaneko for preparation of the manuscript.

REFERENCES

1. Bangsbo J, Gollnick PD, Graham TE, Juel C, Kiens B, Mizuno M and Saltin B (1990) Anaerobic energy production and O$_2$ deficit-debt relationship during exhaustive exercise in humans. *J Physiol* **422**, 539–559.
2. Fitts RH (1994) Cellular mechanisms of muscle fatigue. *Physiol Rev* **74**, 49–94.
3. Greenhaff PL, Campbell-O'Sullivan SP, Constantin-Teodosiu D, Poucher SM, Roberts PA and Timmons LA (2004) Metabolic inertia in contracting skeletal muscle: a novel approach for pharmacological intervention in peripheral vascular disease. *Br J Clin Pharmacol* **57**, 237–243.
4. Nakajima T, Kurano M, Iida H, Takano H, Oonuma H, Morita T, Meguro K, Sato Y, Nagata T and KAATU Training Group (2006) Use and safety of KAATSU training: Results of a national survey. *J KAATSU Training Res* **2**, 5–13.
5. Voet D and Voet JG (2004) Glycolysis. In: *Biochemistry*, 3rd ed. (Voet D, Voet JG, eds.), p 607, J. Wiley & Sons, New York.
6. Yasuda T, Fujita T, Miyagi Y, Kubota Y, Sato Y, Nakajima T, Bemben MG and Abe T (2006) Electromyographic responses of arm and chest muscle during bench press exercise with and without KAATU. *J KAATSU Training Res* **2**, 15–18.

ASSOCIATION OF GLUCOCORTICOID WITH STRESS-INDUCED MODULATION OF BODY TEMPERATURE, BLOOD GLUCOSE AND INNATE IMMUNITY

ストレスによる
体温、血糖、自然免疫の変化と糖質コルチコイドとの関連

chapter 22

Association of glucocorticoid with stress-induced modulation of body temperature, blood glucose and innate immunity
ストレスによる体温、血糖、自然免疫の変化と糖質コルチコイドとの関連

Eisuke Kainuma [a], Mayumi Watanabe [a], Chikako Tomiyama-Miyaji [b], Masashi Inoue [a], Yuh Kuwano [a], HongWei Ren [a], Toru Abo [a],*

[a]Department of Immunology, Niigata University School of Medicine, Niigata 951-8510, Japan
[b]School of Health Sciences, Faculty of Medicine, Niigata University, Niigata 951-8518, Japan
Received 25 August 2008; received in revised form 20 April 2009; accepted 30 April 2009

【キーワード】

ストレス； 糖質コルチコイド； 低体温； 高血糖； 自然免疫； フローサイトメトリー

【要約】

ストレス適応反応のメカニズムを詳細に検証するため、先ず、体温と血糖は、ストレスを受けるとどのように変化するのか注目した。マウスに、6時間拘束ストレスを与えたところ、低体温（39℃ → 33℃）、高血糖（150mg/dl → 350mg/dl）が出現した。また、ストレス適応反応により、血清コルチコステロン値は上昇した（200ng/ml → 最高600ng/ml）。次に、糖質コルチコイド投与により同様の反応が出現するか検証した。ヒドロコルチゾン（5.0および10.0mg/マウス）を投与すると、低体温と高血糖を併発した。そこで、ヒドロコルチゾン投与による免疫学的指標の変化を検証した。免疫抑制として、胸腺萎縮と肝臓におけるB細胞の比率が減少した。一方、特に肝臓における胸腺外分化T細胞とNKT細胞は、ストレス耐性があるリンパ球集団であることが判明した。HSP70（熱ショック蛋白質）のmRNA測定から、ヒドロコルチゾン投与による副腎肥大が示唆された。このような反応のすべて（低体温、高血糖と免疫調整など）は、ヒドロコルチゾン投与が誘発されたが、糖質コルチコイド受容体拮抗剤（RU-486）を前投与することで抑制された。これらの結果から、糖質コルチコイドは、ストレス適応反応における重要なメディエータの1つであることが示唆される。

1. はじめに

身体的・精神的ストレスが、諸疾病の発症に密接に関連すると広く信じられてきた（Cyret et al., 2007; Obrosova, 2002; Nonogaki and Iguchi., 1997）。ストレスと疾病を結びつける因子を考えると、交感神経緊張（Suzuki et al., 1997; Kawamura et al., 1997, 1999; Minagawa et al., 1999, 2000; Mori et al., 2002; Abo and Kawamura, 2002）や糖質コルチコイド分泌（Shimizu et al., 2000; Sagiyama et al., 2004）を挙げることができる。交感神経について、我々は、ストレス適応反応する際の、アドレナリン刺激の影響に特に注目して検証してきた。これまで、体温・血糖および自然免疫に着目して研究してきた（Watanabe et al., 2008）。その結果、αアドレナリン刺激が、低体温、血糖上昇および自然免疫の活性化を誘発することが明らかになり、ストレス適応反応の1つとして新しい免疫（T細胞・B細胞）の減少が確認された。

これらの結果を考慮して、本研究では、特に変化量と経時的変化などについて、アドレナリ

ン以外にストレスを伝達する物質して糖質コルチコイドが、αアドレナリン刺激に類似した反応を誘発させるかを検証した。αアドレナリン刺激と糖質コルチコイドのどちらでも、諸ストレス適応反応（体温・血糖と自然免疫）が、同時に出現するのは、興味深い事実である。

2. 材料と方法

2.1 マウス

C57BL/6（B6）マウスを、日本チャールズ・リバー株式会社（横浜）より購入した。本実験において使用したマウス全ては8-12週齢雄であった。マウスは、新潟大学動物資源飼育施設の室内で、一定温度（25±2℃）一定湿度（50-70%）、12時間 明/暗サイクル（点灯時間 08:00 - 20:00）SPF（特定病原体未感染）環境下で飼育した。

2.2 拘束ストレス

実験群マウスに、2または6時間（09:00-11:00または -15：00）のステンレス製メッシュを用いて拘束ストレスを与えた（Sagiyama et al., 2004）。実験時、マウスは行動の制限は受けたが、自由に呼吸することはできた。本実験は、新潟大学動物実験倫理委員会の承認を得て行なった。

2.3 体温と血糖の測定

マウスの直腸温度をTHERMAC SENSOR（芝浦電子,東京）を用いて測定した。Precision Xtra™（アボットジャパン，千葉）を用いてマウス尾部先端から採取した血液3.5μlの血糖を測定した（Nonogaki and Iguchi, 1997）。

2.4 細胞分離

イソフルラン麻酔したマウスの鎖骨下動脈と静脈より脱血し、肝臓と脾臓を摘出し、肝単核球細胞を定法に従い分離した（Kawamura et al.,1999）。略述すると、摘出した肝臓を200-ゲージステンレススチールメッシュで漉し、5mMのHEPESおよび2%非働化済子牛血清を添加したEagle's MEM培養液中に浮遊させた。培養液で一度洗浄した後、この細胞に100U/mlヘパリンを加え、35%パーコール溶液中に再懸濁させ、2000rpm（424 x g）で15分間比重遠心分離を行なった。分離した細胞塊に溶血溶液（155mM NH$_4$Cl, 10mM KHCO$_3$ 1mM EDTAおよび17mM Tris, pH 7.3）で赤血球（RBC）を溶血させ、再懸濁後、培養液で二度洗浄した。脾臓と胸腺をステンレス・スチールメッシュで濾過して、それぞれ脾臓細胞あるいは胸腺細胞を得た。脾臓細胞を得るため0.2% NaCl溶液を用い赤血球の除去を行なった。

2.5 フローサイトメトリー解析

リンパ球の表現型の解析には二重免疫蛍光染色を行なった（Minagawa et al.,1999）。本実験で用いたモノクローナル抗体を以下記す（BD PharMingen, San Diego, CA）；抗CD3ε（145-2C11）、抗IL-2Rβ（TM-β1）、抗NK1.1（PK136）、抗CD4（RM4-5）、抗CD8α（53-6.7）および抗B220（RA3-6B2）。これらは、いずれもイソチオシアン酸フルオレセイン（FITC）標識とフィコエリトリン（PE）標識されたモノクローナル抗体である。モノクローナル抗体の非特異的結合を防ぐため、抗CD16/CD32（2.4G2）モノクローナル抗体にて前処理行った後、各種標識抗体を加えた。懸濁させたリンパ球（5 x 10^5 – 2 x 10^6/tube）をモノクローナル抗体で染色し、染色したリンパ球をフローサイトメトリー（FACScan）（Becton-Dickinson, Mountain View, CA）を用い解析した。死細胞は、ヨウ化プロピジウムで染色し、前方散乱と側方散乱でのゲーティングを行い除外した。

2.6 ヒドロコルチゾンと糖質コルチコイド受容体遮断薬投与

ヒドロコルチゾン（SAXIZON, 興和創薬（株），東京）をマウス一匹あたり10.0mg（もしくは、5.0もしくは2.5mg）を腹腔内投与し

た。RU-486（糖質コルチコイド受容体とプロゲステロン受容体遮断薬（Mifepristone, Sigma-Aldrich Co., Saint Louis, MO）を生理食塩水に2.0mg/0.1ml（1.5または1.0mg/0.1ml）を懸濁させた（Ashcraft et al., 2008; Jarillo-Luna et al., 2008; Elftman et al., 2007）。マウス一匹あたり、2.0mg（1.5または1.0mg）を腹腔内投与した。

2.7 血清コルチコステロン値測定

心臓採血を行い、4℃、回転速度2500x gにて10分間遠心分離を行なった。血清コルチコステロン値を、標識免疫検定法（RIA）（COAT-A-COUNT、Diagnostic Products Corporation, Los Angeles, CA）を用い測定したが、これにはラット [^{125}I] コルチコステロンを用いた。分析の条件は、感度は5.7ng/ml、分析外の揺れは4.3%、分析内の揺れは5.8%であった。

2.8 RNA総量とRT-PCRの準備

添付マニュアルに従い、ISOGEN（株式会社日本ジーン, 東京）を使用し、摘出した腎臓の一部と副腎からRNA総量を調整した。添付プロトコルに従い、SuperScript™III First-Strand Synthesis System for RT-PCRキット（Invitrogen, Co., Carlsbad, CA）を用いてRNAよりcDNAを得た。HSP70.1およびG3PDHのRT-PCRには、RNA総量50ngを用いた。プライマーと条件は以下の通り。：G3PDH：センスプライマー（5'-GCG AGA CCC CAC TAA CAT CAA ATG-3'）、G3PDHアンチセンスプライマー（5'-CAG TGG ATG CAG GGA TGA TGT TCT-3'）、94℃10分を1回；94℃15秒、60℃30秒そして72℃60秒を30回；7分72℃を1回；HSP70.1：センスプライマー（5'-CTA GCT GCC CAG TTC CCT GGA GAT-3'）；HSP70.1アンチセンスプライマー（5'-AAG CCC AGA ATC CAT TAG CCC TTC-3'）；G3PDHは、同条件で35サイクルである。臭化エチジウムで染色した2%アガロースゲルに泳動後、紫外線照射を行い、PCRの結果を得た。

2.9 統計分析

マウスの体温と血糖の統計解析は、拘束時間（0-2-6h時間）と拘束の有無（対照群、ストレス群）を主要因とした。また、マウスの体温と血糖の解析は、薬物投与後の経時的変化（0-6時間）と試薬の種類（対照群、ヒドロコルチゾン、ヒドロコルチゾン+RU-486）を主要因として、二元配置ANOVA検定と多重比較（シェーファー）検定を用いた（$p < 0.05$）。実験によっては、ヒドロコルチゾン投与後の各時点（0-72h）におけるマウスの各臓器の単核細胞数と血清コルチコステロン値（対照群とストレス群）を主要因として一元配置ANOVA検定を用い、必要ならば、さらに、スチューデントのt検定も用いて解析した（$p < 0.01$）。

結果

3.1 ストレス適応反応

6時間拘束後、マウスを開放した。体温、血糖と血中コルチコステロンを経時的に測定した（Fig. 1）。実験前、拘束マウスの体温は約38.8 ± 0.5℃であったが、ストレス実験後、31.5 - 33.0℃に低下した。(時間, $F_{5,20}$=35.67, $p< 0.001$; グループ, $F_{1,20}$=2880.10, $p< 0.001$; 時間 x グループ, $F_{5,20}$=3.31, $p < 0.05$)（Fig. 1A）。ストレス開放後、このような体温低下は、速やかに回復した（未発表データ）。

対照群のマウスの血糖値は、150mg/dlであった（Fig. 1B）。しかし、マウスに拘束ストレスを与えた後、血糖値は上昇した（280-360mg/dl）（時間, $F_{5,20}$=2.03, $p=0.12$; グループ, $F_{1,20}$=667.73, $p < 0.001$; 時間 x グループ, $F_{5,20}$=4.67, $p < 0.01$）。ストレス開放後、上昇した血糖値は、対照群の値まで回復した。

Figure.1

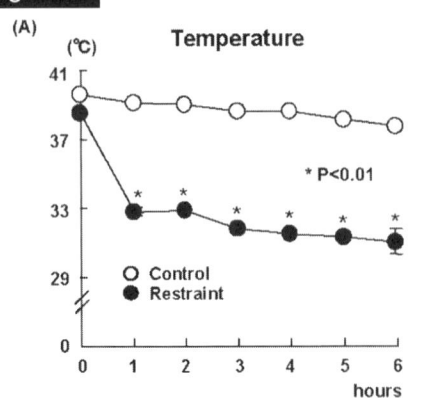

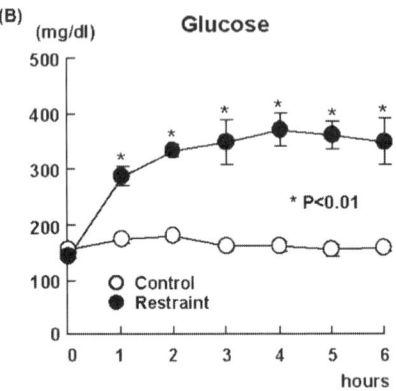

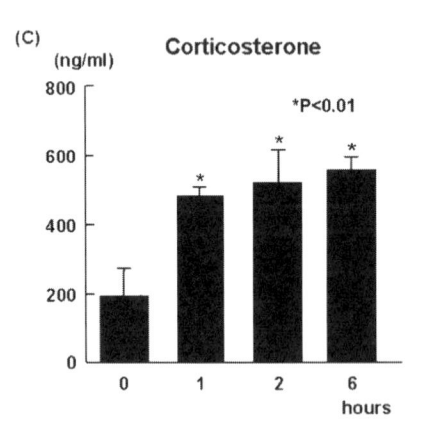

(A) Temperature
(B) Glucose
(C) Corticosterone

ストレスで出現する反応 (A)体温、(B)血糖および(C)血清コルチコステロン マウスに6時間の拘束ストレスを与えた。平均値±1SDは、3匹のマウスを用いて算出した *$p<0.01$

血清コルチコステロン値を測定した (Fig. 1C)。対照群のマウスのコルチコステロン値は、約200 ± 70mg/dlであったが、ストレス群では2および6時間後に、最高500 ± 80mg/dlまで上昇した ($F_{2,8} = 11.66$, $p < 0.01$)。

3.2 糖質コルチコイド投与

拘束ストレス時に類似した反応が、糖質コルチコイド一回投与により誘発されるかを検証した (Fig. 2)。ヒドロコルチゾン投与量を変えて実験した (2.5-10.0mg/匹)。ヒドロコルチゾン投与量が最大時に (10.0mg)、体温低下と血糖値上昇が見られた (Fig. 2A)。このような反応は拘束ストレスの反応に酷似していた。このような反応は2.5mg投与時には見られなかったが、5.0mg投与時には、ある程度見られた (体温:時間、$F_{5,40}=117.01$, $p < 0.001$; グループ, $F_{3,40} = 829.35$, $p < 0.001$; 時間 x グループ, $F_{15,40}=130.78$, $p < 0.001$; 血糖値:時間、$F_{5,40}=214.74$, $p < 0.001$; グループ, $F_{3,40} = 290.41$, $p < 0.001$; 時間 x グループ, $F_{15,40} = 53.54$, $p < 0.001$)。

ヒドロコルチゾン投与量5mgのマウスにおいて、血清コルチコステロン値を測定した (Fig. 2B)。投与後1時間、血清コルチコステロンの高値が見られたが、($F_{3,10}=32.74$, $p<0.001$)、この高値は一過性であり、その後、速やかに低下した。

3.3 糖質コルチコイドによる免疫調整

人間と動物においてストレスにより独特な免疫調整が見られる事実はよく知られている (Sagiyama et al., 2004)。先ず、肝臓、脾臓と胸腺におけるリンパ球を検証した。細胞数は、脾臓において変化を示さず、肝臓においてわずかに減少を示した。最も顕著な変化は、胸腺で見られた。投与後24時間よび72時間の胸腺細胞数は、実験前の3分の1であった (肝臓:$F_{3,7} = 7.77$, $p <0.05$); 脾臓:$F_{3,7} =1.18$, $p=0.42$; 胸腺:$F_{3,7} = 131.90$, $p < 0.001$)。

次に、ヒドロコルチゾンが、リンパ球分画におよぼす影響を検証した (Fig. 4)。CD3およびIL-2Rβ (またはNK1.1) の二重染色を行い、サブセットを同定した (Fig. 4A)。投与後2、4

Figure.2

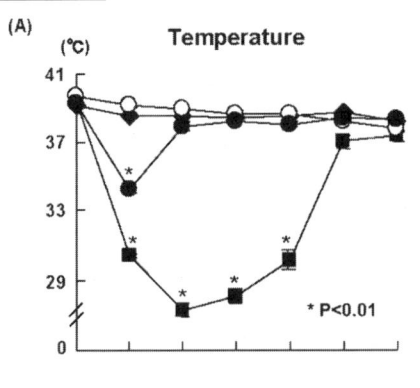

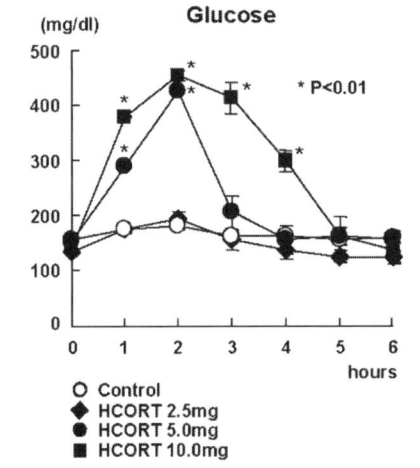

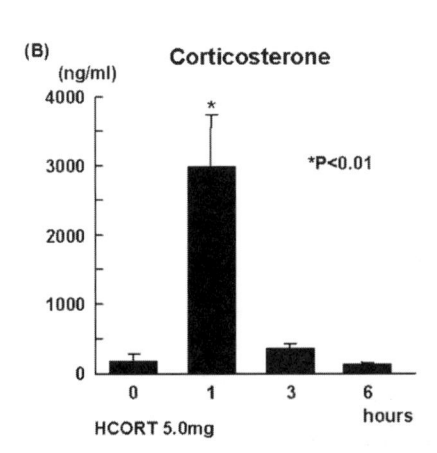

(A)

Temperature

* P<0.01

Glucose

* P<0.01

○ Control
◆ HCORT 2.5mg
● HCORT 5.0mg
■ HCORT 10.0mg

(B) **Corticosterone**

*P<0.01

HCORT 5.0mg

ヒドロコルチゾンの影響 (A)体温の変化とヒドロコルチゾン投与後の血糖値、(B)血清コルチコステロン値 平均値±1SDは、3匹のマウスを用いて算出した *p< 0.01

Figure.3

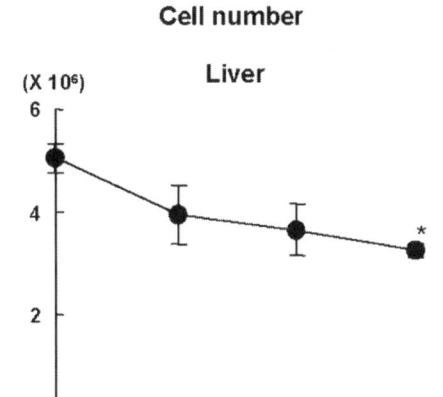

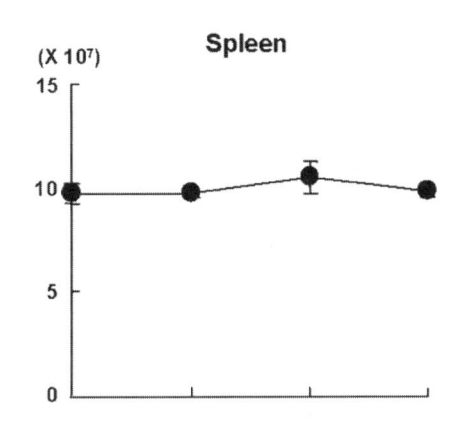

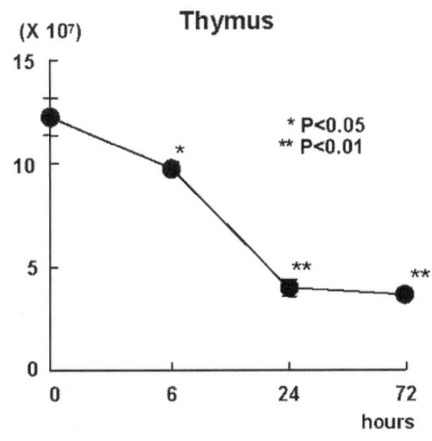

Cell number

Liver

Spleen

Thymus

* P<0.05
** P<0.01

肝臓、脾臓と胸腺における細胞数 平均値±1SDは、3匹のマウスを用いて算出した *p< 0.05, **p< 0.01

Figure.4

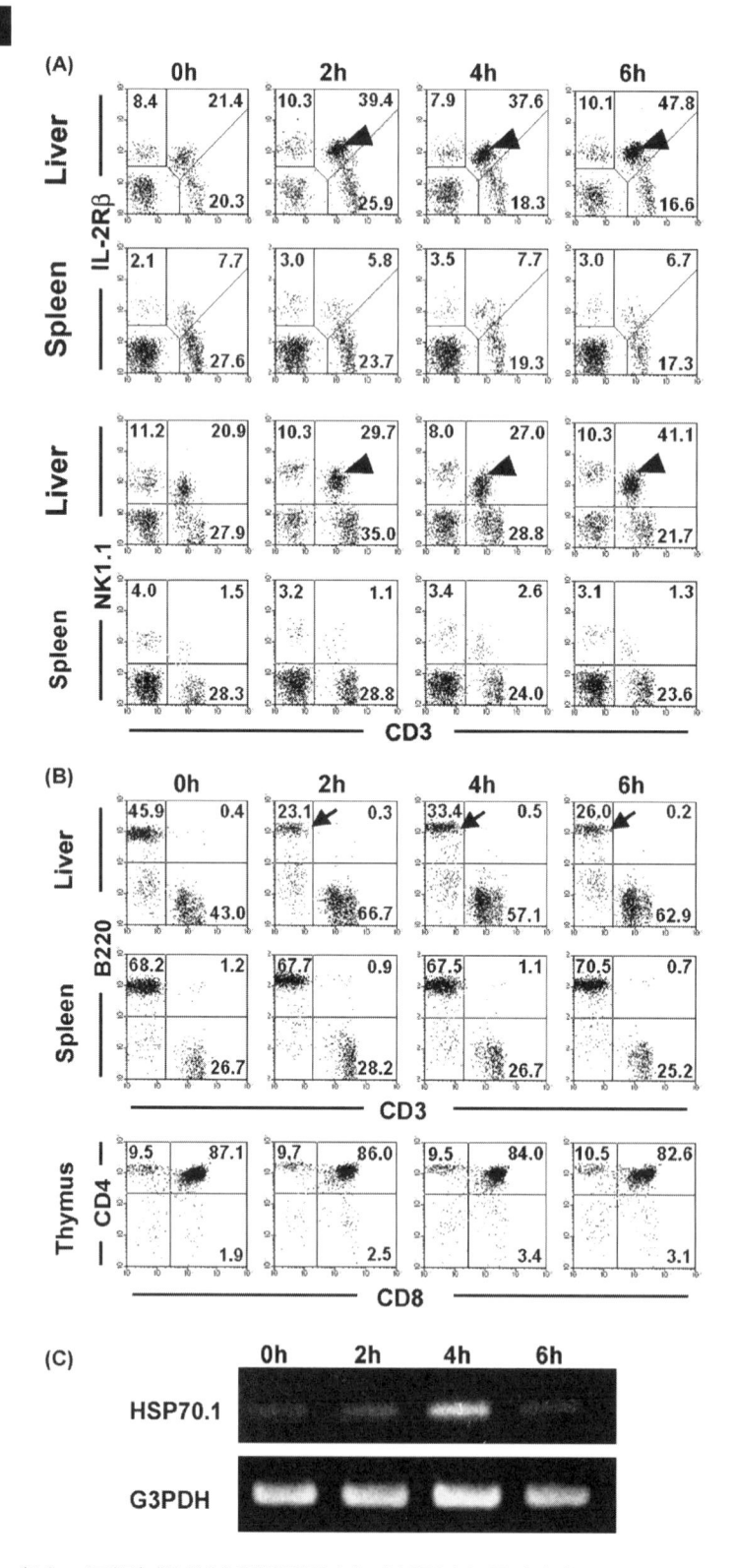

ヒドロコルチゾン（5.0mg/マウス）投与後の免疫学的指標の変化　(A) CD3とIL-2RβおよびCD3とNK1.1の二重染色　(B)肝臓と脾臓におけるCD3とB220の二重染色と胸腺におけるCD4とCD8の二重染色および(C) RT-PCR法によるHSP70.1 mRNAの発現　各分画内の数値は、蛍光陽性細胞の比率を示す　矢印は顕著な変化を認めた箇所である

と6時間、肝臓のIL-2Rβ^+CD3^{int}細胞（胸腺外分化T細胞）とNK1.1$^+$CD3^{int}細胞（NKT細胞）において最も顕著な変化が見られた（矢印）。IL-2Rβ^+CD3^{int}細胞の比率は47.8%に増加し、NK1.1$^+$CD3^{int}細胞の比率は41.0%に増加した。肝臓のIL-2Rβ^+CD3$^-$細胞またはNK1.1$^+$CD3$^-$細胞（ナチュラルキラー細胞）の比率およびIL-2Rβ^-CD3^{high}細胞またはNK1.1$^-$CD3^{high}細胞（胸腺外分化ではないT細胞）に変化は見られなかった。

B220とCD3の二重染色を用いてB細胞（B220$^+$CD3$^-$）を同定できる（Fig. 4B）。肝臓のB細胞の比率が、ヒドロコルチゾン投与により減少した（矢印）。脾臓のB細胞の比率は、ヒドロコルチゾン投与後による変化を示さなかった。胸腺のCD4$^+$8$^+$ダブルポジティブ細胞の比率は免疫抑制の状況下で減少することが知られているが、少なくともヒドロコルチゾン投与後6時間の胸腺では、この現象は見られなかった（Fig. 4B下）。

ストレス関連の反応がHSP70産生を誘導することが知られている（Blake et al.,1991）。そこで、ストレスと関連するHSP70の産生をRT-PCR法を用い測定した（Fig. 4C）。RT-PCRに使用するRNAをヒドロコルチゾン5.0mgを投与したマウスの副腎と腎臓から採取した。ヒドロコルチゾン投与後4時間にHSP70.1発現が顕著であった。

3.4 糖質コルチコイドによる適応反応に対する糖質コルチコイド受容体遮断薬の影響

糖質コルチコイドによる適応反応に、糖質コルチコイド受容体が関与していることを、直接確認するためヒドロコルチゾン投与前に、RU-486を前投与した（Fig. 5）。実験のプロトコルをFig.5Aに、RU-486投与量をグラフの下に示す。

投与量にかかわらずRU-486を前投与する

Figure.5

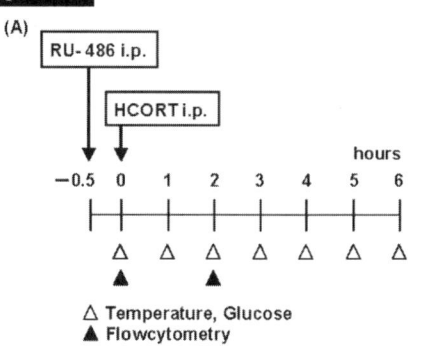

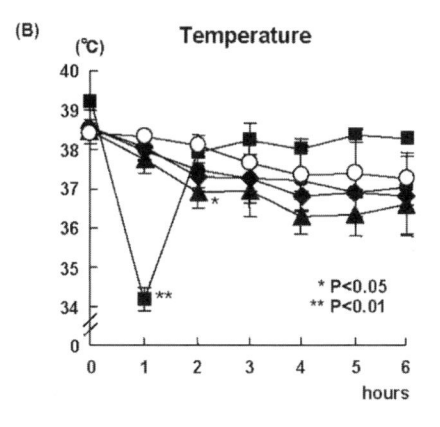

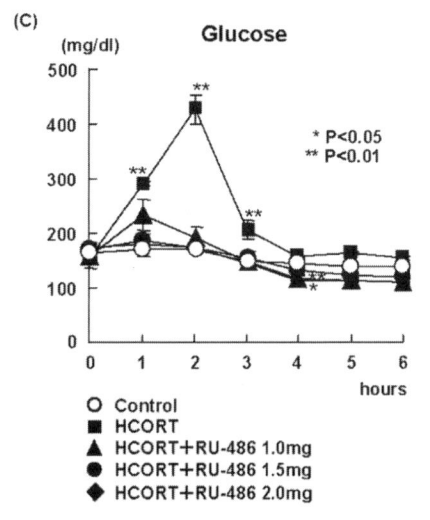

RU-486のプレ投与がヒドロコルチゾン投与による変化に対しておよぼす影響 (A)実験プロトコル(B)体温および(C)血糖　平均値±SDは、3匹のマウスを用いて算出した　*$p<0.05$, **$p<0.01$

と、ヒドロコルチゾン投与（5.0mg）による体温低下および血糖値上昇が軽減されることが明らかになった（体温:時間, $F_{5,50} = 1.89, p = 0.11$;

Figure.6

(A)

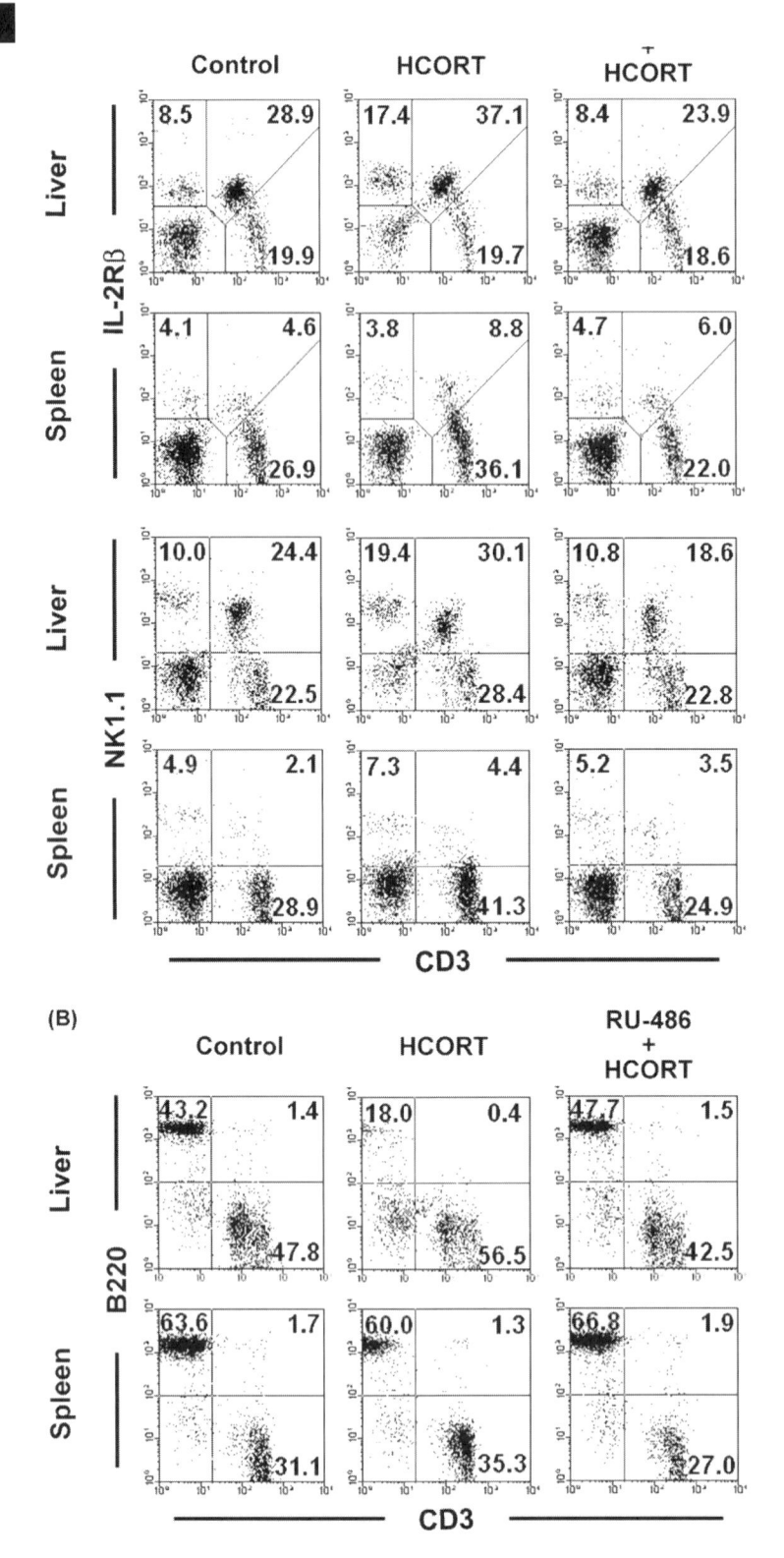

	Control	HCORT	HCORT
Liver (IL-2Rβ / CD3)	8.5 / 28.9 / 19.9	17.4 / 37.1 / 19.7	8.4 / 23.9 / 18.6
Spleen (IL-2Rβ / CD3)	4.1 / 4.6 / 26.9	3.8 / 8.8 / 36.1	4.7 / 6.0 / 22.0
Liver (NK1.1 / CD3)	10.0 / 24.4 / 22.5	19.4 / 30.1 / 28.4	10.8 / 18.6 / 22.8
Spleen (NK1.1 / CD3)	4.9 / 2.1 / 28.9	7.3 / 4.4 / 41.3	5.2 / 3.5 / 24.9

(B)

	Control	HCORT	RU-486 + HCORT
Liver (B220 / CD3)	43.2 / 1.4 / 47.8	18.0 / 0.4 / 56.5	47.7 / 1.5 / 42.5
Spleen (B220 / CD3)	63.6 / 1.7 / 31.1	60.0 / 1.3 / 35.3	66.8 / 1.9 / 27.0

RU-486のプレ投与がヒドロコルチゾン投与による免疫調整に対しておよぼす影響 (A) CD3とIL-2RβとCD3とNK1.1の二重染色(B) CD3とB220の二重染色 各分画内の数値は、蛍光陽性細胞の比率を示す 矢印は顕著な変化を認めた箇所である

グループ, $F_{4,50}$ = 5.94, p < 0.05; 時間 x グループ, $F_{20,50}$=11.15, p<0.001; 血糖値:時間, $F_{5,50}$=254.30, p < 0.001; グループ, $F_{4,50}$=28.22, p < 0.001; 時間 x グループ, $F_{20,50}$ = 41.53, p < 0.001)。

そして、RU-486のストレス関連する免疫反応に対する影響を検証した（Fig. 6）。RU-486を前投与するとヒドロコルチゾン投与による肝臓のIL-2Rβ^+CD3^{int}細胞とNK1.1$^+$CD3^{int}細胞の比率の増加は、軽減されることが明らかになった（Fig. 6A）。同様に、RU-486を前投与するとヒドロコルチゾンによる肝臓のB220$^+$B細胞の比率の減少も、軽減された（Fig. 6B）。

3.5 拘束ストレス適応反応に対する糖質コルチコイド受容体遮断薬の影響

ストレス適応反応は、糖質コルチコイドとレセプター間の相互作用により調整されるのだろうか。このことを検証するため、RU-486（2.0mg）を前投与した後、6時間の拘束ストレスを与える実験を行った（Fig. 7）。その結果、完全ではないもののRU-486を前投与すると、拘束ストレスによる体温低下と血糖上昇が軽減されることが証明された（体温:時間, $F_{3,24}$ =165.46, p < 0.001; グループ, $F_{3,24}$=77.48, p < 0.001;時間 x グループ, $F_{9,24}$=29.12, p < 0.001; 血糖値:時間, $F_{3,24}$=19.80, p< 0.001;グループ, $F_{3,24}$ = 24.36, p<0.001; 時間 x グループ, $F_{9,24}$= 17.65, p < 0.001)。

4. 考察

本研究では、糖質コルチコイド投与が、低体温、高血糖および自然免疫の活性化を同時に誘発することを証明した。このような反応は全て、ストレス適応反応に類似している。換言すると、糖質コルチコイド分泌が、ストレス適応反応の主要な伝達物質である可能性がある。糖質コルチコイド受容体遮断薬（RU-486）を使用して、ヒドロコルチゾン投与による適応反応が、糖質コルチコイド受容体を通じて出現したことを確

Figure.7

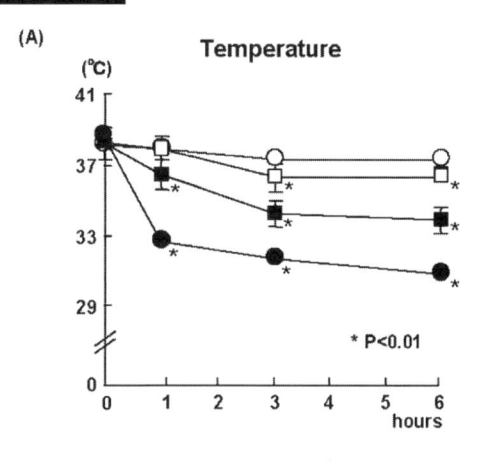

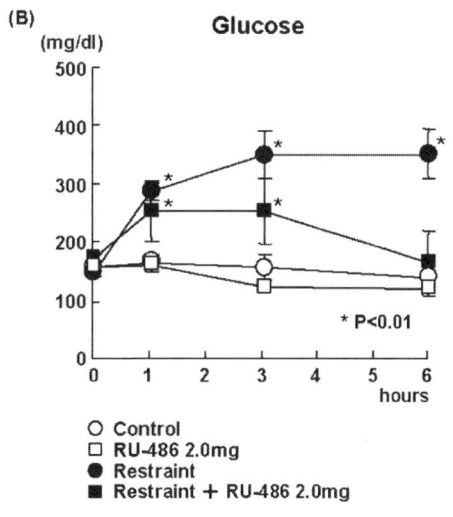

(A) Temperature

(B) Glucose

○ Control
□ RU-486 2.0mg
● Restraint
■ Restraint + RU-486 2.0mg

RU-486のプレ投与が拘束ストレスの影響におよぼす影響　(A)体温(B)血糖値　マウスにRU-486をプレ投与後、6時間拘束ストレスを与えた　平均値±1SDは、3匹のマウスを用いて算出した
**p< 0.01

認した。RU-486を前投与すると、適応反応は3つとも遮断された。この結果は、糖質コルチコイドは、低体温・高血糖および自然免疫の活性化を誘発させる要因の1つであることを示唆する。

以前、我々は、αアドレナリン刺激（アドレナリン）を用いても、低体温・高血糖および自然免疫の活性化が出現する可能性を報告した（Watanabe et al., 2008）。しかし、糖質コルチコイドの影響とαアドレナリンの影響とは同一

ではない。糖質コルチコイドによる反応は、常に、アドレナリンによる反応よりも大きい。体温では、ヒドロコルチゾン10.0mg投与したマウスでは、29℃未満の低体温を示した。一方、アドレナリン25.0μg投与したマウスの体温は37℃であり、対照群マウスの体温は38.8℃であった。最高50.0μgに増量してアドレナリンを投与すると、具合が悪くなったり死亡したりするマウスが続出した。

血糖値でも、アドレナリンと糖質コルチコイドの影響の大きさの相違を確認できた。血糖値は、ヒドロコルチゾンを投与すると最高500mg/dlまで上昇したが、アドレナリンを投与すると400mg/dlまでしか上昇しなかった。つまり、糖質コルチコイドは、αアドレナリンよりもストレス適応反応と関連性が深いと考えられる。本研究では、RU-486を投与すると、ストレス由来の体温低下と血糖値上昇が、不完全ながらも抑制された。この結果は、糖質コルチコイド以外の他の要素（αアドレナリン刺激など）がストレス由来の適応反応と関係していることを示唆する。しかし、このことを推論するにあたり重要であるのは、結果として、不完全ながらもストレス関連反応が抑制されたことである。この結果は、糖質コルチコイドは、ストレス適応反応に対して重要であることを裏打ちするものである。

本研究では、比較的高濃度のヒドロコルチゾンを用いて、拘束ストレス様の適応反応（低体温と高血糖）を誘発させた。この時、血清中糖質コルチコイド値は、通常値を超過したが、その後、非常に迅速に減少した。他方、拘束ストレス実験群の血清中糖質コルチコイド値は、ヒドロコルチゾン投与群の値ほど高くはなかったが長期間持続した。このことから、投与の際には、高濃度のヒドロコルチゾン投与が必要であると考えられる。拘束ストレス時の反応には、糖質コルチコイド以外の他の要素（カテコールアミン、TNFα等）も影響していることを考慮する必要がある。

本実験後半において、ヒドロコルチゾンの免疫に対する影響を検証した。予想通り、ヒドロコルチゾンを高濃度投与すると（10.0mg）、胸腺萎縮が見られた。換言すると、ストレスと糖質コルチコイドが免疫に及ぼす主な影響は、T細胞とB細胞の抑制であったのである。肝臓のB220$^+$B細胞の比率も減少した（Fig. 4B）。しかし、このような抑制の影響は比較的小さく、この時、胸腺のダブルポジティブCD4$^+$8$^+$細胞は減少しなかった（Fig. 4B 下）。興味深いのは、肝臓のIL-2Rβ$^+$CD3^{int}細胞またはNK1.1$^+$CD3^{int}細胞の比率の増加である。このように胸腺外分化T細胞やNKT細胞にはストレス耐性があり、拘束ストレスを受けると、むしろ活性化することは報告されている（Yamamura et al., 1996; Tsukahara et al., 1997; Abo et al., 2007）。これらの結果は、ストレスやヒドロコルチゾン投与により自然免疫が活性化する可能性を示唆するものである。本研究では、ヒドロコルチゾンを投与後4時間に、副腎のHSP70.1 mRNA発現が増加することを示した（Fig. 4C）。そして、糖質コルチコイド受容体遮断薬を投与すると、ヒドロコルチゾンによる自然免疫の増強を抑制できることが確認された。

αアドレナリン刺激（アドレナリン）と糖質コルチコイドとの間で、免疫に対する影響の大きさを比較すると、（胸腺外分化ではない）T細胞・B細胞を抑制するという点において、糖質コルチコイドはαアドレナリンよりも影響が大きかった。しかし、自然免疫増強に対する影響については、糖質コルチコイドもαアドレナリンもほとんど差異はなかった。

最後に、なぜ、ストレス、αアドレナリン刺激もしくはヒドロコルチゾン投与が、低体温と

Figure.8
ストレス反応とそれを伝えるもの

ストレス ➡ 低体温、高血糖[a]

〈伝達物質〉
1) αアドレナリン刺激 → 低体温、高血糖
2) 糖質コルチコイド → 低体温、高血糖

a 短期間ならば、筋肉内の解糖系を刺激して体が瞬発力を利用できるなど、低体温・高血糖は有益であることもある。しかし、ストレスが長期間におよび、このような状況が持続した結果、糖尿病などの慢性病を発症する．

高血糖を同時に誘導するかを考察する必要がある（Fig. 8）。低体温と高血糖は、身体的ストレスや精神的ストレスに悩む患者に、数多く見られるのみならず（Cyr et al., 2007; Obrosova, 2002; Nonogaki and Iguchi, 1997）、糖尿病患者にも（Abraham et al., 2007; Hugo and Ockert, 1992; Katsumichi and Pour, 2007）がん患者にも（Giovannucci, 2007; Dombrowski et al., 2007; Dankner et al., 2007; Ali et al., 2007）見られる。従って、この理由を考察することは重要である。仮説の一つとして、ミトコンドリア機能の抑制が考えられる。ストレスやαアドレナリン刺激が、血管収縮やそれに続いて起こる循環不全（低酸素）誘発した結果、低体温と高血糖が出現する可能性がある。低酸素は、ミトコンドリア機能を抑制する最大の要因である（Devoto et al., 2008; Tuor et al., 1996）。糖質コルチコイドは、ミトコンドリア内で糖質コルチコイド受容体を通じて、ミトコンドリア機能を直接抑制することができるのである（Palmeira et al., 2007; Psarra and Sekeris, 2008; Solakidi et al., 2007; Gavrilova-Jordan and Price, 2007; Sionov et al., 2006a,b）。従って、ミトコンドリアが消費するブドウ糖／ピルビン酸の量が減少した結果、高血糖が生じる可能性がある。いずれにせよ、糖質コルチコイドとαアドレナリン刺激により、低体温、高血糖と自然免疫の活性化が同時に誘発される事実は、興味深い発見である。

資金 文部科学省科学研究費補助金による。
利益相反 なし。

謝辞

本研究は、文部科学省科学研究費補助金による。原稿浄書について金子裕子氏に感謝する。

Association of glucocorticoid with stress-induced modulation of body temperature, blood glucose and innate immunity

Eisuke Kainuma [a], Mayumi Watanabe [a], Chikako Tomiyama-Miyaji [b], Masashi Inoue [a], Yuh Kuwano [a], HongWei Ren [a], Toru Abo [a,*]

[a] Department of Immunology, Niigata University School of Medicine, Niigata 951-8510, Japan
[b] School of Health Sciences, Faculty of Medicine, Niigata University, Niigata 951-8518, Japan

Received 25 August 2008; received in revised form 20 April 2009; accepted 30 April 2009

KEYWORDS
Stress;
Glucocorticoid;
Hypothermia;
Hyperglycemia;
Innate immunity;
Flowcytometry

Summary To know the details of the mechanism on stress-associated responses, attention was first focused on body temperature and blood glucose after stress. Mice were exposed to restraint stress for 6 h. Under this condition, hypothermia (39 °C → 33 °C) and hyperglycemia (150 mg/dl → 350 mg/dl) were induced. Reflecting a stress-associated response, an increase of serum corticosterone (200 ng/ml → up to 600 ng/ml) was observed. It was examined whether an administration of glucocorticoid induced a similar response. An injection of hydrocortisone (5.0 and 10.0 mg/mouse) simultaneously induced hypothermia and hyperglycemia. The effect on immunoparameters by an injection of hydrocortisone was examined. Although immunosuppression was seen as thymic atrophy and a decrease in the proportion of B cells in the liver, extrathymic T cells and NKT cells were found to be stress-resistant lymphocyte populations, especially in the liver. HSP70 mRNA was indicated to increase in the adrenal glands in response to the hydrocortisone injection. All these responses, including hypothermia, hyperglycemia and immunomodulation, induced by the hydrocortisone injection were suppressed by pre-administration of a glucocorticoid receptor antagonist (RU-486). These results suggest that glucocorticoid is one of the important mediators of the stress-associated responses.
© 2009 Elsevier Ltd. All rights reserved.

1. Introduction

It has widely been believed that physical and psychological stresses are intimately related to the onset of many diseases (Cyr et al., 2007; Obrosova, 2002; Nonogaki and Iguchi,

* Corresponding author. Tel.: +81 25 227 2133; fax: +81 25 227 0766.
E-mail address: immunol2@med.niigata-u.ac.jp (T. Abo).

1997). If we consider the connecting factors between stress and diseases, such candidates include the activation of sympathetic nerves (Suzuki et al., 1997; Kawamura et al., 1997, 1999; Minagawa et al., 1999, 2000; Mori et al., 2002; Abo and Kawamura, 2002) and the secretion of glucocorticoid (Shimizu et al., 2000; Sagiyama et al., 2004). With regard to sympathetic nerves, we have intensively characterized the effect of adrenergic stimulation on stress-associated responses. In a previous study, attention was focused on body

0306-4530/$ — see front matter © 2009 Elsevier Ltd. All rights reserved.
doi:10.1016/j.psyneuen.2009.04.021

temperature, blood glucose and innate immunity (Watanabe et al., 2008). As a result, α-adrenergic stimulation was found to induce hypothermia, an increase of blood glucose and activation of innate immunity. Conventional immunity was confirmed to decrease as one of the stress-associated responses.

In light of these findings, in the present study, we examined whether another stress-mediated factor of glucocorticoid induces a similar response to α-adrenergic stimulation, especially with regard to the magnitude and time lag of effects and so on. The simultaneous induction of stress-associated responses between α-adrenergic stimulation and glucocorticoid are of interest in terms of body temperature, blood glucose and innate immunity.

2. Material and methods

2.1. Mice

C57BL/6 (B6) mice were purchased from Charles River Japan (Yokohama, Japan). All mice used were male at 8–12 weeks of age in these experiments. The mice were kept in a room under constant temperature (25 ± 2 °C) and humidity (50–70%) with a 12-h light/dark cycle (light on from 08:00 to 20:00 h). They were fed under specific pathogen-free conditions in the animal facility of Niigata University (Niigata, Japan).

2.2. Restraint stress

Mice assigned to stressed groups were restrained in a wire stainless steel mesh cage for 2 or 6 h (from 09:00 to 11:00 h or 15:00 h) (Sagiyama et al., 2004). Although their movement was limited, they were allowed to breathe freely. All of the experiments were done with the approval of the Animal Ethics Committee of Niigata University.

2.3. Measurement of body temperature and blood glucose

The temperature in the rectum of the mice measured it with THERMAC SENSOR (Shibaura Denki Co., Tokyo, Japan). Blood glucose was measured by 3.5 μl blood of the mice venesection at the tail tip with Precision Xtra TM (Abott Japan Co., Chiba, Japan) (Nonogaki and Iguchi, 1997).

2.4. Cell preparation

Mice anaesthetized with isoflurane were sacrificed by exsanguination from the subclavian artery and vein, and the liver and spleen were removed. Hepatic lymphocytes were prepared as previously described (Kawamura et al., 1999). Briefly, the liver was pressed through 200-gauge stainless steel mesh and suspended in Eagle's MEM medium supplemented with 5 mM HEPES and 2% FCS. After one washing, the pellet was resuspended in 35% Percoll solution containing 100 U/ml heparin and centrifuged at 2000 rpm ($424 \times g$) for 15 min. The pellet was resuspended in red blood cell (RBC) lysis solution (155 mM NH_4Cl, 10 mM $KHCO_3$, 1 mM EDTA, and 17 mM Tris, pH 7.3) and then washed twice with the medium. Splenocytes and thymocytes were obtained by forcing the spleen and thymus, respectively, through stainless steel mesh. Splenocytes were treated with 0.2% NaCl solution to remove RBC.

2.5. Immunofluorescence tests

The phenotype of lymphocytes was identified by two-color immunofluorescence tests (Minagawa et al., 1999). The reagents used for this included anti-CD3ε (145-2C11), anti-IL-2Rβ (TM-β1), anti-NK1.1 (PK136), anti-CD4 (RM4-5), anti-CD8α (53-6.7) and anti-B220 (RA3-6B2) mAbs (BD PharMingen, San Diego, CA). All mAbs were used in fluorescein isothiocyanate (FITC) and phycoerythrin (PE) conjugated forms. To prevent nonspecific binding of mAb, anti-CD16/CD32 (2.4 G2) mAb was added before staining with labeled mAbs. The suspended lymphocytes ($5 \times 10^5 - 2 \times 10^6$/tube) were stained with mAbs and the stained lymphocytes were analyzed with a FACScan (Becton–Dickinson, Mountain View, CA). Dead cells were excluded by forward scatter, side scatter and propidium iodide gating.

2.6. Administration of hydrocortisone and glucocorticoid receptor antagonist

Hydrocortisone (SAXIZON, Kowa Pharmaceutical Co., Tokyo, Japan) was used. Mice were i.p. administered with this agent at a concentration of 10.0 mg/mouse (or 5.0 or 2.5 mg/mouse). RU-486, a glucocorticoid receptor and progesterone receptor antagonist (Mifepristone, Sigma–Aldrich Co., Saint Louis, MO) was suspended at concentration 2.0 mg/0.1 ml (or 1.5 or 1.0 mg/0.1 ml) in physiologic saline (Ashcraft et al., 2008; Jarillo-Luna et al., 2008; Elftman et al., 2007). Mice were i.p. administered with this suspension at concentration of 2.0 mg/mouse (or 1.5 or 1.0 mg/mouse).

2.7. Measurement of serum concentration of corticosterone

Cardiac blood samples were collected and centrifuged at $2500 \times g$ for 10 min at 4 °C. Serum corticosterone levels were determined by radioimmunoassay (RIA) (COAT-A-COUNT, Diagnostic Products Corporation, Los Angeles, CA). The RIA was performed with rat [^{125}I] corticosterone. Sensitivity of the assay was 5.7 ng/ml, the intra-assay variation was 4.3%, the inter-assay was 5.8%.

2.8. Preparation of total RNA and RT-PCR

Total RNAs was prepared from a part of the kidneys and the adrenal glands using ISOGEN (Nippon Gene, Tokyo, Japan) according to the manufacturer's instructions. RNA was converted to cDNA by SuperScript^{tm}III First-Strand Synthesis System for RT-PCR kit (Invitrogen, Co., Carlsbad, CA) using the manufacturer's protocol. RT-PCR for HSP70.1 and that for G3PDH were performed with 50 ng of total RNA by using the following primers and conditions: G3PDH: sense primer, 5'-GCG AGA CCC CAC TAA CAT CAA ATG-3', G3PDH antisense primer, 5'-CAG TGG ATG CAG GGA TGA TGT TCT-3', 1 time at 94 °C for 10 min; 30 times at 94 °C for 15 s, at 60 °C for 30 s and at 72 °C for 60 s; and 1 time at 72 °C for 7 min; HSP70.1: sense primer, 5'-CTA GCT GCC CAG TTC CCT GGA GAT-3'; HSP70.1 antisense primer, 5'-AAG CCC AGA ATC CAT TAG CCC TTC-3'; the same condition for G3PDH except that 35 cycles were employed. The PCR products were visualized on 2% agarose gel stained with ethidium bromide under UV light.

2.9. Statistical analysis

Two-way repeated measure ANOVAs were performed for the analysis of the body temperature or blood glucose in mice by time of restraint stress (from 0 to 2 or 6 h) and group (control and restraint stress) as main factor, also for the analysis of the body temperature or blood glucose in mice by time of reagent treatment (from 0 to 6 h) and group (control, hydrocortisone and hydrocortisone + RU-486) as main factor. The analysis of variance was followed by a Scheffe post hoc analysis when required ($p < 0.05$). In some experiments, One-way repeated measure ANOVAs were performed for the analysis of the number of MNCs in murine various organs by time of hydrocortisone treatment (from 0 to 72 h) and level of serum corticosterone (control and restraint) as main factor. The analysis of variance was followed by a Student's t-test when required ($p < 0.01$).

3. Results

3.1. Stress-induced responses

Mice were exposed to restraint stress for 6 h and then released. Body temperature, blood glucose and blood corticosterone were examined at each point of time (Fig. 1). Primarily, control mice had a high body temperature of around 38.8 ± 0.5 °C, whereas mice exposed to stress showed decreased levels of body temperature between 31.5 and 33.0 °C (Fig. 1A) (time, $F_{5,20} = 35.67$, $p < 0.001$; group, $F_{1,20} = 2880.10$, $p < 0.001$; time × group, $F_{5,20} = 3.31$, $p < 0.05$). After release from the stress, such decreased levels recovered immediately (data not shown).

In the case of blood glucose, control mice had a level of 150 mg/dl (Fig. 1B). However, mice exposed to stress showed elevated levels of glucose (280–360 mg/dl) (time, $F_{5,20} = 2.03$, $p = 0.12$; group, $F_{1,20} = 667.73$, $p < 0.001$; time × group, $F_{5,20} = 4.67$, $p < 0.01$). These levels returned to the control level after the release from stress.

The serum level of corticosterone was then examined (Fig. 1C). In control mice, the level of corticosterone was around 200 ± 70 mg/dl. This level increased up to 500 ± 80 mg/dl at 2 and 6 h of stress ($F_{2,8} = 11.66$, $p < 0.01$).

3.2. Administration of glucocorticoid

It was examined whether a single administration of glucocorticoid evoked a similar response induced by restraint stress (Fig. 2). Various doses (2.5–10.0 mg/mouse) of hydrocortisone were applied in this experiment. At the highest dose (10.0 mg/mouse) of hydrocortisone, body temperature decreased and blood glucose increased (Fig. 2A). These responses were quite similar to those of restraint stress. The dose of 2.5 mg/mouse did not induce such responses, but that of 5.0 mg/mouse induced responses to a certain degree (temperature: time, $F_{5,40} = 117.01$, $p < 0.001$; group, $F_{3,40} = 829.35$, $p < 0.001$; time × group, $F_{15,40} = 130.78$, $p < 0.001$; glucose: time, $F_{5,40} = 214.74$, $p < 0.001$; group, $F_{3,40} = 290.41$, $p < 0.001$; time × group, $F_{15,40} = 53.54$, $p < 0.001$).

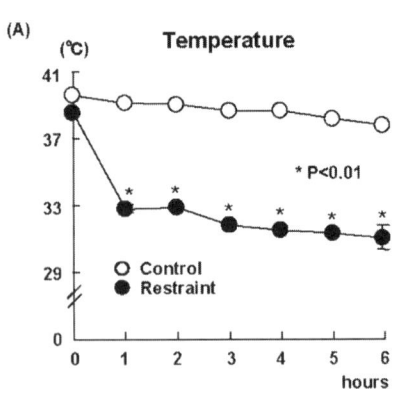

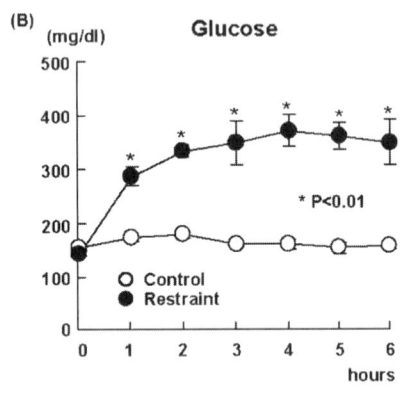

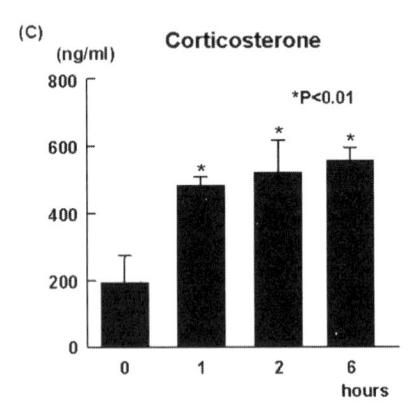

Figure 1 Stress-induced responses. (A) Body temperature, (B) blood glucose, and (C) corticosterone in sera. Mice were exposed to restraint stress for 6 h. The mean value and one SD were produced using 3 mice. $^*p < 0.01$.

When mice were administrated with 5 mg/mouse of hydrocortisone, the sera levels of corticosterone were measured (Fig. 2B). At 1 h after the administration, the high level of corticosterone was detected in serum. ($F_{3,10} = 32.74$,

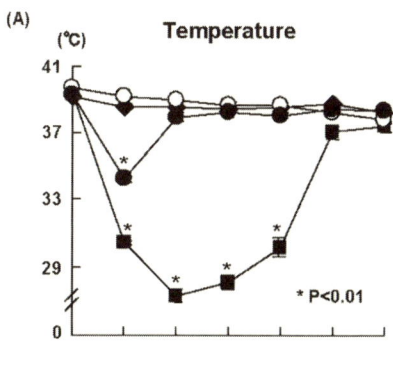

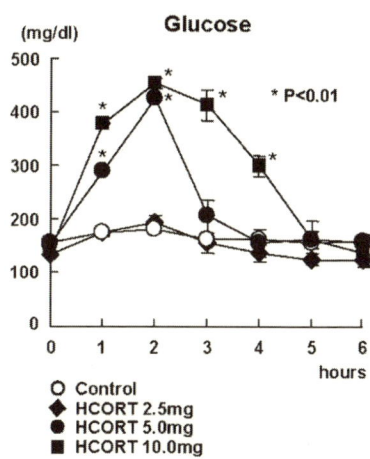

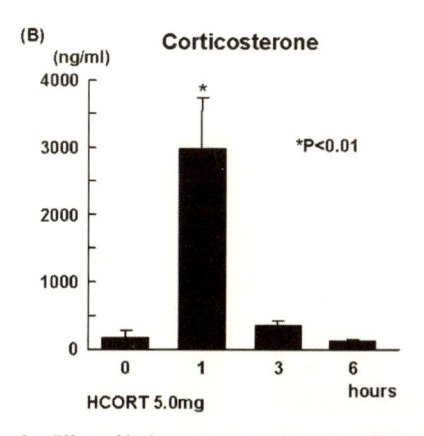

Figure 2 Effect of hydrocortisone. (A) Variation of body temperature and blood glucose after the administration of cortisone, (B) corticosterone in sera. The mean value and one SD were produced using 3 mice. $^*p < 0.01$.

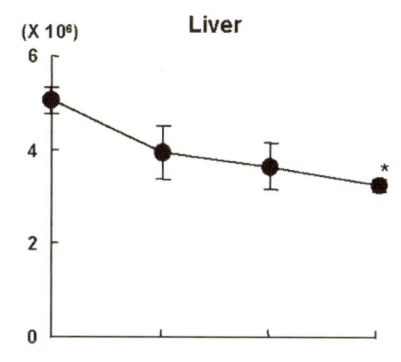

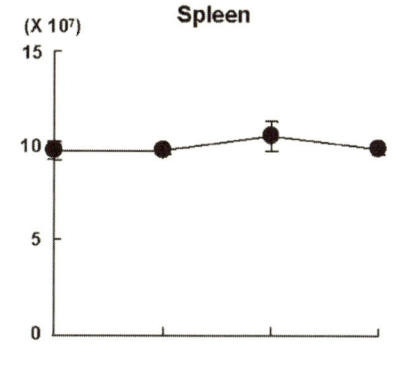

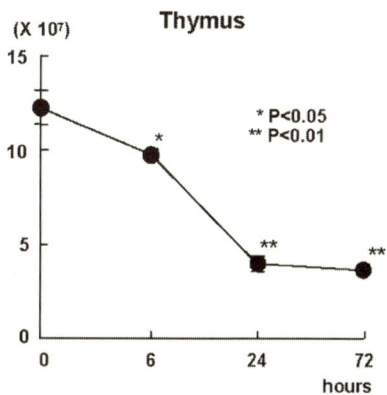

Figure 3 Number of cells yielded by the liver, spleen and thymus. The mean value and one SD were produced using 3 mice. $^*p < 0.05$ and $^{**}p < 0.01$.

$p < 0.001$). However, this level was not continuous but decreased quickly.

3.3. Immunomodulation by glucocorticoid

It is well established that stress induces unique immunomodulation in humans and animals (Sagiyama et al., 2004). It

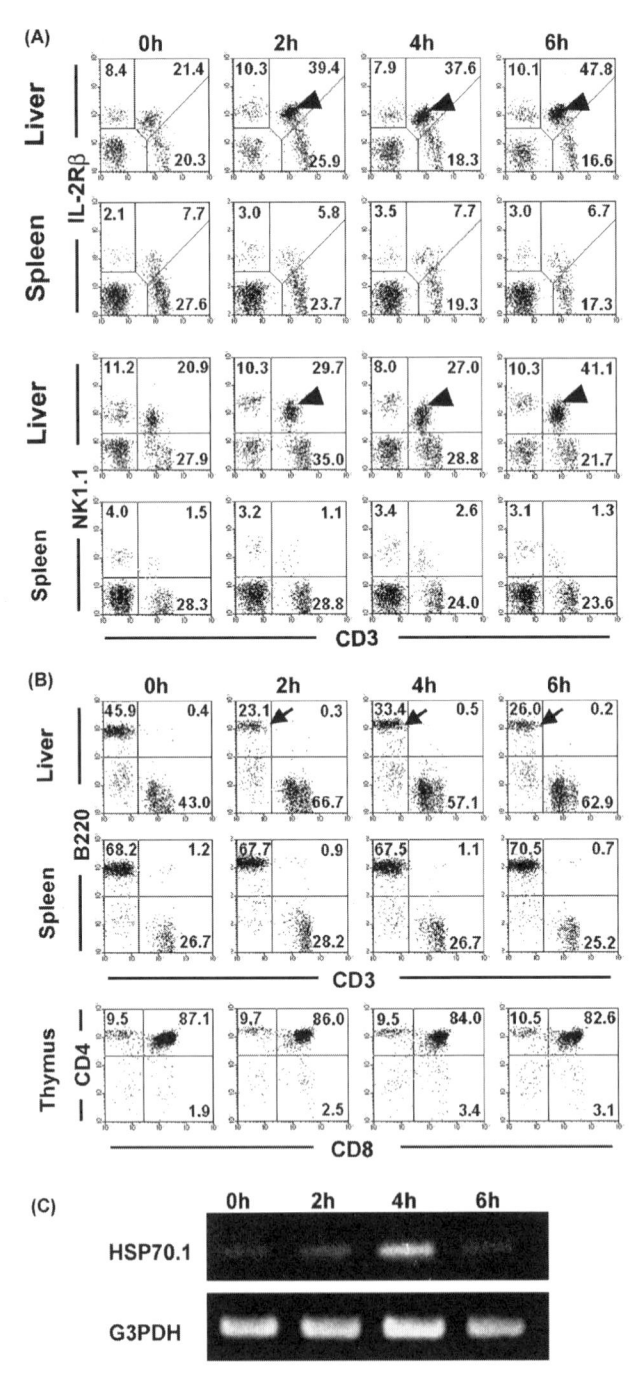

Figure 4 Variation of immunoparameters after the administration of cortisone (5.0 mg/mouse). (A) Two-color staining for CD3 and IL-2Rβ and that for CD3 and NK1.1. (B) Two-color staining for CD3 and B220 in the liver and spleen, and two-color staining for CD4 and CD8 in the thymus. (C) The sign of HSP70.1 mRNA by RT-PCR. Numbers in the squares represent the percentages of fluorescence-positive cells in corresponding areas. Prominent changes are indicated by arrowheads and arrows.

was examined how 5.0 mg/mouse of hydrocortisone mediated immunomodulation (Fig. 3). Lymphocyte yield was first examined in the liver, spleen and thymus. The yield did not vary in the spleen and slightly decreased in the liver. The most prominent change was seen in the thymus, the yield of thymocytes being one-third that of control mice at 24 and 72 h after administration (liver: $F_{3,7} = 7.77$, $p < 0.05$; spleen: $F_{3,7} = 1.18$, $p = 0.42$; thymus: $F_{3,7} = 131.90$, $p < 0.001$).

The effect of hydrocortisone on the distribution of lymphocyte subsets was then examined (Fig. 4). To identify the subsets, two-color staining for CD3 and IL-2Rβ (or NK1.1) was conducted (Fig. 4A). The most prominent change was seen in IL-2Rβ$^+$CD3^{int} cells (i.e., extrathymic T cells) and NK1.1$^+$CD3^{int} cells (i.e., NKT cells) in the liver at 2, 4 and 6 h after administration (indicated by arrowheads). The proportion of IL-2Rβ$^+$CD3^{int} cells increased up to 47.8% and that of NK1.1$^+$CD3^{int} cells increased up to 41.1%. The proportion of IL-2Rβ$^+$ (or NK1.1$^+$) CD3$^-$cells (i.e., NK cells) and that of IL-2Rβ$^-$ (or NK1.1$^-$)CD3^{high} cells (i.e., conventional T cells) in the liver did not significantly change.

B cells were identified as B220$^+$CD3$^-$ cells by two-color staining for B220 and CD3 (Fig. 4B). The proportion of B cells in the liver decreased by the administration of hydrocortisone (indicated by arrows). The proportion of B cells in the spleen remained constant even with such administration. It is known that the proportion of CD4$^+$8$^+$ double-positive cells in the thymus decreases under conditions of immunosuppression. Such a phenomenon was not seen in the thymus by the administration of hydrocortisone at least after 6 h (Fig. 4B bottom).

It is also known that the production of HSP70 is accompanied by stress-associated responses (Blake et al., 1991). Therefore, such production of HSP70 was examined by the RT-PCR method (Fig. 4C). The RNA for RT-PCR was prepared from the adrenal glands and kidneys of mice which were administrated hydrocortisone (5.0 mg/mouse). At 4 h after the administration of hydrocortisone, the expression of HSP70.1 became prominent.

3.4. Effect of glucocorticoid receptor antagonist on glucocorticoid-induced responses

To directly confirm whether glucocorticoid-induced responses were eventually mediated via glucocorticoid receptors, pre-administration of RU-486 was conducted prior to the administration of hydrocortisone (Fig. 5). The experimental protocol is shown in Fig. 5A. The dose of RU-486 is indicated at the bottom of the figure.

It was clearly demonstrated that the pre-administration of RU-486 suppressed the decrease of body temperature and the increase of blood glucose induced by hydrocortisone (5.0 mg/mouse), irrespective of the dose of RU-486 applied (temperature: time, $F_{5,50} = 1.89$, $p = 0.11$; group, $F_{4,50} = 5.94$, $p < 0.05$; time × group, $F_{20,50} = 11.15$, $p < 0.001$; glucose: time, $F_{5,50} = 254.30$, $p < 0.001$; group, $F_{4,50} = 28.22$, $p < 0.001$; time × group, $F_{20,50} = 41.53$, $p < 0.001$).

The effect of RU-486 on stress-associated responses of immunity was then examined (Fig. 6). The increase in the proportion of IL-2Rβ$^+$CD3^{int} cells and NK1.1$^+$CD3^{int} cells induced by hydrocortisone was found to be suppressed by the pre-administration of RU-486 in the liver (Fig. 6A). Similarly, the decrease in the proportion of B220$^+$B cells induced by hydrocortisone was also suppressed in the liver by the pre-administration of RU-486 (Fig. 6B).

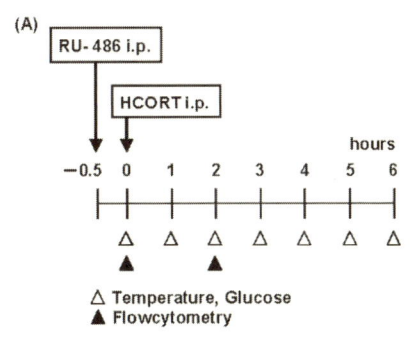

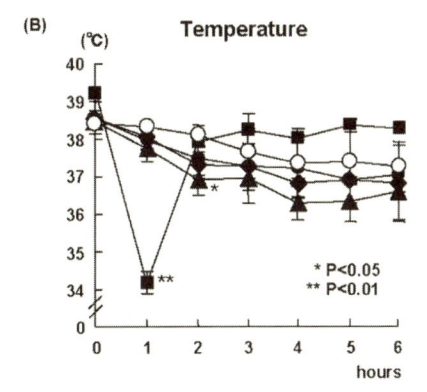

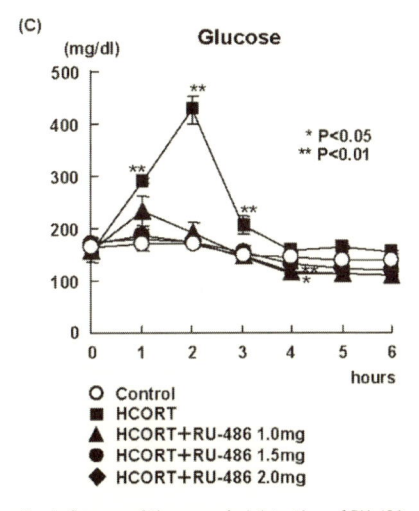

Figure 5 Influence of the pre-administration of RU-486 on the effects induced by the cortisone injection. (A) Experimental schedules, (B) body temperature, and (C) blood glucose. The mean and one SD were produced using 3 mice. $^*p < 0.05$ and $^{**}p < 0.01$.

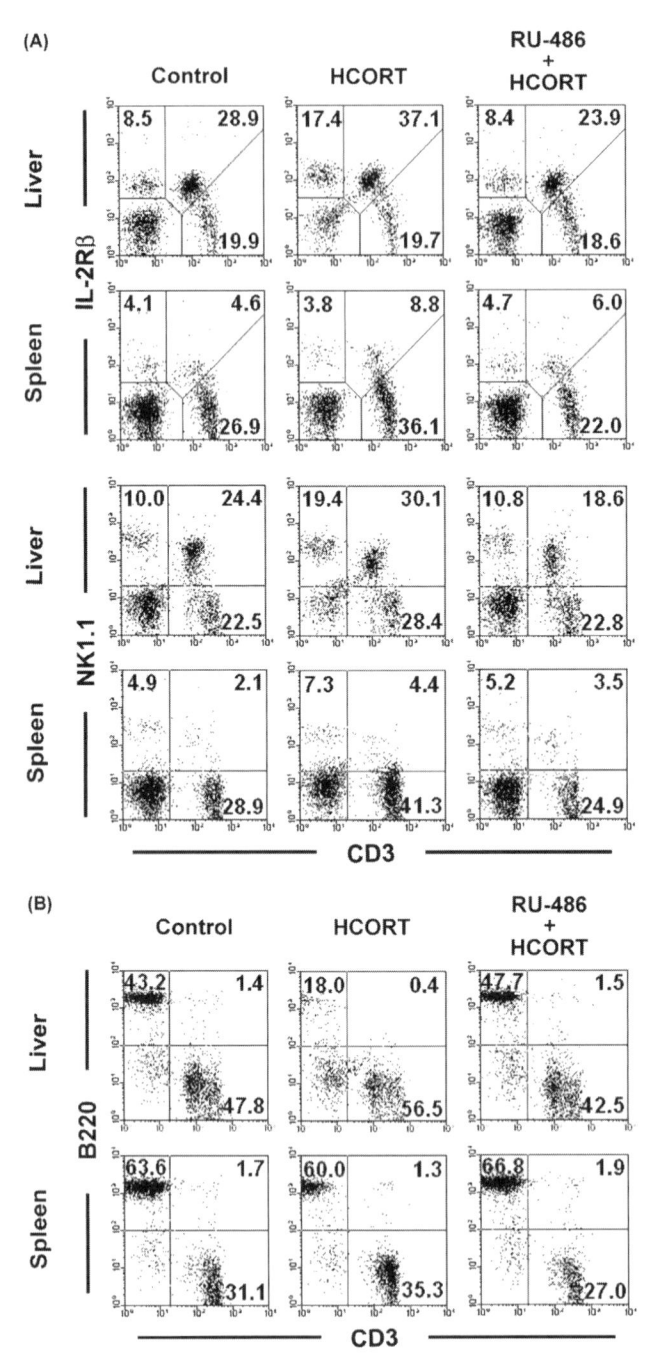

Figure 6 Influence of the pre-administration of RU-486 on the immunomodulation induced by the cortisone injection. (A) Two-color staining for CD3 and IL-2Rβ and that for CD3 and NK1.1, and (B) two-color staining for CD3 and B220. Numbers in the squares represent the percentages of fluorescence-positive cells in corresponding areas. Prominent changes are indicated by arrowheads and arrows.

3.5. Effect of glucocorticoid receptor antagonist on the restraint stress-associated responses

To examine whether stress-associated responses were eventually mediated via the interaction between glucocorticoid and its receptors, pre-administration of RU-486 (2.0 mg/mouse) was conducted prior to the restraint stress (Fig. 7). The stress continued for 6 h. It was demonstrated that pre-administration of RU-486 partially suppressed the decrease of body temperature and the increase of blood glucose induced by the restraint stress (temperature: time, $F_{3,24} = 165.46$, $p < 0.001$; group, $F_{3,24} = 77.48$, $p < 0.001$; time $\times$ group, $F_{9,24} = 29.12$, $p < 0.001$; glucose: time, $F_{3,24} = 19.80$, $p < 0.001$; group, $F_{3,24} = 24.36$, $p < 0.001$; time $\times$ group, $F_{9,24} = 17.65$, $p < 0.001$).

4. Discussion

In the present study, we demonstrated that an administration of glucocorticoid simultaneously induced hypothermia, hyperglycemia and activation of innate immunity. All these responses resembled stress-associated responses. In other words, a secretion of glucocorticoid might be a major mediator of stress-associated responses. To confirm that the present responses induced by the administration of hydrocortisone were mediated via glucocorticoid receptors, glucocorticoid receptor antagonist (RU-486) was used. All three responses were blocked by the pre-administration of RU-486. These results suggest that glucocorticoid is one of the critical factors which induced hypothermia, hyperglycemia and activation of innate immunity.

As shown in our previous study, α-adrenergic stimulation (i.e., adrenaline) has also the potential to induce hypothermia, hyperglycemia and activation of innate immunity (Watanabe et al., 2008). However, the effect of glucocorticoid and that of α-adrenergic stimulation differed. The magnitude of responses induced by glucocorticoid was always greater than that induced by adrenaline. In the case of body temperature, 10.0 mg hydrocortisone/mouse induced hypothermia of less than 29 °C. On the other hand, 25.0 μg adrenaline/mouse induced hypothermia to 37 °C. Control mice showed a body temperature of 38.8 °C. When the dose of adrenaline was increased up to 50.0 μg/mouse, many mice became unhealthy or died.

This difference of magnitude was also true in the case of blood glucose. The maximum dose of hydrocortisone increased blood glucose up to 500 mg/dl, but that of adrenaline increased blood glucose up to 400 mg/dl. In other words, there is a possibility that glucocorticoid might be more seriously associated with stress-associated responses than α-adrenergic stimulation. The partial suppression by RU-486 against the decrease of body temperature and against the increase of blood glucose was induced by the stress in the present study. This result suggests that the other factors (e.g., α-adrenergic stimulus) than glucocorticoid are also associated with the stress-induced phenomena. However, the partial but significant such suppression supports the above-mentioned speculation, namely, an importance of glucocorticoid for the stress-associated responses.

The dose of hydrocortisone which was required to induce the mimic response to restraint stress (i.e., hypothermia and hyperglycemia) was relatively high in this study. In this case, the serum concentration of glucocorticoid increased up to a supra-physiological level but decreased very quickly. On the other hand, the serum level of glucocorticoid induced by the restraint stress was not so high but the increased level was long lasting. It is, therefore, conceivable that a large amount of hydrocortisone was required in the case of administration. We also have to consider the synergic effect of glucocorticoid with other factors (e.g., catecholamines, TNFα, etc) in the actual stress-associated responses.

In a final portion of these experiments, the effects of hydrocortisone on immunity were investigated. As expected, thymic atrophy was induced at the maximum dose (10.0 mg/mouse) of hydrocortisone. Namely, the main effect of stress and glucocorticoid on immunity was the suppression of conventional T and B cells. The proportion of B220$^+$B cells also decreased in the liver (see Fig. 4B). However, all these suppressive effects were relatively small because double-positive CD4$^+$8$^+$ cells in the thymus did not proportionally decrease (see Fig. 4B bottom). An interesting result was the increase in the proportion of IL-2Rβ^+ (or NK1.1$^+$) CD3^{int} cells

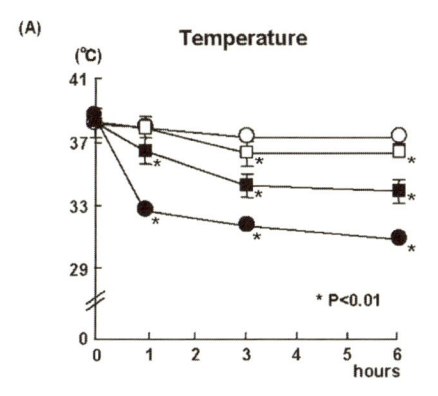

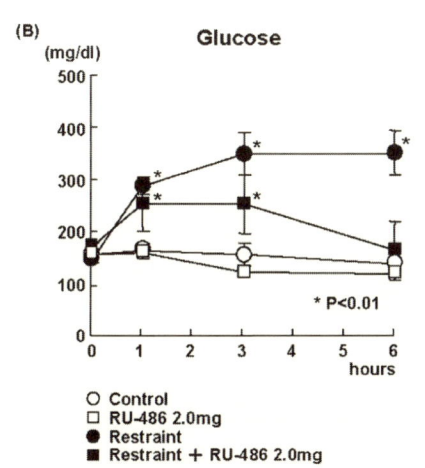

Figure 7 Influence of the pre-administration of RU-486 on the effects induced by restraint stress. (A) Body temperature, (B) blood glucose. Mice were pre-administrated with RU-486 and then exposed to restraint stress for 6 h. The mean value and one SD were produced using 3 mice. **$p < 0.01$

STRESS ⟶ HYPOTHERMIA, HYPERGLYCEMIA [a]

<mediators>

1. α-adrenergic stimulus ⟶ hypothermia, hyperglycemia
2. glucocorticoids ⟶ hypothermia, hyperglycemia

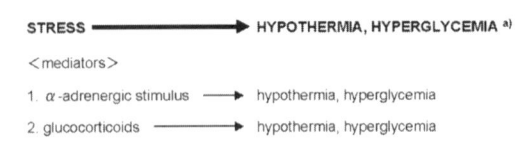

[a] Short-term responses may be beneficial to stimulate glycolysis of the muscles which is responsible for quick moments of the body. However, a continuation of such conditions induced by long-term stress results in chronic diseases including diabetes.

Figure 8 Stress-associated responses and mediators.

in the liver. These extrathymic T cells and NKT cells are known to be stress-resistant and to be rather activated by restraint stress (Yamamura et al., 1996; Tsukahara et al., 1997; Abo et al., 2007). These results suggest that stress and the administration of hydrocortisone can potentially activate innate immunity. The administration of hydrocortisone in this study, was found to increase the sign of HSP70.1 mRNA at 4 h in the adrenal glands (see Fig. 4C). It was confirmed that the augmentation of innate immunity induced by hydrocortisone was inhibited by the use of glucocorticoid receptor antagonist.

If we compare the magnitude of effects on the immunity between glucocorticoid and α-adrenergic stimulation (i.e., adrenaline), the suppressive effect on conventional T and B cells was greater by glucocorticoid than by α-adrenergic stimulation. However, the augmentation effect on the innate immunity was almost the same between glucocorticoid and α-adrenergic stimulation.

Finally, we have to discuss why hypothermia and hyperglycemia are simultaneously induced by stress, α-adrenergic stimulation or hydrocortisone injection (Fig. 8). This question is important because these conditions are frequently seen in many people with physical and psychological stresses (Cyr et al., 2007; Obrosova, 2002; Nonogaki and Iguchi, 1997), in patients with diabetes (Abraham et al., 2007; Hugo and Ockert, 1992; Katsumichi and Pour, 1992) and even in cancer patients (Giovannucci, 2007; Dombrowski et al., 2007; Dankner et al., 2007; Ali et al., 2007). One hypothesis is the suppression of mitochondrial functions. Stress and α-adrenergic stimulation might mediate such effects via vessel contraction and subsequent circulation failure (i.e., hypoxia). Hypoxia is the most serious factor which suppresses mitochondrial functions (Devoto et al., 2008; Tuor et al., 1996). In the case of glucocorticoid, they have the ability to directly suppress mitochondrial functions via glucocorticoid receptors in the mitochondria (Palmeira et al., 2007; Psarra and Sekeris, 2008; Solakidi et al., 2007; Gavrilova-Jordan and Price, 2007; Sionov et al., 2006a,b). Thus, hyperglycemia might concomitantly occur due to less consumption of glucose/pyruvic acid by the mitochondria. In any case, the simultaneous induction of hypothermia, hyperglycemia and activation of innate immunity by both glucocorticoid and α-adrenergic stimulation is an interesting finding.

Role of the funding sources

Funding for this study was provided by a Grant-in-Aid for Scientific Research from the Ministry of Education, Science and Culture, Japan. The funding source had no involvement in study design, in the collection, analysis and in the decision to submit the paper for publication.

Conflict of interest

None declared.

Acknowledgments

This work was supported by a Grant-in-Aid for Scientific Research from the Ministry of Education, Science and Culture, Japan. The authors wish to thank Mrs. Yuko Kaneko for preparation of the manuscript.

References

Abo, T., Kawamura, T., 2002. Immunomodulation by the autonomic nervous system—therapeutic approach for cancer, collagen diseases, and inflammatory bowel diseases. Ther. Apher. 6, 348—357.

Abo, T., Kawamura, T., Kawamura, H., Tomiyama-Miyaji, C., Kanda, Y., 2007. Relationship between diseases accompanied by tissue destruction and granulocytes with surface adrenergic receptors. Immunol. Res. 37, 201—210.

Abraham, N.G., Brunner, E.J., Eriksson, J.W., Robertson, R.P., 2007. Metabolic syndrome: psychosocial, neuroendocrine, and classical risk factors in type 2 diabetes. Ann. NY Acad. Sci. 1113, 256—275.

Ali, N.A., O'Brien Jr., J.M., Blum, W., Byrd, J.C., Klisovic, R.B., Marcucci, G., Phillips, G., Marsh, C.B., Lemeshow, S., Grever, M.R., 2007. Hyperglycemia in patients with acute myeloid leukemia is associated with increased hospital mortality. Cancer 110, 96—102.

Ashcraft, K.A., Hunzeker, J., Bonneau, R.H., 2008. Psychological stress impairs the local $CD8^+$ T cell response to mucosal HSV-1 infection and allows for increased pathogenicity via a glucocorticoid receptor-mediated mechanism. Psychoneuroendocrinology 33, 951—963.

Blake, M.J., Udelsman, R., Feulner, G.J., Norton, D.D., Holbrook, N.J., 1991. Stress-induced heat shock protein 70 expression in adrenal cortex: an adrenocorticotropic hormone-sensitive, age-dependent response. Proc. Natl. Acad. Sci. U.S.A. 88, 9873—9877.

Cyr, N.E., Earle, K., Tam, C., Romero, L.M., 2007. The effect of chronic psychological stress on corticosterone, plasma metabolites, and immune responsiveness in European starlings. Gen. Comp. Endocrinol. 154, 59—66.

Dankner, R., Chetrit, A., Segal, P., 2007. Glucose tolerance status and 20 year cancer incidence. Isr. Med. Assoc. J. 9, 592—596.

Devoto, V.M., Giusti, S., Chavez, J.C., de Plazas, S.F., 2008. Hypoxia-induced apoptotic cell death is prevented by oestradiol via oestrogen receptors in the developing central nervous system. J. Neuroendocrinol. 20, 375—380.

Dombrowski, F., Klotz, L., Bannasch, P., Evert, M., 2007. Renal carcinogenesis in models of diabetes in rats: metabolic changes are closely related to neoplastic development. Diabetologia 50, 2580—2590.

Elftman, M.D., Norbury, C.C., Bonneau, R.H., Truckenmiller, M.E., 2007. Corticosterone impairs dendritic cell maturation and function. Immunology 122, 279—290.

Gavrilova-Jordan, L.P., Price, T.M., 2007. Actions of steroids in mitochondria. Semin. Reprod. Med. 25, 154—164.

Giovannucci, E., 2007. Metabolic syndrome, hyperinsulinemia, and colon cancer: a review. Am. J. Clin. Nutr. 86, 836—842.

Hugo, J.M., Ockert, D.B., 1992. Routine peri-operative management of the diabetic patient. S. Afr. J. Surg. 30, 85—89.

Jarillo-Luna, A., Rivera-Aguilar, V., Martinez-Carrillo, B.E., Barbosa-Cabrera, E., Garfias, H.R., Campos-Rodriguez, R., 2008. Effect of restraint stress on the population of intestinal intraepithelial lymphocytes in mice. Brain Behav. Immun. 22, 265–275.

Katsumichi, I., Pour, P.M., 2007. Diabetes mellitus in pancreatic cancer: is it a causal relationship? Am. J. Surg. 194, 71–75.

Kawamura, H., Kawamura, T., Kokai, Y., Mori, M., Matsuura, A., Oya, H., Honda, S., Suzuki, S., Weerasinghe, A., Watanabe, H., Abo, T., 1999. Expansion of extrathymic T cells as well as granulocytes in the liver and other organs of granulocyte-colony stimulating factor transgenic mice: why they lost the ability of hybrid resistance. J. Immunol. 162, 5957–5964.

Kawamura, T., Toyabe, S., Moroda, T., Iiai, T., Takahashi-Iwanaga, H., Fukuda, M., Watanabe, H., Sekikawa, H., Seki, S., Abo, T., 1997. Neonatal granulocytosis is a postpartum event which is seen in the liver as well as in the blood. Hepatology 26, 1567–1572.

Minagawa, M., Narita, J., Tada, T., Maruyama, S., Shimizu, T., Bannai, M., Oya, H., Hatakeyama, K., Abo, T., 1999. Mechanisms underlying immunologic states during pregnancy: possible association of the sympathetic nervous system. Cell. Immunol. 196, 1–13.

Minagawa, M., Oya, H., Yamamoto, S., Shimizu, T., Bannai, M., Kawamura, H., Hatakeyama, K., Abo, T., 2000. Intensive expansion of natural killer T cells in the early phase of hepatocyte regeneration after partial hepatectomy in mice and its association with sympathetic nerve activation. Hepatology 31, 907–915.

Mori, H., Nishijo, K., Kawamura, H., Abo, T., 2002. Unique immunomodulation by electro-acupuncture in humans possibly via stimulation of the autonomic nervous system. Neurosci. Lett. 320, 21–24.

Nonogaki, K., Iguchi, A., 1997. Stress, acute hyperglycemia, and hyperlipidemia role of the autonomic nervous system and cytokines. Trends Endocrinol. Metab. 8, 192–197.

Obrosova, I.G., 2002. How does glucose generate oxidative stress in peripheral nerve? Int. Rev. Neurobiol. 50, 3–35.

Palmeira, C.M., Rolo, A.P., Berthiaume, J., Bjork, J.A., Wallace, K.B., 2007. Hyperglycemia decreases mitochondrial function: the regulatory role of mitochondrial biogenesis. Toxicol. Appl. Pharmacol. 225, 214–220.

Psarra, A.M., Sekeris, C.E., 2008. Steroid and thyroid hormone receptors in mitochondria. IUBMB Life 60, 210–223.

Sagiyama, K., Tsuchida, M., Kawamura, H., Wang, S., Li, C., Bai, X., Nagura, T., Nozoe, S., Abo, T., 2004. Age-related bias in function of natural killer T cells and granulocytes after stress: reciprocal association of steroid hormones and sympathetic nerves. Clin. Exp. Immunol. 135, 56–63.

Shimizu, T., Kawamura, T., Miyaji, T., Oya, H., Bannai, M., Yamamoto, S., Weerasinghe, A., Halder, R.C., Watanabe, H., Hatakeyama, K., Abo, T., 2000. Resistance of extrathymic T cells to stress and the role of endogenous glucocorticoids in stress associated immuno suppression. Scand. J. Immunol. 51, 285–292.

Sionov, R.V., Kfir, S., Zafrir, E., Cohen, O., Zilberman, Y., Yefenof, E., 2006a. Glucocorticoid-induced apoptosis revisited: a novel role for glucocorticoid receptor translocation to the mitochondria. Cell Cycle 5, 1017–1026.

Sionov, R.V., Cohen, O., Kfir, S., Zilberman, Y., Yefenof, E., 2006b. Role of mitochondrial glucocorticoid receptor in glucocorticoid-induced apoptosis. J. Exp. Med. 203, 189–201.

Solakidi, S., Psarra, A.M., Sekeris, C.E., 2007. Differential distribution of glucocorticoid and estrogen receptor isoforms: localization of GRbeta and ERalpha in nucleoli and GRalpha and ERbeta in the mitochondria of human osteosarcoma SaOS-2 and hepatocarcinoma HepG2 cell lines. J. Musculoskelet. Neuronal Interact. 7, 240–245.

Suzuki, S., Toyabe, S., Moroda, T., Tada, T., Tsukahara, A., Iiai, T., Minagawa, M., Maruyama, S., Hatakeyama, K., Endo, K., Abo, T., 1997. Circadian rhythm of leukocytes and lymphocyte subsets and its possible correlation with the function of autonomic nervous system. Clin. Exp. Immunol. 110, 500–508.

Tsukahara, A., Tada, T., Suzuki, S., Iiai, T., Moroda, T., Maruyama, S., Minagawa, M., Musha, N., Shimizu, T., Hatakeyama, K., Abo, T., 1997. Adrenergic stimulation simultaneously induces the expansion of granulocytes and extrathymic T cells in mice. Biomed. Res. 18, 237–246.

Tuor, U.I., Del Bigio, M.R., Chumas, P.D., 1996. Brain damage due to cerebral hypoxia/ischemia in the neonate: pathology and pharmacological modification. Cerebrovasc. Brain Metab. Rev. 8, 159–193.

Watanabe, M., Tomiyama-Miyaji, C., Kainuma, E., Inoue, M., Kuwano, Y., Ren, H.W., Shen, J.W., Abo, T., 2008. Role of α-adrenergic stimulus in stress-induced modulation of body temperature, blood glucose and innate immunity. Immunol. Lett. 115, 43–49.

Yamamura, S., Arai, K., Toyabe, S., Takahashi, E.H., Abo, T., 1996. Simultaneous activation of granulocytes and extrathymic T cells in number and function by excessive administration of nonsteroidal anti-inflammatory drugs. Cell. Immunol. 173, 303–311.

Internal Environment in Cancer Patients and Proposal that Carcinogenesis is Adaptive Response of Glycolysis to Overcome Adverse Internal Conditions

がん患者の内部環境と提言：
発がんは不利な内部状態を克服する解糖系への適応反応である

Health, 2:781-788, 2010

chapter 23

Internal environment in cancer patients and proposal that carcinogenesis is adaptive response of glycolysis to overcome adverse internal conditions

がん患者の内部環境と提言：
発がんは不利な内部状態を克服する解糖系への適応反応である

Mayumi Watanabe[1], Kenya Miyajima[2], Ittoku Matsui[2], Chikako Tomiyama-Miyaji[3], Eisuke Kainuma[1], Masashi Inoue[1], Hiroaki Matsumoto[1], Yuh Kuwano[1], Toru Abo[1]*

[1]Department of Immunology, Niigata University School of Medicine, Niigata, Japan; *Corresponding Author: immunol2@med.niigata-u.ac.jp
[2]Yushima-Shimizuzaka Clinic, Tokyo, Japan
[3]School of Health Sciences, Faculty of Medicine, Niigata University, Niigata, Japan

【キーワード】

がん；低体温；低酸素；高血糖；解糖；ミトコンドリア

【要約】

近年、我々は研究を重ね、ストレスが低体温と高血糖を同時に誘発することを発見した。低体温と高血糖は、解糖系を利用してエネルギーを速やかに獲得し危機を乗り超えるのに有利である。がん患者の内部環境には、低体温と高血糖が見られることもある。そこで、我々は、低体温と高血糖は、広くがん患者に見られる現象であるか否か研究を進めた。初期および進行がん患者を対象に、血中ガスや体温をはじめとする測定を行った。がん患者の体温では、発がんステージにかかわりなく患者の多くは低体温を示した。さらに、低体温に加えて高血糖も患者群に多く認められた。患者群には、免疫抑制状態と貧血が見られた。患者群の血液ガス分析では、酸素分圧が低く、二酸化炭素分圧が高かった。これらの結果から、患者群に見られる低体温、高血糖および低酸素などの内部環境が、発がんを誘発し、がん細胞分裂を継続させる原因であるという可能性が示唆される。というのは、がん細胞は、解糖系優位のエネルギー産生を行うからだ。低体温、低酸素および高血糖は、解糖系を活性化して、危機状態を回避するのに重要な反応である。しかし、このような反応も長期化すると、ミトコンドリア系抑制を引き起こし、結果として発がんを引き起こす可能性がある。

1. はじめに

がん細胞が、初期に腫瘍塊として現れるのは局所である。しかし、がんは全身をむしばむ疾病ではないかと考える研究者や臨床医は多い。がんが全身をむしばむ疾病であるならば、多くのがん患者に特異的にみられる内部環境を考察する必要がある。がん患者の内部環境を研究し、諸測定項目を分析した。そして、がん患者には低体温と高血糖の両方が見られる場合が多いことが判明した。

これらの結果をふまえ、我々はストレス反応 [1,2] と関連させ、がん患者の研究をすすめた。興味深いことに、ストレスが低体温と高血糖を誘発していた。低体温と高血糖の内部環境は、人間や動物にとって危機状態を回避するのに有益である可能性がある [3]。つまり、迅速に白筋繊維を用いた力を得るには、解糖系から産生されたエネルギーを利用している。解糖系では、エネルギー産生の効率は低い（2ATP/1ブドウ糖）。しかし、解糖系ではATP合成が、ミトコンドリア系に比べ非常に速い（100倍の

速度）[4]。

短期間ならば、低体温と高血糖は、ストレスや危機を逃れるのに都合がよい。しかし、低体温と高血糖は、ミトコンドリア系（酸化的リン酸化）のエネルギー産生にとっては不都合である。低体温と高血糖の患者には、慢性疲労、るいそう、衰弱、耐糖能異常などが見られる。

本研究では、がん患者の内部環境を詳細に検討し、発がんとは生体が不利な内部環境を克服しようとする解糖系への適応現象であるという考え方を提案する。がん細胞が糖代謝を、酸化的リン酸化から解糖へと移行させることを示す証拠は複数ある。そして、がん細胞の細胞質においてミトコンドリアは欠損もしくはごく少数である [5-7]。紫外線、食品添加物、大気汚染といった発がん物質が、原がん遺伝子（プロトオンコジーン）に対しさまざまな突然変異の過程を誘発すると考える研究者は多い [8-12]。しかし、それ以外に、このような突然変異は生体の解糖系への適応であるといった考え方も可能である。偏った生き方は、慢性ストレスの原因ともなる。慢性ストレスが原因で、低体温、低酸素および高血糖といった適応反応が出現している可能性は否定できない。

2. 方法

2.1. 対象

初期および進行がんの患者群の体温を測定した（n=28、54.3 ± 8.0歳）。同年齢層の健常人群の体温も測定した（n=27、45.8 ± 11.0歳）。

さらに、進行がん患者群の体温以外の測定項目の詳細も分析した（n=13）。がん患者群の性別・年齢（52.1 ± 8.7歳）を含む詳細を表にまとめた（Table 1）。患者は、測定時、化学療法も放射線治療も受けていない。測定した健常人群は同年齢層である（n=11、46.7 ± 10.0歳）。

Table 1. 進行がんの患者.

症例	がんの種類	性別	年齢
1	慢性骨髄性白血病	F	68
2	卵巣腫瘍	F	56
3	脳腫瘍	M	50
4	胃がん	F	63
5	耳下腺がん	F	48
6	直腸がん、肺転移	M	58
7	子宮頸がん	F	36
8	直腸がん、肺転移	M	45
9	膀胱がん	M	52
10	肺がん	M	48
11	乳がん	F	56
12	悪性リンパ腫	M	42
13	胃がん	M	55

すべての被験者よりインフォームドコンセントを得た。

2.2. 測定項目

測定分析のため静脈採血を行った。血糖測定にはPrecision Xtra TM（アボットジャパン（株），千葉，東京）を用いた。乳酸値、pH、酸素分圧、二酸化炭素分圧測定にはi-STAT 300F（i-STAT Corporation,NJ,USA）を使用した。

静脈血の血液学的解析として、白血球（WBC）総数測定には、血球計算盤とギムザ染色を用いた。ヘモグロビン（Hb）構成物の測定には、ラウリル硫酸ナトリウム-ヘモグロビン（SLS-Hb）法を、それ以外の測定には血球計算版を用いた。

2.3. 統計学的解析

検定には、スチューデントのt検定、マン・ホイットニーのUテスト、ウエルチのt検定を用いた。

3. 結果

3.1. がん患者における低体温と高血糖

初期及び進行がん患者群（28名）体温測定を行ったところ、低体温と高血糖が見られた。同年齢層の健常人群（27名）の体温測定も行った（Figure 1（a））。健常人群（36.6 ± 0.4℃）と比較するとがん患者群は低体温を示し（36.1 ± 0.5℃）、統計的に有意差が見られた（p < 0.01）。

さらに、進行がん患者群（n=13名）と同年齢層の健常人群（n=11名、Figure 1（b））において、さらに詳細に測定項目を分析した。健常人群（36.5 ± 0.3℃）と比較して、進行がん患者群では（35.9 ± 0.5℃）、低体温が認められた。低体温のみならず、高血糖も、健常人群（106.3の ± 11.1mg/dL）と比較するとがん患者群（125.3の ± 28.5mg/dL）で認められた。

ストレス反応により、低体温と高血糖が同時に出現する。そこで、他のストレスに関連するパラメータについても検討した（Figure 1（b））。一部の進行がん患者では、頻脈（交感神経緊張）や乳酸高値の傾向がみられたが、すべての患者に共通ではなかった（p > 0.05、拍数および乳酸値）。

3.2. がん患者における免疫抑制性と貧血

がん患者群と健常人群における免疫学的指標を測定した（Figure 2（a））。白血球（WBC）は、健常人群（6190 ± 1088/μL）に比較して患者群（4691 ± 1769/μL）では低かった（p < 0.05）。白血球分画では、がん患者群の場合、健常人群に比較すると、顆粒球の比率は高いがリンパ球の比率が低かった（p < 0.01）。単球の比率においては、患者群と健常人群の間に差異は見られなかった。白血球数と分画を用いて各サブセットの絶対数を算出した。リンパ球数において、がん患者群と健常人群との間に最も大きな違いが認められた。患者群のリンパ球数（1334 ± 476/μL）は、健常人群（2387の ± 538μ/L）と比較すると有意に低値を示した（p<0.01）。患者群においてリンパ球数が低値である理由は、白血球総数が低いからである。単球の数と比率においては、健常人群とがん患者

Figure.1

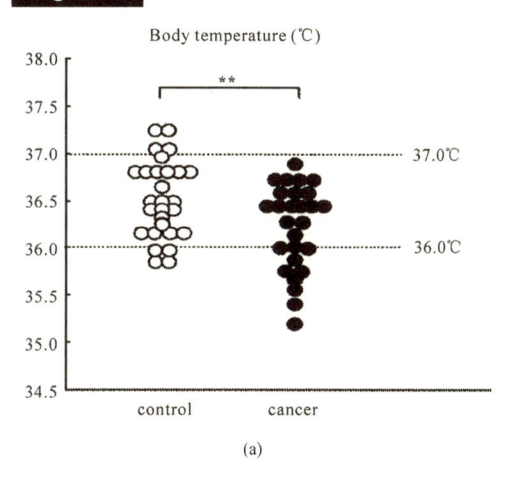

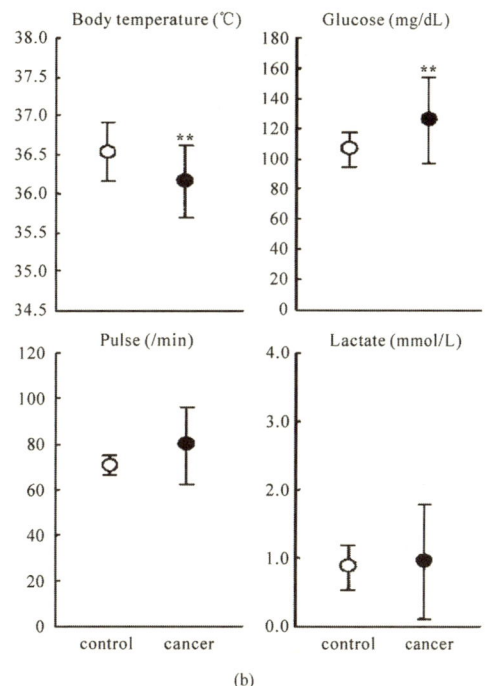

健常人群とがん患者群における体温と諸パラメーターの比較。(a)体温、(b)体温と緒パラメーターの詳細な分析。 実験(a)、健常群(n=27)とがん患者群(n=28)。実験(b)、健常群(n=11)と進行がん(n=13)患者群。体温以外に、血糖値、乳酸値および脈拍数を測定した。体温は、腋窩にて3分間測定を行った(** $p<0.01$)。

Figure.2

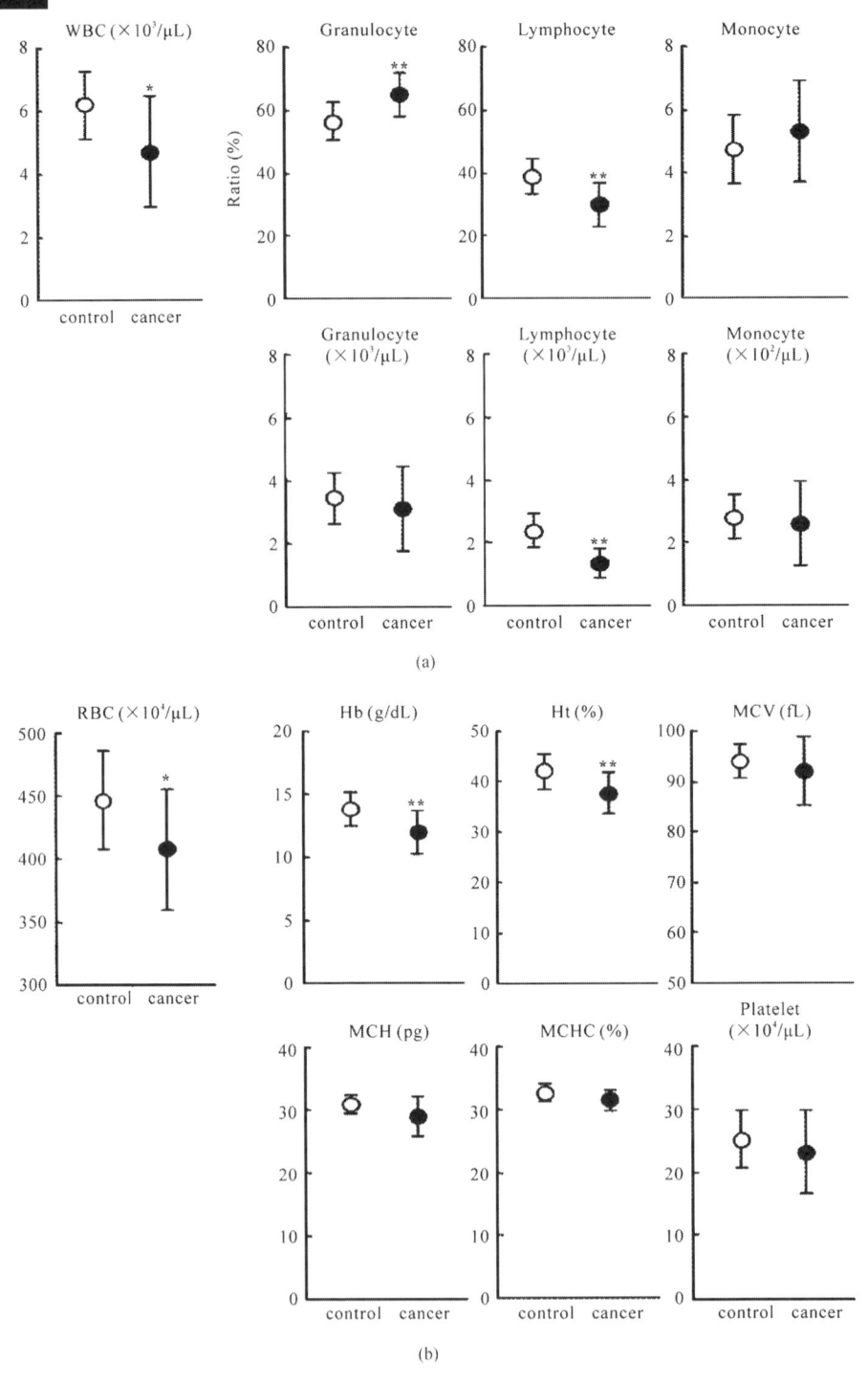

(a)

(b)

血球分析。(a)免疫学的指標、(b)赤血球数とHb値などその他パラメーターの比較の分析。
実験(a)では、それぞれの血球サブセットの絶対数は、白血球総数と白血球分画より算出した。
実験(b)では、赤血球数、Hb値、Ht値、MCV、MCH、MCHCと血小板数を計測した($*p<0.05$、$**p<0.01$)。

群と間で差は認められなかった。

さらに赤血球（RBC）とそれに関連したパラメータについて検討した（Figure 2（b））。白血球総数のみならず赤血球数も、健常人群（$446 ± 39 × 10^4/\mu L$）と比較すると、がん患者群（$407 ± 47 × 10^4/\mu L$）は低値を示した（$p < 0.05$）。Hb値は、健常人群（13.9 ± 1.3g/dL）より患者群（11.9 ± 1.7g/dL）で低値を示した。ヘマトクリット（Ht）値も、健常人群42.0 ± 3.5%）より患者群37.6 ± 4.1%）で低値だった（$p < 0.01$）。赤血球の他のパラメータである赤血球容積（MCV）、平均赤血球ヘモグロビン量（MCH）および平均赤血球ヘモグロビン濃度（MCHC）において、健常人群と患者群との間に、すべて有意差は認められなかった（$p > 0.05$）。同様に、血小板数においても有意差は見られなかった。

3.3. がん患者群における血液ガス分析

進行がん患者群に見られる低体温と貧血が、血液ガス分析のパラメータに影響を及ぼしている可能性がある。そこで、がん患者群の静脈血の解析を行った（Figure 3）。静脈血pHは、患者群（7.36 ± 0.03）は、健常人群（7.40 ± 0.03）より低いことが示された（$p < 0.05$）。血液pHに影響を及ぼす要因には、O_2とCO_2の含有量がある。実際、患者群ではPO_2（mmHg）とSO_2（%）の濃度が、顕著に低値を示した（$p<0.01$、$p<0.05$）。一方、TCO_2（mmol/L）とPCO_2（mmHg）は、患者群で高い傾向があった。BEecf（細胞外液塩基過剰）（mmol/L）は、がん患者群でやや高値であった。

4. 考察

がん患者の多くには、低体温、低酸素および高血糖が同時に見られた。免疫抑制状態としては、顆粒球増加症およびリンパ球減少症を認めた。臨床医は、がん患者が生体に不利な状況

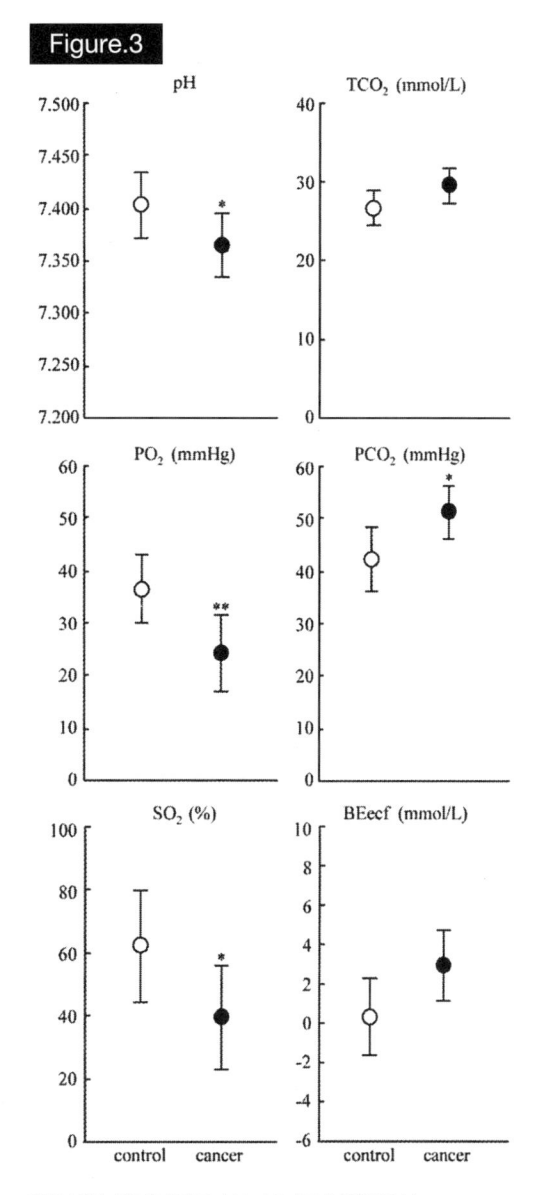

Figure.3

健常人群とがん患者群のpHと血液ガス分析（静脈血）。
(*$p<0.05$、** $p<0.01$)

（低酸素、免疫抑制および貧血）にあることに経験的に気付いているが [13-20]、これらの状況を総合的に研究した医学論文は数少ない。生体がストレス状態にある場合、短期間の低体温、低酸素および高血糖は、危機を脱するのに有益である。しかし、その状態が長期化した場合、この生体の内部環境が発がんを誘発してしまう可能性がある、ということを提言する。こ

Table 2. 2つのエネルギー産生系.

	解糖系	ミトコンドリア系
部位	細胞質	ミトコンドリア
酸素	－もしくは±	＋＋
エネルギー源	ブドウ糖	ピルビン酸（乳酸）ケトン体
体温	低体温（32-36℃）	高体温（＞37℃）
特徴	細胞分裂 瞬発力	細胞分裂の抑制 持続力に使われる
生成の速さ	速い（x 100）	遅い（x 1）
効率	低い（2ATP/グルコース）	高い（36ATP/グルコース）
利用する細胞	精子 がん細胞 再生上皮細胞 骨髄細胞 白筋	心筋 ニューロン 肝細胞 赤筋 その他の各種細胞

Table 3. がん細胞への変化.

	直接的な原因	二次応答	頻度
発がん物質	紫外線 食品添加物 放射線 大気汚染 その他発がん物質	原がん遺伝子または発がん物質による他の遺伝子の突然変異	低い
偏った生き方が原因で生じたストレス	低体温 低酸素 高血糖	原がん遺伝子または「解糖体生命体」への適応として起きた他の遺伝子の突然変異	高い

の考察は、解糖系とミトコンドリア系から構成されるエネルギー産生系［3,4］の知識に基づいたものだ。

約20億年前、解糖系生命体とミトコンドリア系生命体が出会い真核細胞の先祖が発生したと推測されている［21,22］。そして真核細胞は2つのエネルギー生産方法（解糖系とミトコンドリア系）を手に入れた（Table 2）。Table 2のように、2つのエネルギー産生系では、機能、利用方法や特徴は全く異なる。がん患者に見られる内部環境（例えば、低酸素や高血糖などの状態）は、解糖を行うのに都合が良い。

近年、我々はマウスに拘束ストレスを与え、ストレス状況を詳細に分析する研究を行った［1,2］。興味深いことに、ストレス下では低体温と高血糖が起きていることが明らかになった。さらに、カテコラミンや糖櫃コルチコイド投与をすると、すぐさま低体温と高血糖を呈した［2］。短期間ならば、このような低体温や高血糖という内部状態は、解糖系の活性化を通じ白筋繊維は迅速に力を獲得できるので、人間や動物にとって都合がよい［3］。低体温と高血糖は、結果として生体が危機状態に直面した時に、ストレス状態から逃れるために必要な力を産生している。換言すると、低体温や高血糖といった内部状態は、生体が変化に対応するのに失敗したことを意味するのではない。

長期間ストレスにさらされると、低体温や高血糖という内部状態が、ミトコンドリア系を抑制する。ミトコンドリア系は、タンパク質合成のため休みなく力とエネルギーを産生しているのである。従って、ミトコンドリア系が抑制されると、慢性疲労、やせ（衰弱、るいそう）糖尿病をはじめとする疾病が出現する。この概念は、いろいろな病気の発症のメカニズムを理解するのに重要と思われる。

さらに、もう一つ、我々は、低体温、低酸素や高血糖が、発がんと関係している可能性があるという概念を提言する。Table 3に示すように、これまで、研究者や臨床医の間では、発がん物質が、がんを誘発する要因であると信じられてきた。原がん遺伝子が、複数ステップを経て突然変異をした結果、がんが発生すると考えられていたのである。［23-27］。しかし、発がん物質が実際に存在するのは、稀である。長期にわたるストレス由来の内部環境（低酸素と高血糖）が原因で、通常分裂している細胞が、がん細胞（解糖生命体）となる適応反応が出現する。こういった適応反応が出現する場合のストレスは、過労、精神的負荷および肥満といった

生き方の偏りに原因がある可能性がある。発がんの原因は、発がん物質よりも生き方の偏りであると我々は考える。本研究において、がん患者にみられる免疫抑制や貧血は、交感神経緊張によるストレスが原因で出現している可能性が明らかになった［28］。カテコールアミンまたは糖質コルチコイド（視床下部-脳下垂体-副腎系）と白血球サブセット間に相互作用があるという報告がある［29］。

O. Warburgは、がん細胞の細胞質にはミトコンドリアの数が少なく、主に解糖系を利用してエネルギーを産生すると報告した［7］。O. Warburgの見解を裏付ける報告が近年も相次いでいる［30-35］。がん遺伝子は、細胞増殖だけでなく、エネルギー産生系とも関係がある。がん細胞のエネルギー産生が、解糖系優位であるという性質を利用してがん細胞を測定するものが、放射断層撮影法スキャン（PETscan）である［36,37］。エネルギー産生に解糖系を利用する理由は、迅速なエネルギー産生以外にも細胞分裂に必要なエネルギーを得るためである（Table 2）。換言すれば、低体温、低酸素や高血糖とも関連するストレスに対する生体反応は、初期のうちは、アロスタシス（ストレスを克服するための内部環境の変化）と考えられている。しかし、ストレス状態が継続すると、アロスタシス負荷が発生して、適応反応（生体内での「ホメオスタシス」の破綻）として、発がんが起こる。「アロスタシス」の概念は、B.S.McEwen、F.S.Dhabharらが提唱した［38-41］。ストレスの多い生活上の出来事は、アロスタシス負荷と関連するという報告がある［42,43］。

我々は、近年温熱療法装置を利用した研究を行った［44,45］。がん患者にマイルドな温熱療法（最高直腸温38.0℃ 15-30分間）を行ったところ、がんは拡大することなく良好な状況で生存することができた。マイルドな温熱療法で、がんが自然退縮した症例も複数ある［45］。マイルドな温熱療法では、pH、PO_2、PCO_2などの改善がみられた。がん患者にみられる免疫抑制状態や貧血も、軽減された。これらの結果から、がん治療に重要なのは、糖代謝を解糖系からミトコンドリア系（つまり、酸化的リン酸化）へ若干移行させることである可能性が示唆される。局所的で強力な温熱療法（例えば42℃）を行ったところ、がん患者には、効果よりも、むしろ、ひどいストレスが見られた。つまり、がん治療に重要なのは、全身的に内部環境を改善することなのである。だからといって、患者に温熱療法のために、高価な機器の使用を勧める必要はない。がん自然後退のためには、次に挙げる事柄が、最も重要である：就寝時に湯たんぽを使用する、体に良くない生き方（例えば、働きすぎ）を改善する、一日に複数回、深呼吸を行う、食事を見直す、くよくよするのをやめる。

我々は、ここに、以下のことを提言する。ストレス状態は、短期間の危機状態を逃れるには有益である。しかし、ストレス状態の結果として生じる低体温や高血糖は、がん細胞の発生を引き起こす要因となる。換言すると、発がんを「20億年前の解糖生命体」への先祖返りと考えることも可能である。がん細胞の細胞質内のミトコンドリアはごく僅かである。しかし、がん細胞の成長に、ミトコンドリアの機能を無視することはできない［46,47］。J.S. Fang, R.J. GilliesそしてR.A. Gatenは、発がんが進行するのは、低酸素とアシドーシスへの適応反応であり、周辺組織内で、がん細胞と微小環境の間には相互作用が見られるという仮説を提唱している［48,49］。その時、上皮細胞と支持細胞の間のパラクリン（傍分泌）伝達シグナルは、発がんとがんの進行にとって重要であることが知られている［50］。本研究では、実際に、がん患

者には、低酸素、アシドーシスといった全身的な影響が内部環境に起きていることを明らかにすることができた。しかしながら、この概念を裏付けるためには、更なる研究が必要である。現在、低体温、低酸素および高血糖の状況下において、担がんマウスの動物実験やがん細胞培養実験などを行い、研究を継続している。

5. 謝辞

本研究は、文部科学省の科学研究費の支援を受けた。金子裕子氏には原稿浄書、橋本大旗氏と山本香織氏（湯島清水坂クリニック）には臨床研究準備に対して深謝する。

Internal environment in cancer patients and proposal that carcinogenesis is adaptive response of glycolysis to overcome adverse internal conditions

Mayumi Watanabe[1], Kenya Miyajima[2], Ittoku Matsui[2], Chikako Tomiyama-Miyaji[3], Eisuke Kainuma[1], Masashi Inoue[1], Hiroaki Matsumoto[1], Yuh Kuwano[1], Toru Abo[1]*

[1]Department of Immunology, Niigata University School of Medicine, Niigata, Japan;
*Corresponding Author: immunol2@med.niigata-u.ac.jp
[2]Yushima-Shimizuzaka Clinic, Tokyo, Japan
[3]School of Health Sciences, Faculty of Medicine, Niigata University, Niigata, Japan

Received 4 March 2010; revised 16 March 2010; accepted 20 March 2010.

ABSTRACT

In a series of our recent studies, stress was found to induce simultaneously hypothermia and hyperglycemia. These conditions are beneficial to obtain prompt force which depends on the glycolysis pathway and to escape emergency. Since we have noticed that such conditions resemble the internal environment seen in some cancer patients, it was investigated whether such conditions were accompanied with other patients. We selected patients with early and advanced cancer. Body temperature and other parameters including blood gas contents were examined. A difference was seen in body temperature, namely, many patients showed hypothermia, irrespective of cancer stages. Further characterization of other parameters showed that hypothermia and hyperglycemia existed in many patients. They had immunosuppressive state and anemia. Blood gas analysis showed that oxygen contents were low and carbon dioxide contents were high in patients. These results suggest a possibility that the internal environment seen in patients is responsible to induce onset of disease and to maintain their cell growth, because cancer cells have an energy system of predominant glycolysis. Although hypothermia, hypoxia and hyperglycemia are important to activate the glycolysis pathway and to escape from emergency, such responses suppress the mitochondrial pathway for long span and may result in carcinogenesis.

Keywords: Cancer; Hypothermia; Hypoxia; Hyperglycemia; Glycolysis; Mitochondria

1. INTRODUCTION

Many investigators and clinicians have felt that cancer might be a systemic disease although tumor masses are primarily present at local sites. If this is the case, we have to consider specific, common internal environment in cancer patients. In the course of the analysis of many parameters in cancer patients, we noticed that many cancer patients showed simultaneous hypothermia and hyperglycemia.

In light of these findings, we then investigated the internal environment in relation to stress-associated responses [1,2]. Of interest was that both hypothermia and hyperglycemia were induced by stress. Such an internal environment might be beneficial for humans and animals to escape emergencies [3]. Namely, prompt output of force by white muscle fibers depends on the energy production system of glycolysis. Although the efficiency of energy production is low (2 ATP/glucose) in the glycolysis pathway, the ATP synthesis in this system is much quicker ($\times$ 100) than that of the mitochondrial system ($\times$ 1) [4].

In a short span of time, hypothermia and hyperglycemia are therefore good conditions for escape from stress or emergencies. However, these conditions are not appropriate for energy production of the mitochondrial pathway (i.e., oxidative phosphorylation). Many patients with hypothermia and hyperglycemia suffer from general fatigue, emaciated conditions, diabetic disease, etc.

In the present study, we investigated the internal environment in cancer patients in detail and herein propose on adaptation theory, namely, that the onset of cancer is a phenomenon of a glycolytic adaptation response by living beings to overcome deteriorated internal conditions in the body. Cumulative evidence has shown that cancer cells have a shift of glucose metabolism from oxidative phosphorylation to glycolysis, eventually resulting in few or defective mitochondria in the cytoplasm [5-7]. Although many investigators have considered that carcinogens such as ultraviolet rays, food additives, air pollution, etc. [8-12], induce multiple mutation steps in proto-oncogenes, there is an alternative possibility that such mutation is a process of glycolytic adaptation by living beings, namely, cancer cells. Hypothermia, hypoxia and hyperglycemia, which are induced by continuous stress (due to the lifestyle in patients), might be important factors which induce the adaptive response.

2. MATERIALS AND METHODS

2.1. Subjects

Patients with early or advanced cancer were first examined as to body temperature (n = 28). They were 54.3 ± 8.0 years old. Age-matched healthy controls (n = 27), 45.8 ± 11.0 years of age, were also examined.

For detailed analysis of many parameters other than body temperature, patients with advanced cancer (n = 13) were then selected (**Table 1**). Details of the cancer patients are listed in the table, including sex and age (52.1 ± 8.7 years old). At the time of analysis, these patients were receiving neither chemotherapy nor irradiation therapy. Age-matched healthy controls (n = 11), 46.7 ± 10.0 of age, were also examined.

Table 1. Patients with Advanced Cancer.

Case	Type of Cancer	Sex	Age
1	chronic myelogenic leukemia	F	68
2	ovarian cancer	F	56
3	brain cancer	M	50
4	stomach cancer	F	63
5	parotid gland cance	F	48
6	rectum cancer, metastasis to lung	M	58
7	uterus cervical cancer	F	36
8	rectum cancer, metastasis to lung	M	45
9	bladder cancer	M	52
10	lung cancer	M	48
11	breast cancer	F	56
12	malignant lymphoma	M	42
13	stomach cancer	M	55

Informed consent was obtained from all subjects.

2.2. Parameters Tested

Blood for the analysis was obtained from a vein. Blood glucose was measured by Precision Xtra TM (Abott Japan Co., Ltd., Chiba, Japan). Venous blood analysis of lactate and of the levels of pH, O_2 and CO_2 was also performed using i-STAT 300F (i-STAT Corporation, NJ, USA).

To analyze the hematological parameters, leukocyte counts of fresh venous blood were determined by hemocytemeter and were stained by the Giemsa method. The contents of hemoglobin (Hb) and others in the blood were measured by Sodium Lauryl Sulfate (SLS)-Hb methods and hematocytemeter, respectively.

2.3. Statistical Analysis

The difference between the values was determined by Student's t-test, Mann-Whitney's U test and Welch's t-test.

3. RESULTS

3.1. Hypothermia and Hyperglycemia Seen in Cancer Patients

Twenty-eight patients with early or advanced cancer and twenty-seven healthy subjects were examined as to body temperature (**Figure 1(a)**). It was found that there were many persons with hypothermia (36.1 ± 0.5°C) among cancer patients in comparison with healthy persons (36.6 ± 0.4°C), the difference being statistically significant ($p < 0.01$).

We then analyzed many parameters in patients with advanced cancer (n = 13) and age-matched controls (n = 11) (**Figure 1(b)**). Hypothermia was confirmed in these patients with advanced cancer (35.9 ± 0.5°C) in comparison with controls (36.5 ± 0.3°C). In addition to hypothermia, hyperglycemia was also detected in cancer patients (125.3 ± 28.5 mg/dL) in comparison with controls (106.3 ± 11.1 mg/dL).

Since stress-associated responses simultaneously induce hypothermia and hyperglycemia, other stress-associated parameters were also examined in this experiment (**Figure 1(b)**, bottom). Although there was a tendency that some patients with advanced cancer had a high pulse rate (sympathetic nerve activation) and a high level of lactate, these were not common to all patients ($p > 0.05$ in both pulse and lactate).

3.2. Immunosuppressive States and Anemia in Cancer Patients

Immunoparameters were examined in cancer patients and

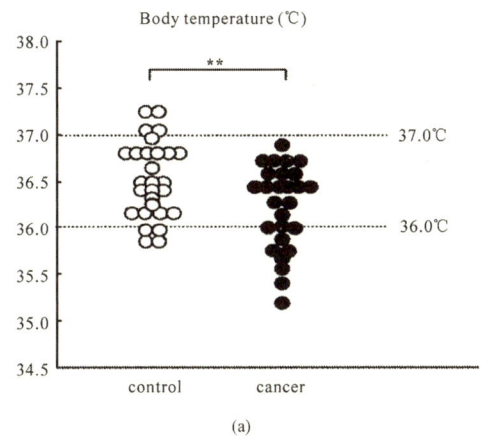

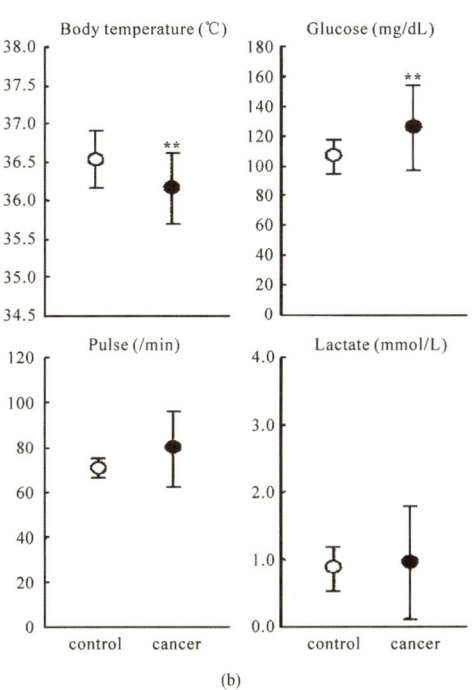

Figure 1. (a) Comparison of body temperature and other parameters between healthy controls and cancer patients. (a). Body temperature, (b). Further analysis of body temperature and others. In experiment (a), healthy controls (n = 27) and cancer patients (n = 28) were examined. In experiment (b), healthy controls (n = 11) and patients with advanced cancer (n = 13) were examined. In addition to body temperature, the levels of glucose and lactate and the pulse rate were examined in this experiment. Body temperature was measured in the axilla for 3 min. ** $p < 0.01$.

healthy controls (**Figure 2(a)**). The total number of white blood cells (WBC) was lower in patients (4691 ± 1769 /μL) than in controls (6190 ± 1088 /μL) ($p < 0.05$). When the ratio of WBC (leukocyte) subsets was enumerated, the ratio of granulocytes was found to be high, while that of lymphocytes was low ($p < 0.01$). The ratio of monocytes was comparable in patients and controls. By calculation, the absolute number of leukocyte subsets was determined. It was found that the most prominent distinction was in lymphocytes, namely, the number of lymphocytes in patients (1334 ± 476 /μL) was extremely low in comparison with the number in controls (2387 ± 538 /μL) ($p < 0.01$). The decrease in the number of leukocytes seen in patients was found to be due to the decrease in the number of lymphocytes. The ratio and number of monocytes were comparable in controls and cancer patients.

The level of red blood cells (RBC) and related parameters was then examined (**Figure 2(b)**). In addition to the decrease in the number of WBC, the number of RBC was found to decrease in cancer patients (407 ± 47 × 10^4/μL) in comparison with controls (446 ± 39× 10^4/μL) ($p < 0.05$). The level of Hb was lower in patients (11.9 ± 1.7 g/dL) than in controls (13.9 ± 1.3 g/dL). The level of hematocrit (Ht) was also lower in patients (37.6 ± 4.1%) than in controls (42.0 ± 3.5%) ($p < 0.01$). Other parameters of RBC, namely, mean red cell volume (MCV), mean corpuscular hemoglobin (MCH) and mean corpuscular hemoglobin concentration (MCHC) were all comparable between controls and patients ($p > 0.05$). This was also the case for the number of platelets.

3.3. Blood Gas Analysis in Cancer Patients

It is conceivable that hypothermia and anemia seen in patients with advanced cancer may influence the parameters as shown by blood gas analysis. Therefore, such analysis using venous blood was conducted (**Figure 3**). It was demonstrated that blood pH was lower in patients (7.36 ± 0.03) than in controls (7.40 ± 0.03) ($p < 0.05$). The major factors influencing blood pH are known to be the levels of O_2 and CO_2 contents. Indeed, the levels of PO_2 (mmHg) and SO_2 (%) were found to be extremely low in patients ($p < 0.01$, $p < 0.05$, respectively). On the other hand, the levels TCO_2 (mmol/L) and PCO_2 (mmHg) tended to be high in patients. BEecf (mmol/L), which shows a base excess in extracellular fluids, was slightly high in cancer patients.

4. DISCUSSION

We herein demonstrated that many cancer patients had hypothermia, hypoxia and hyperglycemia simultaneously. Immunosuppressive states, showing granulocytosis and

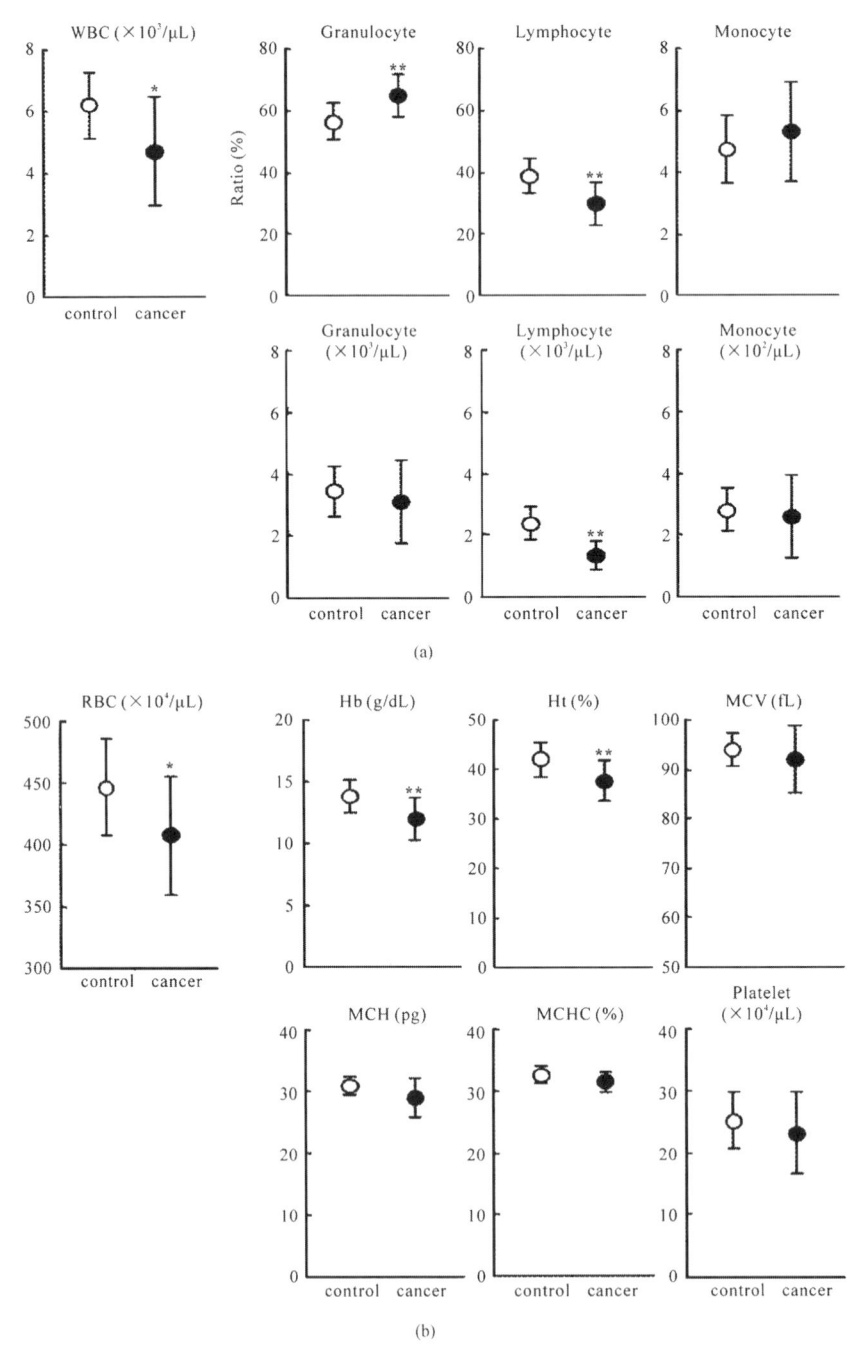

Figure 2. Blood cell analysis. (a) Immunoparameters. (b) Analysis of the number of RBC and the levels of Hb and other parameters. In experiment (a), the absolute number of leukocyte subsets was calculated from the data on the number of WBC and the ratio of leukocyte subsets. In experiment (b), Number of RBC and levels of Hb, Ht, MCV, MCH and MCHC, including the number of platelets, were examined * $p < 0.05$, ** $p < 0.01$.

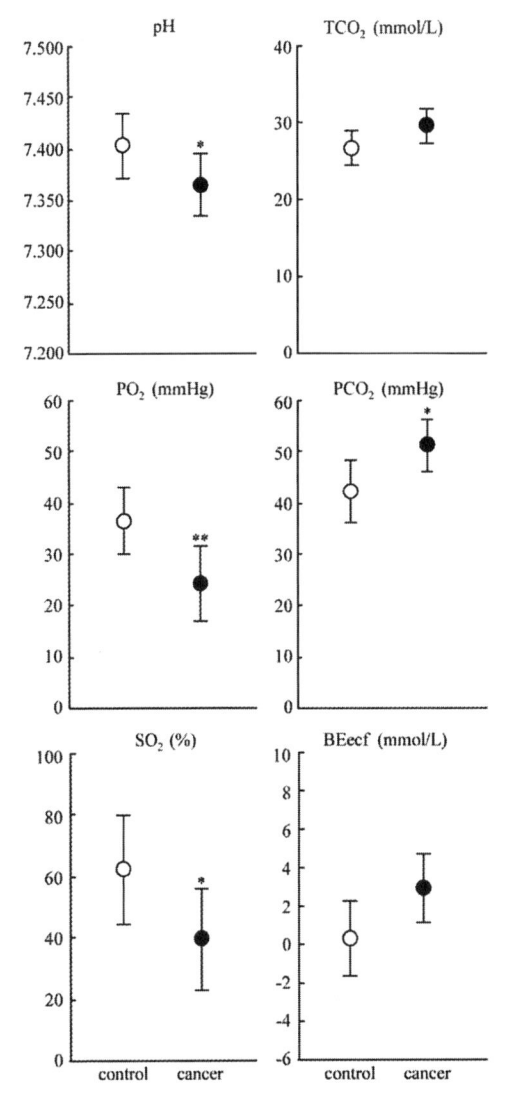

Figure 3. pH and blood gas analysis in healthy controls and cancer patients. Venous blood was used for the analysis. * $p < 0.05$, ** $p < 0.01$.

lymphocytopenia, were also present. Although clinicians are empirically aware of the deteriorated conditions such as hypoxia, immunosuppression and anemia in cancer patients [13-20], as shown by a review of the literature, few studies have been done on the simultaneous identification of all these conditions. We propose the possibility that hypothermia, hypoxia and hyperglycemia are beneficial for stress-exposed persons to escape from emergencies inducing stress for short periods of time, but that such internal environment might become cancer-inducing over a longer period of time. This proposal is based on an understanding of the energy production system comprising the glycolysis and mitochondria pathways [3,4].

It has been speculated that the ancestors of eukaryocytes were generated by a connection between living beings with glycolysis and those with mitochondria at approximately 2 billion years ago [21,22]. Under such situation, eukaryocytes had two energy production methods, namely, the glycolysis and mitochondria pathways (**Table 2**). As shown in this table, the functioning conditions, usage and other characteristics between two pathways are quite different. If we consider the internal environment (*i.e.*, hypoxia and hyperglycemia) seen in cancer patients, these conditions are rather appropriate for the function of glycolysis.

In a recent study, we analyzed in detail the stress-associated conditions in mice exposed to restraint stress [1,2]. Of interest was that such conditions were revealed to be hypothermia and hyperglycemia. In addition, the administration of catecholamines or glycocorticoids also directly induced hypothermia and hyperglycemia [2]. In a short span of time, such internal conditions are beneficial for humans and animals to obtain the prompt force of white muscle fibers via activation of the glycolysis

Table 2. Energy production system.

	Glycolysis Pathway	Mitochondrial Pathway
Site	cytoplasm	mitochondria
Oxgen	- or ±	++
Source	glucose	pyruvic acid (lactate)
		ketone bodies
Temperature	32-36 ℃	> 37 ℃
Usage	cell division	suppression of cell division
	prompt force	continuous force
ATP production	quick (× 100)	slow (× 1)
Efficiency	low (2ATP/glucose)	high (36ATP/glucose)
Cells	sperms	cardiac muscle cells
	cancer cells	neurons
	skin cells	hepatocytes
	bone marrow cells	red muscle cells
	white muscle cells	many other cells

pathway [3]. As a result, such conditions realize the power needed to escape from stressful conditions such as those in emergencies. In other words, the internal conditions of hypothermia and hyperglycemia do not seem to be a failure of our body responses.

If a certain person is exposed to stress for a long time, the internal conditions of hypothermia and hyperglycemia then suppress the mitochondria pathway which produces continuous force and energy for protein synthesis. Such a person might be suffering from general fatigue, emaciated conditions, diabetic disease and other difficulties. This notion seems to be important for understanding the mechanisms involved in the onset of many diseases.

In addition, we propose another possibility of hypothermia, hypoxia and hyperglycemia which may be associated with the onset of malignancy. As shown in **Table 3**, many investigators and clinicians have believed that carcinogens are key factors which induce cancer via the multiple mutation steps of proto-oncogenes [23-27]. However, such carcinogens do not seem to be always present in actual cases. Given this fact, such cases may be rather rare. We propose herein the possibility that the internal environment (*i.e.*, hypoxia and hyperglycemia) induced by continuous stress results in an adaptation response in which normally dividing cells become cancer cells (*i.e.*, living beings with glycolysis). In such cases, stress may be caused by overwork, mental stress, obesity, etc., namely, their lifestyle. We consider that these cases are of higher frequency than those due to carcinogens in carcinogenesis. Immunosuppression and anemia in cancer patients as revealed in the present study might result from such stress via the activation of sympathetic nerves [28]. Interaction of leukocyte subsets with catecholamines or glucocorticoids (hypothalamic-pituitary-adrenal axis) was reported previously [29].

Table 3. Transformation to Cancer Cells.

	Direct Cause	Secondary Response	Frequency
Carcinogens	ultraviolet	mutation of proto-oncogenes or other genes by carcinogens	Less
	food additives		
	radiation		
	air pollution		
	other carcinogens		
Stress from lifestyle	hypothermia	mutation of proto-oncogenes or other genes as adaptation to "living beings of glycolysis"	High
	hypoxia		
	hyperglycemia		

O. Warburg has reported that cancer cells contained a few mitochondria in the cytoplasma and produce energy mainly by the glycolysis pathway [7]. Recent cumulative evidence also supports this earlier observation [30-35]. The functions of oncogenes are eventually related to not only the system of cell-proliferation but also to the system of energy production. The nature of the predominant function of glycolysis in cancer cells is utilized by PET scans [36,37]. The energy produced by glycolysis is used not only to obtain prompt elicitation but also for cell dividing energy (see **Table 2** again). In other words, the initial stress-associated response of hypothermia, hypoxia and hyperglycemia is estimated as allostasis (*i.e.*, change of the internal environment to overcome stress). However, continuous stress then turns to allostatic load and induces the carcinogenesis as adaptation responses (*i.e.*, break of "homeostasis" in our body). These concepts on "allostasis" were proposed by B. S. McEwen, F. S. Dhabhar and their colleagues [38-41]. Stressful life events were reported to be related to such allostatic load [42,43].

In our recent study using hyperthermia equipment [44, 45], many cancer patients could live in good conditions without further tumor enlargement when they exposed to mild hyperthermia (*i.e.*, the maximum rectum temperature is 38.0°C for 15-30 min). In some cases, tumor regression resulted from mild hyperthermia [45]. At this time, the values of pH, PO_2, PCO_2 and other factors improved. Immunosuppression and anemia seen in cancer patients were also alleviated. These results suggest that a slight shift of glucose metabolism from the glycolysis pathway to the mitochondria pathway (*i.e.*, oxidative phosphorylation) might be important to cure malignancy. Local, strong hyperthermia (e.g., 42°C) was not effective and rather acted as severe stress in cancer patients. In other words, systemic improvement of the internal environment is critical to cure malignancies. However, we do not recommend patients to use expensive equipment for hyperthermia. The most important things for spontaneous regression of cancer are as follow: changing harmful lifestyle (e.g., overwork), using hot-water bottle at sleeping time, taking a deep breath several times a day, dietary consideration and control of the fear.

We have herein proposed the possibility that stress-associated conditions are beneficial for humans to escape from emergencies in a short span of time, but that the resulting hypothermia and hyperglycemia act as factors which induce the generation of cancer cells. In other words, the onset of malignancy might be a return to "living beings with glycolysis at 2 billion years ago". Cancer cells eventually contain only a few mitochondria in the cytoplasm. However, we could not neglect a mitochondrial function in tumor cell growth [46,47].

A hypothesis by J. S. Fang, R. J. Gillies and R. A. Gaten was proposed that evolution of carcinogenesis is an adaptation response to hypoxia and acidosis, showing the interaction of cancer cells and microenvironments in the surrounding tissues [48,49]. At that time, a paracrine signaling between epithelial and stromal cells is known to be important for tumor initiation and progression [50]. We were also able to reveal the systemic, internal environment of hypoxia, acidosis and other conditions in actual cancer patients. However, a further research is required to support our proposal definitely. Such research includes an animal experiment using mice with cancer and a cancer cell culture experiment under conditions of hypothermia, hypoxia and hyperglycemia

5. ACKNOWLEDGEMENTS

This work was supported by a Grant-in-Aid for Scientific Research from the Ministry of Education, Science and Culture, Japan. The authors thank Mrs Yuko Kaneko for preparation of the manuscript and Mr Taiki Hashimoto and Ms Kaori Yamamoto (Yushima-Shimizuzaka clinic) for arrangement of the clinical research.

REFERENCES

[1] Watanabe, M., Tomiyama-Miyaji, C., Kainuma, E., et al. (2008) Role of-adrenergic stimulus in stress-induced modulation of body temperature, blood glucose and innate immunity. *Immunology Letters*, **115(1)**, 43-49.

[2] Kainuma, E., Watanabe, M., Tomiyama-Miyaji, C., et al. (2009) Association of glucocorticoid with stress-induced modulation of body temperature, blood glucose and innate immunity. *Psychoneuroendocrinology*, **34(10)**, 1459-1468.

[3] Kainuma, E., Watanabe, M., Tomiyama-Miyaji, C., et al. (2009) Proposal of alternative mechanism responsible for the function of high-speed swimsuits. *Biomedical Research*, **30(1)**, 69-70.

[4] Voet, D. and Voet, J.G. (2004) Glycolysis. In: D. Voet, J.G. Voet, Eds., Biochemistry, 3rd Edition, J. Wiley & Sons, New York, pp. 607-647.

[5] Dang, C.V. and Semenza, G.L. (1999) Oncogenic alterations of metabolism. *Trends in Biochemical Science*, **24(2)**, 68-72.

[6] Shaw, R.J. (2006) Glucose metabolism and cancer. *Current Opinion in Cell Biology*, **18(6)**, 598-608.

[7] Warburg, O. (1956) On the origin of cancer cells. *Science*, **123(3191)**, 309-314.

[8] Nijjar, T., Bassett, E., Garbe, J., et al. (2005) Accumulation and altered localization of telomere-associated protein TRF2 in immortally transformed and tumor-derived human breast cells. *Oncogene*, **24(20)**, 3369-3376.

[9] Rhiemeier, V., Breitenbach, U., Richter, K.H., et al. (2006) A novel aspartic proteinase-like gene expressed in stratified epithelia and squamous cell carcinoma of the skin. *American Journal of Pathology*, **168(4)**, 1354-1364.

[10] Arora, A., Kalra, N., Shukla, Y. (2006) Regulation of p21/ras protein expression by diallyl sulfide in DMBA induced neoplastic changes in mouse skin. *Cancer Letters*, **242(1)**, 28-36.

[11] Ikuta, S., Edamatsu, H., Li, M., Hu, L. and Kataoka, T. (2008) Crucial role of phospholipase C epsilon in skin inflammation induced by tumor-promoting phorbol ester. *Cancer Research*, **68(1)**, 64-72.

[12] Rountree, C.B., Senadheera, S., Mato, J.M., Crooks, G.M. and Lu, S.C. (2008) Expansion of liver cancer stem cells during aging in methionine adenosyltransferase 1A-deficient mice. *Hepatology*, **47(4)**, 1288-1297.

[13] Koksal, Y., Caliskan, U. and Unal, E. (2009) Hypothermia in a child with Hodgkin disease. *Journal of Pediatric Hematology Oncology*, **31(2)**, 136-138.

[14] Nduka, C.C., Puttick, M., Coates, P., Yong, L., Peck, D. and Darzi, A. (2002) Intraperitoneal hypothermia during surgery enhances postoperative tumor growth. *Surgical Endoscopy*, **16(4)**, 611-615.

[15] Cortesi, E., Gascón, P., Henry, D., et al. (2005) Standard of care for cancer-related anemia: improving hemoglobin levels and quality of life. *Oncology*, **68(Suppl 1)**, 22-32.

[16] Heras, P., Argyriou, A.A., Papapetropoulos, S., Karagiannis, S., Argyriou, K. and Mitsibounas, D. (2005) The impact of weekly dosing of epoetin alfa on the haematological parameters and on the quality of life of anemic cancer patients. *European Journal of Cancer Care*, **14(2)**, 108-112.

[17] Mock, V. and Olsen, M. (2003) Current management of fatigue and anemia in patients with cancer. *Seminars in Oncology Nursing*, **19(4 Suppl 2)**, 36-41.

[18] Fairclough, D.L., Gagnon, D.D., Zagari, M.J., Marschner, N. and Dicato, M. (2003) Evaluation of quality of life in a clinical trial with nonrandom dropout: The effect of epoetin alfa in anemic cancer patients. *Quality of Life Research*, **12(8)**, 1013-1027.

[19] Tchekmedyian, N.S. (2002) Anemia in cancer patients: significance, epidemiology, and current therapy. *Oncology*, **16(9 Suppl 10)**, 17-24.

[20] Ishiko, O., Sugawa, T., Tatsuta, I., et al. (1987) Anemia-inducing substance (AIS) in advanced cancer: inhibitory effect of AIS on the function of erythrocytes and immunocompetent cells. *Japanese Journal of Cancer Research*, **78(6)**, 596-606.

[21] Sagan, L. (1967) On the origin of mitosing cells. *Journal of Theoretical Biology*, **14(3)**, 255-274.

[22] Margulis, L. and Stolz, J.F. (1984) Cell symbiosis [correction of symbiosis] theory: status and implications for the fossil record. *Advances in Space Research*, **4(12)**, 195-201.

[23] Osinsky, S., Zavelevich, M. and Vaupel, P. (2009) Tumor hypoxia and malignant progression. *Experimental Oncology*, **31(2)**, 80-86.

[24] Denko, N.C. (2008) Hypoxia, HIF1 and glucose metabolism in the solid tumour. *Nature Reviews Cancer*, **8(9)**, 705-713.

[25] Susnow, N., Zeng, L., Margineantu, D. and Hockenbery, D.M. (2009) Bcl-2 family proteins as regulators of oxidative stress. *Seminars in Cancer Biology*, **19(1)**, 42-49.

[26] Moreno-Sánchez, R., Rodríguez-Enríquez, S., Saavedra, E., Marín-Hernández, A. and Gallardo-Pérez, J.C. (2009) The bioenergetics of cancer: Is glycolysis the main ATP supplier in all tumor cells? *Biofactors*, **35(2)**, 209-225.

[27] Vousden, K.H. and Ryan, K.M. (2009) P53 and metabolism. *Nature Reviews Cancer*, **9(10)**, 691-700.

[28] Abo, T. and Kawamura, T. (2002) Immunomodulation by the autonomic nervous system: Therapeutic approach for cancer, collagen diseases, and inflammatory bowel diseases. *Therapeutic Apheresis*, **6(5)**, 348-357.

[29] Sagiyama, K., Tsuchida, M., Kawamura, H., *et al.* (2004) Age-related bias in function of natural killer T cells and granulocytes after stress: Reciprocal association of steroid hormones and sympathetic nerves. *Clinical and Experimental Immunology*, **135(1)**, 56-63.

[30] Weinberg, R.A. (2007) The Biology of Cancer. 1st Edition, Garland Science, New York.

[31] Kondoh, H. (2008) Cellular life span and the Warburg effect. *Experimental Cell Research*, **314(9)**, 1923-1928.

[32] Nijsten, M.W.N. and van Dam, G.M. (2009) Hypothesis: Using the Warburg effect against cancer by reducing glucose and providing lactate. *Medical Hypotheses*, **73(1)**, 48-51.

[33] Heiden, M.G.V., Cantley, L.C. and Thompson, C.B. (2009) Understanding the Warburg effect: The metabolic requirements of cell proliferation. *Science*, **324(5930)**, 1029-1033.

[34] Máximo, V., Lima, J., Soares, P. and Sobrinho-Simões, M. (2009) Mitochondria and cancer. *Virchows Arch*, **454(5)**, 481-495.

[35] Lee, H.-C. and Wei, Y.-H. (2009) Mitochondrial DNA instability and metabolic shift in human cancers. *International Journal of Molecular Sciences*, **10(2)**, 674-701.

[36] Gambhir, S.S. (2002) Molecular imaging of cancer with positron emission tomography. *Nature Reviews Cancer*, **2(9)**, 683-693.

[37] Vesselle, H., Schmidt, R.A., Pugsley, J.M., *et al.* (2000) Lung cancer proliferation correlates with [F-18] fluorodeoxyglucose uptake by positron emission tomography. *Clinical Cancer Research*, **6(10)**, 3837-3844.

[38] McEwen, B.S. (2000) Allostasis and allostatic load: Implications for neuropsychopharmacology. *Neuropsychopharmacology*, **22(2)**, 108-124.

[39] McEwen, B.S. (2004) Protection and damage from acute and chronic stress, allostasis and allostatic overload and relevance to the pathophysiology of psychiatric disorders. *Annals of the New York Academy of Sciences*, **1032(1)**, 1-7.

[40] Sephton, S.E., Dhabhar, F.S., Keuroghlian, A.S., *et al.* (2009) Depression, cortisol, and suppressd cell-mediated immunity in metastatic breast cancer. *Brain Behavior and Immunity*, **23(8)**, 1148-1155.

[41] Du, J., Wang, Y., Hunter, R., *et al.* (2009) Dynamic regulation of mitochondrial function by glucocorticoids. *Proceedings of the National Academy of Sciences of the United States of America*, **106(9)**, 3543-3548.

[42] Bellingrath, S., Weigl, T. and Kudielka, B.M. (2009) Chronic work stress and exhaustion is associated with higher allostastic load in female school teachers. *Stress*, **12(1)**, 37-48.

[43] Alexander, J.L., Dennerstein, L., Woods, N.F., *et al.* (2007) Role of stressful life events and menopausal stage in wellbeing and health. *Expert Review of Neurotherapeutics*, **7(11 Suppl)**, 93-113.

[44] Tomiyama-Miyaji, C., Watanabe, M., Ohishi, T., *et al.* (2007) Modulation of the endocrine and immune systems by well-controlled hyperthermia equipment. *Biomedical Research*, **28(3)**, 119-125.

[45] Ohishi, T., Nukuzuma, C., Seki, A., *et al.* (2009) Alkalization of blood pH is responsible for survival of cancer patients by mild hyperthermia. *Biomedical Research*, **30(2)**, 95-100.

[46] Deberardinis, R.J., Sayed, N., Ditsworth, D., Thompson, C.B. (2008) Brick by brick: Metabolism and tumor cell growth. *Current Opinion in Genetics and Development*, **18(1)**, 54-61.

[47] Frezza, C. and Gottlieb, E. (2009) Mitochondria in cancer: not just innocent bystanders. *Seminars in Cancer Biology*, **19(1)**, 4-11.

[48] Gillies, R.J. and Gatenby, R.A. (2007) Hypoxia and adaptive landscapes in the evolution of carcinogenesis. *Cancer and Metastasis Reviews*, **26(2)**, 311-317.

[49] Fang, J.S., Gillies, R.D. and Gatenby, R.A. (2008) Adaptation to hypoxia and acidosis in carcinogenesis and tumor progression. *Seminars in Cancer Biology*, **18(5)**, 330-337.

[50] Hu, M. and Polyak, K. (2008) Microenvironmental regulation of cancer development. *Current Opinion in Genetics and Development*, **18(1)**, 27-34.

【著者紹介】

安保　徹
（あぼ　とおる）

新潟大学大学院医歯学総合研究科、国際感染医学講座、免疫学・医動物学分野　教授

［略歴］
- S 35年3月　三厩村立三厩小学校卒業
- S 38年3月　青森市立第一中学校卒業
- S 41年3月　青森県立青森高校卒業
- S 47年3月　東北大学医学部卒業
- S 47年4月　青森県立中央病院　内科研修
- S 49年4月　東北大学歯学部微生物学　助手
- S 54年9月　アメリカ合衆国アラバマ大学留学（5年間）
- S 59年4月　東北大学歯学部微生物学　助手に復職（その後、講師）
- H 3年1月　新潟大学医学部医動物学講座　教授

［主な業績］
- 1980年　ヒトNK細胞抗原CD57に対するモノクローナル抗体（Leu-7）の作製
- 1990年　胸腺外分化T細胞の発見
- 1996年　白血球の自律神経支配の解明
- 1997年　新生児顆粒球増多は肺呼吸開始後の酸素ストレスによって起こる
- 2001年　マラリア感染の防御は胸腺外分化T細胞によって行われる
- 2010年　発ガンは20億年前の解糖系生命体への先祖返り

［所属した学会］
日本免疫学会、日本生体防御学会、日本寄生虫学会、AAI（American Association of Immunologist）

受賞歴
- 1998年　新潟日報文化賞

安保徹の原著論文を読む
膠原病、炎症性腸疾患、がんの発症メカニズムの解明

2013年2月16日　初版第1刷発行

著　者　安保　徹
©2013 T.Abo

発行者　高橋　考

発　行　三和書籍 Sanwa co.,Ltd.

〒112-0013　東京都文京区音羽2-2-2
TEL 03-5395-4630　FAX 03-5395-4632
郵便振替 00180-3-38459
info@sanwa-co.com
http://www.sanwa-co.com/

印刷／製本　日本ハイコム株式会社

乱丁、落丁本はお取替えいたします。定価はカバーに表示しています。
本書の一部または全部を無断で複写、複製転載することを禁じます。
ISBN978-4-86251-147-8 C3047 Printed in Japan

※電子版は「ブックパブ」で購入できます。

三和書籍の好評図書

安保教授の20年にわたる新潟大学での講義録!

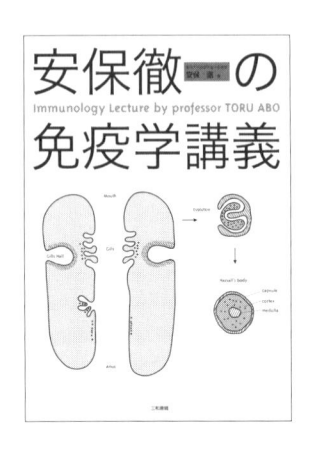

安保徹の免疫学講義
Immunology Lecture by professor TORU ABO

新潟大学教授
安保 徹 著　B5／並製／245ページ／本体6,500円+税

多くの病気はストレスを受けて免疫抑制状態になって発症するが、ストレスをもっとも早く感知するのは免疫系である。末梢血のリンパ球比率やリンパ球総数は敏感にストレスに反応している。しかし、ストレスとリンパ球数の相関を教育現場で学ぶことは少ない。本書は、リンパ球数／顆粒球数が多くの病気の発症メカニズムに関わっていることを詳細に説明するとともに、消炎鎮痛剤の害やそのほかの薬剤の副作用についても解説している。特に自己免疫疾患の治療においては、本書の知識が大いに役立つはずである。

Contents

まえがき／第1章　免疫学総論　part 1／第2章　免疫学総論　part 2／第3章　免疫担当細胞／第4章　B細胞の分化と成熟／第5章　T細胞の種類　part 1／第6章　T細胞の種類　part 2／第7章　主要組織適合抗原　part 1／第8章　主要組織適合抗原　part 2／第9章　サイトカインの働きと受容体／第10章　自然免疫／第11章　膠原病　part 1／第12章　膠原病　part 2／第13章　神経・内分泌・免疫／第14章　免疫系(防御系)と自律神経の関係 part 1／第15章　免疫系(防御系)と自律神経の関係 part 2／第16章　移植免疫／第17章　免疫不全症／第18章　腫瘍免疫学／あとがき／参考文献／索引

好評発売中